Advancements and Innovations in OMFS, ENT, and Facial Plastic Surgery

James C. Melville • Paulo G. Coelho
Simon Young

Editors

Advancements and Innovations in OMFS, ENT, and Facial Plastic Surgery

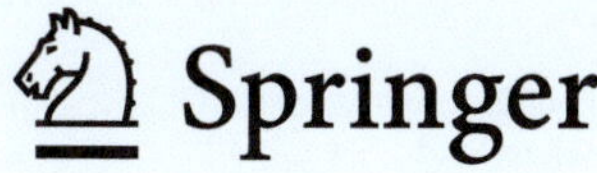 Springer

Editors
James C. Melville (iD)
Department of Oral and
Maxillofacial Surgery
The University of Texas Health Science
Center at Houston
Houston, TX, USA

Paulo G. Coelho (iD)
School of Medicine
New York University
New York, NY, USA

Simon Young (iD)
Department of Oral and
Maxillofacial Surgery
The University of Texas Health Science
Center at Houston
Houston, TX, USA

ISBN 978-3-031-32101-6   ISBN 978-3-031-32099-6   (eBook)
https://doi.org/10.1007/978-3-031-32099-6

This Springer imprint is published by the registered company Springer Nature Switzerland AG
The registered company address is: Gewerbestrasse 11, 6330 Cham, Switzerland

Preface

The craniomaxillofacial structure is an exceptional structure. The face is ultimately who we define ourselves as. With this in mind, three specialties (oral and maxillofacial, otolaryngology, and facial plastic surgery) have emerged to provide care to those who unfortunately need repair of this critical region of the body. This book discusses the advancements and innovations made in the three specialties in order to deliver the most effective patient care. We sought the expertise of the world's leading surgeons to tell this story. Our hope is that the knowledge presented in this book will assist surgeons in providing optimal care for their patients. We hope this book will provide a valuable insight and tool for both the trainee and established surgeon.

Houston, TX, USA   James C. Melville

Acknowledgments

The editors and authors would like to thank the following corporation and individuals for making this book and symposium a reality:

Depuy Synthes, KLS Martin, Stryker, AxoGen Inc., Acumed, AOT, Check Point Surgical, Piezosurgery Inc. Zimmer Biomet.

Alex Herzlinger, Marcus Martin, Brian Hill, Mark Rood, Chris Bastian, Karen Zaderej, Alex Armacost, Mike Green, William Ticoras, Paul Cantin Jr., Monte Gardner, Justin Lyons, JC Pinto, Seth Brusseau, Hunter Cameron, Anthony Brown, Michael Paredes, Jason Nuckols, Dylan Leal, Justin Stefanick, Sean Webster, Veronica Mosby, Tobias Wilken, Sibylle Hirsch, Cyrill Bätscher, and Marta Morawska.

Contents

Contributors

Jumah G. Ahmad Otorhinolaryngology—Head and Neck Surgery, University of Texas Health Sciences Center at Houston, Houston, TX, USA

Ibrahim Alava III Otolaryngology-Head and Neck Surgery, Lyndon B. Johnson General Hospital, Houston, TX, USA

Department of Otorhinolaryngology-Head and Neck Surgery, The University of Texas—McGovern Medical School, Houston, TX, USA

Lior Aljadeff Department of Oral and Maxillofacial Surgery, Section of Oral Oncology, University of Alabama at Birmingham, Birmingham, AL, USA

Salah Al Din Al Azri Maxillofacial Oncology and Microvascular Reconstructive Surgery, Houston, TX, USA

Department of Oral and Maxillofacial Surgery, The University of Texas Health Science Center at Houston, Houston, TX, USA

Ahmed A. Al-Sayed Division of Sleep Surgery, Department of Otolaryngology–Head and Neck Surgery, Stanford University School of Medicine, Stanford, CA, USA

Department of Otolaryngology–Head and Neck Surgery, Faculty of Medicine, King Saud University, Riyadh, Saudi Arabia

Dina Amin Oral and Maxillofacial Surgery, University of Rochester, Rochester, NY, USA

Division of Oral and Maxillofacial Surgery, Emory University School of Medicine, Dallas, TX, USA

Marilyn Andersen Department of Oral and Maxillofacial Surgery, Naval Hospital Twentynine Palms, Twentynine Palms, CA, USA

Michael Andersen Department of Hospital Dentistry, Naval Medical Center San Diego, San Diego, CA, USA

Alfredo Arribas Department of Oral and Maxillofacial Surgery, UTHealth Houston, Houston, TX, USA

Andrew Beech Department of Oral and Maxillofacial Surgery, University of Michigan, Ann Arbor, MI, USA

Department of Oral and Maxillofacial Surgery, Thomas Jefferson University, Philadelphia, PA, USA

Poolak Bhatt Division of Craniofacial and Surgical Care, ASoD, University of North Carolina at Chapel Hill, Chapel Hill, NC, USA

Residency Program in Oral and Maxillofacial Surgery, University of North Carolina Hospitals, Chapel Hill, NC, USA

Jo-Lawrence Martinez Bigcas Department of Otolaryngology Head and Neck Surgery, Kirk Kerkorian School of Medicine at the University of Nevada Las Vegas, Las Vegas, NV, USA

Daniel Boczar, MD Department of Surgery, University of Washington, Seattle, WA, USA

Hilliard T. Brydges Hansjörg Wyss Department of Plastic Surgery, New York University Langone Health, New York, NY, USA

Brian H. Cameron Department of Otorhinolaryngology-Head and Neck Surgery, University of Texas Health Science Center in Houston, McGovern Medical School, Houston, TX, USA

Steve Cannady Division Chief for Head and Neck Surgery, Department of Otorhinolaryngology, University of Pennsylvania, Philadelphia, PA, USA

Srinivasa R. Chandra Oral and Maxillofacial Surgery, Oregon Health Sciences School of Dentistry, Portland, OR, USA

Bo Chen, MD Department of Diagnostic and Interventional Imaging, UTHealth McGovern Medical School, Houston, TX, USA

Allen Cheng Head and Neck Surgical Associates, Oral, Head and Neck Cancer Center Program, Legacy Cancer Institute, Portland, OR, USA

Paulo G. Coelho, MD, DDS, PhD, MBA Department of Biochemistry and Molecular Biology, University of Miami Miller School of Medicine, Miami, FL, USA

Division of Plastic Surgery, Department of Surgery, University of Miami Miller School of Medicine, Miami, FL, USA

Ricardo Rodriguez Colon Hansjörg Wyss Department of Plastic Surgery, New York University Langone Health, New York, NY, USA

Caitlin M. Coviello Department of Otolaryngology—Head and Neck Surgery, Baylor College of Medicine, Houston, TX, USA

Bruce Cronstein, MD Department of Medicine, NYU Grossman School of Medicine, New York, NY, USA

Nagi Demian Oral and Maxillofacial Surgery, University of Texas Health Science Center at Huston, Houston, TX, USA

Neeraja Dharmaraj Bernard and Gloria Pepper Katz Department of Oral and Maxillofacial Surgery, The University of Texas Health Science Center at Houston, School of Dentistry, Houston, TX, USA

Tobias Ettl Department of Oral and Maxillofacial Surgery, University Medical Centre Regensburg, Regensburg, Germany

Elda Fisher Division of Craniofacial and Surgical Care, ASoD, University of North Carolina at Chapel Hill, Chapel Hill, NC, USA

Residency Program in Oral and Maxillofacial Surgery, University of North Carolina Hospitals, Chapel Hill, NC, USA

Roberto L. Flores, MD Hansjörg Wyss Department of Plastic Surgery, NYU Grossman School of Medicine, New York, NY, USA

Abigail Frazier Division of Craniofacial and Surgical Care, ASoD, University of North Carolina at Chapel Hill, Chapel Hill, NC, USA

Residency Program in Oral and Maxillofacial Surgery, University of North Carolina Hospitals, Chapel Hill, NC, USA

Joseph Geiger Oral and Maxillofacial Surgery, DeWitt Daughtry Family Department of Surgery, Miller School of Medicine/Jackson Health System, University of Miami, Miami, FL, USA

Yohaann Ali Ghosh School of Medicine and Dentistry, Griffith University, Gold Coast, Australia

Integrated Prosthetics and Reconstruction, Department of Head and Neck Surgery, Chris O'Brien Lifehouse, Sydney, NSW, Australia

Matthew R. Greives Division of Plastic Surgery, Department of Surgery, McGovern Medical School at the University of Texas Health Science Center, Houston, TX, USA

Shawn Groth Division of Thoracic Surgery, Michael E. DeBakey Department of Surgery, Baylor College of Medicine, Houston, TX, USA

Jeffrey T. Gu Department of Otolaryngology-Head and Neck Surgery, Oregon Health and Science University, Portland, OR, USA

Daniel Hammer Department of Oral and Maxillofacial Surgery, Naval Medical Center San Diego, San Diego, CA, USA

Issa Hanna Department of Oral and Maxillofacial Surgery, UTHealth Houston, Houston, TX, USA

Jeffrey Hartgerink Chemistry and Bioengineering, Rice University, Houston, TX, USA

Undergraduate Studies, Rice University, Houston, TX, USA

Steven Hengen Department of Oral and Maxillofacial Surgery, UTHealth Houston, Houston, TX, USA

Tang Ho Division of Facial Plastic and Reconstructive Surgery, Department of Otorhinolaryngology Head and Neck Surgery, University of Texas Health Science Center in Houston, Houston, TX, USA

Department of Otorhinolaryngology-Head and Neck Surgery, University of Texas Health Science Center in Houston, McGovern Medical School, Houston, TX, USA

Andrew T. Huang Department of Otolaryngology—Head and Neck Surgery, Baylor College of Medicine, Houston, TX, USA

Mohammad S. Jafferji Division of Thoracic Surgery, Michael E. DeBakey Department of Surgery, Baylor College of Medicine, Houston, TX, USA

Jonathon Jundt Bernard and Gloria Pepper Katz Department of Oral and Maxillofacial Surgery, School of Dentistry, The University of Texas Health Science Center at Houston, Houston, TX, USA

Philipp Jürgens Department of Cranio-Maxillofacial Surgery, Leading Medical Center (LMC) Munich, Munich, Germany

Arshad Kaleem Division of Oral and Maxillofacial Surgery, DeWitt Daughtry Family Department of Surgery, Section of Head and Neck Surgical Oncology and Microvascular Reconstructive Surgery, Miller School of Medicine/Jackson Health System, University of Miami, Miami, FL, USA

Head and Neck Oncology/Microvascular Reconstructive Surgery, High Desert Oral and Facial Surgery, El Paso, TX, USA

Ryan Keyho Division of Plastic Surgery, Department of Surgery, McGovern Medical School at the University of Texas Health Science Center, Houston, TX, USA

Roderick Y. Kim Department of Oral and Maxillofacial Surgery, John Peter Smith Hospital, Fort Worth, TX, USA

Natalie A. Krane Division Facial Plastic and Reconstructive Surgery, Department of Otolaryngology-Head and Neck Surgery, Oregon Health and Science University, Portland, OR, USA

Cheuk Sun Edwin Lai Rice University, Houston, TX, USA

Kevin C. Lee Department of Oral and Maxillofacial Surgery, University at Buffalo, New York, NY, USA

Alexis M. Linnebur Carle Foundation Hospital, Urbana, IL, USA

Stanley Yung-Chuan Liu Division of Sleep Surgery, Department of Otolaryngology–Head and Neck Surgery, Stanford University School of Medicine, Stanford, CA, USA

Garren Michael Iida Low Department of Otolaryngology Head and Neck Surgery, Drexel University College of Medicine, Pittsburgh, PA, USA

Department of Otolaryngology Head and Neck Surgery, Allegheny Health Network, Pittsburgh, PA, USA

Myriam Loyo Department of Otolaryngology-Head and Neck Surgery, Oregon Health and Science University, Portland, OR, USA

Victoria A. Manon Bernard and Gloria P. Katz Department of Oral and Maxillofacial Surgery, University of Texas Health Science Center at Houston, Houston, TX, USA

Michael R. Markiewicz Department of Oral and Maxillofacial Surgery, University at Buffalo, Buffalo, NY, USA

Jeffrey S. Marschall Department of Oral and Maxillofacial Surgery, University of Iowa Hospital and Clinics, Iowa City, IA, USA

Robert E. Marx Department of Oral and Maxillofacial Surgery, University of Miami School of Medicine, Florida, USA

James C. Melville, DDS Bernard and Gloria Pepper Katz Department of Oral and Maxillofacial Surgery, School of Dentistry, The University of Texas Health Science Center at Houston, Houston, TX, USA

Department of Oral and Maxillofacial Surgery, The University of Texas Health Science Center at Houston, Houston, TX, USA

Justine Moe Department of Oral and Maxillofacial Surgery, University of Michigan, Ann Arbor, MI, USA

Department of Oral and Maxillofacial Surgery, Thomas Jefferson University, Philadelphia, PA, USA

Marta Morawska Department of Cranio-Maxillofacial Surgery, Advanced Osteotomy Tools (AOT) AG, Basel, Switzerland

Anthony B. Morlandt, MD, DDS, FACS Oral and Maxillofacial Surgery, University of Alabama at Birmingham, Birmingham, Alabama, USA

Vasudev Vivekanand Nayak, MSci, PhD Department of Biochemistry and Molecular Biology, University of Miami Miller School of Medicine, Miami, FL, USA

Annie Nguyen Department of Orthodontics, Montreal Children's Hospital, McGill University Health Centre, Quebec, Canada

Phuong D. Nguyen Division of Plastic Surgery, Department of Surgery, McGovern Medical School at the University of Texas Health Science Center, Houston, TX, USA

Children's Memorial Hermann Hospital, Houston, TX, USA

Justin Odette Dental Department, USS Theodore Roosevelt (CVN 71), San Diego, CA, USA

Ashish Patel Oral, Head and Neck Surgery, Head and Neck Surgical Associates, Portland, OR, USA

Neel Patel Division of Oral and Maxillofacial Surgery, DeWitt Daughtry Family Department of Surgery, Head and Neck Surgical Oncology and Microvascular Reconstructive Surgery, Miller School of Medicine/Jackson Health System, University of Miami, Miami, FL, USA

Zachary S. Peacock Oral and Maxillofacial Surgery, Massachusetts General Hospital (MGH), Boston, MA, USA

Daniel Petrisor Head and Neck Oncologic and Microvascular Reconstructive Surgery, Department of Oral and Maxillofacial Surgery, Oregon Health and Science University, Portland, OR, USA

Matthew J. Recker Department of Neurosurgery, Jacobs School of Medicine and Biomedical Sciences, Buffalo, NY, USA

Renée M. Reynolds Department of Neurosurgery, Jacobs School of Medicine and Biomedical Sciences, Buffalo, NY, USA

Eduardo D. Rodriguez Hansjörg Wyss Department of Plastic Surgery, New York University Langone Health, New York, NY, USA

Dominik Rudecki Department of Oral and Maxillofacial Surgery, UTHealth Houston, Houston, TX, USA

Christopher M. Runyan, MD, PhD Department of Plastic Surgery, Wake Forest University School of Medicine, Winston-Salem, NC, USA

Kunal R. Shetty Otorhinolaryngology—Head and Neck Surgery, University of Texas Health Sciences Center at Houston, Houston, TX, USA

Jonathan Shum Maxillofacial Oncology and Microvascular Reconstructive Surgery, Houston, TX, USA

Department of Oral and Maxillofacial Surgery, The University of Texas Health Science Center at Houston, Houston, TX, USA

The University of Texas Health Science Center at Houston, Houston, TX, USA

Raymond P. Shupak Division of Oral and Maxillofacial Surgery, Geisinger Medical Center, Danville, PA, USA

Department of Oral Medicine and Maxillofacial Surgery, Geisinger Commonwealth School of Medicine, Geisinger Health System, Danville, PA, USA

Parul Sinha Division of Facial Plastic and Reconstructive Surgery, Department of Otorhinolaryngology Head and Neck Surgery, University of Texas Health Science Center in Houston, Houston, TX, USA

Allison Slijepcevic Department of Otolaryngology-Head and Neck Surgery, Atrium Wake Forest Baptist, Wake Forest, NC, USA

Emilio Supsupin Jr, MD Division of Neuroradiology, Department of Radiology, University of Florida College of Medicine - Jacksonville,Jacksonville, FL, USA

Department of Diagnostic and Interventional Imaging, UTHealth McGovern Medical School, Houston, TX, USA

Mari Alina Timoshchuk Department of Oral and Maxillofacial Surgery, School of Dentistry, Louisiana Health Sciences Center, New Orleans, LA, USA

Andrea Torroni, MD, PhD Hansjörg Wyss Department of Plastic Surgery, NYU Grossman School of Medicine, New York, NY, USA

Huy Q. Tran Bernard and Gloria P. Katz Department of Oral and Maxillofacial Surgery, University of Texas Health Science Center at Houston, Houston, TX, USA

Ramzey Tursun Division of Oral and Maxillofacial Surgery, DeWitt Daughtry Family Department of Surgery, Head and Neck Surgical Oncology and Microvascular Reconstructive Surgery Fellowship, Miller School of Medicine/Jackson Health System, University of Miami, Miami, FL, USA

Clinical Surgery, University of Miami, Miami, FL, USA

Oral, Head & Neck Oncologic, University of Miami, Miami, FL, USA

Division of Oral Maxillofacial Surgery, DeWitt Daughtry Family Department of Surgery, Leonard M. Miller School of Medicine, University of Miami, Miami, FL, USA

Microvascular Reconstructive Surgery, University of Miami, Miami, FL, USA

Security Forces Hospital, Riyad, Saudi Arabia

Chi T. Viet Oral and Maxillofacial Surgery, Loma Linda University, Loma Linda, CA, USA

Oral and Maxillofacial Surgery, Loma Linda University, Loma Linda, CA, USA

Jason Wahidi Division of Oral and Maxillofacial Surgery, Department of Surgery, UT Southwestern/Parkland Memorial Hospital, Dallas, TX, USA

Ray Y. Wang Department of Otolaryngology—Head and Neck Surgery, Baylor College of Medicine, Houston, TX, USA

Mark K. Wax Department of Otolaryngology-Head and Neck Surgery, Oregon Health and Science University, Portland, OR, USA

Fayette C. Williams Department of Oral and Maxillofacial Surgery, John Peter Smith Hospital, Fort Worth, TX, USA

Lukasz Witek, MSci, PhD Biomaterials Division, NYU College of Dentistry, New York, NY, USA

Hansjörg Wyss Department of Plastic Surgery, NYU Grossman School of Medicine, New York, NY, USA

Department of Biomedical Engineering, NYU Tandon School of Engineering, Brooklyn, NY, USA

Mark E. Wong Bernard & Gloria Pepper Katz Department of Oral and Maxillofacial Surgery, University of Texas School of Dentistry Houston, Houston, TX, USA

Sarah Anne Wong Oral and Craniofacial Sciences Graduate Program, School of Dentistry, San Francisco, CA, USA

Simon Young Bernard and Gloria Pepper Katz Department of Oral and Maxillofacial Surgery, School of Dentistry, The University of Texas Health Science Center at Houston, Houston, TX, USA

Department of Oral and Maxillofacial Surgery, The University of Texas Health Science Center at Houston, Houston, TX, USA

Waleed Zaid Department of Oral and Maxillofacial Surgery, School of Dentistry, Louisiana Health Sciences Center, New Orleans, LA, USA

Site Director Baton Rouge LSUHSC Oral and Maxillofacial Surgery Department, Our Lady of Lake Regional Medical Center, Baton Rouge, LA, USA

John R. Zuniga Division of Oral and Maxillofacial Surgery, Department of Surgery and Neurology, UT Southwestern/Parkland Memorial Hospital, Dallas, TX, USA

Chapter 1
Innovations in Craniofacial Surgery

Matthew J. Recker, Kevin C. Lee, Renée M. Reynolds, Annie Nguyen, and Michael R. Markiewicz

Introduction

The history of craniofacial surgery speaks to the rapid evolution of the field. The origins of modern craniofacial surgery date back to the 1960s with the work of Paul Tessier [1, 2]. The concept of autogenous bone grafting and his techniques for transcranial and subcranial osteotomies were revolutionary at the time. In the 1980s, the advent of rigid fixation allowed surgeons to perform more extensive and aggressive osteotomies with greater confidence in the stability of their work. In the 1990s, Joseph McCarthy introduced the concept of mandibular distraction allowing for movements of the significantly underdeveloped mandible and soft tissues [3]. Many proponents of distraction soon applied the same concept to other parts of the skull and face. Over the last 15 years, computer-aided surgery has gained popularity and wide acceptance within the surgical community. Each innovation and breakthrough in craniofacial surgery builds on the principles that came before. The works of

M. J. Recker · R. M. Reynolds
Department of Neurosurgery, Jacobs School of Medicine and Biomedical Sciences, Buffalo, NY, USA
e-mail: mrecker@ubns.com; rreynolds@ubns.com

K. C. Lee · M. R. Markiewicz (✉)
Department of Oral and Maxillofacial Surgery, University at Buffalo, New York, NY, USA
e-mail: kcl2136@cumc.columbia.edu; mrm25@buffalo.edu

A. Nguyen
Department of Orthodontics, Montreal Children's Hospital, McGill University Health Centre, Quebec, Canada
e-mail: annie.nguyen@muhc.mcgill.ca

J. C. Melville et al. (eds.), *Advancements and Innovations in OMFS, ENT, and Facial Plastic Surgery*, https://doi.org/10.1007/978-3-031-32099-6_1

Tessier and others before and after him have not been rendered obsolete in the modern era. Rather, today's technology optimizes the results and carries forward the vision of those original pioneers.

Craniosynostosis

Introduction

Craniosynostosis is defined as the premature closure of cranial sutures and can result in abnormal skull development and morphology with sequelae. For centuries, anatomists have recognized a range of skull-shape abnormalities and postulated an association with abnormal cranial sutures [4, 5]. In Virchow's seminal work published in 1851, he defined skull growth patterns related to the fusion of specific cranial sutures and explained that these patterns were due to restriction of skull growth perpendicular to the fused suture [6] (Fig. 1.1). Subsequent work expanded upon Virchow's Law to form our contemporary knowledge of craniosynostosis. We now understand that early sutural fusion initiates compensatory growth in adjacent sutures and within the skull base [7]. In addition to optimizing the cosmetic outcome, the surgical treatment of craniosynostosis is intended to facilitate normal cranial volume expansion and reduce the risk of increased intracranial pressure and subsequent neurodevelopmental delay.

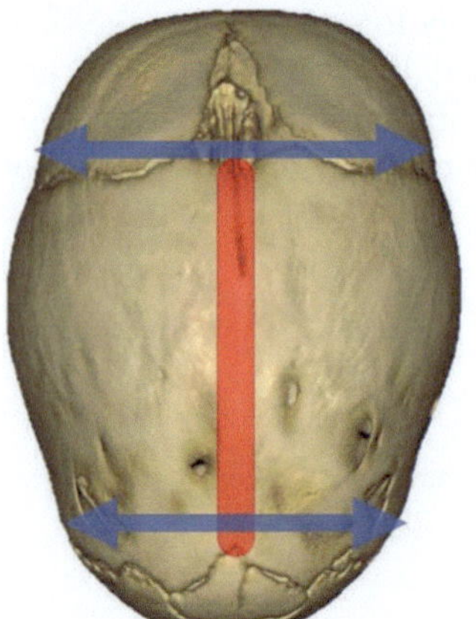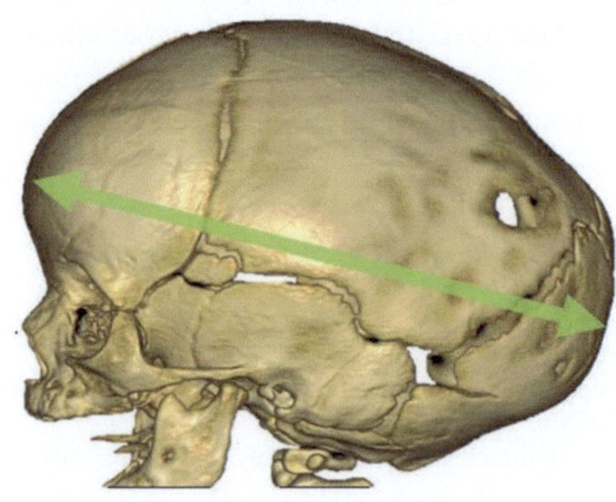

Fig. 1.1 Sagittal synostosis showing arrested growth perpendicular to the fused suture (blue arrows) with compensatory overgrowth parallel to the suture (green arrow)

Epidemiology and Etiology

The incidence of craniosynostosis is estimated to be between 1:2000 and 1:2500 with a male predominance reported between 2:1 and 3:1 [8]. Craniosynostosis can be categorized in several different ways including single versus multi-suture, syndromic versus non-syndromic, and by the specific suture affected. Single suture craniosynostosis is more common with the sagittal suture being the most often affected suture. This accounts for over half of cases. This is followed by unilateral coronal (20–25%), metopic (10%), and lambdoid (2%) craniosynostosis. Non-syndromic cases are typically sporadic events, with no identifiable etiology; however, various risk factors have been implicated such as advanced paternal age and maternal history of smoking [9]. Syndromic cases are related to specific genetic abnormalities and associated syndromes, such as Apert Syndrome (FGFR-2), Crouzon Syndrome (FGFR-2, FGFR-3), Pfeiffer Syndrome (FGFR-1, FGFR-2), Muenke Syndrome (FGFR-3), among others. Syndromic craniosynostosis is more likely to present with multi-suture involvement [8].

Traditional Repair

The treatment of craniosynostosis has undergone a series of trends over decades of evolution. In the late 1800s to mid-1900s, strip craniectomy was used to release the fused suture, but this technique was marred by surgical morbidity and variable cosmetic outcomes due to refusion at craniectomy sites [10, 11]. The evolution of current strategies in management is credited to Tessier after developing cranial vault remodeling in the 1970s, which is the foundation for open techniques used today [12]. Modern open cranial vault expansion encompasses a number of procedures, which are carried out via a coronal incision where portions of the cranium are either removed, remodeled, and replaced with fixation, or remodeled without bony removal. Variations of open cranial vault expansion are tailored to the specific sutures involved and the deformity of the patient. Included in this group are fronto-orbital advancement and posterior vault expansion. These techniques can be carried out with or without the use of distraction osteogenesis. These procedures require consideration of patient age as considerable blood loss can be expected, and operative time and optimal bone thickness to withstand surgical remodeling are pertinent factors. Additionally, the rate of revision surgery is potentially higher in extremely younger patients.

Computer-Aided Surgery

Computer-aided surgery can be divided into five phases (Table 1.1): (1) the *data acquisition phase*, in which all imaging, laser surface scans, clinical information, anthropometric measurements, implant STereoLithography (STL) and measurements are obtained; (2) the *planning phase*, in which computed tomography (CT) data is imported into a proprietary software program for the purposes of virtually planning the surgery; (3) manufacturing phase in which guides, stents, and patient-specific implants are fabricated using 3D printers; (4) *surgical phase,* which is performed utilizing computer-aided design and computer-aided manufacturing (CAD/CAM) derived stereolithographic models, guide-stents, splints, patient-specific implants, and/or intraoperative navigation; and (5) *assessment phase,* in which the accuracy of the treatment plan transfer is evaluated using intraoperative (or postoperative CT imaging). This phase is often neglected; however, it can be used to assess outcomes for the benefit of the patient, the clinician for either critically evaluating their outcomes and technique, or for research purposes (evaluating their outcomes on a larger scale).

Table 1.1 Stages of computer-aided surgery

Step	Tasks	Examples
Data acquisition phase	– Obtain clinical information – Obtain pertinent patient history – Obtain patient imaging – Obtain STL files for potential patient implants	– Laser scanning of teeth, bite, and plaster models – CT scan of hard tissues – Choose hardware manufacturer so STLS files can be imported
Planning phase	– CT scan is imported into software program – Virtual surgery is performed – Virtual implants are manipulated and placed, or patient-specific implants are designed are targeted virtual surgery	– CT scan is imported – Surgery is performed virtually – Osteotomies and movements are simulated – Patient-specific implants are designed
Manufacturing phase	– Patient-specific implants, splints, guides, and hardware are fabricated using 3D printers	– Cutting guides and positioning guides are printed – Stents to reproduce orthognathic movements are printed
Surgical phase	– Surgical phase is carried out in accordance with the virtually planned surgery using guides, stents, and patient-specific implants fabricated during the manufacturing phase	– Surgery is carried out using custom guides – Patient-specific implants are placed
Assessment phase	Using intraoperative navigation and 3D imaging to assess the virtual surgical plan was achieved	– Using intraoperative navigation and postoperative imaging to assess, bony reduction, and implant placement

Computer-Aided Open Repair

Traditionally, open cranial vault remodeling has required manual planning of the craniotomies and osteotomies to remodel the skull. This rather subjective process is dependent on the surgeon's expertise and creative vision to achieve the goal of normal skull shape and volume consistent with age-matched norms and expected growth patterns. Computer-aided surgery has gained popularity in recent years in head and neck surgery, having demonstrated positive impact in orbital reconstruction [13], orthognathic surgery [14], and more. This technology utilizes preoperative CT imaging to virtually plan an ideal surgical outcome prior to surgical intervention. The data from this process is then used to manufacture sterile templates, which are utilized in the operating room to plan the osteotomies and cranial reconstruction [15] (Fig. 1.2). In craniosynostosis, computer-aided surgical planning has been shown to reduce operative time [16], although future research is warranted to describe the impact of this technology on cosmetic and neurologic outcomes in craniosynostosis surgery.

Endoscopic and Minimally Invasive Techniques

In the late 1990s, Barone and Jimenez described their experience using endoscopic strip craniectomy with adjunctive orthotic helmeting as an alternative to open cranial vault expansion. The endoscopic technique utilizes small incisions, under which a burr hole is created. The endoscope is used for visualization as the periosteum is stripped from above the bone, and dura is stripped from below the bone. The suturectomy is then performed using heavy scissors, ultrasonic bone aspiration, or a high-speed drill. This technique results in reduced blood loss and need for blood transfusion, smaller incisions, shorter operative time, and decreased hospital costs compared to open techniques [17]. Since that time, a number of studies have supported the use of endoscopic strip craniectomy in sagittal, metopic, coronal, lambdoid, and multi-suture craniosynostosis with good outcomes. The utility of this technique is limited after 3–6 months of age due to advanced deformity and decreased effectiveness of helmeting. Helmeting carries the benefit of being adjustable over time to optimize three-dimensional growth and is continued until adequate head shape is reached or until 1 year of age.

Although poor outcomes in the historical literature would discourage the use of strip craniectomy, it is important to note the difference in modern techniques. Modern strip craniectomy must be complemented by augmentation of skull growth by orthotic helmeting, springs, or distracting devices [18]. Spring-assisted cranioplasty uses metallic springs of various thickness to exert a constant force to reshape the patient's skull. Both springs and distractors have the advantage of producing more predictable expansion in a known vector and can be used in older children, but require a second operation for removal.

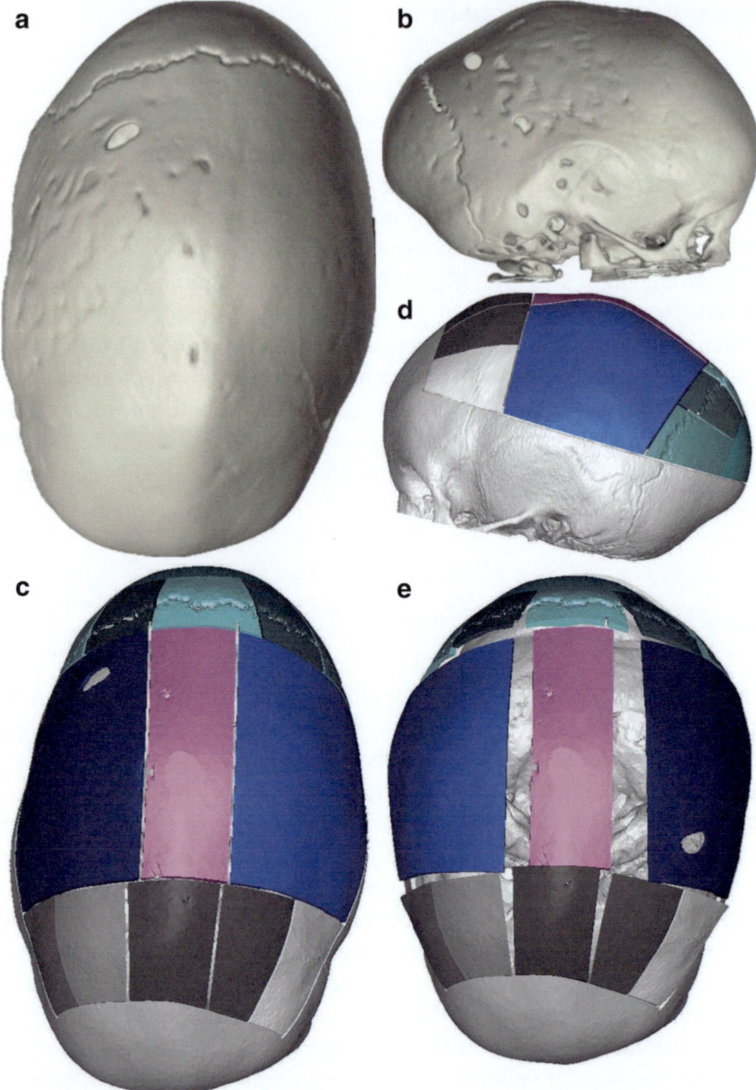

Fig. 1.2 Isolated sagittal synostosis with switch cranioplasty for cranial vault remodeling. (**a**) Bird's eye and (**b**) lateral views of preoperative skull. Segmented skull viewed from (**c**) bird's eye and (**d**) lateral. Planned switch cranioplasty with expansion viewed from (**e**) bird's eye and (**f**) lateral. (**g**) Cutting guide to ensure accurate segmentation and safe distance from (**h**) sagittal sinus. (**i**) Positioning guide for aligning cranial segments allowing for external plating. (**j**, **k**) Bicoronal incision design with subgaleal dissection. (**l**) Cutting guide seated on cranium. (**m**) Cranial segments removed exposing underlying dura. (**n**) Internal view of cranial segments showing "copper beaten" appearance indicating elevated intracranial pressure. (**o**) Bony segments fixated according to virtual plan and (**p**) reapplied to patient. Two-year postoperative result as viewed from (**q**) lateral, (**r**) frontal, (**s**) bird's eye. (Reproduced with permission from Markiewicz MR, Recker MJ, Reynolds RM. Management of Sagittal and Lambdoid Craniosynostosis Open Cranial Vault Expansion and Remodeling. Oral Maxillofac Surg Clin North Am. 2022;34 (3):395–419)

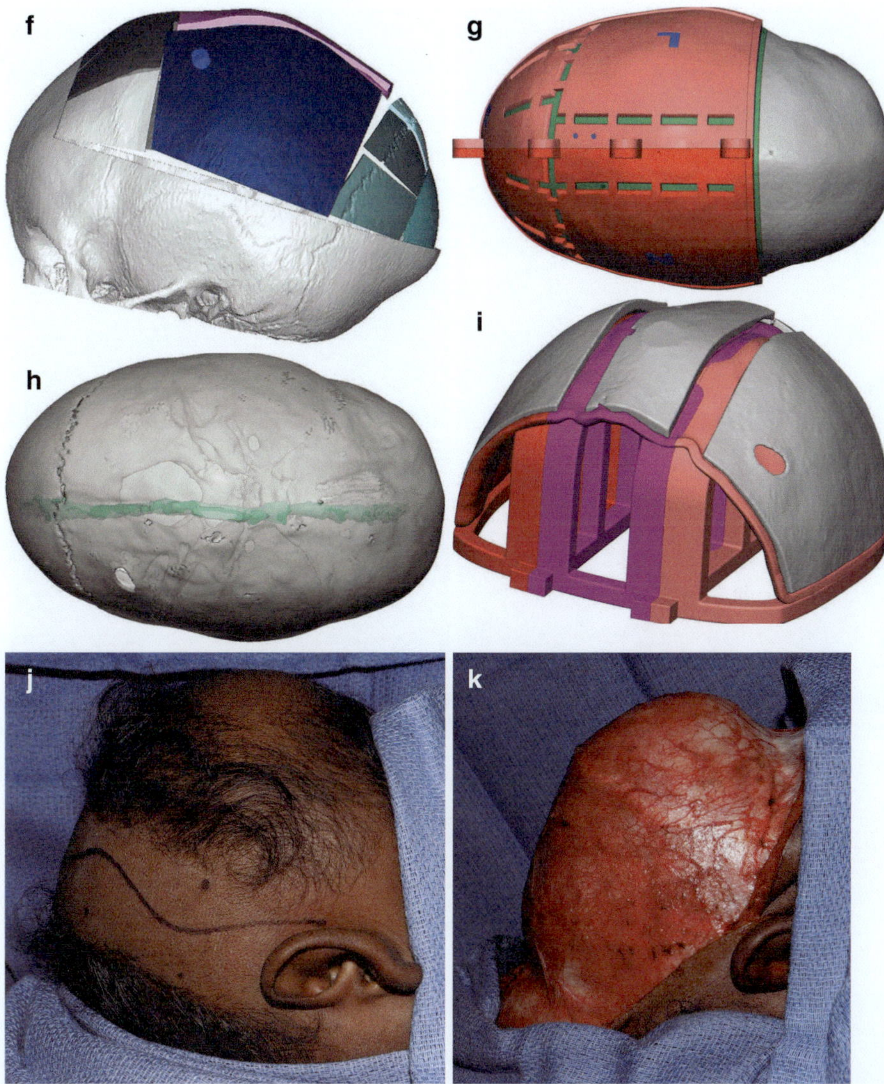

Fig. 1.2 (continued)

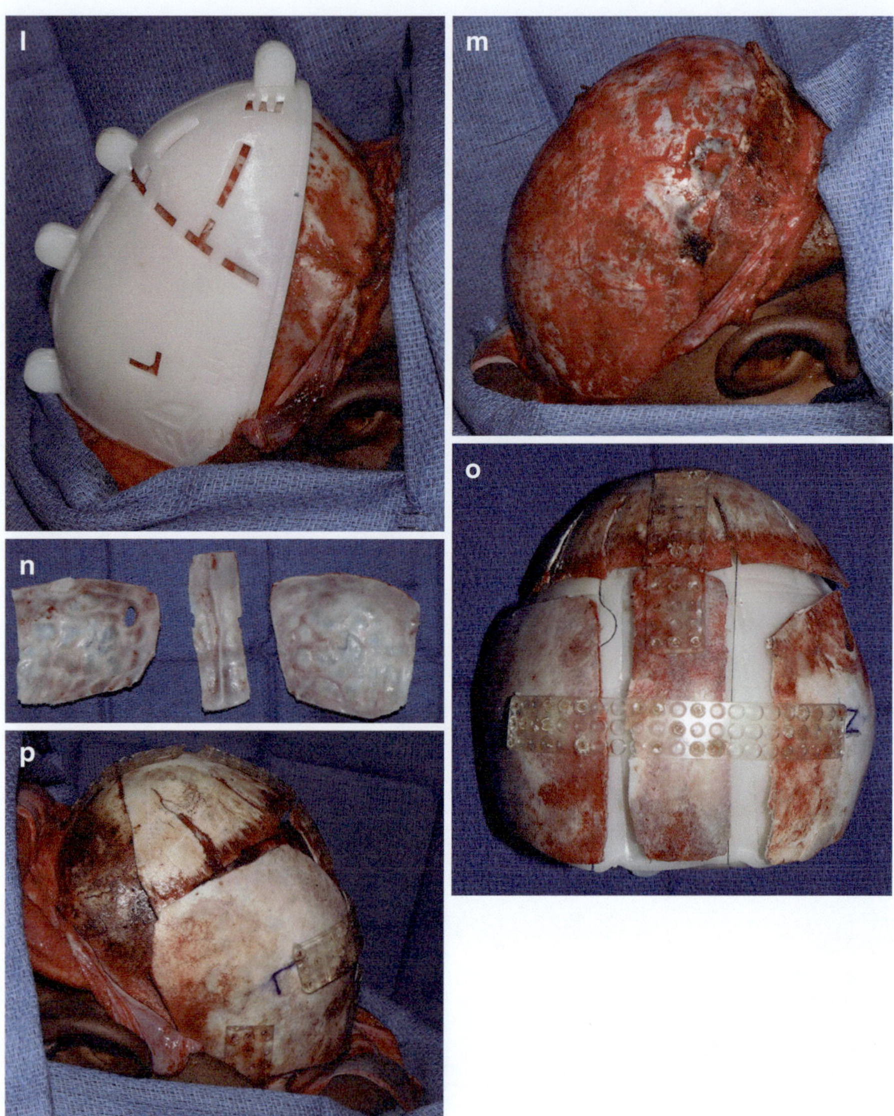

Fig. 1.2 (continued)

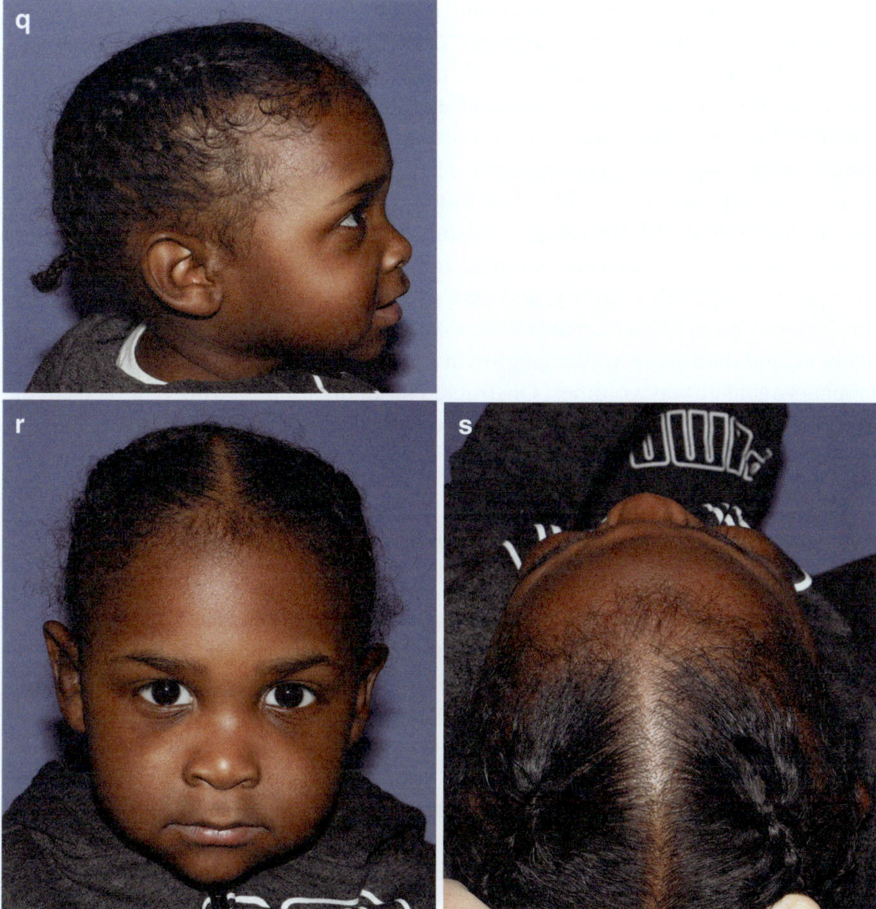

Fig. 1.2 (continued)

Midface Advancement

Introduction

Craniofacial dysostosis refers to the syndromic form of craniosynostosis that includes premature fusion of not only the cranial sutures but also the sutures of the anterior skull base [19]. Notably, Apert, Crouzon, Carpenter, and Pfeiffer syndromes are included in this family of malformations. Autosomal dominant defects in various fibroblast growth factor receptors (FGFRs) have been identified and implicated in the pathogenesis of these syndromes. Unlike that of Apert and other such syndromes, the defects in Crouzon are largely limited to the head and face.

Restricted skull base growth in craniofacial dysostosis results in severe midface hypoplasia. This manifests as a concave "dish-face" profile, maxillary constriction, a high-arched palate, and a parrot-beak deformity of the nose [20]. The shallow orbits, which create a striking degree of exophthalmos, are also a consequence of premature fusion at the cranial base. Bicoronal synostosis contributes to the brachycephalic head shape and hypertelorism. There are a variety of functional considerations in these patients. As with other forms of craniosynostosis, it is important to evaluate for increased intracranial pressures and brain growth restriction. Concern for either would mandate early surgical release of the involved sutures. Proptosis can expose the eyeball to injury, and care should be taken to ensure that the cornea is protected. Vision likewise needs to be assessed early on. Infants are obligate nasal breathers, and the severe midfacial growth restriction can cause decreased nasal and nasopharyngeal airway volumes. Obstructed nasal breathing during oral feeds in the neonatal period can lead to failure to thrive and poor weight gain.

Traditional Midface Reconstruction in the Syndromic Patient

The management of patients with syndromic craniosynostosis varies by center; however, the generally accepted sequencing involves cranio-orbital surgery in infancy, midface advancement in mid-childhood, and orthognathic surgery for occlusal correction after skeletal maturity [19]. Global midface advancement is achieved with a LeFort III osteotomy. If the supraorbital ridges are judged to be well-positioned, a Monobloc advancement can be deferred. The goals of the LeFort III operation are to normalize the projection of the inferior orbital rim, zygoma, and maxilla. Obtaining a good Class 1 occlusal relationship is not a consideration at this time as the dental discrepancies can be subsequently corrected in adulthood with orthodontics and a LeFort I. The LeFort III procedure was originally described as a single-staged procedure; however, with the advent of craniofacial distraction osteogenesis, there has been a strong preference toward progressively distracting the segments following craniofacial disjunction. Compared to the conventional approach, midface distraction has been shown to reduce morbidity and relapse [21]. Distraction also allows for larger advancements. Immediate rigid fixation permits only 6–10 mm of stable advancement, whereas up to 20 mm are possible with distraction [20].

Contemporary Treatment

Modern technology has improved the safety and predictability of the subcranial LeFort III osteotomy. Piezoelectric devices allow for better protection of the orbital soft tissues. The high-frequency vibrations that are transmitted to the metal instrument tip selectively cut mineralized tissues without collateral thermal damage to the bone. Compared with mechanical saws, piezo devices have been shown to improve the speed and safety of the LeFort III procedure [22]. With respect to planning, the simulated movements on computer-aided surgery translate to more accurate intra-operative movements (Fig. 1.3). For distraction, internal distractor guides can be fabricated to ensure that the desired vectors are achieved [23]. Surgical guides can also be made for the pterygoid plate and nasofrontal junction osteotomes (Fig. 1.4). The predicted movements have become so reliable in all planes of space that some

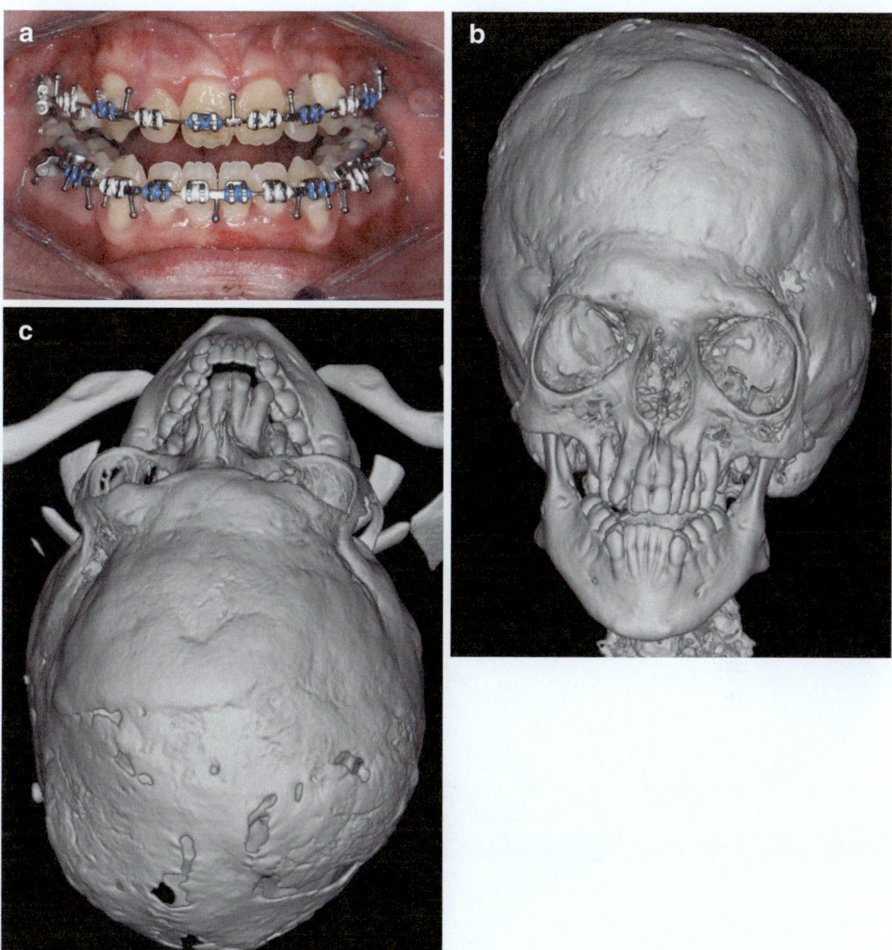

Fig. 1.3 Computer-assisted planning of LeFort III distraction with augmentation cranioplasty. Preoperative (**a**) occlusion and (**b, c**) CT scan of head and face showing cranial defects and deficient bitemporal and biparietal volume. (**d**) Planned orientation of internal distractors to achieve (**e, f**) final expected position of midface. (**g, h**) Heat map of bone to optimize the location of predictive holes. (**i, j**) Design of custom cranioplasty implant using normative data to provide volume and coverage. (Reproduced with permission from Schlieder D, Markiewicz MR. Craniofacial Syndromes: The Le Fort III Osteotomy for Correction of Severe Midface Hypoplasia. Atlas Oral Maxillofac Surg Clin North Am. 2022;30 (1):85–99)

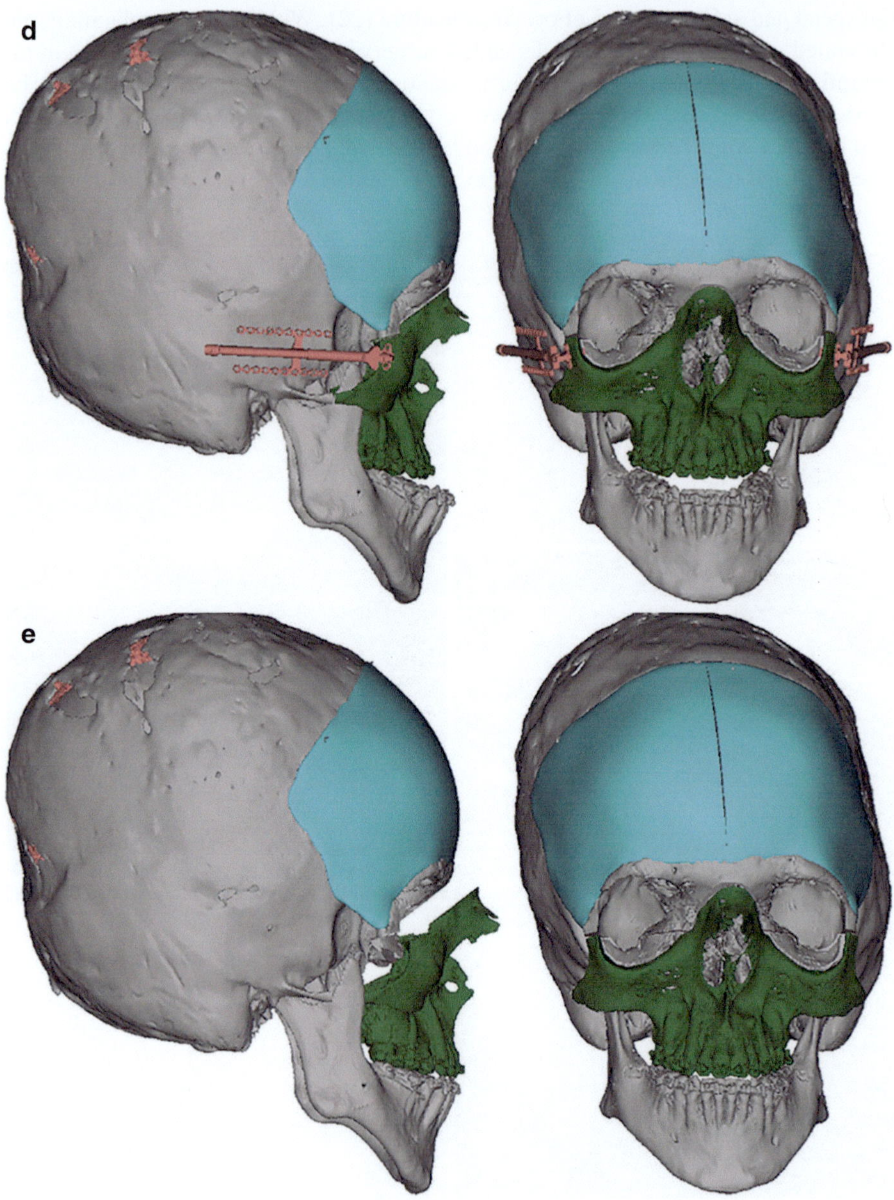

Fig. 1.3 (continued)

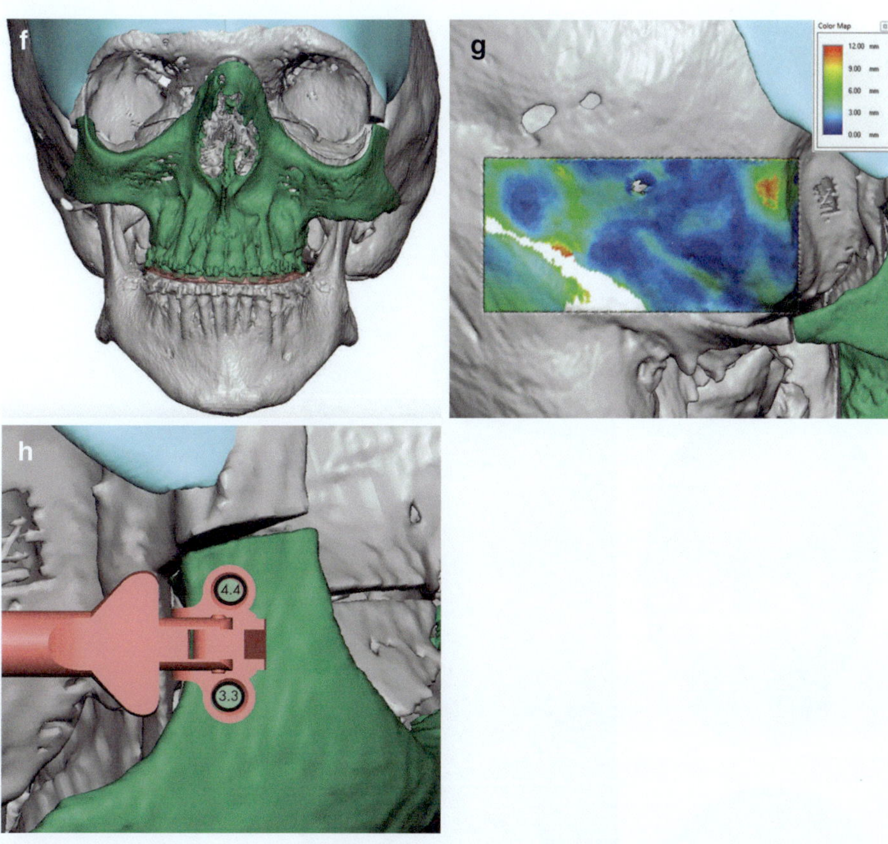

Fig. 1.3 (continued)

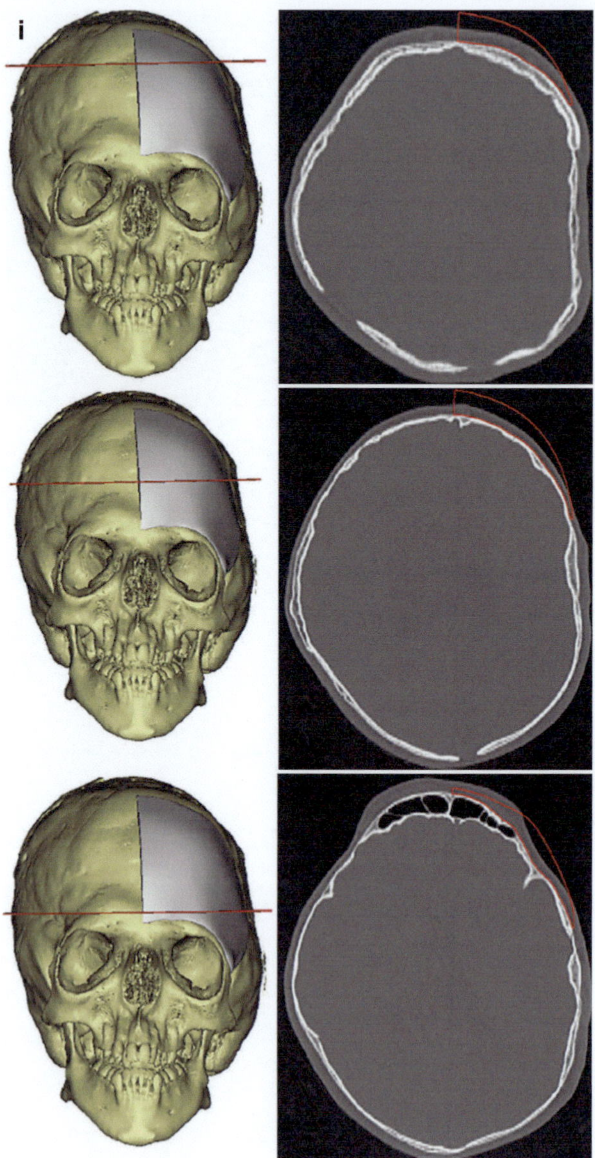

Fig. 1.3 (continued)

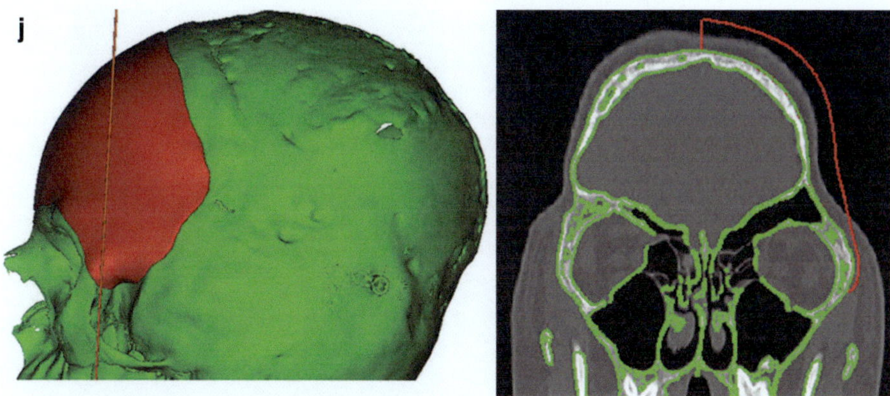

Fig. 1.3 (continued)

surgeons are performing simultaneous LeFort I and III advancements [24]. When the midface and the maxilla are simultaneously and independently osteotomized, less movement is required for each piece to reach proper occlusion. This is useful for cases of soft tissue restriction or when a single-staged surgery is desired. Finally, virtual planning allows surgeons to design and guide unconventional osteotomies that would be difficult to execute in a free-hand style. This has led to the creation of "modified" LeFort II/III osteotomies through a combined transoral and transconjunctival approach [25]. The concealed access of these modified procedures spares the morbidity and external scarring of a coronal flap, although they do not permit for nasofrontal advancement.

Pierre Robin Sequence

Introduction

Pierre Robin sequence, or Robin sequence (RS), is a rare congenital anomaly characterized by a clinical triad of micrognathia, glossoptosis, and upper airway obstruction [26]. In RS, the precipitating event of an underdeveloped mandible initiates the subsequent cascade of tongue base retropositioning, possible palatal clefting, and respiratory and/or feeding difficulties. The cleft palate of RS is generally U-shaped and wider than that seen with other cleft conditions. Furthermore, the RS mandible is morphologically abnormal with a shorter ramus and a more oblique symphysial angle [27]. RS may occur in isolation or as part of an underlying genetic syndrome. Isolated RS comprises between 20% and 40% of cases [28, 29]. The precise etiology of mandibular retrognathia in these isolated cases is unknown but may be related to sporadic mutations of the SOX9 gene; however, this has not been proven with convincing data [30]. Because no single genetic locus has been found to be consistently altered across patients, isolated RS may also stem from environmental

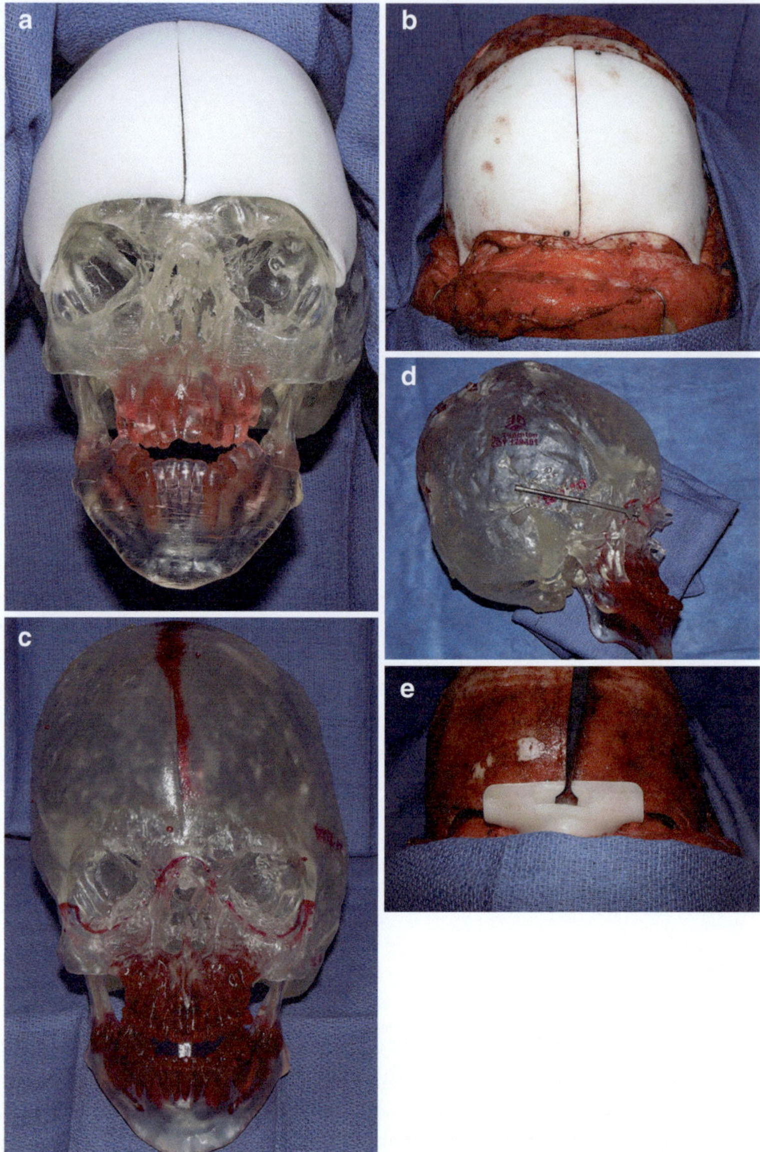

Fig. 1.4 Intraoperative implants and guides. Cranioplasty implants (**a**) fit to model and (**b**) patient. (**c**) Stereolithographic model showing pertinent anatomy and planned osteotomies. (**d**) Internal distractor fit to model. (**e**) Nasofrontal osteotome guide ensuring safe orientation away from anterior skull base. Imaging (**f**) immediately after distractor placement and (**g**) after completion of distraction. (**h**) Excellent postop occlusion obtained with skeletal advancement. (Reproduced with permission from Schlieder D, Markiewicz MR. Craniofacial Syndromes: The Le Fort III Osteotomy for Correction of Severe Midface Hypoplasia. Atlas Oral Maxillofac Surg Clin North Am. 2022;30 (1):85–99)

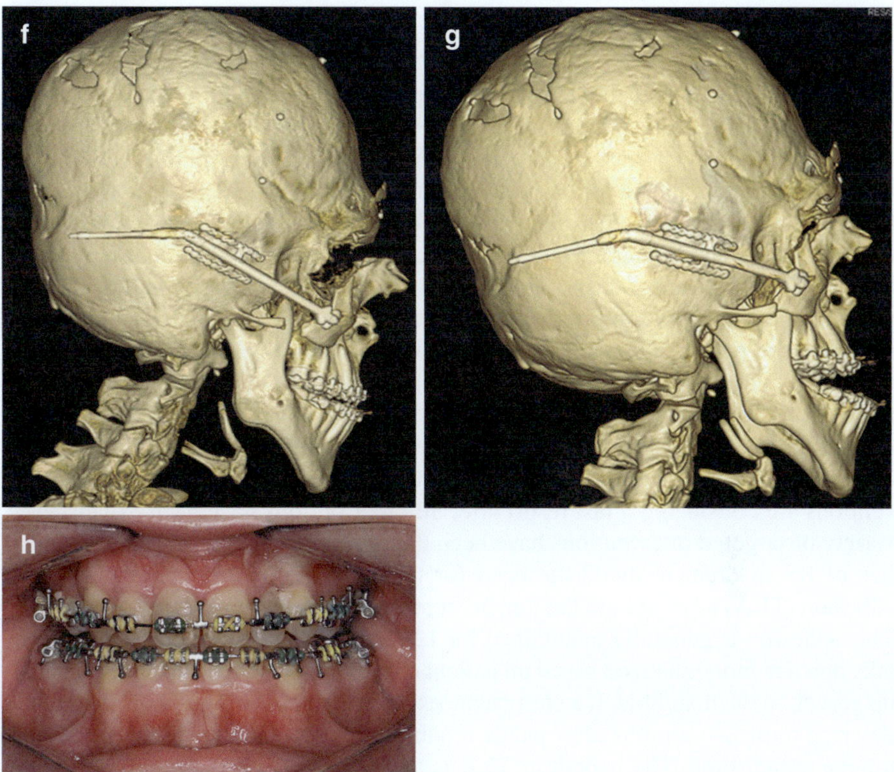

Fig. 1.4 (continued)

influences of intrauterine growth restriction [31]. This environmental theory would account for the postnatal catch-up growth observed with some patients. On the contrary, syndromic patients with RS are believed to present with a primary mandibular growth disorder. Stickler syndrome followed by velocardiofacial syndrome are most commonly associated with RS, although over 50 named syndromes are known to present with features of RS. It is important to note that some researchers have found that neither isolated nor syndromic RS patients exhibit meaningful catch-up growth. This discordance highlights the fact that, although the clinical consequences of micrognathia are well-known, the precise etiology and long-term trajectory of RS are poorly understood.

Traditional Repair

Infants with RS can present along a broad spectrum of respiratory and feeding difficulties, and surgical interventions are aimed at improving these issues. Nonoperative measures for relieving airway obstruction include prone positioning, positive airway pressure, and intubation. It is important to verify tongue base collapse with endoscopy and rule out other potential confounding conditions such as hypotonia, central apneas, and laryngomalacia. In the authors' experience, the decision to treat the mandible in cases of suspected RS is not always straightforward especially in the setting of multiple contributing comorbidities. In patients who have multifactorial drivers of poor weight gain and disordered breathing, tracheostomy and gastrostomy tube placement reliably provide a definitive means of ensuring spontaneous respirations and adequate nutrition.

The routine and permanent use of tracheostomy and gastrostomy tubes should not be the treatment of choice to circumvent oropharyngeal collapse. These interventions are considered a last resort after all other options have been exhausted. A variety of targeted interventions have been developed to treat the anatomic anomalies of RS in order to avoid the need for tracheostomy/gastrostomy. Tongue–lip adhesion (TLA) aims to hold the tongue in protrusion by pexying it to the lower lip. This adhesion is generally maintained for 12 months; however, the exact timing of take down is individualized based on patient requirement and the capacity for catch-up growth in the mandible. If a cleft palate exists, the release of the TLA is generally deferred until 2–3 months after palate repair assuming that it is safe to detach the tongue at that time. The benefit of TLA is that the effects are immediate, and the procedure is well-tolerated with little need for specialized home care afterwards. The literature supports the use of TLA for cases of mild obstructive sleep apnea (OSA); however, recent experiences out of high-volume craniofacial centers have demonstrated that mandibular distraction osteogenesis (MDO) consistently outperforms TLA across all endpoints [32]. MDO treats the primary deformity by lengthening and projecting the mandible. MDO involves performing a posterior body osteotomy, applying mechanical distractors, transporting the free segments, and allowing for bony consolidation of the intervening callous. Following a brief latency period (often unnecessary in infants), the distraction is generally performed at a rate of 1 to 2 mm per day until the patient becomes slightly overcorrected and prognathic. We use the relationship of the upper and lower alveolar ridges as a guide to judge lower jaw position. The distractor arms are removed once distraction is completed; however, a secondary procedure is still required to take out the remaining hardware after a couple months of consolidation.

Mandibular distraction, as first described by McCarthy, was initially performed using external devices with transcutaneous pins. In the early 1990s, external distractors were the standard method for mandibular distraction. These external devices are still used in select circumstances with the main advantage being that the distraction vector can be altered and adjusted during the period of activation. In resource-limited settings given their reusability, reduced surgical time, and lower overall treatment costs, external distractors are often still employed. Although infants generally tolerate the external appliance, the multiple pin sites are susceptible to infection and postremoval scarring. In the late 1990s and early 2000s, external distractors were largely supplanted by lower-profile internal distractors with percutaneous distraction arms. These semi-buried devices have a unidirectional ratchet that prevents backwards activation and provides a safety mechanism against inadvertent movements. The limitations to these appliances are that the vector cannot be altered once the device is buried and that removal requires a revisit to the operating room to uncover and retrieve the device.

Contemporary Treatment

As in other areas of craniofacial surgery, computer-aided surgical planning has drastically improved the technique and safety of MDO. The accuracy of computer-assisted distraction cannot be understated. A series out of Spain found that their final screw placement was consistently within 1 mm of their plan and that angular deviations of their osteotomy line were less than 4 degrees off-axis [33]. This confirms the notion that surgeons are able to reliably and accurately execute their virtual plan. Dental complications of MDO are well-known and some are certainly unavoidable given the limited availability of bone stock and age at which RS patients are treated [34]. Computer-aided surgical planning allows surgeons to plan the osteotomies away from tooth buds and the inferior alveolar nerve to optimize tooth development. Multiangular osteotomies can be designed for this purpose. Likewise, the predictive holes can be registered and pre-drilled through the same osteotomy cutting guide in order to minimize trauma to the developing structures. The thickness of the bone can be measured to guide appropriate screw selection. Although MDO is performed with a straight-line advancement, computer-aided surgical planning assists with choosing the optimal vector and with matching this vector on both sides of the mandible. When the distraction is simulated, the MDO gap can be measured, and the duration of activation can be predicted. Stereolithographic models are used to preoperatively adapt the footplates for ease and time-savings (Fig. 1.5). To the best of our knowledge, custom-milled or printed internal distractors are not commercially available at this time; however, patient-specific distraction hardware may be in the pipeline as such devices would further reduce surgical deviation from the proposed plan.

Some of the challenges with computer-aided surgical planning, in addition to the cost of the technology, include data acquisition and manufacturing lead time. CT scans are required to capture the cross-sectional anatomy, and the exposure of infants to ionizing radiation is a valid concern. In our experience, infants often need intubation and general anesthesia to eliminate motion artifact especially, because repeating a CT for poor image quality is difficult to justify when the anatomy can be visualized and the sole purpose is to obtain accurate surgical guides. Many RS infants also have difficult airways that require high-risk intubations by skilled

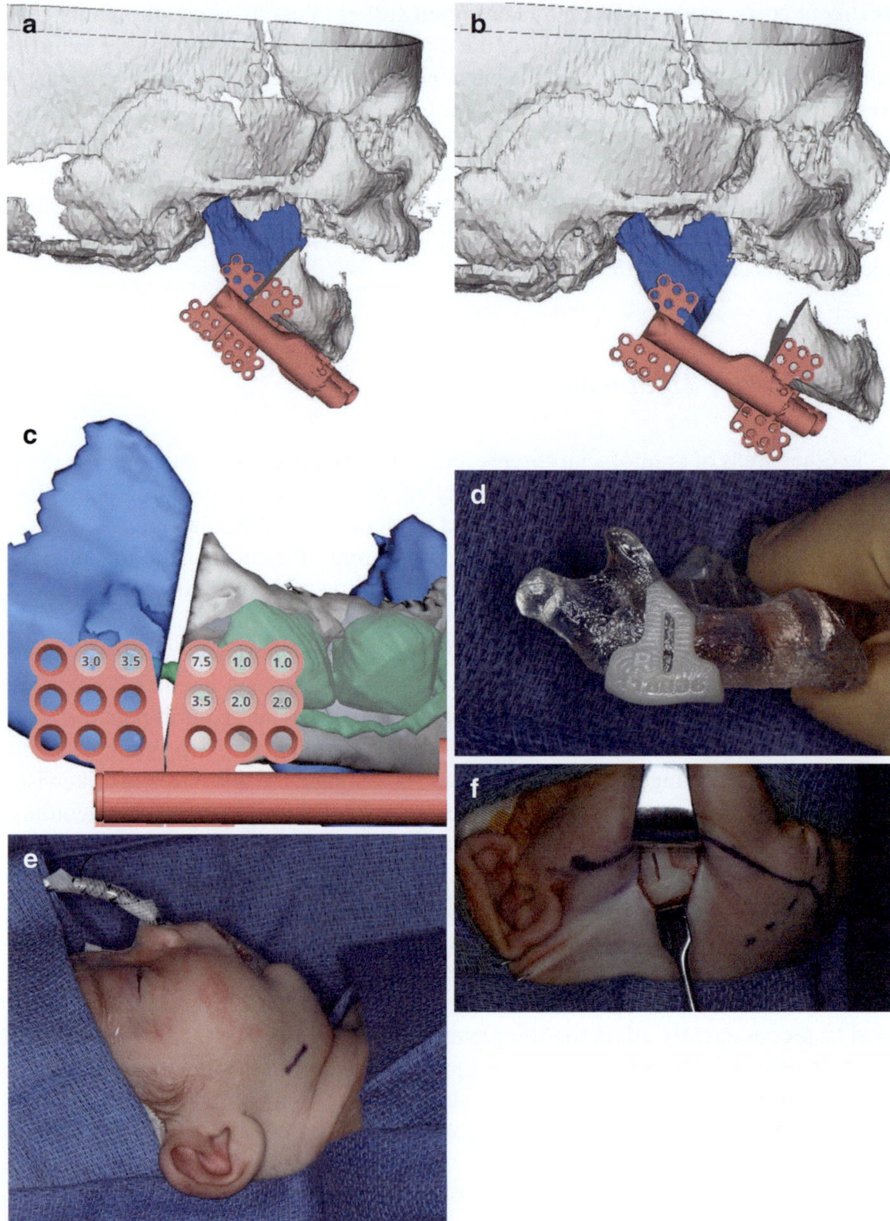

Fig. 1.5 Patient with Robin sequence (RS) planned for mandibular distraction. (**a**, **b**) Internal distractors placed virtually with simulated movement. (**c**) Oblique osteotomy planned away from tooth buds with depth measurements of pertinent anatomy. (**d**) Cutting guide registered on patient model. (**e**) Preoperative markings showing planned incision. (**f**, **g**) Intraoperative access with excellent guide fit and distractor adaptation. (**h**) Immediate postoperative result showing distractor arms exiting anteriorly. (**i**) Symmetric advancement with overcorrection to Class III relationship. (**j**) Improved mandibular projection appreciated at the time of distractor removal

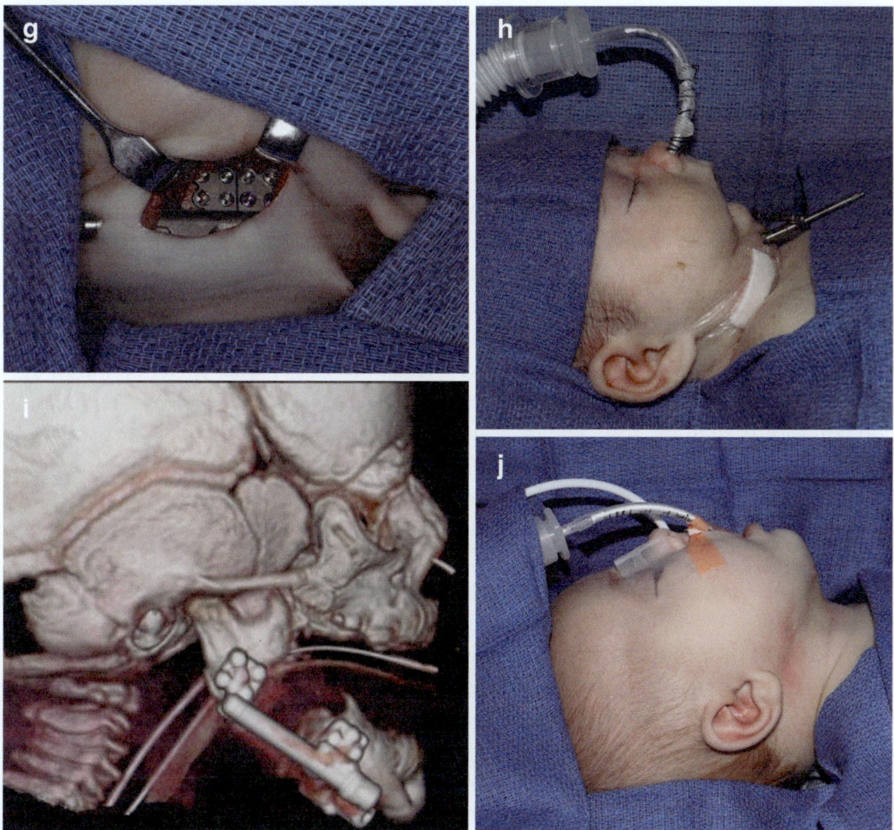

Fig. 1.5 (continued)

specialists. As a result, extubating these patients after CT is not always advisable. Finally, although the lead-time for obtaining patient models and guides has decreased in recent years, at least 7 days is generally required between planning session and surgery date. In most cases, this period of time is not prohibitive to using computer-aided surgical technology, and with the expansion of in-house printing capabilities at more and more centers, we anticipate that the manufacturing time will continue to shorten.

Hemifacial Microsomia and Treacher Collins Syndrome

Introduction

Both hemifacial microsomia (HFM) and Treacher Collins syndrome (TCS) are congenital conditions arising from the abnormal development of the first and second branchial arches. HFM, which is better termed craniofacial microsomia, is the second most common congenital anomaly of the face following cleft lip and palate. The term Goldenhar syndrome is used in the presence of internal organ and vertebral alterations. The incidence of HFM lies between 1 in 3000 and 5000 births. The precise etiology of HFM is unknown; however, the prevailing theory implicates an in-utero vascular event affecting the stapedial artery, which in turn results in massive tissue injury in the characteristic distribution. Experiments provoking a stapedial artery hematoma in mouse embryos have successfully replicated the HFM phenotype [35]. The branchial arches are derived from neural crest cells, and failed migration is thought to also play a role in the pathogenesis. There is also a potential genetic contribution to HFM, as higher rates of HFM have been identified among first degree relatives and an autosomal dominant inheritance pattern has been observed. Classically, HFM affects boys more commonly than girls, and although 10% of cases have a bilateral presentation, the right side is affected more severely and commonly than the left. The reasons for this pattern are poorly understood. The OMENS classification of HFM is the most commonly used nomenclature for stratifying disease severity. The OMENS system encompasses the anatomic spectrum of craniofacial deformities seen in HFM, namely, the orbit, mandible, ear, facial nerve, and soft tissue.

TCS, also known as mandibulofacial dysostosis, likewise manifests as an underdevelopment of the first two branchial arches. TCS is much rarer than HFM, arising in 1 in 50,000 births, and is most frequently caused by mutations to the TCOF1 gene, which is inherited in an autosomal dominant fashion. Despite their similarities, there are a few distinguishing features between HFM and TCS. TCS is always bilateral with fairly symmetric facial hypoplasia. The malar depression, sunken cheek appearance, and downward slating of the palpebral fissures are much more profound in TCS. TCS also has a higher rate of palatal clefting and transverse maxillary constriction, whereas in HFM there is a tendency to see Tessier 7 clefting and macrostomia from failed fusion of the maxillary and mandibular processes. Although the Kaban–Pruzansky classification of mandibular deficiency is integrated as part of the OMENS classification for HFM, the Kaban–Pruzansky classification is also an acceptable taxonomy for describing the TCS mandible given the morphologic similarities.

Traditional Repair

A wide range of severities exists for both HFM and TCS. In infancy, the early treatment goals are aimed at relieving airway obstruction, correcting orofacial clefts, and addressing any vision and hearing abnormalities. Some surgeons will elect to intervene and operate on the facial bones during active growth with the intent of minimizing psychosocial stress and intercepting growth to limit the magnitude of secondary craniofacial deformities. Similar to other dentofacial deformities, definitive skeletal and soft tissue correction are best postponed until after skeletal maturity. Maxillomandibular growth is completed around 16–18 years with skeletal maturity being reached later for boys than girls. The cranium and orbit generally can be corrected earlier, at around age 10, because skull growth is complete at that time. Likewise, for HFM, the growth of an unaffected ear is completed at around 7 years, so auricular reconstruction of the malformed ear can be done any time after then.

Similar to RS infants, OSA secondary to mandibular retrognathia is treated with either TLA, MDO, or tracheostomy. Because severe expressions of HFM and TCS present with an absent ramus-condyle unit (RCU), MDO may not be feasible in infancy given the poor retromolar bone stock. Therefore, it may be prudent to obtain a plain film prior to submitting the patient to a CT for surgical planning. Among children with grade 2b and 3 mandibular morphology, Kaban and Pruzansky have traditionally recommended early mandibular reconstruction to keep pace with normative growth. Their preference toward early intervention was motivated by the aforementioned reasons with the thought that doing so would simplify subsequent corrections at maturity. Furthermore, without staging the reconstruction, the soft tissue envelope in adulthood may not be able to accommodate the sudden stretch required to make the necessary skeletal movements. Still, despite the intuitive logic, the benefits of early interceptive surgery have yet to be proven [36].

At the time of Kaban and Pruzansky's publication, RCU reconstruction had primarily been achieved with costochondral grafting. The rib graft is a relatively simple harvest and does not require any additional imaging outside of a chest X-ray. If the periosteal sleeve of the rib is preserved and reapproximated in children, a neo-rib can regenerate to fill the donor defect. Costochondral grafts in younger patients have the purported benefit of conferring growth potential so long as care is taken to ensure that the cartilaginous cap remains attached. Unfortunately, the overwhelming consensus is that costal cartilage growth is unpredictable [37]. Some believe the amount of growth is a function of the size of the cartilaginous cap that is attached to the graft.

In the early 1990s, when distraction of the maxillofacial complex gained popularity, vertical ramus distractors became another popular option for RCU reconstruction. As with mandibular distractors, the first such devices were externally fixated. Some patients planned for distraction may require an initial bone graft to create a surface to attach the posterior foot plate. Mandibular distraction for HFM and TCS often requires a multivector or a curvilinear pathway to simultaneously advance, vertically lengthen, and counterclockwise rotate the mandible. In the absence of a glenoid fossa, it may be hard to ensure that the transported bone reaches a suitable landing point. It is often the case that the distracted condylar segment ends up far away from the external auditory meatus in a position too medial and anterior to give any meaningful function.

The orbito-zygomatic complex is another region that maxillofacial surgeons are often challenged with reconstructing. The rudimentary malar bones can be osteotomized and advanced, raised, and lateralized to improve projection. A split calvarial bone graft is often used for augmentation because of its good take, low absorption rates, and existing availability through the same coronal access used to approach the upper midface [38]. Iliac crest bone can also be harvested to but is less preferred.

Contemporary Treatment

The dilemmas posed by the challenging morphology of HFM and TCS patients have motivated surgeons and engineers to develop creative solutions that are no more invasive than the aforementioned treatment options. Currently, ramus distraction can be simulated digitally as discussed in the previous section (Fig. 1.6). In the

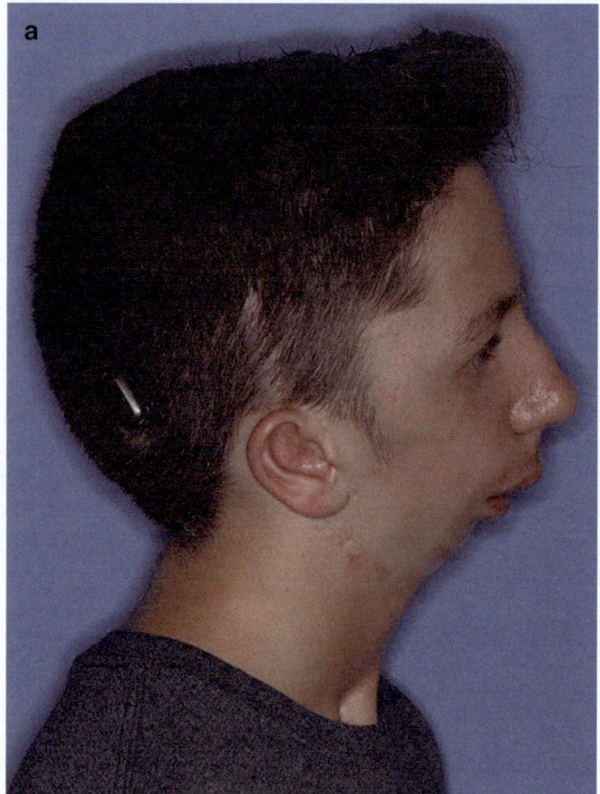

Fig. 1.6 Patient with Nager syndrome presenting with deficient rami and microretrognathia. (**a, b**) Preoperative profile view and skeletal anatomy. (**c**) Simulated movement using curvilinear distractor. (**d**) Ramus cutting guide with predictive holes. (**e, f**) Intraoperative fit of cutting guide and distractor with (**g**) stereolithographic model for verification. (**h, i**) Clinical result following the completion of mandibular distraction. (**j, k**) Second-stage maxillary surgery and genioplasty planned at the time of distractor removal to correct occlusion and further improve chin projection. (**l, m**) Final pre- and postoperative results showing improved midface and chin projection

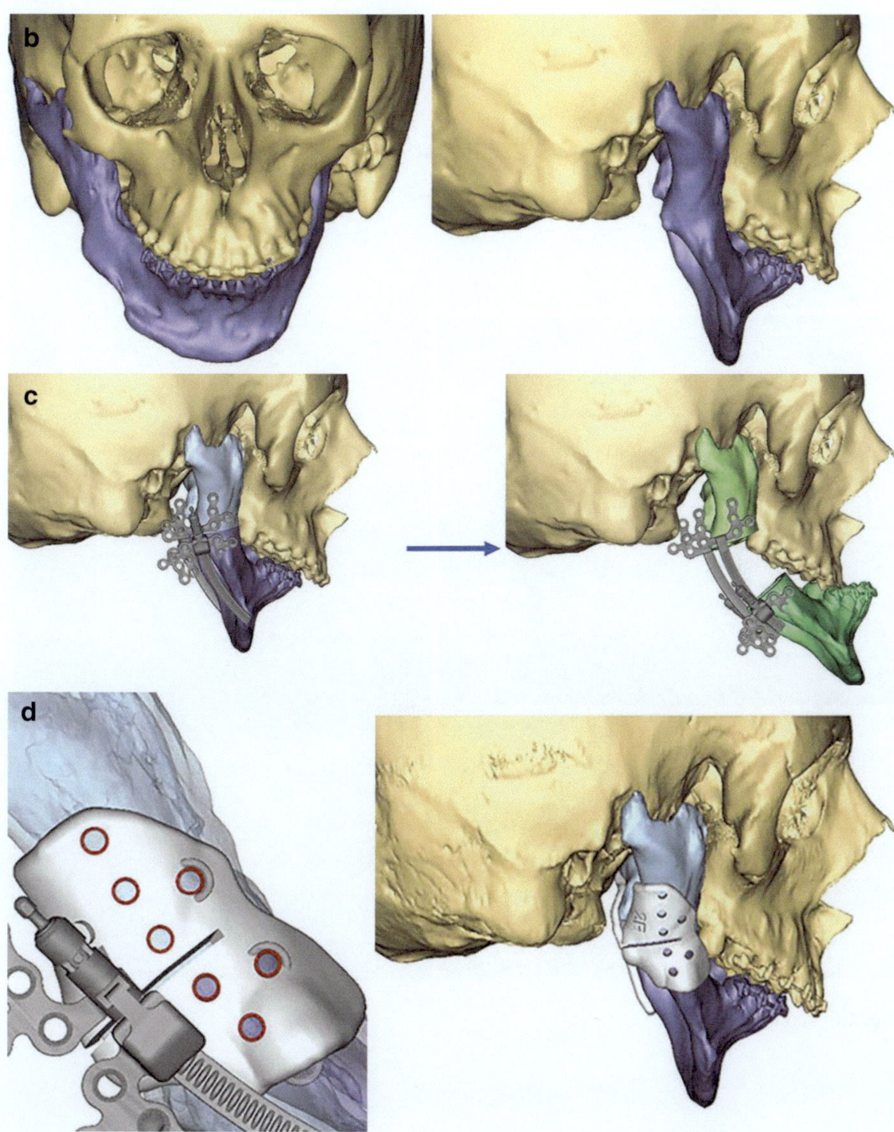

Fig. 1.6 (continued)

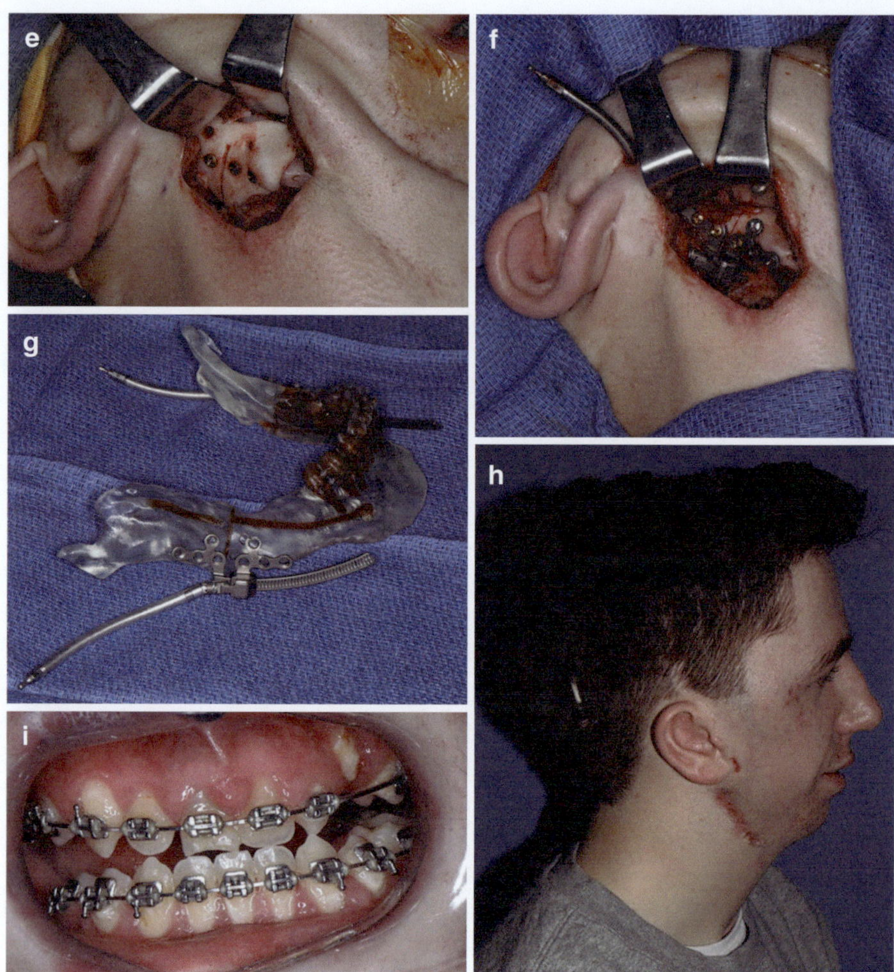

Fig. 1.6 (continued)

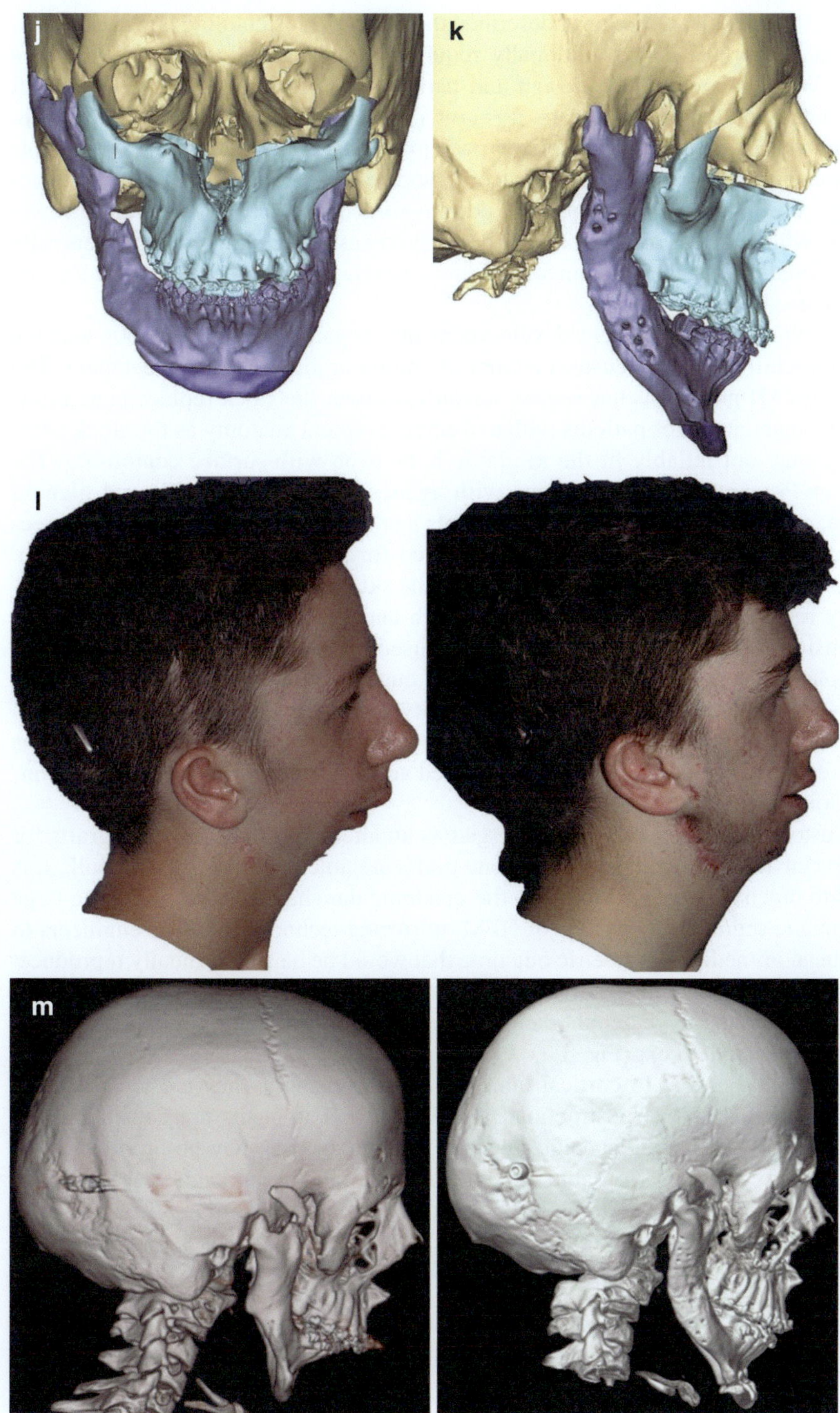

Fig. 1.6 (continued)

1950s, Trauner and Obwegeser described the inverted L osteotomy; however, a transcervical approach was traditionally required to achieve the necessary exposure [39]. With computer-aided design and patient-specific cutting guides, bone graft templates, and fixation hardware, it is now possible to perform the inverted L osteotomy via a completely transoral approach [40]. This is a useful options for patients with enough soft tissue stretch to accommodate large counterclockwise advancements. The inverted L technique also permits surgeons to perform these large movements with less fear of lengthening the pterygomasseteric sling which is generally considered an unstable movement and prone to relapse in the context of the sagittal split osteotomy.

Another relatively recent development that began in the early 2000s was the commercially available custom temporomandibular joint (TMJ) replacement. The custom TMJ prosthesis has several advantages over the stock replacement and is almost mandatory for patients with extremely atypical anatomy as the stock prosthesis may not reliably fit the available bone even with surface contouring. For Kaban–Pruzansky type 3 patients with agenesis of both the RCU and glenoid fossa, extended custom TMJ replacements can be designed to independently recreate the missing anatomy without the need for preceding bony reconstruction. Large, broad footplates can be adapted to the skull base and shaped to simultaneously recreate the both the zygomatic arch and glenoid fossa [41]. Long distal extensions off condylar component can be used to reach suitable bone in the parasymphyseal region. These unconventional custom joint replacements have been shown to have excellent mechanical stability and to drastically improve maximal incisal opening [41]. The extended custom joint is a welcomed solution for cases where the RCU anatomy is underdeveloped and inadequate for distraction or conventional orthognathic osteotomies.

Custom facial implants have emerged as an alternative to onlay bone grafts for midfacial augmentation. Although bone grafts are able to add reasonable bulk, it is hard to precisely contour them into the quadrangular shape needed to replace large zygomatic segments. For cases of HFM, mirroring technology allows engineers to create an immediate symmetric outcome that would be hard to manually reproduce. In our experience, the most frequently used materials for alloplastic implants include silicone, polyetheretherketone (PEEK), titanium, and high-density porous polyethylene (MedPor) (Fig. 1.7). PEEK implants are thermally resistant and biomechanically similar to cortical bone, and unsurprisingly, they are the preferred material for cranial reconstruction. Although PEEK implants are considered the gold standard of patient-specific implants, their high cost may be prohibitive for some. MedPor is an affordable alternative that is also remarkably stable. Unlike PEEK, MedPor implants are porous in nature and conducive to rapid fibovascular ingrowth, which is thought to improve long-term stability but also complicate subsequent removal [42, 43].

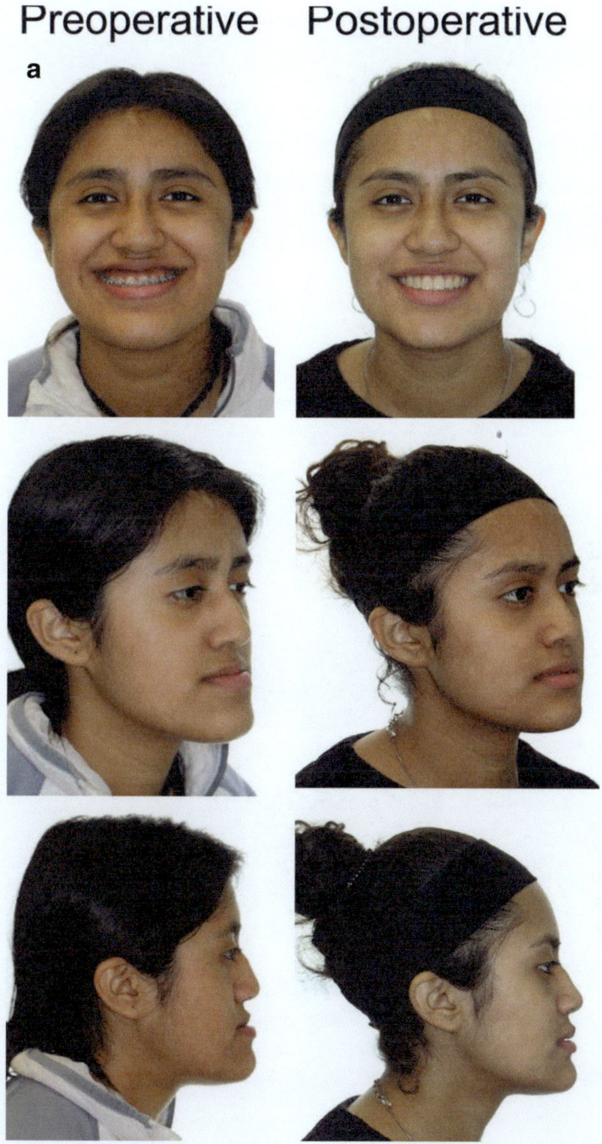

Fig. 1.7 Orthognathic surgery combined with custom silicone implant malar augmentation. Pre- and postoperative (**a**) facial and (**b**) intraoral photos. (**c**) Orthognathic surgical plan. (**d**, **e**) Frontal view showing implant height, lateral view showing implant projection. (**f**, **g**) Patient-specific implants are fixated after LeFort I osteotomy with care taken to avoid impinging on the infraorbital nerve. (Implantech Associates, Inc.; Ventura, CA). Pre- and postoperative side profile views of patient (**h**)

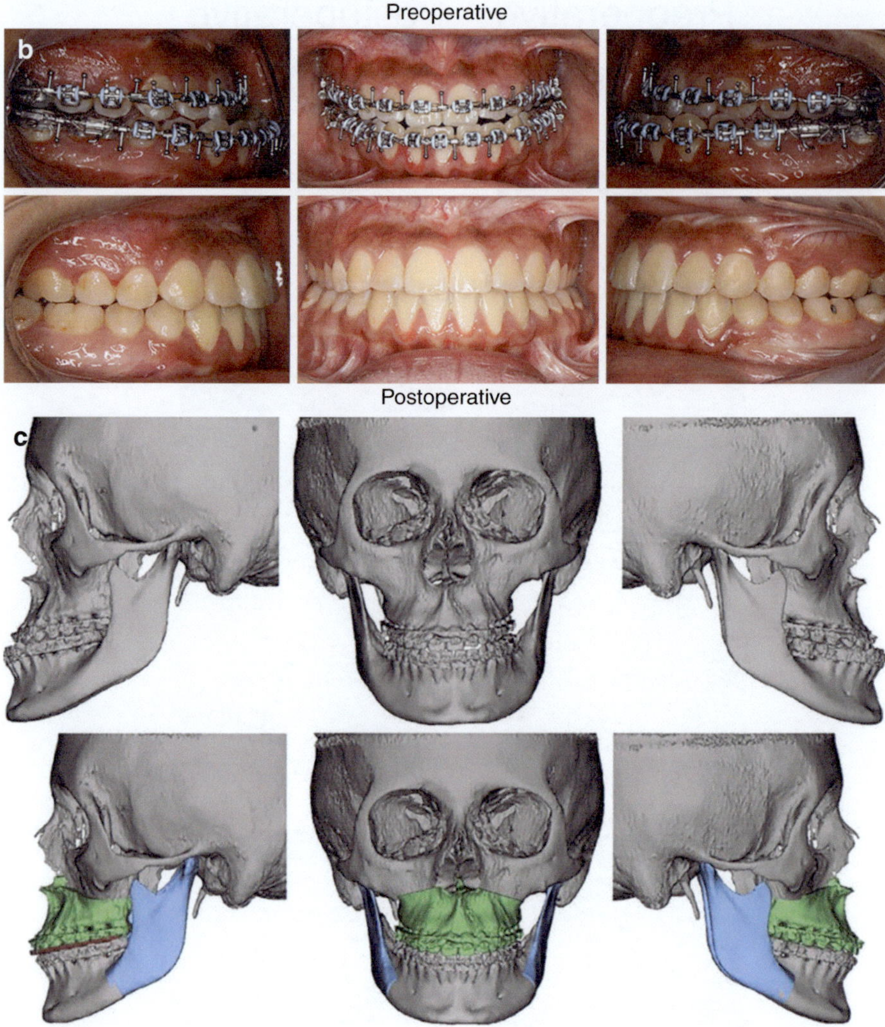

Fig. 1.7 (continued)

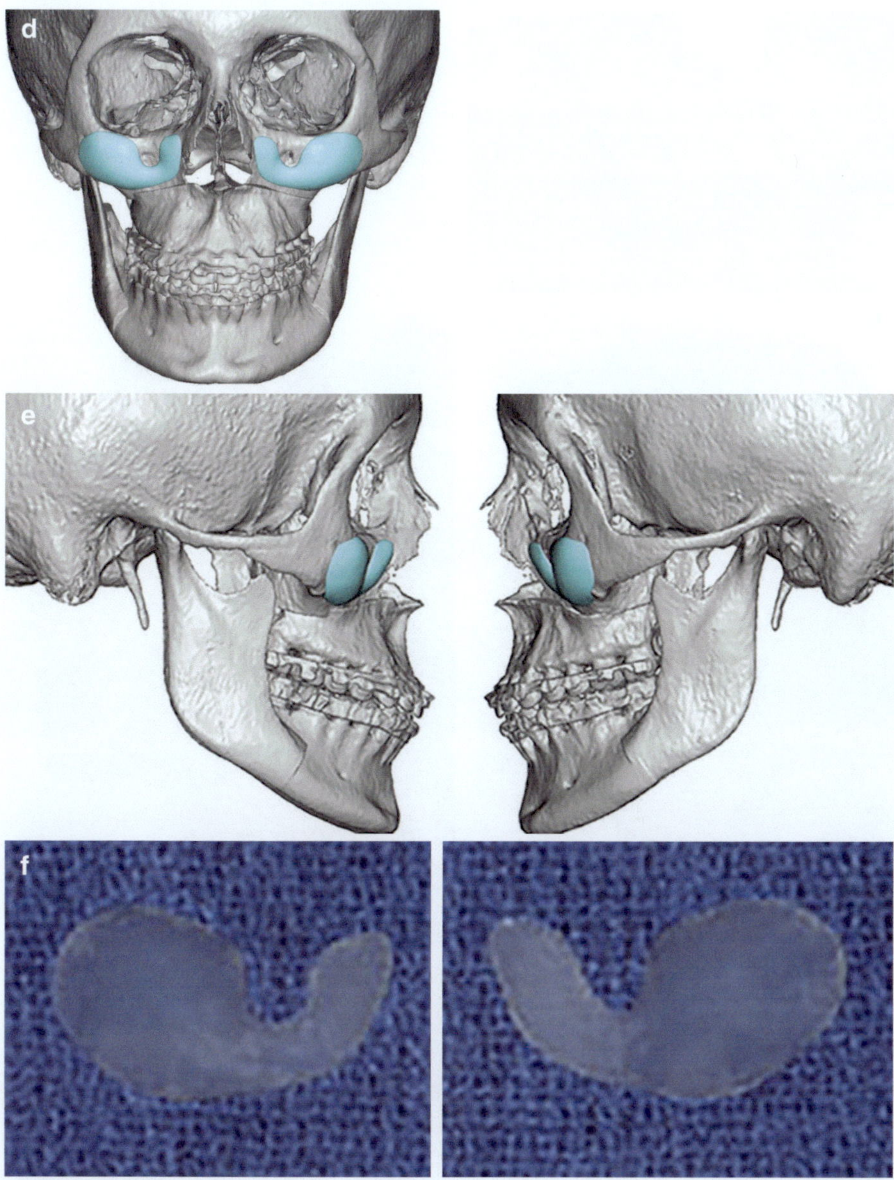

Fig. 1.7 (continued)

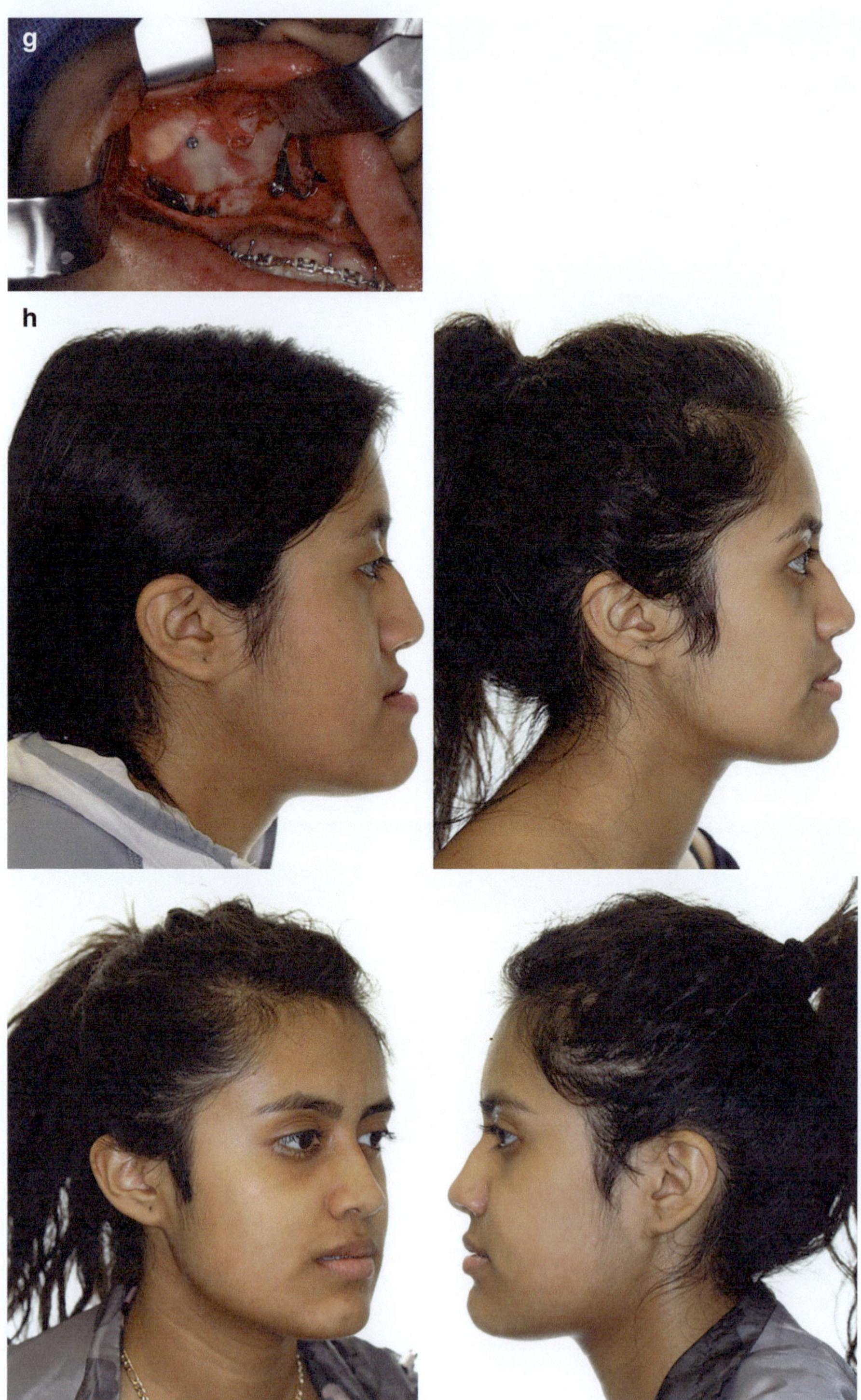

Fig. 1.7 (continued)

Summary and Outlook

In conclusion, the benefits of modern technology have extended into the field of craniofacial surgery. The original osteotomies described by Tessier and Obwegeser are still used today; however, we are now able to execute them with an unprecedented level of precision and confidence. The acceptable margin of deviation from the surgical plan has narrowed thanks in large part to patient-specific guides and implants. Computer-aided surgical technology is becoming more commonplace, and medical centers are beginning to realize the associated healthcare value that it brings as the cost of doing business decreases. Consequently, we anticipate that there will be a drive to decentralize manufacturing. High-volume centers will likely reduce their reliance on outsourcing and seek to develop on-site point of care planning and printing. This in-house service is already in place at many centers and has been shown to be cheaper with a shorter lead-time [44].

Although we are able to manipulate and predict the location of the bony skeleton, the quality of our soft tissue simulations still does not reach a level of usefulness. Likewise, one of the primary challenges of craniofacial surgery is being able to operate in the fourth dimension. We need to understand and predict the effects of surgery on growth and the effects of growth on surgery. In the future, computational frameworks may provide insight into these problems. Overall, it is important to recognize that continued progress in this field relies on the cooperative multidisciplinary efforts of all professionals caring for patients with craniofacial differences.

References

1. Tessier P. Total facial osteotomy. Crouzon's syndrome, Apert's syndrome: oxycephaly, scaphocephaly, turricephaly. Ann Chir Plast. 1967;12(4):273–86.
2. Tessier P, Guiot G, Rougerie J, Delbet JP, Pastoriza J. Cranio-naso-orbito-facial osteotomies. Hypertelorism. Ann Chir Plast. 1967;12(2):103–18.
3. McCarthy JG, Schreiber J, Karp N, Thorne CH, Grayson BH. Lengthening the human mandible by gradual distraction. Plast Reconstr Surg. 1992;89(1):1–8; discussion 9–10, 1.
4. A V. De Humani Corporis Fabrica. Basel: Oporinus; 1543.
5. Dc G. Curygua Universale e Perfetta. Venetia: Ziletta; 1583.
6. Virchow R. Uber den Cretinismus, namentlich in franken, und uber pathologische schadelformen. Verh Phys Med Ges Wurz. 1851;2:241.
7. Delashaw JB, Persing JA, Broaddus WC, Jane JA. Cranial vault growth in craniosynostosis. J Neurosurg. 1989;70(2):159–65.
8. Di Rocco F, Arnaud E, Renier D. Evolution in the frequency of nonsyndromic craniosynostosis. J Neurosurg Pediatr. 2009;4(1):21–5.
9. Hackshaw A, Rodeck C, Boniface S. Maternal smoking in pregnancy and birth defects: a systematic review based on 173 687 malformed cases and 11.7 million controls. Hum Reprod Update. 2011;17(5):589–604.
10. Lannelongue M. De la craniectomie dans la microcephalie. CR Seances Acad Sci. 1890;110:1382.
11. Lane L. Pioneer craniectomy for relief of mental imbecility due to premature sutural closure and microcephalus. J Am Med Assoc. 1892;18(2):49–50.

12. Pattisapu JV, Gegg CA, Olavarria G, Johnson KK, Ruiz RL, Costello BJ. Craniosynostosis: diagnosis and surgical management. Atlas Oral Maxillofac Surg Clin North Am. 2010;18(2):77–91.
13. Bly RA, Chang SH, Cudejkova M, Liu JJ, Moe KS. Computer-guided orbital reconstruction to improve outcomes. JAMA Facial Plast Surg. 2013;15(2):113–20.
14. Hsu SS, Gateno J, Bell RB, Hirsch DL, Markiewicz MR, Teichgraeber JF, et al. Accuracy of a computer-aided surgical simulation protocol for orthognathic surgery: a prospective multicenter study. J Oral Maxillofac Surg. 2013;71(1):128–42.
15. Mardini S, Alsubaie S, Cayci C, Chim H, Wetjen N. Three-dimensional preoperative virtual planning and template use for surgical correction of craniosynostosis. J Plast Reconstr Aesthet Surg. 2014;67(3):336–43.
16. Andrew TW, Baylan J, Mittermiller PA, Cheng H, Johns DN, Edwards MSB, et al. Virtual surgical planning decreases operative time for isolated single suture and multi-suture craniosynostosis repair. Plast Reconstr Surg Glob Open. 2018;6(12):e2038.
17. Barone CM, Jimenez DF. Endoscopic craniectomy for early correction of craniosynostosis. Plast Reconstr Surg. 1999;104(7):1965–73; discussion 74–5.
18. Berry-Candelario J, Ridgway EB, Grondin RT, Rogers GF, Proctor MR. Endoscope-assisted strip craniectomy and postoperative helmet therapy for treatment of craniosynostosis. Neurosurg Focus. 2011;31(2):E5.
19. Posnick JC, Ruiz RL, Tiwana PS. Craniofacial dysostosis syndromes: stages of reconstruction. Oral Maxillofac Surg Clin North Am. 2004;16(4):475–91.
20. Derderian C, Seaward J. Syndromic craniosynostosis. Semin Plast Surg. 2012;26(2):64–75.
21. Bradley JP, Gabbay JS, Taub PJ, Heller JB, O'Hara CM, Benhaim P, et al. Monobloc advancement by distraction osteogenesis decreases morbidity and relapse. Plast Reconstr Surg. 2006;118(7):1585–97.
22. Gleizal A, Bera JC, Lavandier B, Beziat JL. Piezoelectric osteotomy: a new technique for bone surgery-advantages in craniofacial surgery. Childs Nerv Syst. 2007;23(5):509–13.
23. Gray R, Gougoutas A, Nguyen V, Taylor J, Bastidas N. Use of three-dimensional, CAD/CAM-assisted, virtual surgical simulation and planning in the pediatric craniofacial population. Int J Pediatr Otorhinolaryngol. 2017;97:163–9.
24. Hammoudeh JA, Goel P, Wolfswinkel EM, Fahradyan A, Vartanian E, Garg R, et al. Simultaneous midface advancement and orthognathic surgery: a powerful technique for managing midface hypoplasia and malocclusion. Plast Reconstr Surg. 2020;145(6):1067e.
25. Fariña R, Valladares S, Raposo A, Silva F. Modified Le fort III osteotomy: a simple solution to severe midfacial hypoplasia. J Craniomaxillofac Surg. 2018;46(5):837–43.
26. Robin P. Glossoptosis due to atresia and hypotrophy of the mandible. Am J Dis Child. 1934;48(3):541–7.
27. Zellner EG, Reid RR, Steinbacher DM. The Pierre Robin mandible is hypoplastic and morphologically abnormal. J Craniofac Surg. 2017;28(8):1946–9.
28. Izumi K, Konczal LL, Mitchell AL, Jones MC. Underlying genetic diagnosis of Pierre Robin sequence: retrospective chart review at two children's hospitals and a systematic literature review. J Pediatr. 2012;160(4):645–50.e2.
29. Lee KC, Eisig SB, Carrao V, Chuang S-K, Perrino MA. Which factors affect length of stay and readmission rate in mandibular distraction osteogenesis? J Oral Maxillofac Surg. 2019;77(8):1681–6.
30. Selvi R, Priyanka AM. Role of SOX9 in the etiology of Pierre-Robin syndrome. Iran J basic Med Sci. 2013;16(5):700–4.
31. Bütow K-W, Zwahlen RA, Morkel JA, Naidoo S. Pierre Robin sequence: subdivision, data, theories, and treatment—part 3: prevailing controversial theories related to Pierre Robin sequence. Ann Maxillofac Surg. 2016;6(1):38–43.
32. Zhang RS, Hoppe IC, Taylor JA, Bartlett SP. Surgical management and outcomes of Pierre Robin sequence: a comparison of mandibular distraction osteogenesis and tongue-lip adhesion. Plast Reconstr Surg. 2018;142(2):480–509.

33. Vanesa V, Irene MP, Marta AS, Francisco José PF, Miguel BS, Mireia RM, et al. Accuracy of virtually planned mandibular distraction in a pediatric case series. J Craniomaxillofac Surg. 2021;49(2):154–65.
34. Peacock ZS, Salcines A, Troulis MJ, Kaban LB. Long-term effects of distraction osteogenesis of the mandible. J Oral Maxillofac Surg. 2018;76(7):1512–23.
35. Poswillo D. The pathogenesis of the first and second branchial arch syndrome. Oral Surg Oral Med Oral Pathol. 1973;35(3):302–28.
36. Nagy K, Kuijpers-Jagtman AM, Mommaerts MY. No evidence for long-term effectiveness of early osteodistraction in hemifacial microsomia. Plast Reconstr Surg. 2009;124(6):2061–71.
37. Perrott DH, Umeda H, Kaban LB. Costochondral graft construction/reconstruction of the ramus/condyle unit: long-term follow-up. Int J Oral Maxillofac Surg. 1994;23(6 Pt 1):321–8.
38. Freihofer H. Variations in the correction of Treacher Collins syndrome. Plast Reconstr Surg. 1997;99:647.
39. Trauner R, Obwegeser H. The surgical correction of mandibular prognathism and retrognathia with consideration of genioplasty. I. Surgical procedures to correct mandibular prognathism and reshaping of the chin. Oral Surgery Oral Medicine Oral Pathol. 1957;10(7):677–89; contd.
40. Franco PB, Farrell BB. Inverted L osteotomy: a new approach via intraoral access through the advances of virtual surgical planning and custom fixation. J Oral Maxillofac Surg. 2016;2(1):1–9.
41. Briceno WX, Milkovich J, El-Rabbany M, Caminiti MF, Psutka DJ. Reconstruction of large defects using extended temporomandibular joint patient-matched prostheses. J Oral Maxillofac Surg. 2022;80(6):1018–32.
42. Wellisz T. Clinical experience with the medpor porous polyethylene implant. Aesthet Plast Surg. 1993;17(4):339–44.
43. Ridwan-Pramana A, Wolff J, Raziei A, Ashton-James CE, Forouzanfar T. Porous polyethylene implants in facial reconstruction: outcome and complications. J Cranio-Maxillofac Surg. 2015;43(8):1330–4.
44. Bergeron L, Bonapace-Potvin M, Bergeron F. In-house 3D model printing for acute Cranio-maxillo-facial trauma surgery: process, time, and costs. Plast Reconstr Surg Glob Open. 2021;9(9):e3804.

Chapter 2
Advancements and Innovations in Cleft Surgery

Ryan Keyho, Matthew R. Greives, and Phuong D. Nguyen

Current Standards in Cleft Care

Current standard cleft lip and palate repair today involves multiple techniques depending on the specific type of deformity, surgeon experience, and training bias. Techniques for palate repair include Von Langenbeck bipedicle flaps, Bardach flaps, Veau–Wardill–Kilner Pushback, Furlow double opposing Z-plasty, and more recently, the inclusion of tissue augmentation with buccal flaps. Likewise, multiple techniques for cleft lip repair have been described with the two current most common being the rotation advancement and anatomic subunit repair techniques. Though there have historically been many modifications to cutaneous lip markings and designs, more recently, there has been emphasis on providing nasal floor closure and prevention of anterior oral nasal fistulas. In earlier descriptions of the rotation advancement technique, the "M" and "L" flaps have been used to provide anterior nasal floor closure and sagittal projection of the cleft nose. Newer strategies have been developed to create oral nasal separation at the time of the index lip surgery.

R. Keyho · M. R. Greives
Division of Plastic Surgery, Department of Surgery, McGovern Medical School at the
University of Texas Health Science Center, Houston, TX, USA
e-mail: ryan.j.keyho@uth.tmc.edu; matthew.r.greives@uth.tmc.edu

P. D. Nguyen (✉)
Division of Plastic Surgery, Department of Surgery, McGovern Medical School at the
University of Texas Health Science Center, Houston, TX, USA

Children's Memorial Hermann Hospital, Houston, TX, USA
e-mail: phuong.nguyen@uth.tmc.edu

Oronasal Fistula Complications and Prevention by Surgical Techniques

A well-described complication after cleft palate repair is an oronasal fistula. These can be symptomatic with increased air escape creating hypernasality and oral nasal regurgitation. Fistulas may occur due to wound dehiscence, with increased risk with high tension during closure, trauma to the flaps, hematomas, infections, or other sources of tissue ischemia. The morbidity of an oronasal fistula varies and depends on the size and significance. A recent meta-analysis estimated the incidence of oronasal fistula following primary cleft palate repair at an incidence of 4.9% [1]. Reports of fistula incidence during international mission trips, however, was significantly higher at 35.4% [2, 3]. Children in low-resource settings have been shown to have higher complication rates than children in high-resource settings. Regression analysis has demonstrated that older age at palatoplasty and Veau class III and IV are associated with post-palatal fistulas [2].

Multiple attempts at classification and standardization of description of oronasal fistulas have been created. Perhaps the most widely used, the Pittsburgh classification system aims to provide a clinically structured approach to defining the fistula anatomy divided into seven types. This anatomically based numerical fistula classification system is categorized as: type I, bifid uvula; type II, soft palate; type III, junction of the soft and hard palate; type IV, hard palate; type V, junction of the primary and secondary palates (for Veau IV clefts); type VI, lingual alveolar; and type VII, labial alveolar (Fig. 2.1) [4, 5]. This numerical distinction improves communication and clarifies ambiguities in reporting in the literature. More recently, others have added descriptions that belie whether the fistula is midline, lateral, or subtotal [6].

Although some fistulas may be managed in a conservative manner, larger fistulas may progress to cause significant speech deficits and velopharyngeal insufficiency. Fistula repair is aimed at improving symptomatic regurgitation and speech clarity. Orthodontic maxillary arch expansion is usually completed prior to closure attempts. Anterior and alveolar fistulas (type VI and VII) may be addressed at the time of alveolar bone grafting. A multitude of techniques have been described for fistula repair [7]. Generally, when feasible, one should attempt a two-layered closure with nasal lining and oral lining in order to prevent flap contraction and recurrence. This may require remobilizing the original flaps versus tissue augmentation such as with buccal flaps. Overall, the decision regarding how to treat fistulas will depend on the severity and classification of the fistula and the degree of velopharyngeal dysfunction present [8].

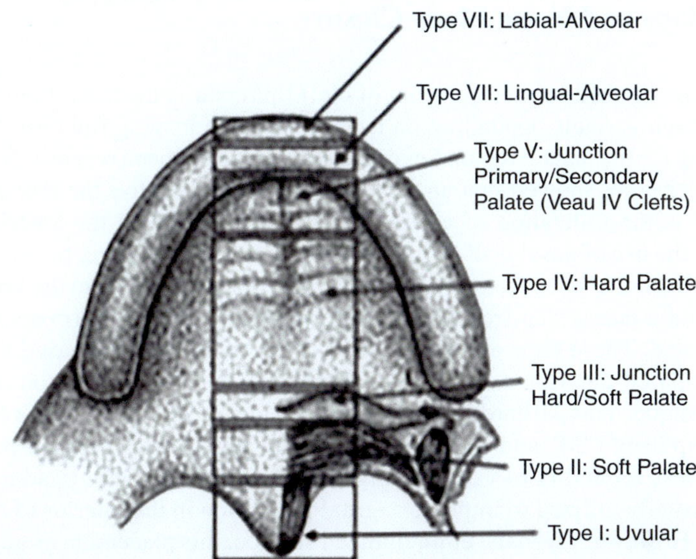

Fig. 2.1 Pittsburgh classification of palatal fistulas. (used with permission from Anderson BJ, Fallah KN, Lignieres AA, Moffitt JK, Luu KL, Cepeda A Jr., Doringo IL, Nguyen PD, Teichgraeber JF, Greives MR. Predictive Factors for Velopharyngeal Insufficiency Following Primary Cleft Palate Repair. Cleft Palate Craniofac J. 2022 Jul;59(7):825–832. doi: 10.1177/10556656211026861. Epub 2021 Aug 16. PMID: 34396792)

Tissue Augmentation with Buccal Mucosal Flaps

Several studies have evaluated the use of tissue augmentation, specifically buccal mucosal flaps for velopharyngeal insufficiency following primary palatoplasty repair. Buccal myomucosal flaps provide additional tissue with or without fat pad transfer for tissue lengthening of the nasal and oral lining and allow for a reduction in scar contracture along the soft and hard palate by providing vascularized tissue at the site of repair [9].Tissue augmentation strategies have been shown to be a good source for improving speech by lengthening the palate following primary palatoplasty repair. These flaps may reduce morbidity by decreasing dead space and reducing tension on the palatal closure. More recently, there has been growing experience with the use of tissue augmentation at the time of primary palatal repair to optimize healing and functional outcomes [10].

Nasal Flaps and Nasal Floor Closure

An often overlooked but central tenet of cleft lip repair is the nasal floor closure. This has been variable depending on technique, often leaving full closure of the nasal lining for the palatal repair. Several techniques have been recently described. Mittermiller et al. showed that an effective option to decrease the risk of fistula formation is the utilization of a one or two-layer closure of the anterior nasal floor with the use of nasal wall lining flaps [11]. In this procedure, the medial flap is created from the mucoperiosteum and mucoperichondrium from the vomer and septum, and a lateral flap from the mucoperiosteum of the piriform aperture are approximated. These flaps are often more vascular and have increased thickness when compared anterior nasal floor closure with the classic rotation advancement technique. This Millard technique utilizes medial and lateral flaps elements from the lip itself ("M" and "L" flaps), which are relatively diminutive in surface area with less reliability of vascularity given the narrow pedicle. In addition, the L flap is usually utilized to improve sagittal projection in the interior of the nasal vestibule. However, given the epithelialized surface, this placement as augmentation of the nasal mucosa pits "unlike" with "like." Lastly, the M flap is usually only substantial enough to reconstruct the most anterior nasal sill, while leaving the posterior nasal floor unrepaired. Proponents of the complete nasal lining closure technique describe improved outcomes for both unilateral and bilateral complete cleft lip and palate repair patients by decreasing the alveolar fistula rate when compared to medial and lateral flap closure, while also increasing the ease of future bone grafting due to complete closure of the nasal floor [11]. Mendoza and Perez describe a technique for reconstruction of the nasal floor concurrently with cheiloplasty in unilateral cleft lip and palate patients. Their procedure involved the use of two nasal mucosal flaps, medial and lateral, repositioned anatomically to close the nasal floor. Among the 358 patients that underwent repair with this technique, 6% had asymmetry of the nasal base less than 1 mm, 5% had nasal fistulas, and 1% required revision [12]. An inferior turbinate flap has also been described to create the nasal lining to repair oronasal fistulas [13]. In our current practice, we aim to perform complete closure of the nasal floor using a superiorly based medial flap from mucoperiosteum of the septum and a superiorly based lateral flap from the mucoperiosteum of the inferior turbinate (Fig. 2.2). This is performed at the index cleft lip procedure in both unilateral and bilateral cases. Flaps are dissected using a cottle elevator in a subperiosteal/chondral level after extension of incision at the inferior aspect of the turbinate and septum, respectively. The nasal floor is reconstructed from posterior to anterior using a Vicryl suture. The main advantage of this procedure at this time is adequate surgical exposure and reduction of subsequent oronasal fistula. Additionally, this provides improvement of symmetry of the alar bases and pyriform (Fig. 2.3).

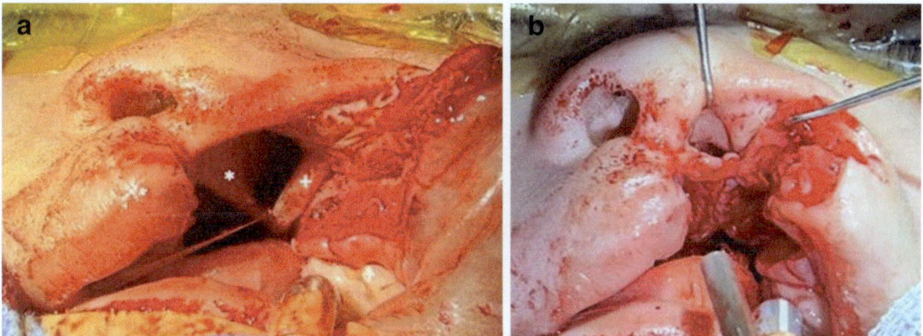

Fig. 2.2 (a) Nasal floor closure in left unilateral complete cleft lip and palate with medial septal mucosal (*) and lateral inferior turbinate (+) mucoperiosteal flaps. (b) Complete nasal floor closure

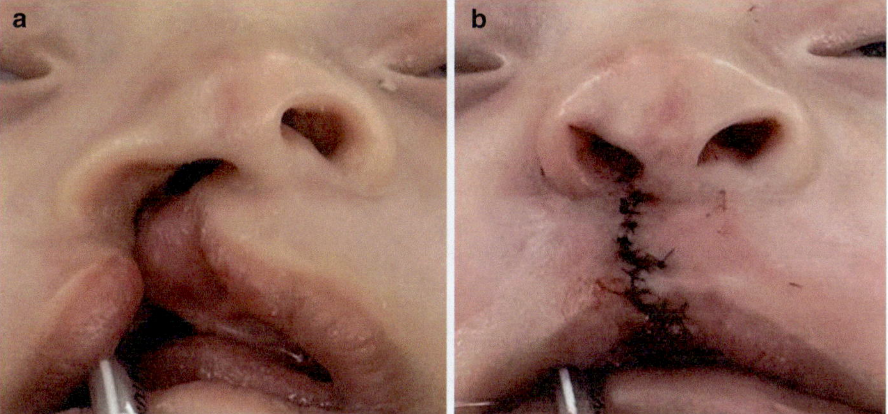

Fig. 2.3 (a) Preoperative worm's eye view of right unilateral complete cleft lip, palate, and alveolus. Note inferiorly displaced pyriform and nasal ala. (b) Postoperative repair of cleft lip with complete closure of nasal floor using medial septal mucosal and lateral inferior turbinate flap. Note improved symmetry and position of pyriform and nasal ala

Modified Von Langenbeck Approach

A modified Von Langenbeck approach to cleft palate repair using an anterior triangle flap was described by Stewert et al. [14]. The triangular flap consists of oral mucosa as a turnover flap and is intended for secondary palate repair only with closure of the anterior nasal mucosa. The Von Langenbeck flaps then are approximated in standard fashion for the oral lining. The proposed advantage of this approach allows for reduced tension at the anterior aspect of the cleft and may be particularly useful for Veau 2 clefts. In their review of their experience, 0 of 192 patients who underwent this technique developed an oronasal fistula [14].

Hard Palate Closure Timing

Several groups have reported on outcomes of the use of primary vomerine flaps (VF) to assist in closure of the anterior hard palate at the time of lip repair, particularly Sommerlad [15]. A single-layer vomer flap of the hard palate has been advocated to reduce the need for a lateral incision. However, there has been suggestion that the vomerine dissection may cause restricted midfacial growth. Hay et al. reviewed their outcomes utilizing vomerine flap closure with a 10-year follow-up specifically evaluating for midface development and hypoplasia. When comparing those with VF versus non-VF patients, there was no statistically significant difference in maxillary growth when assessed cephalometrically [15].

Maggiulli et al. investigated the effects of VF closure of the hard palate at the time of lip repair compared with nonclosure of the hard palate among patients with unilateral cleft lip and palate with respect to the subsequent alveolar arch gap at the time of palate repair at 6 months. The decrease of alveolar arch gap width in the VF group was significantly more than the decrease in the non-VF group, with no significant decrease in the anterior and posterior arch width or anteroposterior length of the hard palate [16].

Buccal Fat Pad and Buccal Flap

The implementation of tissue augmentation to lengthen the palate and fill dead space has been a concept championed for several decades [17]. Initial indications of using buccal myomucosal flaps (BMMF) as an adjunct for decreasing wound tension with double opposing z-plasties has evolved into many iterations for both primary palate repair, secondary fistula repair, and palatal lengthening in velopharyngeal insufficiency (VPI) [17]. BMMFs are random patterned flaps that can be quickly harvested from either cheek. Optimization of the flaps include adhering to the 3:1 length to width ratio, keeping a wide base at the pedicle between the retromolar trigone and the maxillary tuberosity, and maintenance of a thin flap of approximately 3 mm in thickness to reduce venous congestion [17, 18] (Fig. 2.4). These flaps may have multiple geometric insets and can be utilized either in unilateral or in bilateral form [19]. In our series, we assessed outcomes for cleft patients with VPI who had a conversion Furlow palatoplasty alone (FA) or conversion Furlow with buccal flaps (FB) after primary straight-line repair of the palate [19]. Of these 77 patients, 16 (21%) had an FB. The FA group had a 7% postoperative fistula rate ($n = 4$) with no postop fistulas in the FB group. Both demonstrated a decrease in hypernasality and total parameter scores postoperatively. As such, we feel that the use of buccal flaps in revision Furlow palatoplasty may decrease risk of postoperative complications.

More recently, pedicled buccal fat pads have been utilized to aid in oral mucosal healing and augmenting tissue bulk [20]. Compared to other options of VPI repair

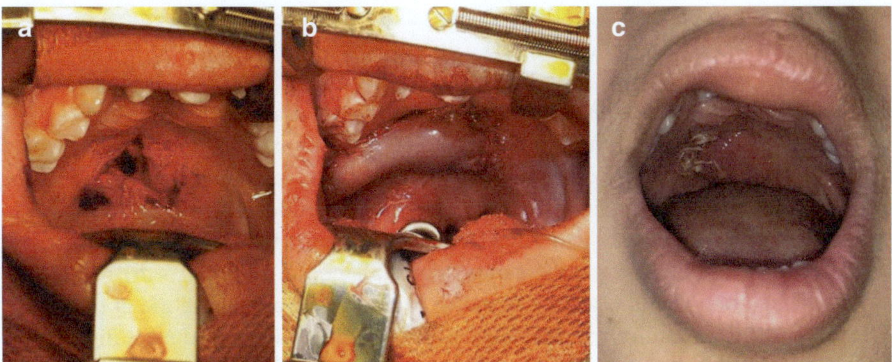

Fig. 2.4 (**a**) Oronasal palatal fistula following straight line cleft palate repair. (**b**) R sided buccal musculomucosal flap for fistula closure after inset. (**c**) Healed buccal flap 1 month following division of pedicle

including double opposing z-plasty, pharyngeal flap surgery, and sphincter pharyngoplasty, buccal fat pad augmentation helps to release tension on the oral mucosal flap by providing an additional source of vascularized tissue on the soft palate without the restriction of closure of the buccal mucosa as in a BMMF. An anatomic study demonstrated that buccal fat pads can provide coverage from the soft palate to the posterior third of the hard palate and across the midline [21]. Approximately three-fourths of the flaps are also able to cover the mid hard palate, though none were extensive enough to cover the anterior hard palate. Park et al. reviewed their experience in correcting VPI in cleft patients using either double opposing z-plasty (DOZ) either alone or with the aid of buccal fat pad (BFP). They report that BFPs reduced the tension of the DOZ mucosal flap and maximized palatal lengthening and muscle repositioning (7.5 ± 2.1 mm vs. 4.4 ± 1.7 mm, respectively). This promoted velopharyngeal closure in patients with moderate and moderate-to-severe velopharyngeal insufficiency. With these tissue augmentation adjuncts, the surgeon's armamentarium for optimizing palate repair has greatly increased. A recent study proposed a decision-tree algorithm for identifying when to utilize BFPs and buccal myomucosal flaps [22].

Growth Factors for Alveolar Bone Grafting

Bone grafting of the alveolus is traditionally performed at the age of mixed dentition to (a) align the alveolar arches and (b) provide sufficient bone stock for eruption of the canine. A recent literature review has advocated for secondary alveolar bone grafting (SABG) at an earlier age (4–7 years) before the eruption of lateral incisors over the later group (8–12 years) before the eruption of maxillary permanent canines. This review demonstrated that 6/7 of the studies in their inclusion criteria concluded that early SABG provided a better outcome than late SABG with regard to bone volume, surgical complication, maxillary permanent canine impaction rate, and anterior incisor crown length [23].

Alveolar bone grafting has traditionally utilized autologous cancellous bone from the iliac crest. Although this has been the gold standard, drawbacks of donor site morbidity and anatomic size limitation have drawn pursuance of alternative methods of bone grafting. Several studies have investigated the use of growth factors for bone grafting in cleft lip and palate repair. Recent investigations into using rhBMP-2 in combination with demineralized bone matrix as an alternative to autologous alveolar bone grafting have challenged the status quo. Makar et al. found that rhBMP-2 with demineralized bone matrix as an alternative to traditional alveolar bone grafting provides decreased morbidity but does have possible risks of increased swelling. As this product remains an off-label use, this group proposed that it is implemented for patients with tenuous soft tissues when the likelihood of graft failure is high. In their small case series, all of their patients who underwent BMP-2/DBM grafting generated bone in the cleft [24]. Liang et al. conducted a review of six different bone graft substitutes and evaluated the evidence behind their usage, efficacy, and cost. These bone substitutes were as follows: hydroxyapatite, demineralized bone matrix (DBM), β-tricalcium phosphate (TCP), calcium phosphate, recombinant human bone morphogenetic protein-2 (rhBMP-2), and rhBMP7. They found that BM, TCP, rhBMP-2, and rhBMP7 were the most extensively studied substitutes in terms of alveolar cleft repair; however, much of the evidence was level III or below. Specifically, rhBMP-2 was the best studied and had comparable efficacy to iliac crest bone graft (ICBG) for bone regeneration volume and density. The literature indicated that rhBMP-2 was found to have a 3% complication rate compared to 2.6% in ICBG patients. Common postoperative complaints included oral edema, mouth pain, and oral erythema. No studies have shown increased risk of malignancy following use of rhBMP-2.

A systematic review by Uribe et al. identified five articles that evaluated bone volume formation in rhBMP-2 groups versus control groups. Although the bone volume formation was slightly higher in the rhBMP-2 group over the control group (61.11% vs. 59.12%), the average bone height formation was higher in the control group compared to the rhBMP-2 group (75.4% vs. 61.5%). However, the risk of bias in the articles may pose some limitations to the validity of the results [25].

In perhaps the largest single institution review, Hammoudeh et al. performed a comparative analysis of rhBMP-2 with demineralized bone matrix compared to iliac crest bone graft for secondary alveolar graft in cleft lip and palate patients in a review of 501 cases [26]. There were 258 rhBMP-2/DBM procedures and 243 iliac crest bone graft procedures on 414 patients over a 12-year period. Canine tooth eruption in the cleft site through the graft were similar between the groups, whereas 23/228 (10.0%) rhBMP-2/DBM patients and 28/242 (11.6%) required repeat surgery for alveolar cleft repair. Although 36 patients in the rhBMP-2 group had facial swelling, this was not felt to provide significant morbidity. The major advantages of the rhBMP-2/DBM technique is the avoidance of a secondary donor site and its inherent morbidity, as well as reduction in pain. RhBMP-2 has a long-standing record of effect of bone formation and may offer a viable alternative to traditional iliac crest bone grafting. However, prior to adoption of widespread implementation, long-term data on potential side effects need to be ascertained.

ERAS Protocol Innovations in Cleft Patients

Postoperative pain control following cleft lip and palate repair has undergone significant scrutiny in recent years. Enhanced Recovery After Surgery (ERAS) protocols have become pervasive across surgical disciplines. ERAS was first introduced in 2001 by a group in Northern Europe among patients undergoing colonic resection with the goal of reducing postoperative morbidity in relation to pain [27]. Over the last two decades, a multitude of ERAS protocols have since been utilized to improve patient outcomes across various postoperative surgical populations. ERAS protocols include patient-centered, evidence-based pain management plans organized by multidisciplinary care teams. Recent advances in ERAS protocols for cleft lip and palate postoperative patients have been tailored to minimize the use of opioids and subsequently decrease the length of stay and complication rates. An ERAS protocol that seeks to minimize the use of opioids for postoperative palatoplasty patients was described by Hush et al. This protocol included: Gabapentin 10 mg/kg/dose q8, acetaminophen 10 mg/kg/dose q4 PRN, and Ketorolac 0.5 mg/kg/dose IV q6 PRN for severe pain (max of 3 doses). Alternatively, a regime of Ibuprofen 10 mg/kg/dose q6 for mild–moderate pain was available. Postoperatively, a daily regimen of gabapentin, acetaminophen, and ibuprofen were prescribed as needed [28]. Overall application of ERAS led to a 95.7% reduction in narcotic administration and a 31.7% decrease in LOS when compared to controls. Our group utilized an ERAS protocol for palatoplasty patients that had a multimodality regime of Morphine 0.05–0.1 mg/kg IV q1 PRN and acetaminophen 10 mg/kg IV q6 scheduled during the immediate postoperative period. Depending on postoperative pain, acetaminophen or ibuprofen 10 mg/kg PO q6 PRN (FLACC score 1–5) or oxycodone 0.1 mg/kg PO q4–6 PRN (FLACC pain score 6–10) was administered. Patients in the ERAS protocol received significantly less mg of morphine on postoperative Day 1 through 4 than those on the ad lib pathway. Return visits to the hospital for pain management following primary palatoplasty decreased from 7.1% to 0% with the ERAS protocol [29].

These recent studies indicate that while currently limited in the pediatric population, multimodal ERAS protocols can provide safe and effective pain control regimens for postoperative cleft patients while mitigating the need for opiates. These protocols lead to decreased morbidity and shorter lengths of inpatient stay.

Conclusions

Cleft care continues to evolve both in technique and in management. Nasal floor closure and the use of tissue augmentation to palatal repair have given the surgeon a greater armamentarium while improving patient outcomes and quality of life. The use of alternatives to iliac crest bone grafting, namely rhBMP2 and demineralized bone matrix, offers a tantalizing option that would preclude donor site morbidity. Lastly, ERAS protocols have minimized the use of opioids and demonstrated to improve pain management and shorten length of stay.

References

1. Bykowski MR, Naran S, Winger DG, Losee JE. The rate of Oronasal fistula following primary cleft palate surgery: a meta-analysis. Cleft Palate Craniofac J. 2015;52(4):e81–7; [cited 2022 Mar 6]. https://pubmed.ncbi.nlm.nih.gov/25322441/.
2. Daniels KM, Yu EY, Maine RG, Corlew S, Bing S, Hoffman WY, et al. Palatal fistula risk after primary palatoplasty: a retrospective comparison of humanitarian operations and tertiary hospitals. Lancet. 2015;386(9993):532; [cited 2022 Mar 6]. https://pubmed.ncbi.nlm.nih.gov/26313085/.
3. Daniels KM, Yang Yu E, Maine RG, Heng Y, Yang L, Shi B, et al. Palatal fistula risk after primary palatoplasty. Cleft Palate Craniofac J. 2018;55(6):807–13. [cited 2022 Mar 6]. https://pubmed.ncbi.nlm.nih.gov/28001101/.
4. Smith DM, Vecchione L, Jiang S, Ford M, Deleyiannis FW, Ann Haralam M, et al. The pittsburgh fistula classification system: a standardized scheme for the description of palatal fistulas. Cleft Palate Craniofac J. 2007;44(6):590–4; [cited 2022 Mar 6]. https://pubmed.ncbi.nlm.nih.gov/18177198/.
5. Anderson BJ, Fallah KN, Lignieres AA, Moffitt JK, Luu K-L, Cepeda A, et al. Predictive factors for velopharyngeal insufficiency following primary cleft palate repair. Cleft Palate Craniofac J. 2021;59(7):825–32; [cited 2022 Mar 8]. https://pubmed.ncbi.nlm.nih.gov/34396792/.
6. Fayyaz GQ, Gill NA, Ishaq I, Aslam M, Chaudry A, Ganatra MA, et al. Pakistan comprehensive fistula classification. Plast Reconstr Surg. 2019;143(1):140e–51e; [cited 2022 Mar 6]. https://pubmed.ncbi.nlm.nih.gov/30431540/.
7. Rothermel AT, Lundberg JN, Samson TD, Tse RW, Allori AC, Bezuhly M, et al. A toolbox of surgical techniques for palatal fistula repair. Cleft Palate Craniofac J. 2020;58(2):170–80; [cited 2022 Mar 8]. https://pubmed.ncbi.nlm.nih.gov/32806926/.
8. Hu S, Levinson J, Rousso JJ. Revision surgery of the cleft palate. Semin Plast Surg. 2020;34(2):120–8; [cited 2022 Mar 7]. https://pubmed.ncbi.nlm.nih.gov/32390780/.
9. Ayyash AM, Anstadt EE, Dvoracek LA, Marji FP, Lee JY, Losee JE, et al. An intraoperative salvage after transection of the greater palatine artery during cleft palate repair. J Craniofac Surg. 2020;31(2):e133–5; [cited 2022 Mar 10]. https://pubmed.ncbi.nlm.nih.gov/31934976/.
10. Anstadt EE, Bruce MK, Ford M, Jabbour N, Pfaff MJ, Bykowski M, et al. Tissue augmenting palatoplasty for the treatment of velopharyngeal insufficiency. Cleft Palate Craniofac J. 2021;59(12):1461; [cited 2022 Mar 18]. https://pubmed.ncbi.nlm.nih.gov/34787006/.
11. Mittermiller PA, Sethi H, Morbia RP, Johns D, Baylan J, Lorenz HP, et al. Anatomical nasal lining flaps for closure of the nasal floor in unilateral and bilateral cleft lip repairs reduce fistulas at the alveolus. Plast Reconstr Surg. 2018;142(6):1549–56; [cited 2022 Mar 13]. https://pubmed.ncbi.nlm.nih.gov/30188474/.
12. Mendoza M, Pérez A. Anatomical closure technique of the nasal floor for patients with complete unilateral cleft lip and palate. J Plast Surg Hand Surg. 2013;47(3):196–9; [cited 2022 Mar 18]. https://pubmed.ncbi.nlm.nih.gov/23547535/.
13. Rahpeyma A, Khajehahmadi S. Inferior turbinate flap for nasal-side closure of palatal fistula in cleft patients. Plast Reconstr Surg Glob Open. 2015;2(12):e265; [cited 2022 Mar 20]. https://pubmed.ncbi.nlm.nih.gov/25587499/.
14. Stewart TL, Fisher DM, Olson JL. Modified von Langenbeck cleft palate repair using an anterior triangular flap: decreased incidence of anterior oronasal fistulas. Cleft Palate Craniofac J. 2009;46(3):299–304. https://doi.org/10.1597/07-185.1; [cited 2022 Mar 17].
15. Hay N, Patel B, Haria P, Sommerlad B. Maxillary growth in cleft lip and palate patients, with and without vomerine flap closure of the hard palate at the time of lip repair. Cleft Palate Craniofac J. 2018;55(9):1205–10. https://doi.org/10.1177/1055665618764960; [cited 2022 Mar 9].
16. Maggiulli F, Hay N, Mars M, Worrell E, Green J, Sommerlad B. Early effect of vomerine flap closure of the hard palate at the time of lip repair on the alveolar gap and other maxillary

dimensions. Cleft Palate Craniofac J. 2014;51(1):43–8; [cited 2022 Mar 6]. https://pubmed.ncbi.nlm.nih.gov/23651320/.

17. Mann RJ, Fisher DM. Bilateral buccal flaps with double opposing z-plasty for wider palatal clefts. Plast Reconstr Surg. 1997;100(5):1139–43; [cited 2022 Mar 14]. https://pubmed.ncbi.nlm.nih.gov/9326774/.

18. Franco D, Rocha D, Arnaut M, Freitas R, Alonso N. Versatility of the buccinator myomucosal flap in atypical palate reconstructions. J Craniomaxillofac Surg. 2014;42(7):1310–4; [cited 2022 Mar 16]. https://pubmed.ncbi.nlm.nih.gov/24787083/.

19. Ligneres A, Anderson B, Alimi O, Cepeda A, Teichgraeber JF, Nguyen PD, Greives MR. Do buccal flaps improve velopharyngeal insufficiency in conversion Furlow palatoplasty for patients with cleft palate? Plast Reconstr Surg. 2022;8(9 Suppl):67–8; [cited 2022 Mar 16]. https://www.ncbi.nlm.nih.gov/pmc/articles/PMC7553451/.

20. Qiu CS, Fracol ME, Bae H, Gosain AK. Prophylactic use of buccal fat flaps to improve oral mucosal healing following furlow palatoplasty. Plast Reconstr Surg. 2019;143(4):1179–83; [cited 2022 Mar 15]. https://pubmed.ncbi.nlm.nih.gov/30921142/.

21. Whitehouse H, Schwaiger M, Nicholas R, Fallico N, Atherton DD. A cadaveric study of the buccal fat pad: implications for closure of palatal fistulae and donor-site morbidity. Plast Reconstr Surg. 2020;146(6):1331–9; [cited 2022 Mar 24]. https://pubmed.ncbi.nlm.nih.gov/33234964/.

22. Qamar F, McLaughlin MM, Lee M, Pringle AJ, Halsey J, Rottgers SA. An algorithmic approach for deploying buccal fat pad flaps and buccal myomucosal flaps strategically in primary and secondary palatoplasty. Cleft Palate Craniofac J. 2022:105566562210848; [cited 2022 Mar 24]. https://pubmed.ncbi.nlm.nih.gov/35262434/.

23. Fahradyan A, Tsuha M, Wolfswinkel EM, Mitchell K-AS, Hammoudeh JA, Magee W. Optimal timing of secondary alveolar bone grafting: a literature review. J Oral Maxillofac Surg. 2018;77(4):843–9; [cited 2022 Mar 24]. https://pubmed.ncbi.nlm.nih.gov/30576671/.

24. Makar KG, Buchman SR, Vercler CJ. Bone morphogenetic protein-2 and demineralized bone matrix in difficult bony reconstructions in cleft patients. Plast Reconstr Surg Glob Open. 2021;9(6):e3611; [cited 2022 Mar 26]. https://pubmed.ncbi.nlm.nih.gov/34168938/.

25. Uribe F, Alister JP, Zaror C, Olate S, Fariña R. Alveolar cleft reconstruction using morphogenetic protein (rhbmp-2): a systematic review and meta-analysis. Cleft Palate Craniofac J. 2020;57(5):589–98; [cited 2022 Mar 26]. https://pubmed.ncbi.nlm.nih.gov/31698953/.

26. Hammoudeh JA, Fahradyan A, Gould DJ, Liang F, Imahiyerobo T, Urbinelli L, et al. A comparative analysis of recombinant human bone morphogenetic protein-2 with a demineralized bone matrix versus iliac crest bone graft for secondary alveolar bone grafts in patients with cleft lip and palate. Plast Reconstr Surg. 2017;140(2):318e–25e; [cited 2022 Mar 26]. https://pubmed.ncbi.nlm.nih.gov/28746285/.

27. Brown JK, Singh K, Dumitru R, Chan E, Kim MP. The benefits of enhanced recovery after surgery programs and their application in cardiothoracic surgery. Methodist Debakey Cardiovasc J. 2018;14(2):77–88; [cited 2022 Mar 28]. https://pubmed.ncbi.nlm.nih.gov/29977464/.

28. Hush SE, Brady C, Soldanska M, Williams JK. Expanded analysis of a modified enhanced recovery protocol in cleft palatoplasty. Cleft Palate Craniofac J. 2020;57(10):1190–6; [cited 2022 Mar 28]. https://pubmed.ncbi.nlm.nih.gov/32567352/.

29. Moffitt JK, Cepeda A, Ekeoduru RA, Teichgraeber JF, Nguyen PD, Greives MR. Enhanced recovery after surgery protocol for primary cleft palate repair: improving transition of care. J Craniofac Surg. 2021;32(1):e72–6; [cited 2022 Mar 28]. https://pubmed.ncbi.nlm.nih.gov/32897976/.

Chapter 3
Novel Cancer Immunotherapies and Molecular Biomarkers in Head and Neck Cancer

Sarah Anne Wong, Neeraja Dharmaraj, Victoria A. Manon, Simon Young (ID), and Chi T. Viet

Introduction

Head and neck squamous cell carcinoma (HNSCC) is the sixth most common cancer worldwide, with over 60,000 new cases in the United States each year [1]. HNSCC includes distinct disease sub-types, each located in different anatomic locations, with different etiology, patient demographics, and molecular profiles. Oral squamous cell carcinoma (OSCC) is a distinct sub-type that has remained particularly treatment resistant. Even when compared to other subsets of HNSCC, such as oropharyngeal cancer, OSCC remains one of the deadliest, without significantly improved outcomes in recent years. Furthermore, OSCC is on the rise. In the last 20 years, the OSCC incidence has increased by two-thirds, most dramatically in young patients, and has resulted in 400,000 new annual cases globally [2]. Of the

S. A. Wong
Oral and Craniofacial Sciences Graduate Program, School of Dentistry,
University of California, San Francisco, CA, USA
e-mail: Sarah.Wong@ucsf.edu

N. Dharmaraj · V. A. Manon
Bernard and Gloria Pepper Katz Department of Oral and Maxillofacial Surgery, The University of Texas Health Science Center at Houston, School of Dentistry,
Houston, TX, USA
e-mail: Neeraja.Dharmaraj@uth.tmc.edu; Victoria.A.Manon@uth.tmc.edu

S. Young
Department of Oral and Maxillofacial Surgery, The University of Texas Health Science Center at Houston, Houston, TX, USA
e-mail: Simon.Young@uth.tmc.edu

C. T. Viet (✉)
Department of Oral and Maxillofacial Surgery, Loma Linda University School of Dentistry,
Loma Linda, CA, USA
e-mail: cviet@llu.edu

© The Author(s), under exclusive license to Springer Nature Switzerland AG 2023
J. C. Melville et al. (eds.), *Advancements and Innovations in OMFS, ENT, and Facial Plastic Surgery*, https://doi.org/10.1007/978-3-031-32099-6_3

30,000 Americans newly diagnosed with OSCC each year, half will die of this disease, resulting in approximately one death per hour [3]. This high mortality is compounded by significant morbidity due to OSCC treatment that often results in cosmetic and functional deformities affecting patients' ability to eat, taste, speak, and relate to others. Taken together, the significant burden of this disease necessitates the development of improved diagnostic tools and targeted treatment options.

In 2001, the completion of the human genome project launched the era of personalized medicine. It was believed that the genetic code could be utilized to develop specific biomarker panels for use in determining a patient's individual cancer risk and in identifying dysregulated molecular pathways with the ultimate goal of developing targeted therapies to address the disease. This approach has proved successful in several cancer fields such as breast cancer, where commercially available genomic tests have been used to predict patient risk of recurrence, guide treatment, and improve patient survival, especially in young women with metastatic cancer [4].

Biomarkers have also served as a powerful tool for specific HNSCC sub-types such as oropharyngeal cancer (OPSCC). Unlike OSCC, OPSCC is primarily caused by the human papilloma virus (HPV) (>70% of cases). Since HPV-positive OPSCC patients have a significantly higher 3-year survival rate (82.4%) than their HPV-negative counterparts (57.1%), it has become standard-of-care for patients to be tested for overexpression of *p16*, a biomarker for HPV infection, and risk-stratified according to this marker [5]. Recent studies have also shown that therapies targeting HPV-positive OPSCC can increase survival to 90% even in the setting of treatment de-escalation [6]. In contrast, HPV does not play a significant role in the etiology or prognosis of OSCC, even in young nonsmokers [7], and no biomarker similar to *p16* exists for OSCC.

OSCC biomarker research trails behind that of other cancers. Until recently, there were no biomarkers available that effectively distinguished low- versus high-risk OSCC patients of the same stage. The need for OSCC biomarkers is highlighted by the fact that up to 80% of new OSCC cases are early stage (I/II) without regional lymph node involvement or distant metastasis [8]. However, despite early diagnosis, the 5-year mortality risk for these patients remains at 40–60% [3, 8]. Treatment of early stage I/II OSCC remains highly variable with treatment options ranging from surgery alone to a combination of surgery plus adjuvant treatments such as elective neck dissection (END), radiation (RT), chemoradiation (chemoRT), or immunotherapy. At present, patients' risk of recurrence and mortality as well as their need for adjuvant therapy has been determined solely by clinicopathologic features such as tumor grade, depth of tumor invasion, margin status, the presence of perineural invasion (PNI), or lymphovascular invasion (LVI). Unfortunately, these clinicopathologic features alone do not accurately determine disease risk. Ideal diagnostic tools will need to combine both nonmolecular and molecular features in order to more accurately predict individual risk and prescribe optimal treatment (Fig. 3.1).

Immunotherapy offers a promising new modality for cancer treatment and has become an emerging standard-of-care for many different types of cancer, including melanoma, lung, and HNSCC [9]. Drugs of this class work by bolstering the host immune response to promote tumor detection and destruction. Unlike conventional

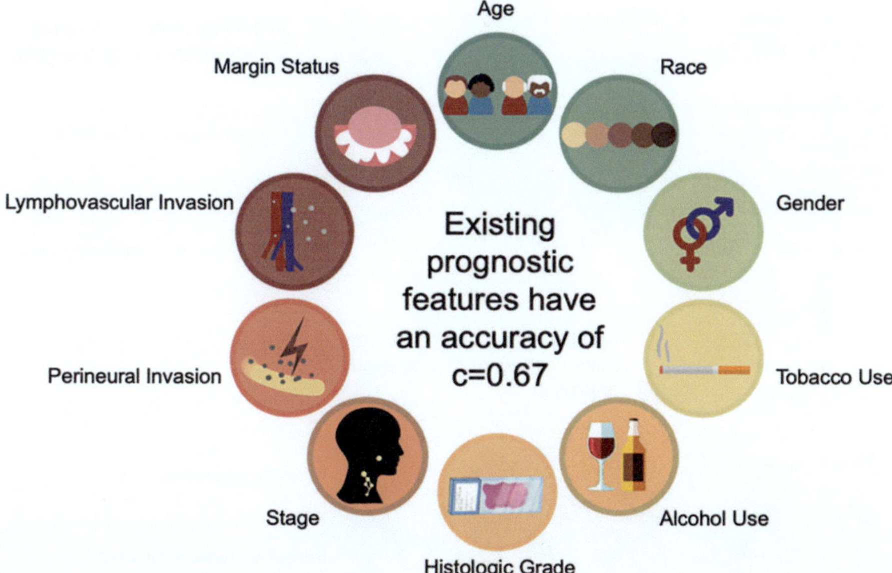

Fig. 3.1 HNSCC patient risk has been determined solely by clinicopathologic features, which include age, race, gender, tobacco history, alcohol use, histologic grade, tumor stage, perineural invasion, lymphovascular invasion, and margin status. However, use of clinicopathologic features alone has demonstrated poor prognostic success with a concordance (c)-index of 0.67. Notably, the c-index has been shown to significantly increase (as high as 0.915) when clinicopathologic features are combined with the patient's molecular fingerprint

treatments, immunotherapy can potentially generate a specific and long-lasting anti-tumor effect. However, clinical success rates remain low (15–20%), and there is significant risk of systemic toxicity from immune-related adverse events (irAEs) due to often-required high dose and frequency of treatment. Indeed, as the field moves toward combined immunotherapy and combinations of immune- and radiation therapy, the risk of severe and potentially fatal irAEs has increased. Thus, there is significant need for the development of innovative strategies that not only increase the effectiveness of current immunotherapies but also reduce their potential systemic toxicities [9].

The tumor immune microenvironment (TIME) is the "front line" for tumor–immune interactions and is the critical locus for immunotherapy activity. HNSCC, caused either by HPV-infection or carcinogens, is known to have a highly immunosuppressive TIME. A large milieu of immune suppressive cells is known to be present, including myeloid-derived suppressor cells (MDSCs) that inhibit T-cell activation and proliferation, regulatory T-cells (Treg) that suppress effector T-cells, and anti-inflammatory (M2) macrophages. Furthermore, tumor cells are known to highly express anti-inflammatory cytokines such as TGF-β, IL-1, and VEGF as well as checkpoint molecules PD-1/PD-L1, CTLA-4, and TIM-3 (Fig. 3.2). Together, this immunosuppressive TIME neutralizes or kills tumor-infiltrating

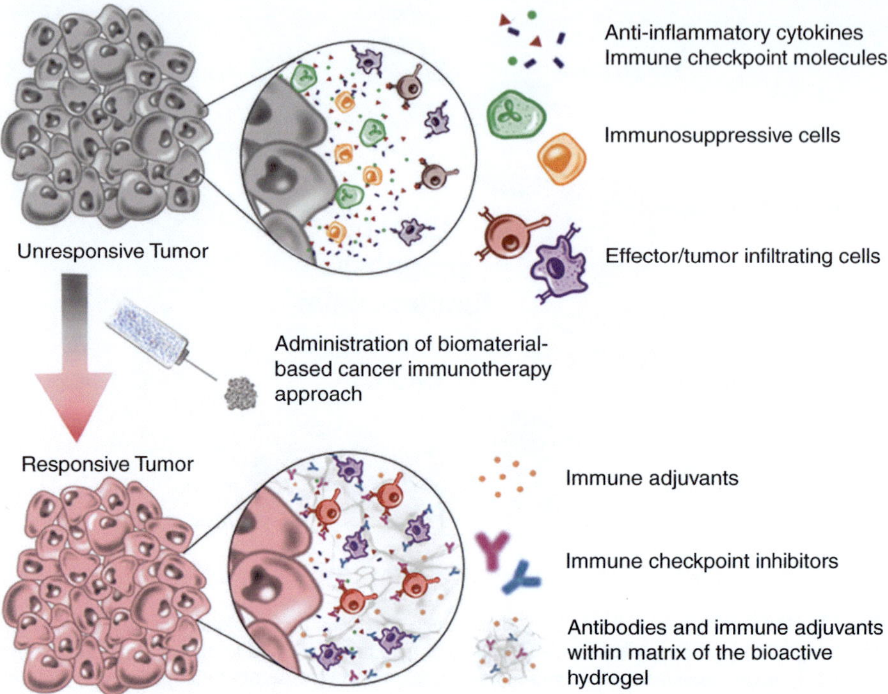

Fig. 3.2 The local tumor immune microenvironemnt (TIME) is highly immunosuppressive due to the presence of immunosuppressive cells (regulatory T cells, myeloid-derived suppressor cells, anti-inflammatory/M2 macrophages), anti-inflammatory cytokines (TGF- β, IL-1, VEGF), and checkpoint molecules (PD-1/PD-L1, CTLA-4, TIM-3). Together, these factors render immune cells ineffective, resulting in failed immuno- and radiotherapy. Biomaterials enable the localized delivery of immunotherapeutics, which directly combat the immunosuppressive tumor microenvironment and promote a long-lasting, anti-tumor effect while reducing systemic toxicity. Immunotherapeutics include checkpoint inhibitors (nivolumab, pembrolizumab), small molecule inhibitors (L-NIL), and cancer vaccines (mesoporous silica rod (MSR)-based vaccines). Biomaterials have the potential to deliver all of the above and even mimic immunmotherapy drugs themselves, thus reducing the necessity for the addition of external agents or factors

effector T-cells and renders immunotherapy and standard radiotherapy ineffective. In response, biomaterials-based platform technologies for immunomodulation of the adverse TIME are quickly emerging as a powerful tool for the treatment of cancer. The wide variety of biomaterial systems now include lipid nanocarriers, synthetic nanoparticles and microparticles, implantable or injectable scaffolds, and hydrogels [10]. With biomaterials enabling precision drug delivery and localization through spatial and temporal control, the versatile use of biomaterials is immense [10]. Specifically, injectable biomaterials for the targeted delivery of localized, controlled-release immunotherapeutics not only holds promise in minimizing systemic exposure and reducing toxicity but also has the potential to reverse the immunosuppressive TIME while stimulating a localized anti-tumor effect (Fig. 3.2).

Advances made in recent years have the potential to transform all phases of patient care, from innovations in patient diagnosis with the discovery of novel biomarkers and the development of noninvasive biopsy techniques to advances in cancer treatment with the development of vaccines, immunomodulatory drugs, and injectable biomaterials. We review these advances and more in this chapter.

Advances in OSCC Biomarker Research

Researchers have sought to create a multigene risk score that allows clinicians to better tailor treatment for OSCC patients. To date, these studies have sought to use differences in gene expression, gene amplification and deletion, methylation, and microRNA (miRNA) as potential biomarkers. For the majority of these studies, the primary goal has been to prevent overtreatment by predicting patient risk for neck metastasis and their need for END. Since neck metastasis cannot be detected clinically or via imaging in >20% of early-stage OSCC patients and this risk of occult metastasis portends poor survival without prophylactic neck lymphadenectomy, it has become routine for surgeons to perform END on all patients, even if this means overtreatment in 80% of patients and significant concomitant morbidity such as shoulder dysfunction, nerve damage, and lymphedema [11].

Initially, molecular signatures of disease showed limited clinical success, predominantly because studies sought to identify global markers of multiple head and neck cancer subtypes. However, narrowing the focus to only one sub-type, allows for identification of a more accurate molecular signature. One example of this is a large biomarker study published in 2004 that identified a unique 102-gene signature by comparing changes in gene expression patterns in patients with and without neck metastasis [12, 13]. The initial study showed that the 102-gene signature was 86% accurate in predicting neck metastasis, but the subsequent multicenter validation study showed a negative predictive value (NPV) of 72% for all stages of OSCC and OPSCC [11]. Notably, the NPV increased to 89% when the patient cohort was limited to only early stage (I/II) OSCC patients. This finding not only highlights the importance of evaluating head and neck cancer by sub-type but also the promising potential of using molecular biomarkers for early-stage patients.

The majority of biomarker studies have not focused on early-stage OSCC patients. However, this patient population has the potential to benefit most from biomarker-based evaluation. Unlike late-stage (III/IV) OSCC patients who routinely receive triple-modality therapy (surgery, radiation, and chemotherapy), treatment recommendations for early-stage OSCC patients are highly variable due to the lack of accurate and individualized metrics to measure risk. To address this variability in disease outcome, recent studies have focused on identifying biomarkers that distinguish high- versus low-risk early-stage OSCC patients. Yoon et al. published a study focusing on early-stage OSCC patients that used differences in miRNA patterns to predict 5-year survival [3]. The group discovered a 3 miRNA signature and combined this with tumor-node-metastasis (TNM) classification and histologic grade to create a risk score with a concordance (c)-index of 0.832.

Shifting the focus to epigenetic biomarkers, epigenetics (i.e., DNA methylation) has been shown to play the most prominent role in regulating OSCC progression. Numerous studies have demonstrated how methylation leads to genomic instability and the dysregulation of key genes involved in OSCC etiology [8, 14, 15]. For example, an epigenome-wide association study (EWAS) demonstrated how methylation inactivates a number of critical tumor suppressor genes in head and neck cancer patients [16]. Initially, these epigenetic-based studies demonstrated poor prognostic success due to the use of heterogeneous study populations that included both early- and late-stage OSCC patients as well as patients with cancer at different subsites (i.e., oral cavity, oropharynx, hypopharynx, larynx). Additionally, these studies relied only on molecular data without including clinicopathologic features to determine risk.

A recent study, however, demonstrated clinical significance and prognostic potential when using epigenetic biomarkers to predict 5-year mortality in early-stage (I/II) OSCC patients. In this study, patients' mortality risk scores were determined by combining both molecular and nonmolecular features. The molecular panel consisted of a 12-gene methylation signature. Notably, all 12 genes had been previously linked to patient survival in other cancers. However, 11 of the 12 had never been previously linked to OSCC. The study's nonmolecular panel consisted of the following clinicopathologic features: age, race, sex, tobacco use, alcohol use, histologic grade, stage, perineural invasion (PNI), lymphovascular invasion (LVI), and margin status. When assessing 5-year mortality using patients' clinicopathologic features alone, the c-index from this study was 0.67, which was not different from previous studies using clinicopathologic features to predict risk (Fig. 3.1). Importantly, the c-index increased to 0.915 when the clinicopathologic features were combined with the 12-gene molecular panel [8]. This data highlights the critical role of molecular biomarkers in determining patient risk and demonstrates how utilizing molecular information as part of a risk score has the potential to mitigate overtreatment in low-risk patients while preventing undertreatment in high-risk patients. Work is currently being done to validate this risk score with a larger multi-institutional cohort.

Noninvasive Biopsy Techniques for OSCC Diagnosis

One advantage of treating OSCC is that the oral cavity is easily accessible and, thus, lends itself well to the development of noninvasive biopsy techniques. Such techniques would allow frequent sample harvesting not only for initial diagnosis but also to monitor treatment response and recurrence. Importantly, samples harvested via these techniques could allow for risk score calculation prior to surgery. Since it is standard of care for adjuvant treatments to occur within several weeks of surgery, it is essential that the patient's risk score be calculated beforehand if it is to play a role in determining the need for adjuvant treatment. Collecting samples via noninvasive biopsy at the time of diagnosis allows for this to occur, in contrast to waiting for data from formalin-fixed, paraffin-embedded (FFPE) tissue samples following tumor resection, which could result in the delay of potentially necessary treatment.

Studies have sought to use saliva, brush swabs, and circulating tumor cells (CTC) to noninvasively collect OSCC cell samples at the time of diagnosis (Fig. 3.3). Unfortunately, saliva has not proven to be a viable option as the concordance of methylation patterns between saliva and cancer tissue has been highly variable [17]. However, a preliminary study using noninvasive brush swabs has shown a high concordance with cancer tissue ($r = 0.913$) and no significant differences in DNA yield between tissue and brush swab samples [18]. Methylation data resulting from this noninvasive technique can be used to calculate molecular risk at the time of diagnosis and has high clinical relevance and translational potential. Additional studies have sought to use circulating tumor cells (CTCs) as an early marker of metastatic disease. The presence of CTCs has been associated with treatment resistance, locoregional recurrence, and reduced progression-free survival [19]. Work is being done to identify molecular phenotypes of CTCs that indicate patient prognosis and response to treatment [19, 20].

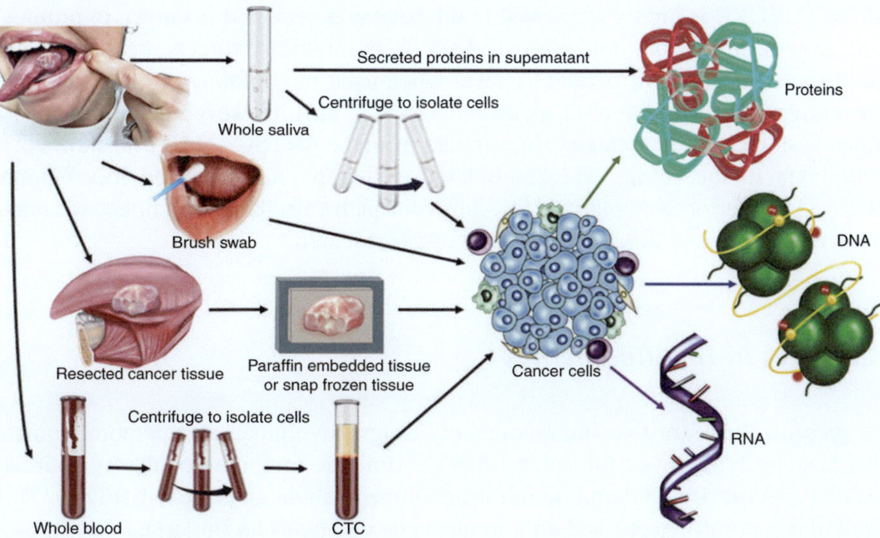

Fig. 3.3 Several noninvasive biopsy techniques have been developed for head and neck squamous cell carcinoma (HNSCC) biomarker research. These techniques include the use of saliva, brush swabs, and circulating tumor cells (CTC's) for cancer cell collection. Due to the minimally invasive nature of these techniques, they can be used repeatedly to monitor treatment response and easily collected at the point-of-care. Moreover, cells harvested using noninvasive techniques of sufficient quantity and quality for biomarker analysis, which plays a critical role in predicting individual patient risk and determining the appropriate level of adjuvant treatment

Advances in Head and Neck Cancer Treatment

Current adjuvant treatment for head and neck cancer includes radiation, chemotherapy, and immunotherapy. Among the recent advances in this field are the use of repurposed drugs to overcome drug resistance in common chemotherapies and the development of new immunomodulatory drugs, cancer vaccines, and biomaterial-based delivery systems in the immunotherapy field.

Cisplatin is currently first-line chemotherapy for advanced-stage HNSCC patients, either in combination with radiation for patients with good performance or alone for those with limited performance [21]. Unfortunately, cisplatin resistance has been shown to significantly reduce patient survival. Although the mechanism of cisplatin resistance is complex and poorly understood, studies have indicated that DNA methylation may play a critical role. Cisplatin-sensitive and cisplatin-resistant patient tumors have distinct methylation profiles, and gene methylation patterns can be used as a biomarker of cisplatin-resistance [22]. Decitabine is a hypomethylating drug that has been used in clinical trials to treat hematological and solid malignancies [23, 24]. In preclinical HNSCC models, it has been shown to restore cisplatin sensitivity, inhibit tumor growth, and reduce cancer-related pain.

Cetuximab is another common chemotherapy drug with reported drug resistance. It is a chimeric monoclonal antibody that binds and inhibits the epidermal growth factor receptor (EGFR), which has been repeatedly linked to the progression of HNSCC. EGFR is highly expressed in the head and neck and is known to promote cell growth, migration, and survival. Due to its inhibitory effects, cetuximab has been shown to improve patient survival when used in combination with intensive chemotherapy for recurrent or metastatic HNSCC [25]. However, cetuximab resistance is an increasing concern. Recent data from the ARTSCAN III trial shows that cetuximab in the setting of chemoradiation therapy for advanced locoregional HNSCC is inferior to cisplatin [26]. Numerous pathways have been linked to cetuximab resistance, and this area warrants further research.

Advances in Immunotherapy

At present, there are two immunotherapy drugs, nivolumab and pembrolizumab, that have been approved for use in HNSCC. Both are immunomodulatory antibodies that specifically bind and inhibit programmed cell death protein 1 (PD-1). This protein is naturally expressed on immune cells and plays an important role in promoting self-tolerance, suppressing T-cell activity, and preventing autoimmune disease. However, in the context of cancer, stimulation of PD-1 by cancer cells can lead to tumor evasion of immune attack. By blocking the immune checkpoint protein, PD-1, nivolumab and pembrolizumab have been shown to increase survival rates and improve patient outcomes, especially when combined with radio- or chemotherapy [27]. Unfortunately, these therapies are currently only used in the setting of recurrent or metastatic cancer and have only been effective in 12–20% of HNSCC cases. This may be due, in part, to the immunosuppressive tumor-immune microenvironment (TIME) associated with HNSCC [28]. To overcome this challenge, biomaterial-based cancer immunotherapy platforms have emerged as a way for investigators to improve conventional immunotherapeutic strategies. The ability of biomaterial platforms to provide spatiotemporal control over the delivery of multiple bioactive molecules and/or cells to direct cell behavior has generated further advances in immunotherapy [10] (Fig. 3.2). Development of immunocompetent preclinical models of HNSCC has played a critical role in this field [29].

Innovations in Biomaterials for Controlled-Release Immunotherapy

Mesoporous silica rod (MSR)-based biomaterial vaccines form structures that provide a microenvironment that support and modulate immune cells in vivo. MSR-based vaccines have also been shown to confer long-term immunity and protect against tumor rechallenge in multiple preclinical models as previously reviewed [30]. These studies illustrate the potential of MSR-based cancer vaccines to generate a potent anti-tumor effector T-cell response in situ. Dharmaraj et al., in an orthotopic syngeneic model of OSCC, assessed the efficacy of a mesoporous silica rod (MSR) cancer vaccine targeting HPV-16 E7. While the mEER model that constantly expresses the E7 antigen showed increased efficacy, the MOC2-E6E7 model exhibited tumor growth delay and a modest prolonged survival [31]. Synthetic cyclic dinucleotides (CDNs) are a new class of immunotherapeutics that induce strong anti-tumor responses in preclinical models through the Stimulator of Interferon Genes (STING) pathway [32]. In fact, STING-agonist therapy using CDNs have been considered as an "intratumoral in situ vaccine" to convert cold tumors into hot tumors. However, CDN monotherapy has shown poor efficacy in preclinical models of HNSCC, requiring multiple injections and concurrent administration of immune checkpoint antibodies [33]. Leach et al. developed a novel peptide hydrogel-based platform for intratumoral CDN delivery, called "STINGel" based on the ability of biomaterials to allow for controlled release of drugs. MultiDomain Peptide (MDP) is an easily syringe-deliverable carrier hydrogel that self-assembles to form a nanofibrous matrix. The localized delivery of CDN from this matrix in STINGel improved the overall survival in MOC2-E6E7 murine model of HNSCC compared to controls as shown in Fig. 3.4 [34]. It is well established that the pro-tumorigenic enzyme inducible nitric oxide synthase (iNOS) is highly upregulated in several cancers and promotes conditions favorable to tumor growth [35, 36]. iNOS promotes activation of immunosuppressive tumor-infiltrating myeloid-derived suppressor cells (MDSCs) [37]. The small molecule drug, N6-(1-iminoethyl)-L-lysine (L-NIL), has been used to selectively inhibit iNOS and regulate downstream effects that favor tumor growth [35]. Therefore, the ability to modulate iNOS activity at the tumor site

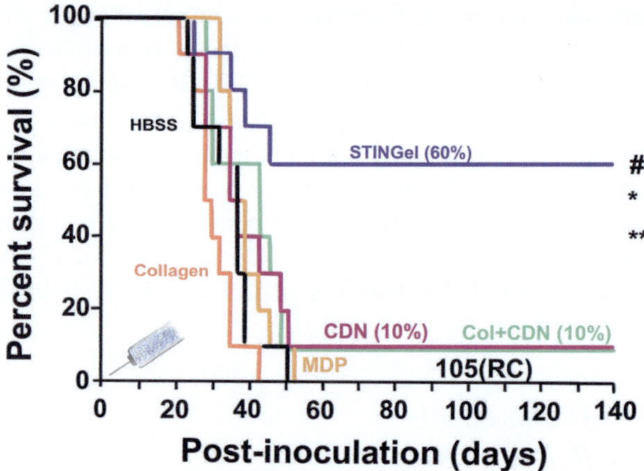

Fig. 3.4 Survival of the different experimental groups based on euthanasia timepoints resulting from excessive tumor burden. The total experimental period was 140 days post-tumor cell *inoculation*. The 3(IJ) on the x-axis refers to timepoint for intra-tumoral injection, and 105(RC) refers to timepoint for survivor rechallenge. Whereas 60% of the STINGel-treated *C57BL/6 mice* survived until the endpoint of the study, all control group (HBSS, MDP gel, and collagen gel) mice were euthanized prior to reaching the endpoint due to excessive tumor burden. Only 10% of CDN alone and collagen+CDN treated mice survived (lines overlaid on plot). *$p < 0.0282$ vs. CDN, **$p < 0.0064$ versus MDP gel, #$p < 0.0498$ versus Collagen + CDN. (Adapted from [34])

is beneficial for cancer immunotherapy. Additionally, we observed modest improvements with STINGel treatments, which address only immune stimulation and not immune suppression, explaining failure of the system in models with significant MDSCs. Based on the above research, a drug-mimicking hydrogel, LNIL-MDP, was designed to mimic the small molecule inhibitor of inducible iNOS, L-NIL. Specifically, the hydrogel was designed to be a novel anticancer biomaterial without addition of any external agents/factors [38]. The "L-NIL-MDP" hydrogel had comparable bioactivity to L-NIL and was able to inhibit iNOS and affect tumor biology over an extended period of time when loaded with CDN as the formulation termed "SynerGel" [39]. Leach et al. demonstrated the feasibility of biomaterial-based immunotherapy platforms like STINGel and the next-generation material SynerGel as strategies for increasing the efficacy of CDN immunotherapies.

Conclusion

Despite the capricious nature of HNSCC, significant advances have been made that affect all stages of patient care (Fig. 3.5). Risk stratification techniques now exist that integrate new molecular biomarker data with clinicopathologic features, allowing for more accurate treatment decisions for early-stage cancer patients. Noninvasive biopsy techniques, such as brush swabs, have been found to be just as effective in harvesting tissue samples of sufficient quantity and quality for risk score

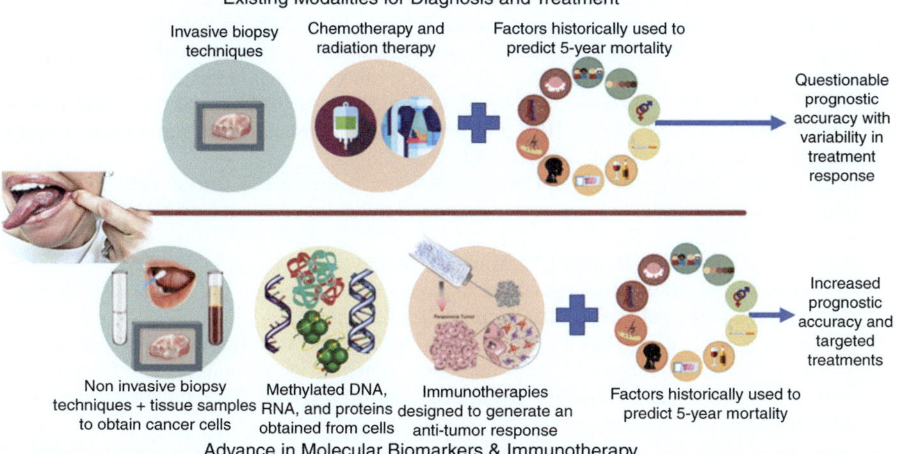

Fig. 3.5 Numerous advances have developed throughout all stages of HNSCC patient care. Whereas diagnosis previously depended solely on clinicopathologic features and used paraffin-embedded tissue samples harvested at the time of tumor resection to determine adjuvant treatment, we are now able to more accurately determine individual patient risk by combining molecular biomarker analysis with clinicopathologic features and obtain this information prior to surgery through noninvasive biopsy techniques. With regard to treatment, patients have primarily been limited to chemo- and radiation therapy, which carry significant systemic toxicity. Advances in immunotherapy now provide the potential for a long-lasting anti-tumor effect. The localized delivery of these drugs via biomaterials has enabled a targeted immune response while reducing systemic toxicity. Together, these advances have the potential for significant clinical impact

analysis. Drug repurposing of demethylating drugs has the potential to reverse cisplatin-resistance. Cancer vaccines targeting "driver" oncogenes show promising therapeutic potential. Injectable biomaterials demonstrate not only the therapeutic power of using localized, controlled-release drug delivery to reduce systemic toxicity and improve treatment response, but can also serve as drug mimetics themselves. The studies reviewed here highlight the critical role of intra- and inter-university collaborations and the profound discoveries that can result from these endeavors. Future areas of study include the use of biomarkers to monitor treatment response and the development of biomaterials for the controlled-release of numerous immunotherapies.

References

1. SEER Surveillance Epidemiology and End Results Fast Facts. [cited Feb 12 2022]. https://seer.cancer.gov/statfacts/html/oralcav.html.
2. Gulland A. Oral cancer rates rise by two thirds. BMJ. 2016;355:i6369.
3. Yoon AJ, Wang S, Kutler DI, Carvajal RD, Philipone E, Wang T, et al. MicroRNA-based risk scoring system to identify early-stage oral squamous cell carcinoma patients at high-risk for cancer-specific mortality. Head Neck. 2020;42(8):1699–712.

4. Fan C, Oh DS, Wessels L, Weigelt B, Nuyten DS, Nobel AB, et al. Concordance among gene-expression-based predictors for breast cancer. N Engl J Med. 2006;355(6):560–9.
5. Ang KK, Harris J, Wheeler R, Weber R, Rosenthal DI, Nguyen-Tan PF, et al. Human papillomavirus and survival of patients with oropharyngeal cancer. N Engl J Med. 2010;363(1):24–35.
6. Viet CT, Dierks EJ, Cheng AC, Patel AA, Chang SC, Couey MA, et al. Transoral robotic surgery and neck dissection for HPV-positive oropharyngeal carcinoma: importance of nodal count in survival. Oral Oncol. 2020;109:104770.
7. Bragelmann J, Dagogo-Jack I, El Dinali M, Stricker T, Brown CD, Zuo Z, et al. Oral cavity tumors in younger patients show a poor prognosis and do not contain viral RNA. Oral Oncol. 2013;49(6):525–33.
8. Viet CT, Yu G, Asam K, Thomas CM, Yoon AJ, Wongworawat YC, et al. The REASON score: an epigenetic and clinicopathologic score to predict risk of poor survival in patients with early stage oral squamous cell carcinoma. Biomark Res. 2021;9(1):42.
9. Cohen EEW, Bell RB, Bifulco CB, Burtness B, Gillison ML, Harrington KJ, et al. The Society for Immunotherapy of Cancer consensus statement on immunotherapy for the treatment of squamous cell carcinoma of the head and neck (HNSCC). J Immunother Cancer. 2019;7(1):184.
10. Leach DG, Young S, Hartgerink JD. Advances in immunotherapy delivery from implantable and injectable biomaterials. Acta Biomater. 2019;88:15–31.
11. van Hooff SR, Leusink FK, Roepman P, Baatenburg de Jong RJ, Speel EJ, van den Brekel MW, et al. Validation of a gene expression signature for assessment of lymph node metastasis in oral squamous cell carcinoma. J Clin Oncol. 2012;30(33):4104–10.
12. Roepman P, Kemmeren P, Wessels LF, Slootweg PJ, Holstege FC. Multiple robust signatures for detecting lymph node metastasis in head and neck cancer. Cancer Res. 2006;66(4):2361–6.
13. Roepman P, Wessels LF, Kettelarij N, Kemmeren P, Miles AJ, Lijnzaad P, et al. An expression profile for diagnosis of lymph node metastases from primary head and neck squamous cell carcinomas. Nat Genet. 2005;37(2):182–6.
14. Viet CT, Jordan RC, Schmidt BL. DNA promoter hypermethylation in saliva for the early diagnosis of oral cancer. J Calif Dent Assoc. 2007;35(12):844–9.
15. Viet CT, Schmidt BL. Methylation array analysis of preoperative and postoperative saliva DNA in oral cancer patients. Cancer Epidemiol Biomarkers Prev. 2008;17(12):3603–11.
16. Guerrero-Preston R, Michailidi C, Marchionni L, Pickering CR, Frederick MJ, Myers JN, et al. Key tumor suppressor genes inactivated by "greater promoter" methylation and somatic mutations in head and neck cancer. Epigenetics. 2014;9(7):1031–46.
17. Arantes L, De Carvalho AC, Melendez ME, Lopes CA. Serum, plasma and saliva biomarkers for head and neck cancer. Expert Rev Mol Diagn. 2018;18(1):85–112.
18. Viet CT, Zhang X, Xu K, Yu G, Asam K, Thomas CM, et al. Brush swab as a noninvasive surrogate for tissue biopsies in epigenomic profiling of oral cancer. Biomark Res. 2021;9(1):90.
19. Tada H, Takahashi H, Kuwabara-Yokobori Y, Shino M, Chikamatsu K. Molecular profiling of circulating tumor cells predicts clinical outcome in head and neck squamous cell carcinoma. Oral Oncol. 2020;102:104558.
20. Tada H, Takahashi H, Kawabata-Iwakawa R, Nagata Y, Uchida M, Shino M, et al. Molecular phenotypes of circulating tumor cells and efficacy of nivolumab treatment in patients with head and neck squamous cell carcinoma. Sci Rep. 2020;10(1):21573.
21. Pignon JP, le Maitre A, Maillard E, Bourhis J, Group M-NC. Meta-analysis of chemotherapy in head and neck cancer (MACH-NC): an update on 93 randomised trials and 17,346 patients. Radiother Oncol. 2009;92(1):4–14.
22. Viet CT, Dang D, Achdjian S, Ye Y, Katz SG, Schmidt BL. Decitabine rescues cisplatin resistance in head and neck squamous cell carcinoma. PloS One. 2014;9(11):e112880.
23. Stewart DJ, Issa JP, Kurzrock R, Nunez MI, Jelinek J, Hong D, et al. Decitabine effect on tumor global DNA methylation and other parameters in a phase I trial in refractory solid tumors and lymphomas. Clin Cancer Res. 2009;15(11):3881–8.

24. Cashen AF, Schiller GJ, O'Donnell MR, DiPersio JF. Multicenter, phase II study of decitabine for the first-line treatment of older patients with acute myeloid leukemia. J Clin Oncol. 2010;28(4):556–61.
25. Cohen MH, Chen H, Shord S, Fuchs C, He K, Zhao H, et al. Approval summary: cetuximab in combination with cisplatin or carboplatin and 5-fluorouracil for the first-line treatment of patients with recurrent locoregional or metastatic squamous cell head and neck cancer. Oncologist. 2013;18(4):460–6.
26. Gebre-Medhin M, Brun E, Engstrom P, Haugen Cange H, Hammarstedt-Nordenvall L, Reizenstein J, et al. ARTSCAN III: a randomized phase III study comparing chemoradiotherapy with cisplatin versus cetuximab in patients with locoregionally advanced head and neck squamous cell cancer. J Clin Oncol. 2021;39(1):38–47.
27. Kujan O, van Schaijik B, Farah CS. Immune checkpoint inhibitors in oral cavity squamous cell carcinoma and oral potentially malignant disorders: a systematic review. Cancers (Basel). 2020;12(7):1937.
28. Watermann C, Pasternack H, Idel C, Ribbat-Idel J, Bragelmann J, Kuppler P, et al. Recurrent HNSCC Harbor an immunosuppressive tumor immune microenvironment suggesting successful tumor immune evasion. Clin Cancer Res. 2021;27(2):632–44.
29. Li Q, Dong H, Yang G, Song Y, Mou Y, Ni Y. Mouse tumor-bearing models as preclinical study platforms for oral squamous cell carcinoma. Front Oncol. 2020;10:212.
30. Nguyen TL, Choi Y, Kim J. Mesoporous silica as a versatile platform for cancer immunotherapy. Adv Mater. 2019;31(34):e1803953.
31. Dharmaraj N, Piotrowski SL, Huang C, Newton JM, Golfman LS, Hanoteau A, et al. Antitumor immunity induced by ectopic expression of viral antigens is transient and limited by immune escape. Onco Targets Ther. 2019;8(4):e1568809.
32. Corrales L, Glickman LH, McWhirter SM, Kanne DB, Sivick KE, Katibah GE, et al. Direct activation of STING in the tumor microenvironment leads to potent and systemic tumor regression and immunity. Cell Rep. 2015;11(7):1018–30.
33. Moore E, Clavijo PE, Davis R, Cash H, Van Waes C, Kim Y, et al. Established T cell-inflamed tumors rejected after adaptive resistance was reversed by combination STING activation and PD-1 pathway blockade. Cancer Immunol Res. 2016;4(12):1061–71.
34. Leach DG, Dharmaraj N, Piotrowski SL, Lopez-Silva TL, Lei YL, Sikora AG, et al. STINGel: controlled release of a cyclic dinucleotide for enhanced cancer immunotherapy. Biomaterials. 2018;163:67–75.
35. Sikora AG, Gelbard A, Davies MA, Sano D, Ekmekcioglu S, Kwon J, et al. Targeted inhibition of inducible nitric oxide synthase inhibits growth of human melanoma in vivo and synergizes with chemotherapy. Clin Cancer Res. 2010;16(6):1834–44.
36. Fukumura D, Kashiwagi S, Jain RK. The role of nitric oxide in tumour progression. Nat Rev Cancer. 2006;6(7):521–34.
37. Jayaraman P, Parikh F, Lopez-Rivera E, Hailemichael Y, Clark A, Ma G, et al. Tumorexpressed inducible nitric oxide synthase controls induction of functional myeloid-derived suppressor cells through modulation of vascular endothelial growth factor release. J Immunol. 2012;188(11):5365–76.
38. Leach DG, Newton JM, Florez MA, Lopez-Silva TL, Jones AA, Young S, et al. Drugmimicking Nanofibrous peptide hydrogel for inhibition of inducible nitric oxide synthase. ACS Biomater Sci Eng. 2019;5(12):6755–65.
39. Leach DG, Dharmaraj N, Lopez-Silva TL, Venzor JR, Pogostin BH, Sikora AG, et al. Biomaterial-facilitated immunotherapy for established oral cancers. ACS Biomater Sci Eng. 2021;7(2):415–21.

Chapter 4
Advancements and Innovations in Otologic Surgery: Endoscopic and Exoscopic Ear Surgery

Jumah G. Ahmad, Kunal R. Shetty, and Ibrahim Alava III

Introduction

Otologic surgery involves very precise dissection of microscopic structures to eradicate pathology, reconstruct anatomy, and restore function. To be done safely and efficiently, high magnification and appropriate illumination are required. Traditionally, this has been achieved using binocular microscopy, the workhorse of otologic surgery. The middle ear space is complex with many hidden recesses in all directions. These spaces are challenging to visualize with the fundamental limitations of the microscope as its optics remain outside the body at a distance to the tissue of interest. This means that the field of view is limited by the narrowest part of the ear canal and that attaining a wider field of view requires destructive measures such as removal of soft tissue and bone. The endoscope is ideal when utilizing small surgical corridors to access the hidden recesses of the middle ear by bypassing the narrow ear canal and bringing the optics only centimeters from the tissue of interest, in turn obviating the need for destructive measures for visualization. Additionally, the microscope presents challenges as it relates to surgeon ergonomics and comfort, requiring prolonged periods of neck flexion. Trainee education is also hindered because the operator has a three-dimensional view, and the observer is

J. G. Ahmad · K. R. Shetty
Otorhinolaryngology—Head and Neck Surgery, University of Texas Health Sciences Center at Houston, Houston, TX, USA
e-mail: Jumah.G.Ahmad@uth.tmc.edu; Kunal.R.Shetty@uth.tmc.edu

I. AlavaIII (✉)
Otolaryngology-Head and Neck Surgery, Lyndon B. Johnson General Hospital, Houston, TX, USA

Department of Otorhinolaryngology-Head and Neck Surgery, The University of Texas—McGovern Medical School, Houston, TX, USA
e-mail: Ibrahim.Alava@uth.tmc.edu

© The Author(s), under exclusive license to Springer Nature Switzerland AG 2023
J. C. Melville et al. (eds.), *Advancements and Innovations in OMFS, ENT, and Facial Plastic Surgery*, https://doi.org/10.1007/978-3-031-32099-6_4

only offered a two-dimensional image via the teaching head. The discrepancy in views makes for a frustrating teaching and learning experience. The digital extra-corporeal scope, or exoscope, is complementary to the endoscope and was designed to replace the operating microscope. When compared with the microscope, it provides an immersive surgical view with improved ergonomics and an enhanced teaching experience since all parties have the same high-definition three-dimensional view in an ergonomically favorable neutral neck position. In this chapter, we discuss the advances in visualization for otologic surgery, particularly endoscopic and exo-scopic ear surgery.

Endoscopic Ear Surgery

In the 1990s, Jean-Marc Thomassin, Dennis Poe, and Muaaz Tarabichi described new otologic applications of endoscopy, including management of cholesteatomas and perilymphatic fistulas [1, 2]. In 1997, Tarabichi et al. published outcomes of endoscopic management of acquired cholesteatoma in 38 adult patients; 36 of which underwent transcanal endoscopic ear surgery. Twenty-nine out of 30 were disease free at 1 year, 10/13 were disease free at 2 years, and 4/6 were disease free at 2 years on surgical second look exploration. He concluded that transcanal endo-scopic resection of cholesteatoma is safe and effective [3]. He later published long-term outcome data of 101 ears operated on using the endoscope with up to 5 years of follow-up. Three cases were converted into postauricular tympanomastoidec-tomy. There were no iatrogenic facial nerve injuries. Bone thresholds were stable, except in one patient with perilymphatic fistula. Six ears required revision surgery, and nine required office-based minor procedures. He concluded that minimally invasive management and surveillance of cholesteatoma had long-term results that compared well to those of postauricular methods [4].

Although it was often met with skepticism throughout the decades, the endo-scope has emerged as a powerful surgical tool for minimally invasive surgery, allowing access to hidden recesses for visualization, excision, or correction of pathologies without unnecessary disruption of overlying soft tissue or bone [5]. Many surgical fields within otolaryngology adopted the endoscope as an essential tool in their armamentarium, including rhinology and laryngology (Fig. 4.1). The field of otology is currently undergoing a similar evolution, advancing the endo-scope's utility from observational to operative [6].

Although binocular microscopy has been the workhorse of otologic surgery, the endoscope has gained significant attention and integrated adoption in recent years. Otoendoscopy is the use of rigid endoscopes to examine the ear. Endoscopes were first used in otology solely to describe ear anatomy [7, 8]. Outside of the operating room, the endoscope can be used during examination of the outer and middle ear and for debridement of complex mastoid cavities. Endoscopic ear surgery is the use of rigid endoscopes to perform otologic surgery. The binocular microscope provides a great three-dimensional view for line-of-sight surgery but has a significantly

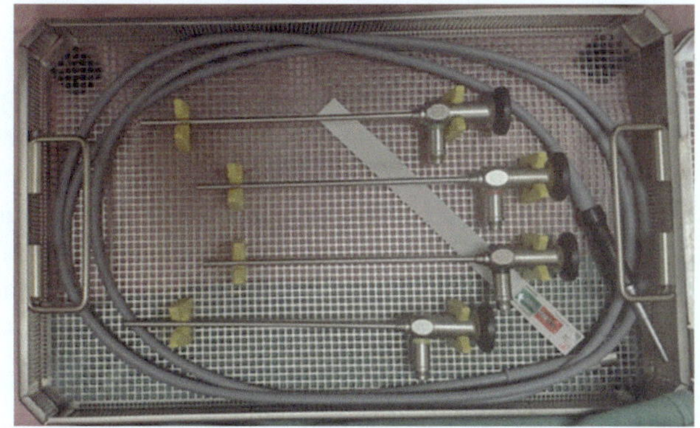

Fig. 4.1 Endoscopic Sterilization Tray with Silicon Holders: Standard set of rigid endoscopic telescopes (0-degree, 30-degree, 45-degree, 70-degree) with light source

limited views of the spaces and recesses of the middle ear, rendering transcanal cases difficult especially when the external ear canal is small or tortuous (e.g., pediatric cases). The binocular microscopic transcanal view is also limited by the size of the speculum being used. Therefore, bony resection (e.g., mastoidectomy) is needed to visualize and access complex middle ear disease using binocular microscopy.

An endoscope can be used to perform transcanal ear surgery with superior visualization and access that cannot be obtained by the limited line-of-sight binocular microscope. Unlike the line-of-sight surgery with the microscope and a speculum, the endoscope has a fisheye lens that is brought very close to the anatomic structures of interest, provides a wide-angle view, and displays a high-definition image of anatomy that cannot be appreciated even on the best binocular microscope. By providing superior transcanal operative access, a postauricular incision can be avoided when the disease is complex but limited to the middle ear. The benefits extend beyond the lack of an incision to avoiding the need for a mastoidectomy in certain cases thereby not disrupting the natural supply and demand of atmospheric gases and maintaining normal middle ear pressure equilibrium. These benefits in turn decrease patient morbidity, operative times, and surgical cost.

Transcanal endoscopic ear surgery has demonstrated comparable outcomes in the management of cholesteatoma, tympanic membrane perforations, and otosclerosis as compared to microscopic approaches, while utilizing less invasive surgical corridors and reducing the need for postauricular incisions [9, 10]. When a postauricular approach is required, the endoscopic-assisted transmastoid approach can avoid a canal wall down mastoidectomy in cases of cholesteatoma. The superior visualization offered by the endoscope provides the surgeon increased confidence when performing stapedectomy. A systematic review of the literature on total endoscopic stapedectomy demonstrated comparable safety and efficacy outcomes when compared to traditional approaches [11]. The endoscope also has utility in treatment of superior canal dehiscence, facial nerve decompression, and various petrous apex and skull base lesions including glomus tumors, meningiomas, and vestibular schwannomas [12–16]. In well-trained hands, endoscopic ear surgery is safe and effective with results similar to those achieved with traditional otomicroscopic techniques [17].

Zero-Degree Endoscopy

Performing an endoscopic exploratory tympanotomy with a 0° endoscope provides a view of the entire tympanic membrane and structures within the mesotympanum without any bony removal. Mesotympanic structures that can be seen include the chorda tympani, entire ossicular chain, tympanic portion of the facial nerve, cochleariform process, cochlear promontory, round window, pyramidal eminence, and stapes tendon. With adequate experience, tympanoplasty, ossicular chain reconstruction, and stapedectomy can be performed entirely endoscopically.

Angled Endoscopy

Using angled endoscopes allows for the visualization of the remaining middle ear spaces and their contents including the epitympanum, retrotympanum, protympanum, and hypotympanum.

Visual access to the epitympanic spaces including the entire attic and supratubal recess are possible, areas that traditionally are very difficult to see without a canal wall down procedure when the pathology is anterior in its location and extension. Access to the aditus ad antrum is possible with angled instruments to perform a limited dissection toward the mastoid. The cog can be seen and identified as a bony ridge connecting to the tegmen, separating the posterior and proper epitympanum from the supratubal recess and anterior epitympanic air cells. The horizontal semicircular canal can also be seen in this space using an angled endoscope directed superiorly.

Transcanal access to the retrotympanum is made possible including the sinus tymapni, which is an area that is challenging to see even in a canal wall down approach to the retrotympanum. Detailed view of microscopic structures bordering the sinus tympani can be obtained such as the ponticulus anteriorly and the subiculum posteriorly.

The hypotympanum can be accessed with detailed views of the funiculus, which is a ridge of bone connecting the cochlear promontory to the hypotympanic air cells, under which is the sub-cochlear air cell tunnel, which can provide access to the petrous apex and internal auditory canal using curved dissection instruments.

Anteriorly, access to the protymapnum allows for clearance of disease extending toward the eustachian tube to confidently confirm patency. The carotid artery can also be seen pulsating here if dehiscent.

Without the endoscope, angled instruments are required to blindly scoop out disease from these spaces. Middle ear mirrors are used at times to peek into these spaces, but the quality is too limited and insufficient for safe and complete dissection. The higher magnification obtained with the endoscope provides details of these spaces not achieved by binocular microscopy.

Transmastoid Endoscopic Ear Surgery

If mastoidectomy is performed via postauricular approach to clear out remnant disease not accessible by transcanal approach, the external canal skin is not violated and remains separate. Once all bony removal is complete during the mastoidectomy (smaller mastoidectomy compared with a traditional microscopic transmastoid approach), a 30° endoscope can be used to visualize and clear all disease from the mastoid antrum toward the middle ear. It is important to drape a gauze sponge along the posterior wall of the mastoid cavity to stabilize the endoscope, so it does not skid back and forth in an unstable manner, freeing the other hand for dissection. This transmastoid endoscopic debridement of complex disease obviates the need for a canal wall down procedure and all its associated disadvantages including: an open cavity requiring longer healing times, continuous ear drainage, accumulation of keratin debris, frequent follow-up for lifelong mastoid bowl maintenance, vertigo attacks following cleanings and temperature or pressure changes, shallow middle ear space making ossicular chain reconstruction difficult, inferior hearing outcomes, difficulty in fitting a hearing aid, and the necessity for dry ear precautions. Accessing the aditus ad antrum and epitympanum through canal wall up mastoidectomy to remove extensive cholesteatoma reduces the number of canal wall down mastoidectomies performed [18]. Second look tympanotomies can also be performed to assess and explore the middle ear for any residual disease if any concerns arise postoperatively.

Underwater Endoscopic Ear Surgery

Underwater endoscopic ear surgery is a novel technique in the otologic surgical armamentarium that will be increasingly relevant in the coming years. This technique involves filling the middle ear with fluid to surround and protect the inner ear. The main setting to consider underwater surgery is when trying to delicately dissect around the inner ear in a bloody surgical field. It provides enhanced visualization and decreased potential for thermal injury and pneumolabyrinth when managing inner ear fistulae. The relative protective effect is provided by surrounding the inner ear with fluid of a similar salt composition to that within the inner ear. It has been demonstrated that Ringer's solution is very similar in its content to the perilymph in the scala tympani [19]. In 2016, Anagiotos A et al. published a retrospective study on 15 patients with residual hearing who underwent cochlear implantation after having filled the middle ear and mastoid cavity with body-temperature Ringer solution and compared the outcomes with a cohort of historical controls. They noted a significant difference in the hearing outcomes with improved hearing as compared to a dry insertion. This implies that if the inner ear is manipulated when surrounded by a solution of similar composition and temperature, there may be a relatively increased preservation of function [20].

The most developed current application of underwater ear surgery is the management of cholesteatoma and resultant fistulae. Yamauchi et al. published on the technique in 2017 and subsequently published a case series in 2021 demonstrating its effectiveness in eradicating disease and resolving symptoms while preserving auditory function [21, 22]. Cholesteatoma is complicated by fistulae of the inner ear in 5–10% of cases in the western literature. The most common location is in the lateral semicircular canal followed by the cochlea and oval window. This is followed by the superior and the posterior semicircular canals [23]. A systematic review by Lim et al. in 2017 [24], showed that there are generally poor levels of evidence for management of cholesteatomatous labyrinthine fistula. The key question of whether there are any differences in hearing outcomes in removing versus leaving the cholesteatoma matrix over the fistula remained without a clear answer. Although there is no confirmatory data, removing the disease is intuitive to decrease ongoing inner ear inflammatory burden. The question of steroids has also been debated. There is a trend toward improved hearing in the literature with intravenous steroids on induction. There is no harm in using topical steroids on pledgets when dissecting cholesteatoma matrix off the inner ear structures. There is no clear evidence for continued postoperative use of steroids [25]. It is likely wise to use some form of steroids given the inflammatory pathophysiology of the disease if there are no contraindications. Hearing and specifically bone conduction results are better when the membranous labyrinth is not violated, intravenous steroids are used on induction, and when the fistula is in the semicircular canal rather than vestibule and cochlea since the involved hair cells are further away from the fistula when located in a semicircular canal.

There is still debate regarding differences in hearing outcomes with plugging or resurfacing fistulae. There is a trend toward plugging off the semicircular canal as it gives the surgeon more confidence in the repair and implies less ongoing labrynthitis when managing the cholesteatoma. For many decades, the approach to managing fistulae has been debated. There have been no comparative or randomized studies to suggest a superior approach. The method of choice has been based on institutional or surgeon preference and concurrent patient pathology. There has been a range of descriptions from canal wall up and canal wall down mastoidectomy to radical mastoidectomy, and more recently endoscopic approaches. The technique for the underwater endoscopic management of cholesteatoma and resultant fistula or superior semicircular canal dehiscence repair is via canal wall up transmastoid approach. A zero-degree 2.7 mm or 4 mm 18 cm endoscope with an endoscrub sheath attachment is used with Ringer's solution warmed to body temperature for irrigation +/− added steroids. The endoscope is stabilized on a gauze placed over the sigmoid sinus. It is important to note that when performing endoscopic ear surgery underwater, there is about a 30% magnifying effect in anatomy when compared to endoscopic ear surgery in the same position in a dry ear [26]. However, the image is much clearer as the irrigation is constantly clearing debris and blood from the field. These considerations are important when beginning to perform these cases in order to compensate for these factors. Dissection begins with continuous irrigation via the endoscrub, and a round or sickle knife is used to dissect and remove cholesteatoma matrix to identify the area of bony erosion and the underlying fistula. Cholesteatoma matrix is then carefully removed from within the fistula to ultimately clear all disease from within the inner ear. A composite tragal cartilage graft is then used to cover the defect, and then, the area is resurfaced using bone pate harvested during the mastoidectomy. Regarding drawbacks to underwater ear surgery, one of the main questions that has yet to be addressed is whether there are any long-term hearing effects from high-volume irrigation through large fistulae and resultant rapid perilymph volume exchange.

Another application of underwater endoscopic ear surgery is transmastoid superior semicircular canal dehiscence repair. This technique is via standard canal wall down mastoidectomy followed by a transition to an underwater dissection to identify, dissect, and open the superior semicircular canal to plug it with fascia in order to close the third window. The area is then resurfaced with bone pate and covered with perichondrium. This technique has been demonstrated to be successful with resolution of symptoms and minimal changes in bone conduction lines [21]. Other settings to consider the underwater endoscopic approach include the need to dissect disease medial to the facial nerve in the retrofacial recess where there may be concern for possible nearby inner ear fistula and if trying to avoid aerosolization when there is concern for airborne infectious disease.

With the continued refinement of underwater endoscopic ear surgery, existing techniques are constantly being enhanced, and new techniques are being developed. A novel technique developed in Japan describes transcanal endoscopic hydromastoidectomy by filling the external auditory canal with Ringer solution and drilling attic and antral dissections using a curved round coarse diamond bur attached to an otological drill underwater. When cases are selected carefully, this can be effective and can avoid the morbidity associated with postauricular incisions [27]. Another well-described technique is that of piezoelectric surgery, which is powered through the passage of an electric current through a ceramic medium, creating ultrasonic oscillations that are transmitted to a vibrating tip. It has been around for 15–20 years and initially used in dental, orthodontic, and maxillofacial surgery. It has been brought to otorhinolaryngology in the form of applications in rhinoplasty and otologic surgery. The device produces low-frequency ultrasonic frequencies in the region of 25 to 30 kilohertz with microvibrations to perform clean bony cuts without disturbing soft tissue structures. Since the introduction of this technology to otologic surgery, the question has been whether this poses injury to the inner ear. This has been debated, and there have been case series demonstrating that it is safe in preserving hearing function but also more recent evidence suggesting that its use over the cochlea can cause outer and inner hair cell damage [28–31]. Its application in stapedectomy seems to have suboptimal results when compared to use of the microdrill and CO_2 laser in higher frequencies of hearing [32]. This implies that the ultrasonic range in which the piezosurgical device is operating may be transmitting energy and causing some damage to the inner ear. Additionally, a study demonstrated that use of this device on the malleus produced decreased auditory brainstem responses, cautioning its use around the ossicles [33]. In conclusion, this can be a very useful tool when dissecting in the attic and antrum providing clearer visualization when compared to underwater drilling, produces very neat bone cuts, and provides very nice dissections around cholesteatoma. However, it should be used with caution around the ossicles and the inner ear. In cases of inner ear tumors where hearing preservation is not possible, piezoelectric surgery can be employed for clean translabyrinthine and transcochlear dissections to gain access to the tumor for removal with simultaneous cochlear implantation for tinnitus suppression and possible hearing rehabilitation [34].

Resident Training and Teaching

As the endoscope becomes widely adopted in otologic surgery and trends across multiple centers, trainees will see less canal wall down mastoidectomies for chronic ear disease. This may require a redefinition of the procedures needed to fulfill training program requirements. Endoscopic ear surgery will, however, facilitate excellent training by providing high-definition images of anatomic structures and relationships. It also allows the teacher to clearly see what the trainee is performing as they both have the same view. This is in contrast to binocular microscopy where the person operating has a three-dimensional view while the side teaching port generally only provides a two-dimensional image in most microscopes, restricting certain views (e.g., the annulus, the drop off of the bony canal, etc.). This limits the amount of safe teaching that can be allowed before the teaching surgeon must take over. Although endoscopy provides a significantly enhanced trainee otologic surgical experience, there is a steep learning curve and fewer opportunities for training in residency and fellowship. Despite the steep learning curve, endoscopic ear surgery offers several advantages over the microscope, and with the rise in the demand for minimally invasive approaches, there is a clear role for the endoscope in the future of otologic surgery. Identifying strategies to improve the training process for the novice and experienced otolaryngologist is paramount [35].

Disadvantages of Endoscopic Ear Surgery

The disadvantages of endoscopic ear surgery are inherent to the use of the endoscope and, therefore, are the same disadvantages that Dr. David Kennedy heard when he introduced endoscopic sinus surgery in the United States in the mid-1980s [36] (Table 4.1). Since the surgeon must use one hand to hold and operate the endoscope at all times, endoscopic surgery is limited to one-handed dissection. This requires a more advanced skill set to perform a given task such as placement and positioning of grafts and prostheses. In one-handed surgery, the surgeon must rely on native tissue for countertraction when dissecting since the other hand is occupied by the endoscope. Visualization can also be challenging in the setting of a bloody surgical field since the surgeon cannot have a suction in the other hand. Another

Table 4.1 Endoscopic ear surgery

Advantages
• Wide-angle view of field
• Enhanced depth of view
• Ergonomically advantageous with heads up view
• Line of sight easily manipulated
• Increased illumination of surgical field
• Can reduce necessity of surgical dissection and destruction of soft tissue
• Low cost of use
• Excellent tool for teaching with video monitor
Disadvantages
• Inherent learning curve with use
• Limitations with scope size in small ear canals
• Does not permit surgeon use of two hands
• Decreased instrumentation armamentarium compatible with endoscopic otologic surgery

limitation of endoscopic surgery is the lack of depth perception where in contrast to binocular microscopy, the endoscope provides a static two-dimensional image with a single-lens camera. Lastly, there is limited specialized instrumentation designed for endoscopic ear surgery [37]. However, rhinologists today have no issue with one-handed surgery and dissection, using high-definition screens and two-dimensional camera systems, and instrumentation has been developed and become highly specialized to access all the sinuses. These are skillsets that can be developed and issues that can be worked around over time and with experience as the endoscope is integrated into otologic surgery.

Setup and Safety

Endoscopic ear surgery requires more equipment in an already crowded operating room. When adapting the use of the endoscope in otologic surgery, one should plan and standardize the operating room layout ahead of time taking into consideration the laterality of the operation. The binocular microscope, the endoscope tower, and the associated instruments for both should be in the room and available for every case even if not being used. This way, when a second system is needed, it will always be available at a moment's notice. Screens should be available for nearly every person in the operating room. The surgeon should have a screen across the field at eye level, and the scrub technician should have another screen at eye level to anticipate the surgeon's needs and efficiently provide the needed instruments.

Before incorporating use of the endoscope to one's otologic surgery practice, it is imperative to understand the risks of ear endoscopy. All endoscopes used are rigid and, therefore, capable of impaling important surrounding structures. This is especially important when using angled endoscopes where the trajectory image displayed is different from that of the endoscope shaft. The endoscope sizes used in ear surgery range from 2.7 to 4 mm in diameter and 11 to 18 cm in length [38]. When selecting a size, one should consider the size of the ear canal and the quality of image needed. The length should be long enough to provide adequate hand working space but not too long that it decreases stability. It should be noted that larger diameter endoscopes transmit higher light intensity. The light transmitted by the endoscope into the middle ear can transmit heat up to 117° Fahrenheit within 60 s, which can burn and melt away structures such as the tympanic membrane and chorda tympani in seconds [39]. It is recommended to always keep the fiber-optic light source intensity no greater than 50% during endoscopic ear surgery to reduce thermal injury to outer and middle ear anatomy. The external and middle ear can be rapidly cooled by removing the endoscope, irrigating, and suctioning [40]. It is also important to limit the amount of antifog solution used given its potential for ototoxicity similar to that of gentamicin on ABR (auditory brainstem response) shifts shown by Nomura et al. in guinea pig models [8]. The surgeon should wipe the tip of the endoscope with a wet saline sponge after applying the antifog solution to minimize the amount introduced into the middle ear.

Endoscope holders have utility in endoscopic ear surgery; however, risk of injury to the patient should be considered. If two hands are being used for dissection, the endoscope held in a static fixed position using a holder, and the patient's head moves due to light sedation, then there is high risk to impale middle ear contents with the endoscope and cause significant harm [38]. There will not be enough time to release the endoscope and remove it from the ear safely before injury has occurred. Since paralysis is typically avoided in ear surgery for nerve monitoring, this is a significant concern. Physical restraint such as head pinning during lateral skull base cases mitigates the risk of injury and frees the surgeon's second hand for additional instrumentation or suctioning to facilitate more efficient surgery with better visualization.

Incorporating the Endoscope into Practice

Incorporating the endoscope into practice can be a daunting task as the learning curve is quite steep. It is recommended to do this process in a stepwise fashion by first using the endoscope during chronic ear surgery after the microscopic dissection to examine the middle ear, retrotympanum, epitympanum, protympanum, and hypotympanum looking for hidden disease. Practice can be achieved by examining the antrum through the ear canal and through the mastoid cavity. One should always start with a 0° endoscope to learn the lay of the land before examining with angled endoscopes [41]. Next, it is recommended to start with simple transcanal cases to get comfortable with the setup and to get the operating room team comfortable with the new configuration. These can be otoendoscopic exams of the tympanic membrane prior to starting a microscopic case, cerumen removal, myringotomy with tube placement, exploratory tympanotomy, and myringoplasty. As the endoscope is incorporated into more complex cases, one can start the tympanomeatal flap with the microscope and then complete the elevation using the endoscope to enhance and fine tune endoscopic skills while remaining efficient. If the surgeon is right-handed, it is recommended to start with left ear cases since they are easier because the operating hand works around the anterior overhang, and most chronic ear disease is found posteriosuperior, which can be naturally and directly reached with the right hand in a left ear. Whereas if a right-handed surgeon is operating on a right ear, the endoscope and instruments will have to cross making the case more challenging and more difficult to learn. As one gains more experience through these methods, a slow transition can be made by working less with the microscope and more with the endoscope.

The Future of Endoscopic Ear Surgery

As endoscopic ear surgery becomes a relevant part of otologic surgical practice, exposure to trainees will be critical. More prospective studies need to be performed to better establish the outcomes of endoscopic technique. Safety studies particularly as they relate to heat effects will be of significant importance. Instrument development for greater quality and more consistent dissections will be needed. Education through available courses will enhance skillsets using fresh cadaveric temporal bones and three-dimensionally printed ears for practice.

Use of the Exoscope in Otologic Surgery

The extracorporeal video microscope or exoscope is a recent addition to the microsurgical armamentarium and was designed to replace the operative microscope [42]. The exoscope consists of a high-definition or 4 K video camera with optical and/or digital zoom and a fiber-optically delivered or LED light source. This system is suspended above the surgical field with a manually actuated articulating holder or robotic arm, which transmits a three-dimensional image to a high-resolution monitor placed at eye level directly across from the surgeon. The exoscope's advantages over the binocular microscope include a large field of view; longer focal length creating ample working space; more manageable and maneuverable with ability to easily adjust the surgical view; the ability to share the surgeon's view with all operating room personnel; enhanced surgical ergonomics and comfort; decreased cost; less obstructive of the surgical field; better for teaching; and better image quality, magnification, depth perception, and lighting [43] (Table 4.2). The exoscope has been successfully used in cochlear implantation, mastoidectomies, vestibular schwannoma resections, temporal lobe encephaloceles, and cholesteatomas.

A disadvantage of exoscopes is lack of training opportunities as is expected with new and emerging technology. With experience, however, there does not appear to

Table 4.2 Exoscopic ear surgery

Advantages
• Higher depth of field than microscope at same working distance
• Allows three-dimensional visualization of surgical field
• Ergonomically advantageous with heads up view
• Less bulky and intrusive allowing more surgical working area
• Allows use of both hands
• Excellent tool for teaching with video monitor
Disadvantages
• Inherent learning curve with use
• Increased cost of use
• Must use 3D glasses for use
• Unit not as widely institutionally available

be significant differences in operating time or complication rates when comparing the exoscope to the microscope [44, 45]. Other disadvantages include reduced image resolution at higher magnifications and decreased illumination in narrow surgical corridors, supporting the idea that the exoscope is best paired with use of the endoscope in these circumstances [42].

Surgical Ergonomics

Traditional microscopic surgery is associated with unfavorable ergonomics. Binocular microscopy, even with armrests, Trendelenburg positioning, and a decreased 250-mm focal length places strain on the neck, shoulders and back during prolonged dissection. The stack height of the microscope increases the distance between the end of the oculars to the surgical field, requiring a static posture with the neck flexed and outstretched arms. The stack also obstructs the view of the surgical field for operating room personnel and requires a static posture with the neck flexed and arms stretched forward. Furthermore, the nature of microscopic surgery necessitates frequent adjustments intraoperatively. A 2015 study found that surgeons used the microscope handgrip controls to change focal length, zoom, or position an average of once every 114 s, which accounted for 8% of the total case time. Remarkably, surgeons modified several behaviors in order to prevent loss of alignment and further need for microscopic readjustment, such as avoiding looking away from the oculars during handoffs, maintaining unergonomic body postures, and even operating using a nonfocused view or at the edge of the field of view [46].

The endoscope and exoscope offer operating conditions with relaxed posture and enhanced body mechanics [18]. By utilizing a video monitor placed at eye level directly across from the user, the endoscope and exoscope allow the surgeon to view the surgical field while maintaining proper natural neck joint alignment, avoiding stress on the cervical and thoracic spine [47]. These three-dimensional systems have been associated with a significant increase in surgeons' rating of ergonomic comfort and decrease in back and eye strain, and may reduce asthenopia and subsequent difficulties in concentration that can accompany prolonged microscopic ocular use [48, 49].

Conclusion

Endoscopic ear surgery is a major paradigm shift in the management of middle ear disease. It is difficult, but the advantages of wide field view via transcanal approach justify the steep and slow learning curve. One should use both the microscope and endoscope together when starting to learn and incorporate endoscopic ear surgery into practice. Lastly, the exoscope is an advantageous alternative to the microscope for ear surgery as it provides a higher quality immersive visual experience and superior ergonomics.

References

1. Thomassin JM, Duchon-Doris JM, Emram B. Endoscopic ear surgery. Initial evaluation. Ann Otolaryngol Chir Cervicofac. 1990;107(8):564–70.
2. Poe DS, Bottrill ID. Comparison of endoscopic and surgical explorations for perilymphatic fistulas. Am J Otol. 1994;15(6):735–8.
3. Tarabichi M. Endoscopic management of acquired cholesteatoma. Am J Otol. 1997;18:544. https://doi.org/10.1016/j.otohns.2008.05.179.
4. Tarabichi M. Endoscopic management of cholesteatoma: long-term results. Otolaryngol Head Neck Surg. 2000;122(6):874–81. https://doi.org/10.1016/S0194-59980070017-9.
5. Kapadiya M, Tarabichi M. An overview of endoscopic ear surgery in 2018. Laryngoscope Investig Otolaryngol. 2019;4:365–73.
6. Ridge SE, Shetty KR, Lee DJ. Current trends and applications in endoscopy for otology and neurotology. World J Otorhinolaryngol Head Neck Surg. 2021a;7(2):101–8. https://doi.org/10.1016/j.wjorl.2020.09.003; Published 2021 Feb 6.
7. Mer SB, Derbyshire AJ, Brushenko A, Pontarelli DA. Fiberoptic endotoscopes for examining the middle ear. Arch Otolaryngol. 1967;85:387–93.
8. Nomura Y. Effective photography in otolaryngology-head and neck surgery: endoscopic photography of the middle ear. Otolaryngol Head Neck Surg. 1982;90:395–8.
9. Tseng CC, Lai MT, Wu CC, Yuan SP, Ding YF. Comparison of the efficacy of endoscopic tympanoplasty and microscopic tympanoplasty: a systematic review and meta-analysis. Laryngoscope. 2017;127(8):1890–6. https://doi.org/10.1002/lary.26379; Epub 2016 Nov 9.
10. Hoskison EE, Harrop E, Jufas N, Kong JHK, Patel NP, Saxby AJ. Endoscopic stapedotomy: a systematic review. Otol Neurotol. 2021;42(10):e1638–43. https://doi.org/10.1097/MAO.0000000000003242.
11. Hall AC, Mandavia R, Selvadurai D. Total endoscopic stapes surgery: systematic review and pooled analysis of audiological outcomes. Laryngoscope. 2020;130(5):1282–6. https://doi.org/10.1002/lary.28294; Epub 2019 Sep 30.
12. Totten DJ, Smetak MR, Manzoor NF, Perkins EL, Cass ND, Hatton K, Santapuram P, O'Malley MR, Haynes DS, Bennett ML, Rivas A. Endoscope-assisted superior semicircular canal dehis-

cence repair: single institution outcomes. Ann Otol Rhinol Laryngol. 2021;131:743. https://doi.org/10.1177/00034894211041223; Epub ahead of print.

13. Jufas N, Bance M. Endoscopically-assisted transmastoid approach to the geniculate ganglion and labyrinthine facial nerve. J Otolaryngol Head Neck Surg. 2017;46(1):53. https://doi.org/10.1186/s40463-017-0231-1. PMID: 28830539; PMCID: PMC5567439.

14. Marchioni D, Gazzini L, Bonali M, Bisi N, Presutti L, Rubini A. Role of endoscopy in lateral skull base approaches to the petrous apex. Eur Arch Otorhinolaryngol. 2020;277(3):727–33. https://doi.org/10.1007/s00405-019-05750-9; Epub 2019 Dec 2.

15. Fermi M, Ferri G, Bayoumi Ebaied T, Alicandri-Ciufelli M, Bonali M, Badr El-Dine M, Presutti L. Transcanal endoscopic management of Glomus tympanicum: multicentric case series. Otol Neurotol. 2021;42(2):312–8. https://doi.org/10.1097/MAO.0000000000002929.

16. Isaacson B, Killeen DE, Bianconi L, Marchioni D. Endoscopic assisted lateral skull base surgery. Otolaryngol Clin North Am. 2021;54(1):163–73. https://doi.org/10.1016/j.otc.2020.09.020.

17. Emre IE, Cingi C, Bayar Muluk N, Nogueira JF. Endoscopic ear surgery. J Otolaryngol. 2020;15(1):27–32. https://doi.org/10.1016/j.joto.2019.11.004.

18. Ridge SE, Shetty KR, Lee DJ. Heads-up surgery: endoscopes and exoscopes for otology and neurotology in the era of the COVID-19 pandemic. Otolaryngol Clin North Am. 2021b;54(1):11–23. https://doi.org/10.1016/j.otc.2020.09.024.

19. Acta Oto-Laryngologica. Physical properties, chemical composition and electrophysiologic aspects of labyrinthine fluids and their significance for cochlear and vestibular functions. A critical discussion and a table-form presentation (appendix). Acta Otolaryngol. 1966;62(sup218):25–76. https://doi.org/10.3109/00016486609125420.

20. Anagiotos A, Beutner D, Gostian AO, Schwarz D, Luers JC, Hüttenbrink KB. Insertion of cochlear implant electrode array using the underwater technique for preserving residual hearing. Otol Neurotol. 2016;37(4):339–44. https://doi.org/10.1097/MAO.0000000000000989.

21. Yamauchi D, Hara Y, Hidaka H, Kawase T, Katori Y. How I do it: underwater endoscopic ear surgery for plugging in superior canal dehiscence syndrome. J Laryngol Otol. 2017;131(8):745–8. https://doi.org/10.1017/S0022215117001104; Epub 2017 May 23.

22. Yamauchi D, Honkura Y, Kawamura Y, Shimizu Y, Sunose T, Hara Y, Ohta J, Suzuki J, Kawase T, Katori Y. Underwater endoscopic ear surgery for closure of Cholesteatomatous labyrinthine fistula with preservation of auditory function. Otol Neurotol. 2021;42(10):e1669–76. https://doi.org/10.1097/MAO.0000000000003241.

23. Rosito LPS, Canali I, Teixeira A, Silva MN, Selaimen F, Costa SSD. Cholesteatoma labyrinthine fistula: prevalence and impact. Braz J Otorhinolaryngol. 2019;85(2):222–7. https://doi.org/10.1016/j.bjorl.2018.01.005; Epub 2018 Mar 9.

24. Lim J, Gangal A, Gluth MB. Surgery for Cholesteatomatous labyrinthine fistula. Ann Otol Rhinol Laryngol. 2017;126(3):205–15. https://doi.org/10.1177/0003489416683193; Epub 2017 Jan 10.

25. Jang CH, Jo SY, Cho YB. Matrix removal of labyrinthine fistulae by non-suction technique with intraoperative dexamethasone injection. Acta Otolaryngol. 2013;133:910–5.

26. Kakehata S, Ito T, Yamauchi D. Approach to the inner ear by "underwater" endoscopic ear surgery: its utilization and prospects. In: Innovations in endoscopic ear surgery. Singapore: Springer; 2020. https://doi.org/10.1007/978-981-13-7932-1.

27. Nishiike S, Oshima K, Imai T, Uetsuka S. A novel endoscopic hydro-mastoidectomy technique for transcanal endoscopic ear surgery. J Laryngol Otol. 2019;133(3):248–50. https://doi.org/10.1017/S002221511900046X.

28. Salami A, Dellepiane M, Proto E, Mora R. Piezosurgery in otologic surgery: four years of experience. Otolaryngol Head Neck Surg. 2009a;140(3):412–8. https://doi.org/10.1016/j.otohns.2008.11.013.

29. Crippa B, Dellepiane M, Mora R, Salami A. Stapedotomy with and without piezosurgery: 4 years' experience. J Otolaryngol Head Neck Surg. 2010;39(2):108–14.

30. Salami A, Dellepiane M, Ralli G, Crippa B, Mora R. Effects of piezosurgery on the cochlear outer hair cells. Acta Otolaryngol. 2009b;129(5):497–500. https://doi.org/10.1080/00016480802311049.

31. Pawlowski KS, Koulich E, Cuda D, Wright CG, Stabilini E, Roland PS. Effects of cochlear drilling with piezosurgery medical device in rats. Laryngoscope. 2011;121(1):182–6. https://doi.org/10.1002/lary.21166.
32. Cuda D, Murri A, Mochi P, Solenghi T, Tinelli N. Microdrill, CO2-laser, and piezoelectric stapedotomy: a comparative study. Otol Neurotol. 2009;30(8):1111–5. https://doi.org/10.1097/MAO.0b013e3181b76b08.
33. Siu JM, Negandhi J, Harrison RV, Wolter NE, James A. Ultrasonic bone removal from the ossicular chain affects cochlear structure and function. J Otolaryngol Head Neck Surg. 2021;50(1):23. https://doi.org/10.1186/s40463-021-00491-4. PMID: 33810814; PMCID: PMC8017701.
34. Ma AK, Patel N. Endoscope-assisted partial cochlectomy for Intracochlear schwannoma with simultaneous cochlear implantation: a case report. Otol Neurotol. 2020;41(3):334–8. https://doi.org/10.1097/MAO.0000000000002539.
35. Barber SR, Chari DA, Quesnel AM. Teaching endoscopic ear surgery. Otolaryngol Clin North Am. 2021;54(1):65–74. https://doi.org/10.1016/j.otc.2020.09.005.
36. Kennedy DW. Functional endoscopic sinus surgery: technique. Arch Otolaryngol. 1985;111:643. https://doi.org/10.1001/archotol.1985.00800120037003.
37. Kozin ED, Lee DJ. Basic principles of endoscopic ear surgery. Oper Tech Otolaryngol Head Neck Surg. 2017;28:2. https://doi.org/10.1016/j.otot.2017.01.001.
38. Ryan P, Wuesthoff C, Patel N. Getting started in endoscopic ear surgery [published correction appears in J Otol. 2020 Dec;15(4):180]. J Otol. 2020;15(1):6–16. https://doi.org/10.1016/j.joto.2018.10.002.
39. Kozin ED, Lehmann A, Carter M, et al. Thermal effects of endoscopy in a human temporal bone model: implications for endoscopic ear surgery. Laryngoscope. 2014;124:E332–9.
40. Ito T, Kubota T, Takagi A, et al. Safety of heat generated by endoscope light sources in simulated transcanal endoscopic ear surgery. Auris Nasus Larynx. 2016;43:501. https://doi.org/10.1016/j.anl.2015.12.014; [Epub ahead of print].
41. Kozin ED, Lee DJ, Pollak N. Getting started with endoscopic ear surgery. Otolaryngol Clin North Am. 2021;54(1):45–57. https://doi.org/10.1016/j.otc.2020.09.009.
42. Smith S, Kozin ED, Kanumuri VV. Initial experience with 3-dimensional exoscope-assisted transmastoid and lateral skull base surgery. Otolaryngol Head Neck Surg. 2019;160:364. https://doi.org/10.1177/0194599818816965.
43. Ricciardi L, Chaichana KL, Cardia A. The exoscope in neurosurgery: an innovative "point of view". A systematic review of the technical, surgical, and educational aspects. World Neurosurg. 2019;S1878-8750(19):30080–4. https://doi.org/10.1016/j.wneu.2018.12.202.
44. Mamelak AN, Nobuto T, Berci G. Initial clinical experience with a high-definition exoscope system for microneurosurgery. Neurosurgery. 2010;67:476. https://doi.org/10.1227/01.NEU.0000372204.85227.BF.
45. Garneau JC, Laitman BM, Cosetti MK. The use of the exoscope in lateral skull base surgery: advantages and limitations. Otol Neurotol. 2019;40:236. https://doi.org/10.1097/MAO.0000000000002095.
46. Eivazi S, Afkari H, Bednarik R. Analysis of disruptive events and precarious situations caused by interaction with neurosurgical microscope. Acta Neurochir. 2015;157:1147. https://doi.org/10.1007/s00701-015-2433-5.
47. Capone AC, Parikh PM, Gatti ME. Occupational injury in plastic surgeons. Plast Reconstr Surg. 2010;125:1555. https://doi.org/10.1097/PRS.0b013e3181d62a94.
48. Zhang Z, Wang L, Wei Y. The preliminary experiences with three-dimensional heads-up display viewing system for vitreoretinal surgery under various status. Curr Eye Res. 2019;44:102. https://doi.org/10.1080/02713683.2018.1526305.
49. Wong AK, Davis GB, Joanna NT. Assessment of three-dimensional high-definition visualization technology to perform microvascular anastomosis. J Plast Reconstr Aesthet Surg. 2014;67:967. https://doi.org/10.1016/j.bjps.2014.04.001.

Chapter 5
Anatomic (AI) and Functional/Molecular Imaging (FMI) in the Diagnosis and Treatment of Head and Neck Pathologies

Emilio Supsupin Jr and Bo Chen

Introduction

This chapter illustrates the complementary role of anatomic (AI) and functional/molecular imaging (FMI) in the accurate diagnosis and management of head and neck pathologies. Advances in AI and FMI have directed the workup for accurate diagnosis of various head and neck pathologies and guided appropriate treatment. The potential role of imaging in evaluation of treatment response and further management is also addressed.

Imaging of Head and Neck Pathologies

This is not an exhaustive nor all-inclusive discussion of head and neck pathologies. However, AI and FMI play a critical role in the diagnosis and/or treatment of the representative pathologies selected in this discussion.

E. Supsupin Jr (✉)
Division of Neuroradiology, Department of Radiology, University of Florida College of Medicine - Jacksonville, Jacksonville, FL, USA

Department of Diagnostic and Interventional Imaging, UTHealth McGovern Medical School, Houston, TX, USA
e-mail: Emilio.P.Supsupin@uth.tmc.edu; Emilio.Supsupin@jax.ufl.edu

B. Chen
Department of Diagnostic and Interventional Imaging, UTHealth McGovern Medical School, Houston, TX, USA
e-mail: Bo.Chen@uth.tmc.edu

© The Author(s), under exclusive license to Springer Nature Switzerland AG 2023
J. C. Melville et al. (eds.), *Advancements and Innovations in OMFS, ENT, and Facial Plastic Surgery*, https://doi.org/10.1007/978-3-031-32099-6_5

Atypical Skull Base Osteomyelitis (ASBO)

Skull base osteomyelitis (SBO) is rare but can be a potentially life-threatening infection [1–5]. The diagnosis can be challenging [6]. Radiologic evaluation plays a critical role in the diagnosis and management of SBO [6]. With aggressive management, greater than 90% survival rate in ASBO was reported at 18-month follow-up, although up to one-third of patients had neurologic sequelae [2].

SBO occurs in two forms: typical (TSBO) and atypical (ASBO) [6]. TSBO classically occurs in elderly diabetic patients, resulting from necrotizing otitis externa from Pseudomonas species [1, 3]. On the contrary, ASBO has a predilection to the central skull base and is not preceded by otologic pathology [2, 3, 5]. Patients are generally middle-aged to elderly with underlying diabetes or other immunocompromised conditions (HIV, chronic steroid use, etc.) [2]. Seventy percent of patients with ASBO had a predisposing factor affecting bone vascularization, including diabetes (45%) [7]. Gram-positive bacteria (including *Staphylococcus*) are more common than *Pseudomonas* species [2, 3]. The most common symptoms of ASBO are headache and cranial neuropathies [2]. Fever is uncommon and is found only in 20% of cases [2].

ASBO Imaging

Unenhanced computed tomography (CT) is often first line in the imaging workup of suspected head and neck infections [6]. The study of choice for finding cortical bone erosion is high-resolution thin-slice CT with bone algorithm reformatted in multiple planes [6].

Complementary to CT, magnetic resonance imaging (MRI) of the skull base is superior for evaluating soft-tissue infiltration, marrow involvement, and intracranial complications related to SBO [3, 6]. To fully evaluate the skull base and surrounding structures, a combination of MR sequences is necessary [6]. This includes T1, T2, STIR, diffusion weighted imaging (DWI), and T1-weighted fat-saturated contrast-enhanced images [6].

The soft-tissue abnormality in the nasopharynx may be the dominant feature, which can be indistinguishable from an infiltrative neoplasm [6]. In osteomyelitis affecting the bone marrow, loss of normal fat signal in the marrow space causes T1 hypointensity and STIR hyperintensity [4, 6, 8, 9]. The affected marrow shows heterogeneous gadolinium enhancement [4, 6, 8, 9].

Nuclear medicine imaging served as a cornerstone for evaluation of SBO before CT and MRI [10]. The various radionuclide studies supply functional and metabolic information that can help confirm and localize infection of the skull base and can be complementary to clinical findings and anatomic imaging to monitor treatment response [6].

[18F] Fluorodeoxyglucose-Positron Emission Tomography (FDG-PET) detects increased glucose metabolism [6]. FDG is nonspecific and accumulates at sites of high glucose demand, including active infection, inflammatory, post-operative, or neoplastic processes [6, 8]. Advantages of FDG-PET/CT over other nuclear medicine studies include wider availability, shorter imaging time, and higher spatial resolution [6]. It can complement other modalities in determining the extent of infection in confirmed cases of SBO and maybe useful for evaluation of treatment response [6, 8]. A recent study showed similar diagnostic sensitivity of [18F] FDG-PET/CT and MRI [11]. However, PET-CT had better specificity (71.0% vs. 28.5%) in finding infection [11].

Technetium Tc99m methylene diphosphonate (Tc99m MDP) can show increased osteoblastic bone activity that occurs in response to infection [6]. There is abnormal increased tracer uptake in bone on all three phases (immediate blood flow, blood pool [5–10 min], and delayed phase [3–4 h]) [6]. Isolated soft-tissue infection will be differentiated by a normal delayed phase [6]. Delayed-phase single photon emission computed tomography (SPECT) improves anatomic localization [6]. However, a bone scan lacks specificity for infection and may show abnormal activity in non-infectious processes such as malignancy, trauma, recent surgery, and noninfectious inflammatory conditions [6]. In the setting of osteomyelitis, a bone scan can remain abnormal even after satisfactory treatment due to bone healing and remodeling [1, 2, 12, 13].

Gallium-67 citrate (Ga-67) scan targets acute-phase reactants like lactoferrin and bacterial siderophores [6]. It has a high specificity for infection and complements bone scan [6]. Gallium-67 citrate (Ga-67) binds to white blood cells engaged in the immune response to infection [6]. A normal Ga-67 scan reliably excludes SBO, even with an abnormal bone scan. An increased uptake on a Ga-67 scan confirms infection [6].

Ga-67 scan plays an important role in monitoring of treatment response, converting to normal findings after successful treatment [6]. Persistent increased uptake suggests residual infection [6]. The scan can be repeated to monitor antibiotic response until findings become normal [12, 14]. Long scan time requiring delayed images up to 48–72 h is the major limitation of a Ga-67 scan [6].

A technetium-labeled white blood cell scan is less commonly used. However, like a Ga-67 scan, it has a high specificity in the initial diagnosis of SBO [1, 6, 15, 16]. A tagged white blood cell study can confirm healing after completion of antibiotic therapy [1, 6, 15, 16].

The imaging findings in ASBO are illustrated in Fig. 5.1a–d and summarized in Box 5.1. Stroke can be a devastating complication of ASBO when left untreated or when diagnosis is delayed or missed (Fig. 5.2).

Box 5.1 Imaging Findings in ASBO
- Loss of normal fatty marrow signal in the central skull base
- Periclival soft tissue infiltration and abnormal enhancement
- Mastoid effusion from Eustachian tube obstruction
- Slight increase in DWI signal

Nasopharyngeal Carcinoma (NPCA)

NPCA (nasopharyngeal carcinoma) is a leading form of cancer in certain regions of the world such as the Cantonese population of Southern China and Hong Kong where the reported incidence is as high as 20 cases per 100,000 person-years [17, 18]. It is a rare cancer worldwide with incidence rates of less than 1 case per 100,000 person-years in north America and Europe [17, 18]. It is an aggressive head and neck cancer with high incidence of locoregional spread and of distant metastasis at presentation. NPCA has a relatively high incidence of systemic metastasis (up to 41%) when compared to other head and neck cancers [18]. NPCA may spread into the parapharyngeal soft tissues, skull base, or intracranial structures [18]. The nasopharynx has a rich lymphatic plexus. Seventy-five percent of patients present with enlarged cervical nodes, 80% of whom have bilateral involvement [18].

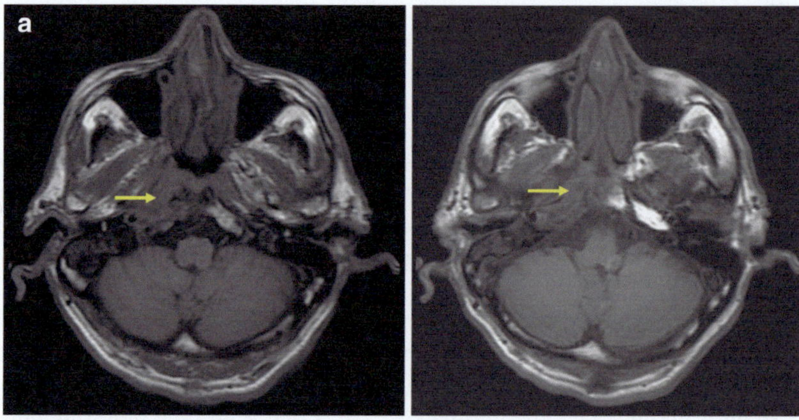

T1-weighted MRI depicting loss of normal fatty marrow signal in the central skull base with periclival soft tissue infiltration (arrows)

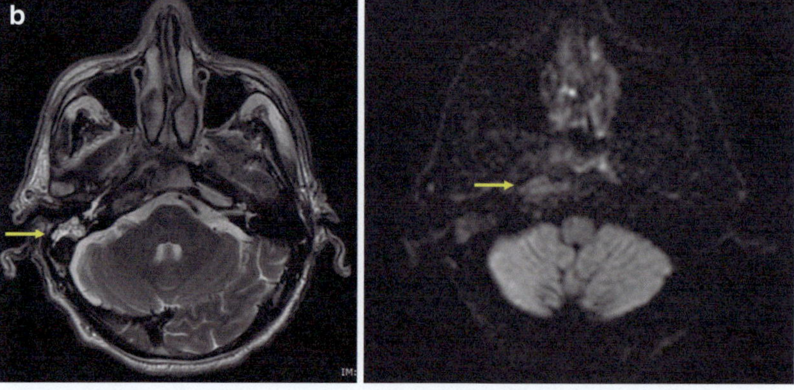

T2-weighted MRI showing right mastoid effusion due to Eustachian tube obstruction (arrow)

Slightly increased signal on diffusion weighted imaging (arrow)

Fig. 5.1 **(a–d)** 62-year-old male with uncontrolled diabetes (DM 2) with neck pain

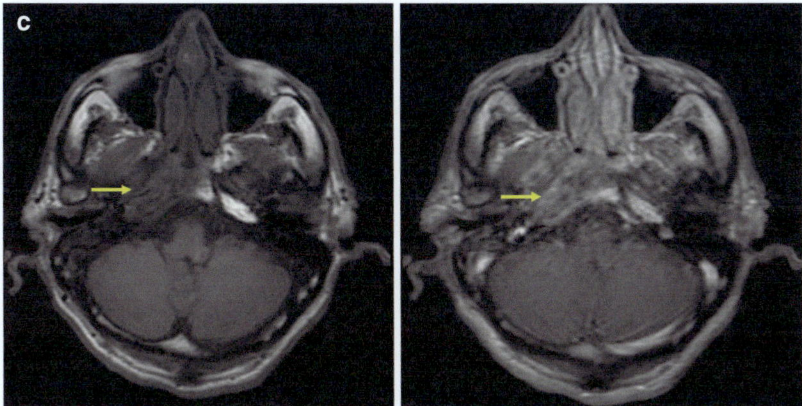

Periclival soft tissue infiltration with abnormal enhancement in the central skull base on T1 postcontrast MRI

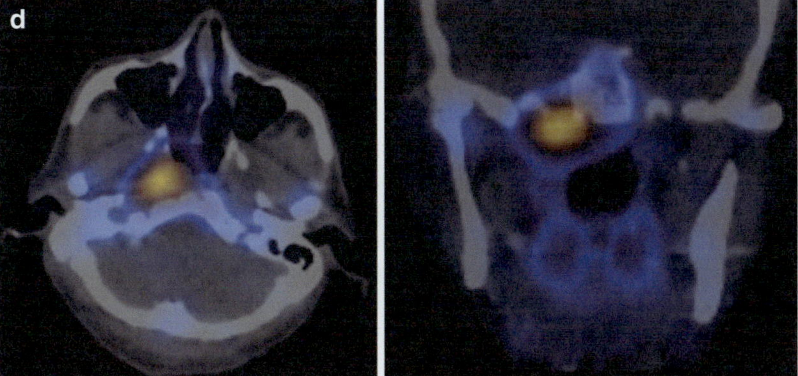

SPECT/CT with tagged WBC scan: Fused images show the location of the abnormality in the right retropharyngeal soft tissue compatible with infection – atypical skull base osteomyelitis.

Fig. 5.1 (continued)

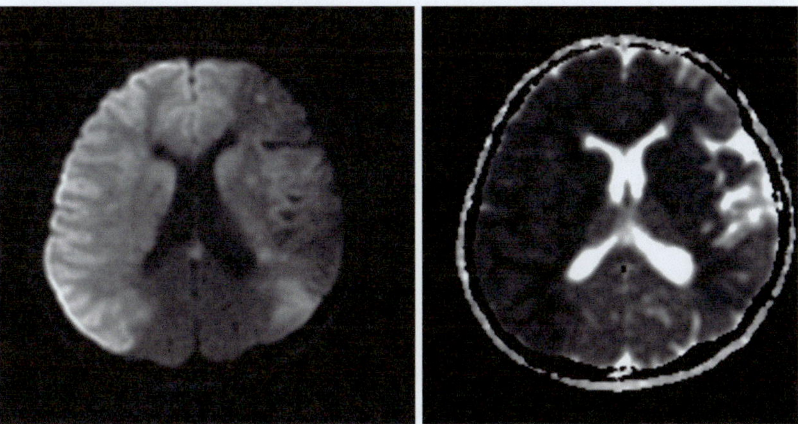

Fig. 5.2 Massive bilateral hemispheric strokes as a complication of untreated atypical skull base osteomyelitis (ASBO)

Determination of tumor extension and delineation of target volume rely on imaging [17, 18]. The main treatment of NPCA is radiotherapy and chemotherapy because of its specific anatomic location and excellent response to radiation [18]. Staging of patients with NPCA is the basic step to successful treatment [18]. TNM stage is the major prognostic factor of patient survival in NPCA [18]. The correct diagnosis of tumor extension and the delineation of target volume depend on imaging [18].

NPCA Imaging

MRI and FDG-PET have complementary roles. MRI contributes to T staging, whereas FDG-PET/CT has greater efficacy for N and M staging [17, 18]. In the future, PET/MRI may play a significant role in the treatment of NPCA by combining the benefits of PET and MRI [17].

MRI plays a significant role in diagnosis, staging, treatment planning, and prognostication. It has a high sensitivity, specificity, and accuracy of 100%, 93%, and 95%, respectively, in diagnosing NPCA [19]. These figures are comparable to endoscopy with biopsy, with corresponding values of 95%, 100%, and 98% [19]. MRI can provide a more accurate evaluation of the extent of primary tumor [17, 18]. Because of its superior spatial and soft-tissue contrast resolution, MRI is the imaging modality of choice to delineate the extent of the primary tumor [20, 21]. MRI can identify retropharyngeal lymph nodes misdiagnosed on CT as soft-tissue infiltration [18].

The various metabolic parameters from FDG-PET scans gathered before treatment provide valuable prognostic information [17]. FDG-PET and FDG-PET/CT have the potential to change management in patients with NPCA when compared to conventional imaging because of their superior ability to detect nodal and distant metastases [22, 23]. FDG-PET/CT is limited by its lack of contrast resolution in identifying retropharyngeal nodes that merged with adjacent primary tumor or to discriminate direct tumor invasion from retropharyngeal metastasis [17] [18]. However, for finding cervical lymph node metastasis, FDG-PET/CT may be more accurate than MRI [17, 18].

A combination of Epstein–Barr virus (EBV) DNA levels and FDG-PET can effectively monitor patients during follow-up to detect recurrence and can help in planning treatment and assessing prognosis in recurrent cases [17].

Fig. 5.3a–c illustrate the role of PET/CT in the accurate staging of NPCA.

Carotid Body Tumors (CBTs)

The carotid body (CB) is a structure within the adventitia of the common carotid artery at the inferomedial aspect of the carotid bifurcation [24]. CB has several functions, including regulation of heart rate and blood pressure, and acts as a chemoreceptor and baroreceptor [25].

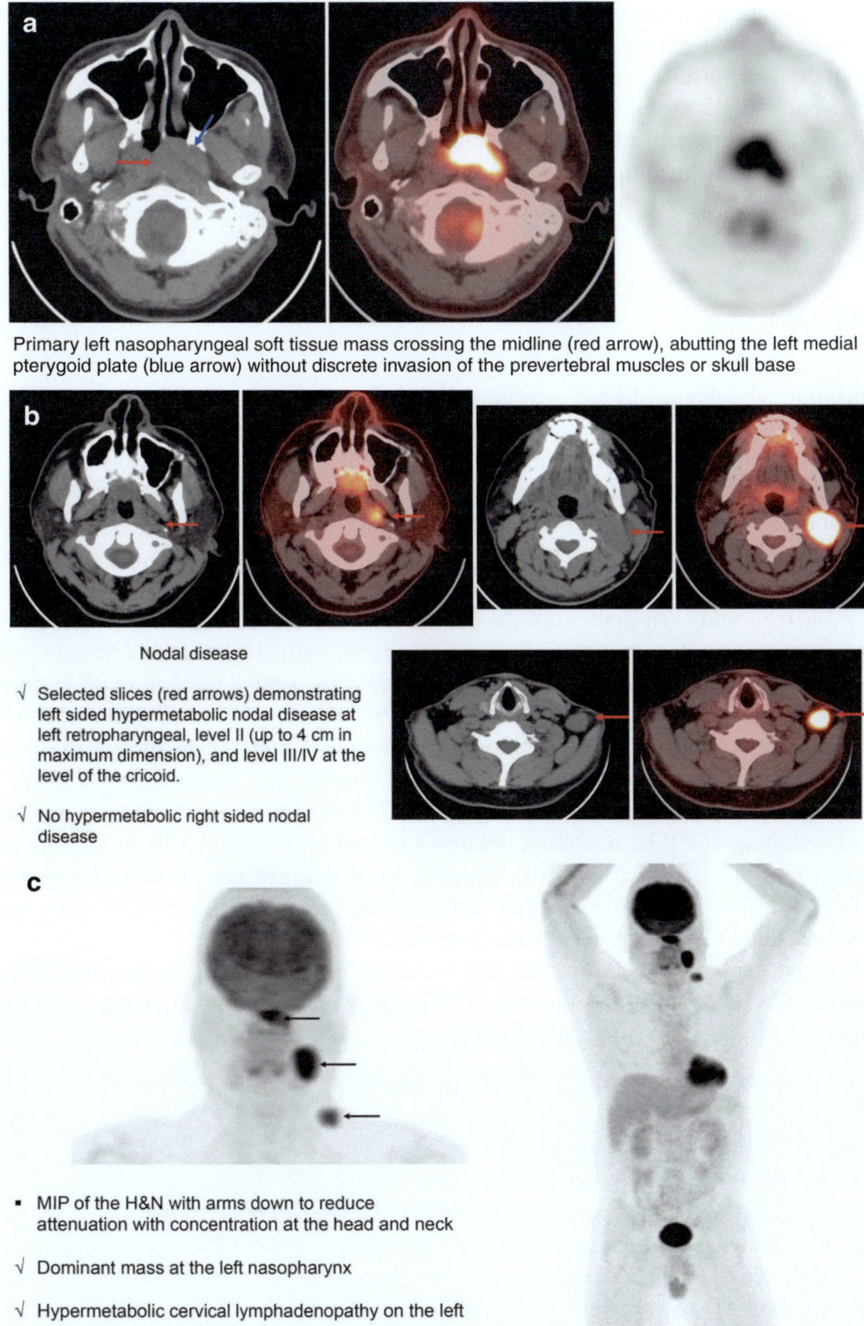

Fig. 5.3 (**a**) PET/CT depicting a biopsy proven EBV + nasopharyngeal cancer in a 53-year-old East Asian male with palpable left-sided lymphadenopathy. (**b**) PET/CT showing the extent of nodal disease ipsilateral to the primary mass. (**c**) PET showing the extent of nodal disease with no distant metastasis

Paraganglioma (carotid body tumor) is the most common pathology of the carotid body [26]. Carotid body tumor (CBT) is rare [27]. They are mostly benign, but malignant forms can be seen in up to 5% of patients [28]. Despite being rare, CBTs constitute most of the head and neck paragangliomas [29]. Accurate staging of CBT is particularly important because the malignant potential of tumor is not predictable from histology [30]. Malignancy is proved based on locoregional or distant metastasis [30].

CBT Imaging

Conventional imaging like ultrasound, CT, MRI, and arteriography are used for diagnosis of CBTs [30]. CBT is depicted on imaging as an avidly enhancing soft-tissue mass at the carotid bifurcation. Larger lesions have typical findings of splaying of the carotid bifurcation, avid enhancement, and characteristic "salt and pepper" appearance due to slowly flowing blood products and vascular flow-voids [27]. These tumors are readily visualized with current CT and MR imaging modalities [27]. However, distant metastases can be missed in malignant forms [30].

^{123}I-MIBG and ^{111}In-pentetreotide scintigraphy have been used in paragangliomas, in whole body scanning with high specificity [30]. However, the sensitivity was low in smaller lesions because of limitations in the spatial resolution of gamma cameras [30]. Recently, ^{68}Ga-DOTA peptides, PET tracers for somatostatin receptor imaging, have been used in neuroendocrine tumors with higher sensitivity and specificity, providing better resolution and quantification by PET technology [31, 32].

A small study showed that ^{68}Ga-DOTATATE PET–CT is a valuable diagnostic tool for staging of CBTs, detecting unknown lesions and changing the management of patients [30]. It is also useful in showing expression of somatostatin receptors and opportunity for peptide receptor radionuclide therapy (^{177}Lu-DOTATATE) for both metastatic CBT and pheochromocytoma [30].

Fig. 5.4a and Box 5.2 illustrate and summarize the imaging findings of CBT, respectively. Fig. 5.4b shows the role of ^{68}Ga-DOTATATE PET–CT in the accurate diagnosis of malignant (metastatic) CBT.

Box 5.2 Imaging Findings in CBT
- Avidly enhancing, hypervascular mass at the carotid bifurcation
- Splaying of the internal and external carotid arteries ("Lyre sign")
- Classic salt (bright signal from slow flow and blood products) and pepper (flow-voids) appearance
- Uptake of somatostatin-rich metastatic disease on ^{68}Ga-DOTATATE PET-CT scan

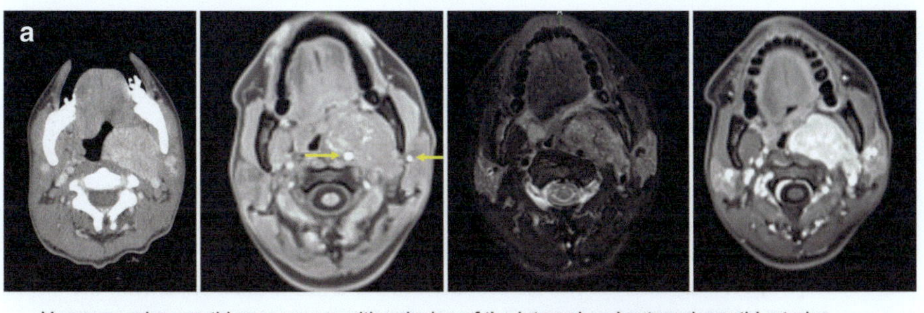

Hypervascular carotid space mass with splaying of the internal and external carotid arteries (yellow arrows). There are flow-voids within the mass with "salt and pepper" appearance. Findings consistent with carotid body tumor (paraganglioma). Plan – for resection

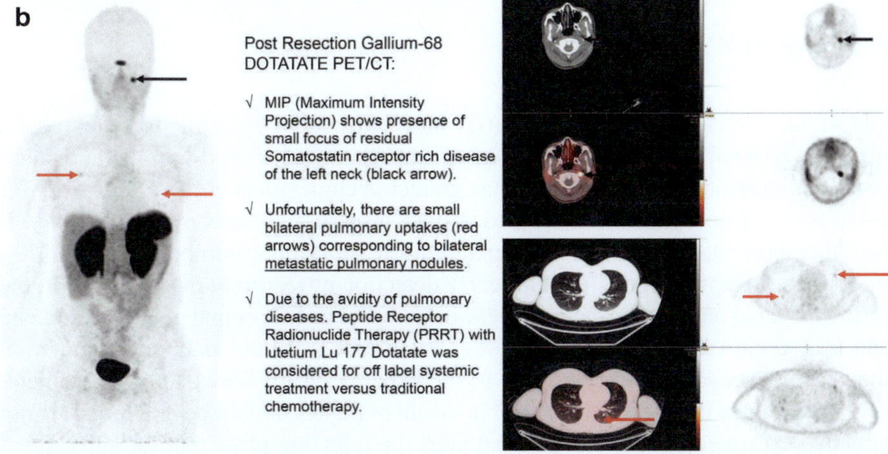

Fig. 5.4 (**a**) 20-year-old female with neck mass. (**b**) Metastases in malignant carotid body tumor

Squamous Cell Carcinoma (SCC) with Perineural Tumor Spread (PTS)

Many cutaneous, mucosal, and salivary malignancies carry high potential of perineural spread of disease. The most common nerves affected are the trigeminal and facial nerves (85% and 25%, respectively) due to the larger surface that they innervate [33]. The most affected trigeminal nerve branch is V2, but multiple branches of different cranial nerves can be involved due to anatomic contiguity. Certain tumor types such as mucoepidermoid carcinoma, adenoid cystic carcinoma, desmoplastic variant of melanoma, and squamous cell carcinoma are the most common culprits. Based on ACR (American College of Radiology) criteria, MRI of the skull base and brain with contrast are considered appropriate for evaluation of cranial neuropathy due to superior soft-tissue contrast, as well as less artifact from potential dental hardware. Typical primary MRI appearance of perineural spread of tumor is enhancement along the course of a thickened nerve with obliteration of fat at foraminal openings or the pterygopalatine fossa [34]. Secondary MRI signs include denervation atrophy of the innervated muscles with edema and enhancement during the early part of the process and muscular atrophy with fat replacement in the chronic phase. While perineural tumor spread may be asymptomatic, uncontrolled disease can carry significant debilitating clinical presentation such as neuropathic pain or motor dysfunction due to the affected nerve. The prognostic value of perineural spread of disease varies along histologic types and location with worse prognosis in certain scenarios [35, 36]. Both anterograde and retrograde tumor spread can occur [37] Retrograde spread of disease into the skull base foramina are more difficult to treat [38].

Imaging SCC with PTS

FDG-PET/CT is often used for initial and subsequent imaging for therapeutic response of head and neck tumors including melanoma, parotid tumors, and squamous cell carcinoma [39]. PET/CT has greater accuracy than either CT or MRI for assessment of nodal involvement and distant disease and synchronous primary. It can alter both staging and therapy planning in substantial number of cases [40]. Following therapy, PET/CT enables early detection of recurrent disease [41]. In the setting of head and neck cancers, linear or curvilinear FDG uptake within the head and neck region should be investigated, particularly along the anatomical course of the trigeminal and facial nerves due to their increased likelihood for involvement. MIP (maximum intensity projection) in all three planes should be examined. If not already performed, the radiologist can alert the referring physician for subsequent MRI evaluation of the area of abnormality on PET/CT to delineate the affected nerve and potential for local treatment.

Fig. 5.5 illustrates the role of MRI and FDG-PET/CT in the anatomic and functional depiction of perineural spread of squamous cell carcinoma along the trigeminal nerve.

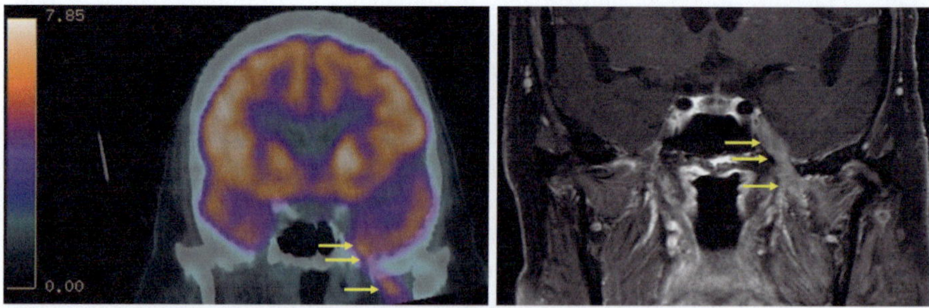

Increased FDG uptake corresponding to abnormal thickening and cord-like enhancement along the left trigeminal nerve distribution (arrows)

Fig. 5.5 Perineural spread of disease along the trigeminal nerve in a patient with squamous cell carcinoma

FDG-PET/CT does require patient preparation. The patient's blood glucose level must be controlled through diet, temporary refraining from exercise, and medications because the FDG molecule is a glucose analog.

Papillary Thyroid Cancer (PTC): Imaging and Treatment

Well-differentiated thyroid cancers including papillary and follicular and Hurthle cell variants constitute over 90% of the primary thyroid cancers [42]. The well-differentiated cell types carry an excellent prognosis. Most of these are discovered incidentally on cross-sectional evaluation of the neck with CT or MRI. For the initial evaluation of the thyroid abnormalities, neck ultrasound and CT of the neck are considered appropriate by the ACR. Neck ultrasound offers superior spatial resolution with the ability for real-time intervention (such as a primary mass and nodal biopsy without radiation). The classic sonographic appearance is a solid mass with irregular margins and internal vascularity with punctuate calcification [43]. CT evaluates the regional nodal disease, which can have variable appearance including cystic or solid feature or calcification [44]. The primary treatment is surgical resection with possible cervical nodal dissection.

After surgical treatment, majority of the patients undergo further evaluation for potential radioactive iodine ablation, which has been in practice since the 1940s. The purpose of the radioactive iodine treatment is to ablate the residual thyroid tissue to facilitate cancer surveillance via thyroglobulin and to treat iodine avid disease, which may be microscopic [45]. After surgery, iodine-based imaging with either low dose I-131 or low dose I-123 can be performed to evaluate for residual local and whole-body abnormalities and deemed appropriate for suspected recurrence of differentiated thyroid cancer and appropriate for early imaging after treatment of differentiated thyroid cancer.

The iodine-based functional studies have the advantage to assess the amount of residual disease after surgery and allow for dose calculation for the I-131 therapy, which carries the beta radiation, allowing for the local destruction of the cells that take up iodine. Iodine-based therapy can be performed for various stages of papillary thyroid cancer but particularly the advanced stages, which confer better survival [46].

Taking advantage of the long half-life and larger dose of the I-131 for treatment, post ablation images with gamma radiation offer a complete evaluation of the burden of disease in the body, as illustrated by the case example (Fig. 5.6a, b). Excellent anatomic details can be delineated with SPECT/CT. Surveillance whole-body iodine-based imaging can be performed and correlated with serum thyroglobulin and sonographic evaluation.

Iodine-based imaging requires several inconvenient preparations including discontinuation of certain thyroid medications or Thyrogen shots to achieve the proper thyroid-stimulating hormone (TSH) level, special low-iodine diet, evaluation of interfering medications including iodinated contrast for CT, and caution in the setting of potential pregnancy.

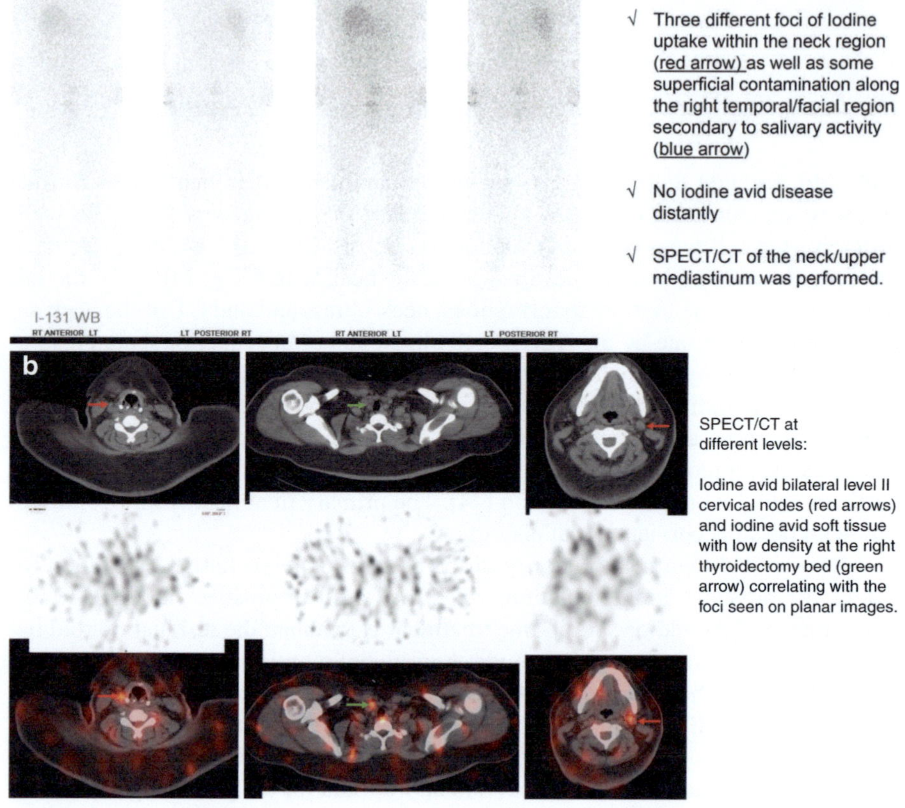

Fig. 5.6 (**a**) Postablation I-131 scan after 7 days. (**b**) Postablation SPECT/CT

Parathyroid Adenoma: Imaging and Localization

Parathyroid Adenoma is the most common cause of primary hyperparathyroidism, accounting for vast majority of cases, (75–85%) [47]. Preoperative identification of the abnormality has altered the approach of curative parathyroidectomy [48]. Majority of adenomas are posterior to the thyroid gland, but ectopic adenoma can be seen in the mediastinum, retropharyngeal region, carotid sheath, or intrathyroid. Based on the current ACR appropriateness criteria, initial evaluation of primary, secondary and tertiary, and recurrent primary hyperparathyroidism can be performed with neck ultrasound, CT of the neck with and without contrast (4D protocol) and functional imaging with SPECT/CT, which are all deemed appropriate.

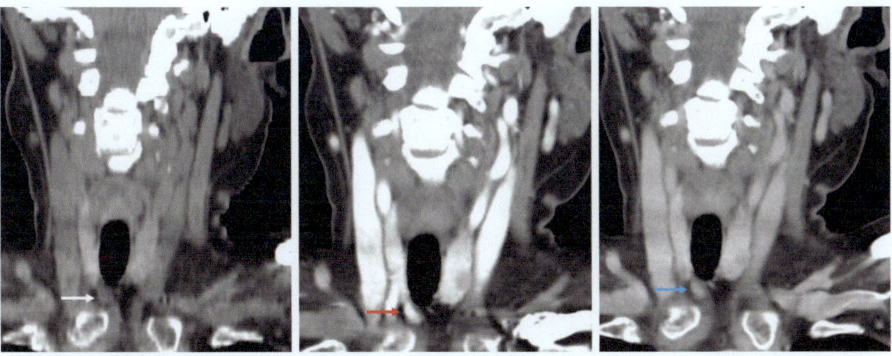

Typical parathyroid adenoma on 4D CT: hypoattenuating nodule (white arrow) below the inferior pole of the right thyroid lobe with enhancement on arterial phase (red arrow) and washout on delayed phase (blue arrow)

Fig. 5.7 Parathyroid adenoma

The abnormality appears on ultrasound as a hypervascular homogeneously hypoechoic nodule distinct from the thyroid gland with feeding vessel seen on Doppler. On 4D CT, the classic pattern is a hypodense soft tissue mass separate from the thyroid gland in the noncontrast images with avid arterial enhancement and washout in the delayed phase (Fig. 5.7).

Various protocols of radiotracer with SPECT/CT can be performed including dual time Tc-99m Sestamibi, dual tracer techniques with Tc-99m Sestamibi with I-123, and Tc-99m Sestamibi and Tc-99m Pertechnetate. The dual time Tc-99m Sestamibi is the most employed technique (Fig. 5.8a, b). While the protocol can vary, our institution performs a planar image of the skull base to the superior mediastinum at 20 min and 2 h, and a SPECT/CT is done of the same region at 20 min for anatomical localization of the abnormality. PET/CT is novel modality for investigation of this pathology.

With the improving accuracy of preoperative imaging, the earlier surgical paradigm has shifted to minimally invasive parathyroidectomy, which yields superior results [49].

In addition to the anatomical evaluation of SPECT/CT, the abnormal gland can be localized intraoperatively with a handheld probe if both the study and the operation are planned closely in time. The relative duration of functional imaging and the heterogeneous quality of the CT portion of the functional study can be improved.

Just as the advent of the functional imaging and 4D CT has changed the surgical planning, the imaging paradigms remain in flux and constantly challenged by data. Recent studies have advocated for the use of 4D CT over functional imaging [50].

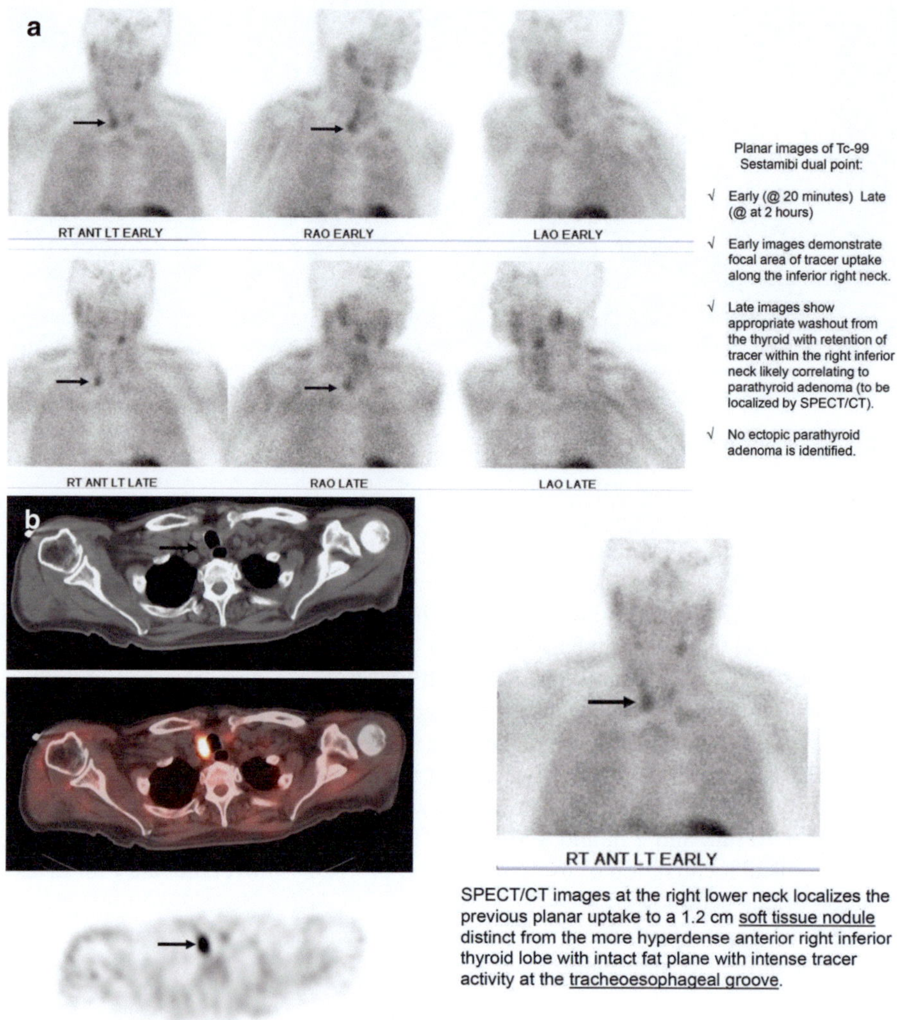

Fig. 5.8 (**a**) Parathyroid localization by Tc-99–Sestamibi. (**b**) Parathyroid localization by SPECT/CT

Conclusion

We highlighted the complementary role of AI and FMI in the accurate diagnosis and management of various head and neck pathologies. The advantages and limitations of imaging modalities are addressed. Appropriate use of imaging may help improve patient outcomes.

References

1. Carfrae MJ, Kesser BW. Malignant otitis externa. Otolaryngol Clin N Am. 2008;41(3):537–49, viii-ix.
2. Johnson AK, Batra PS. Central skull base osteomyelitis: an emerging clinical entity. Laryngoscope. 2014;124(5):1083–7.
3. Chang PC, Fischbein NJ, Holliday RA. Central skull base osteomyelitis in patients without otitis externa: imaging findings. AJNR Am J Neuroradiol. 2003;24(7):1310–6.
4. Borges A. Imaging of the central skull base. Neuroimaging Clin N Am. 2009;19(4):669–96.
5. Clark MP, Pretorius PM, Byren I, Milford CA. Central or atypical skull base osteomyelitis: diagnosis and treatment. Skull Base. 2009;19(4):247–54.
6. Chapman PR, Choudhary G, Singhal A. Skull base osteomyelitis: a comprehensive imaging review. AJNR Am J Neuroradiol. 2021;42(3):404–13.
7. Ridder GJ, Breunig C, Kaminsky J, Pfeiffer J. Central skull base osteomyelitis: new insights and implications for diagnosis and treatment. Eur Arch Otorhinolaryngol. 2015;272(5):1269–76.
8. Bag AK, Chapman PR. Neuroimaging: intrinsic lesions of the central skull base region. Semin Ultrasound CT MR. 2013;34(5):412–35.
9. Alleyne CH Jr, Vishteh AG, Spetzler RF, Detwiler PW. Long-term survival of a patient with invasive cranial base rhinocerebral mucormycosis treated with combined endovascular, surgical, and medical therapies: case report. Neurosurgery. 1999;45(6):1461–3. discussion 1463–1464.
10. Mendelson DS, Som PM, Mendelson MH, Parisier SC. Malignant external otitis: the role of computed tomography and radionuclides in evaluation. Radiology. 1983;149(3):745–9.
11. Kulkarni SC, Padma S, Shanmuga Sundaram P. In the evaluation of patients with skull base osteomyelitis, does 18F-FDG PET CT have a role? Nucl Med Commun. 2020;41(6):550–9.
12. Chakraborty D, Bhattacharya A, Gupta AK, Panda NK, Das A, Mittal BR. Skull base osteomyelitis in otitis externa: the utility of triphasic and single photon emission computed tomography/computed tomography bone scintigraphy. Indian J Nucl Med. 2013;28(2):65–9.
13. Strashun AM, Nejatheim M, Goldsmith SJ. Malignant external otitis: early scintigraphic detection. Radiology. 1984;150(2):541–5.
14. van Kroonenburgh A, van der Meer WL, Bothof RJP, van Tilburg M, van Tongeren J, Postma AA. Advanced imaging techniques in Skull Base osteomyelitis due to malignant otitis externa. Curr Radiol Rep. 2018;6(1):3.
15. Adams A, Offiah C. Central skull base osteomyelitis as a complication of necrotizing otitis externa: imaging findings, complications, and challenges of diagnosis. Clin Radiol. 2012;67(10):e7–e16.
16. Rozenblum-Beddok L, Verillaud B, Paycha F, et al. (99m)Tc-HMPAO-leukocyte scintigraphy for diagnosis and therapy monitoring of skull base osteomyelitis. Laryngoscope Investig Otolaryngol. 2018;3(3):218–24.
17. Mohandas A, Marcus C, Kang H, Truong MT, Subramaniam RM. FDG PET/CT in the management of nasopharyngeal carcinoma. AJR Am J Roentgenol. 2014;203(2):W146–57.
18. Wang-Sheng Chen J-JL, Hong L, Xing Z-B, Wang F, Li C-Q. Comparison of MRI, CT and 18F-FDG PET/CT in the diagnosis of local and metastatic of nasopharyngeal carcinomas: an updated meta-analysis of clinical studies. Am J Transl Res. 2016;8(11):4532–47.
19. King AD, Vlantis AC, Bhatia KS, et al. Primary nasopharyngeal carcinoma: diagnostic accuracy of MR imaging versus that of endoscopy and endoscopic biopsy. Radiology. 2011;258(2):531–7.
20. Ng SH, Chan SC, Yen TC, et al. Staging of untreated nasopharyngeal carcinoma with PET/CT: comparison with conventional imaging work-up. Eur J Nucl Med Mol Imaging. 2009;36(1):12–22.
21. King AD, Ma BB, Yau YY, et al. The impact of 18F-FDG PET/CT on assessment of nasopharyngeal carcinoma at diagnosis. Br J Radiol. 2008;81(964):291–8.

22. Chang MC, Chen JH, Liang JA, Yang KT, Cheng KY, Kao CH. Accuracy of whole-body FDG-PET and FDG-PET/CT in M staging of nasopharyngeal carcinoma: a systematic review and meta-analysis. Eur J Radiol. 2013;82(2):366–73.
23. Law A, Peters LJ, Dutu G, et al. The utility of PET/CT in staging and assessment of treatment response of nasopharyngeal cancer. J Med Imaging Radiat Oncol. 2011;55(2):199–205.
24. Lack EE, Armed Forces Institute of Pathology (US), Universities Associated for Research and Education in Pathology. Tumors of the adrenal gland and extra-adrenal paraganglia. Washington, DC: Published by the Armed Forces Institute of Pathology Under the Auspices of Universities Associated for Research and Education in Pathology; 1997.
25. Kliewer KE, Cochran AJ. A review of the histology, ultrastructure, immunohistology, and molecular biology of extra-adrenal paragangliomas. Arch Pathol Lab Med. 1989;113(11):1209–18.
26. Mafee MF, Raofi B, Kumar A, Muscato C. Glomus faciale, glomus jugulare, glomus tympanicum, glomus vagale, carotid body tumors, and simulating lesions. Role of MR imaging. Radiol Clin N Am. 2000;38(5):1059–76.
27. Nguyen RP, Shah LM, Quigley EP, Harnsberger HR, Wiggins RH. Carotid body detection on CT angiography. AJNR Am J Neuroradiol. 2011;32(6):1096–9.
28. Sajid MS, Hamilton G, Baker DM, Joint Vascular Research G. A multicenter review of carotid body tumour management. Eur J Vasc Endovasc Surg. 2007;34(2):127–30.
29. Wasserman PG, Savargaonkar P. Paragangliomas: classification, pathology, and differential diagnosis. Otolaryngol Clin N Am. 2001;34(5):845–62. v-vi.
30. Simsek DH, Sanli Y, Kuyumcu S, Basaran B, Mudun A. (68)Ga-DOTATATE PET-CT imaging in carotid body paragangliomas. Ann Nucl Med. 2018;32(4):297–301.
31. Ambrosini V, Campana D, Bodei L, et al. 68Ga-DOTANOC PET/CT clinical impact in patients with neuroendocrine tumors. J Nucl Med. 2010;51(5):669–73.
32. Mojtahedi A, Thamake S, Tworowska I, Ranganathan D, Delpassand ES. The value of (68) Ga-DOTATATE PET/CT in diagnosis and management of neuroendocrine tumors compared to current FDA approved imaging modalities: a review of literature. Am J Nucl Med Mol Imaging. 2014;4(5):426–34.
33. Panizza BJ. An overview of head and neck malignancy with perineural spread. J Neurol Surg B Skull Base. 2016;77(2):81–5.
34. Ong CK, Chong VF. Imaging of perineural spread in head and neck tumours. Cancer Imaging. 2010;10:S92–8.
35. Liebig C, Ayala G, Wilks JA, Berger DH, Albo D. Perineural invasion in cancer: a review of the literature. Cancer. 2009;115(15):3379–91.
36. Majoie CB, Hulsmans FJ, Verbeeten B Jr, Castelyns JA, Oldenburger F, Schouwenburg PF, Andries Bosch D. Perineural tumor extension along the trigeminal nerve: magnetic resonance imaging findings. Eur J Radiol. 1997;24(3):191–205.
37. Amit M, Eran A, Billan S, Fridman E, Na'ara S, Charas T, Gil Z. Perineural spread in noncutaneous head and neck cancer: new insights into an old problem. J Neurol Surg B Skull Base. 2016;77(2):86–95.
38. Bakst RL, Glastonbury CM, Parvathaneni U, Katabi N, Hu KS, Yom SS. Perineural invasion and perineural tumor spread in head and neck cancer. Int J Radiat Oncol Biol Phys. 2019;103(5):1109–24.
39. Paes FM, Singer AD, Checkver AN, Palmquist RA, De La Vega G, Sidani C. Perineural spread in head and neck malignancies: clinical significance and evaluation with 18F-FDG PET/CT. Radiographics. 2013;33(6):1717–36.
40. Mak D, Corry J, Lau E, Rischin D, Hicks RJ. Role of FDG-PET/CT in staging and follow-up of head and neck squamous cell carcinoma. Q J Nucl Med Mol Imaging. 2011;55(5):487–99.
41. Wong RJ, Lin DT, Schoder H, Patel SG, Gonen M, Wolden S, Kraus DH, et al. Diagnostic and prognostic value of [(18)F-fluorodeoxyglucose positron emission tomography for recurrent head and neck squamous cell carcinoma]. J Clin Oncol. 2002;20(20):4199–208.
42. Hoang JK, Branstetter BFT, Gafton AR, Lee WK, Glastonbury CM. Imaging of thyroid carcinoma with CT and MRI: approaches to common scenarios. Cancer Imaging. 2013;13:128–39.

43. Shin JH. Ultrasonographic imaging of papillary thyroid carcinoma variants. Ultrasonography. 2017;36(2):103–10.
44. Bin Saeedan M, Aljohani IM, Khushaim AO, Bukhari SQ, Elnaas ST. Thyroid computed tomography imaging: pictorial review of variable pathologies. Insights Imaging. 2016;7(4):601–17.
45. Carballo M, Quiros RM. To treat or not to treat: the role of adjuvant radioiodine therapy in thyroid cancer patients. J Oncol. 2012;2012:707156.
46. Yang Z, Flores J, Katz S, Nathan CA, Mehta V. Comparison of survival outcomes following postsurgical radioactive iodine versus external beam radiation in stage IV differentiated thyroid carcinoma. Thyroid. 2017;27(7):944–52.
47. Piciucchi S, Barone D, Gavelli G, Dubini A, Oboldi D, Matteuci F. Primary hyperparathyroidism: imaging to pathology. J Clin Imaging Sci. 2012;2:59.
48. Khan AA, Hanley DA, Rizzoli R, Bollerslev J, Young JE, Rejnmark L, Bilezikian JP, et al. Primary hyperparathyroidism: review and recommendations on evaluation, diagnosis, and management. A Canadian and international consensus. Osteoporos Int. 2017;28(1):1–19.
49. Udelsman R, Lin Z, Donovan P. The superiority of minimally invasive parathyroidectomy based on 1650 consecutive patients with primary hyperparathyroidism. Ann Surg. 2011;253(3):585–91.
50. Kattar N, Migneron M, Debakey MS, Haidari M, Pou AM, McCoul ED. Advanced computed tomographic localization techniques for primary hyperparathyroidism: a systematic review and meta-analysis. JAMA Otolaryngol Head Neck Surg. 2022;148:448–56.

Chapter 6
Advancements and Innovations in Sleep Surgery

Stanley Yung-Chuan Liu and Ahmed A. Al-Sayed

Introduction

Obstructive sleep apnea (OSA) is a complex condition that afflicts all ages. Upper airway surgery is an important treatment option. Sleep surgery has evolved with improved understanding of facial skeletal development and sleep physiology. Evolving skeletal techniques and upper airway stimulation (UAS) are effective extrapharyngeal interventions with high success rate. With more emphasis on the timing of interventions in growing individuals, there is also the likelihood of reducing risk of OSA in adulthood [1].

Another advance in the treatment paradigm of sleep surgery is focus on precision. The selection and sequence of procedure(s) should follow a systematic and organized method [2]. The Powell–Riley protocol [3] was introduced in the early 1990s to limit unnecessary surgery through physical examination including pharyngoscopy, polysomnography (PSG), and lateral cephalometry. The protocol acknowledged the commonality of multi-level airway collapse in OSA patients. Surgical options in Phase I of the protocol consisted of nasal surgeries,

S. Y.-C. Liu (✉)
Division of Sleep Surgery, Department of Otolaryngology–Head and Neck Surgery, Stanford University School of Medicine, Stanford, CA, USA
e-mail: ycliu@stanford.edu

A. A. Al-Sayed
Division of Sleep Surgery, Department of Otolaryngology–Head and Neck Surgery, Stanford University School of Medicine, Stanford, CA, USA

Department of Otolaryngology–Head and Neck Surgery, Faculty of Medicine, King Saud University, Riyadh, Saudi Arabia
e-mail: alsayed@stanford.edu

© The Author(s), under exclusive license to Springer Nature Switzerland AG 2023
J. C. Melville et al. (eds.), *Advancements and Innovations in OMFS, ENT, and Facial Plastic Surgery*, https://doi.org/10.1007/978-3-031-32099-6_6

tonsillectomy, uvulopalatopharyngoplasty, genioglossus advancement, and hyoid myotomy with suspension. Phase II, which is maxillomandibular advancement (MMA), was reserved for incompletely treated OSA after re-evaluation by PSG 6-months following Phase I. The rationale behind the protocol was based on a 60% surgical response with Phase I surgery, and therefore, a majority not needing MMA.

The Stanford sleep surgery protocol since 2015 [4] reflects the reality that all treatment modalities, from medical to surgical, are on a continuum of care (Fig. 6.1). Classic Phase I procedures can follow MMA in indicated patients. Surgery to relieve nasal obstruction can help improve adherence to medical management such as positive airway pressure therapy. More important than individual surgical success is the overall treatment efficacy for every patient. The aim of this chapter is to provide an overview of this updated protocol and discuss the latest innovations in sleep surgery. A few highlights include the role of drug-induced sedation (sleep) endoscopy (DISE), the advent of UAS, and precision in both patient selection and procedure accuracy in skeletal surgery.

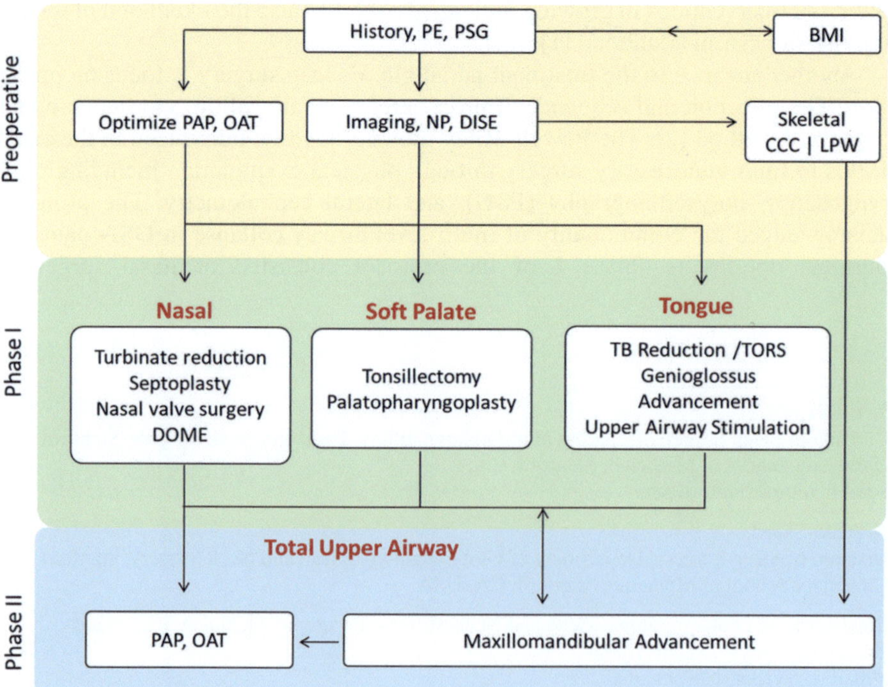

Fig. 6.1 The updated Stanford sleep surgery protocol

Nasal Surgeries

The internal nasal valve represents the area of highest resistance in the upper airway. The internal nasal valve is composed of the nasal septum, the upper lateral cartilage, the head of the inferior turbinate, and the nasal floor. Airway patency can be enhanced by correcting a septal deviation, upper lateral stabilization, inferior turbinate reduction, or expansion of the nasal floor. Improving nasal patency decreases the associated sequence of mouth breathing, posterior tongue collapse, and hypopharyngeal narrowing. Treating nasal obstruction does not cure OSA. However, it improves continuous positive airway pressure (CPAP) compliance and sleep quality of life (QoL) [5]. A narrow nasal floor is a previously under-recognized cause of nasal obstruction and failure of nasal surgeries [6]. Nasal obstruction early on in life leads to a facial growth pattern characterized by transverse maxillary deficiency. This is associated with nasal obstruction later in life and predisposes to sleep-disordered breathing, nasal surgery failure, and CPAP intolerance.

Maxillary Expansion—"Rhinognathic Surgery"

The dissociation of adult and pediatric OSA is artificial. The underpinnings and development of OSA follow a continuum across age. Orofacial growth is influenced by many upper airway variables with nasal airflow playing a critical role. Mouth breathing and an abnormal position of the tongue in the oral cavity occurs when skeletal growth is at a maximum early in life, leading to a decrease in growth stimulation of intermaxillary cartilage [7]. That, in turn, leads to a high-arched palate and predisposes to sleep apnea later in life [8]. Furthermore, the dysfunction in facial growth has secondary consequences on the maxillomandibular position, and such changes have a negative feedback impact on the support of the muscles of the upper airway. Hence, skeletal development influences dental occlusal angle, facial aesthetics, and upper airway patency [9].

Ideally, transverse maxillary hypoplasia (TMH) is addressed while facial growth is still active [10]. There is strong evidence demonstrating the resolution of persistent pediatric OSA post adenotonsillectomy with maxillary expansion [11]. The need for a similar treatment in adults was observed by Christian Guilleminault of Stanford University [12, 13]. However, such as the cribriform plate, parts of the temporal bone, and zygoma. Excessive force applied to these areas can result in cerebrospinal fluid leakage, transient hearing loss, and facial asymmetry.

Craniomaxillofacial surgeons conventionally perform surgically assisted rapid palatal expansion (SARPE) for adult TMH, which combines LeFort I level osteotomies, pterygoid disjunction, and a tooth-anchored expander. However, there are a couple of drawbacks to this technique: [1] the LeFort I osteotomies are not enough for transverse expansion; therefore, a midpalatal suture split is required.

However, [2] even with multipiece osteotomies, the tooth-anchored expander exerts the lateralizing forces on the dentoalveolar segments, thus lateralizing the teeth more so than the split maxilla. Consequently, the SARPE does not adequately address the nasal floor, the key area in sleep-disordered breathing in adults [14].

The need to expand the maxilla of adults in a predictable, fast, and stable manner is clear. In fact, most surgical interventions for OSA focus on the Anterior-Posterior (AP) dimension of the airway. Even with expansion pharyngoplasty, where the goal is to expand the palatopharyngeus and palatoglossus muscles, the expansion is limited by the width of the maxilla. Hence, skeletal maxillary expansion would be the only procedure that addresses the lateral dimension of the skeleton. Physiologically, the improvement in nasal breathing during sleep expands upper airway dilator muscles (Fig. 6.2) [6, 15]. Maxillary expansion has both structural and physiological contributions to a wider airway during sleep. It is important to note distraction osteogenesis maxillary expansion (DOME) is not meant to be a single procedure. Rather, in a patient-specific fashion, DOME has continually evolved to convert a high-arched palate to a *dome*-shaped palate [13]. Over time, with virtual surgical planning, Lefort guides to be used for nasal endoscopic approaches, and improved orthodontic anchorage devices, DOME is a patient-specific approach to address nasal breathing during sleep. DOME has become an integral part of the revised Stanford sleep surgery protocol. As the technique was refined over time, it is possible nowadays to perform the procedure in a minimally invasive nasal endoscopic approach (MINI-DOME) [16].

In this section, we will be reviewing the indications, contraindications, patient selection, diagnostic workup, specific risks, patient consent, anesthetic considerations, required equipment, procedural steps, complications, and postoperative care of DOME and MINI-DOME.

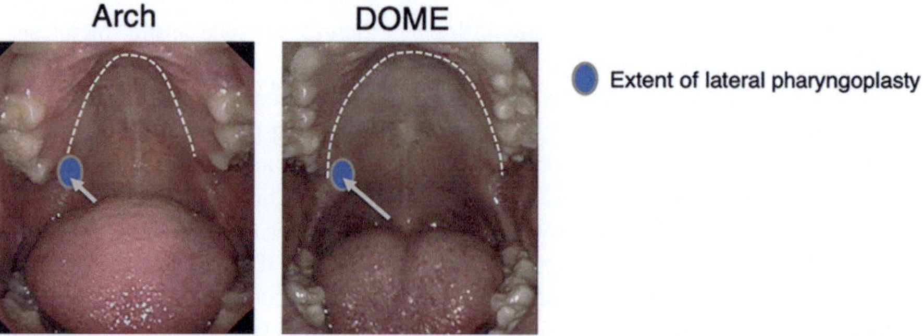

Fig. 6.2 Distraction Osteogenesis Maxillary Expansion (DOME) increases the transverse dimension of the maxilla, which provides more space for the tongue to rest in the oral cavity. Additionally, it allows for greater pharyngoplasty expansion

Indications and Contraindications

DOME is recommended generally for adults with OSA who have any or more of the following features: (1) TMH with or without crossbite, (2) persistent nasal obstruction after nasal surgery with mild OSA and a high-arched palate, and (3) moderate to severe OSA with a high-arched palate as a phased procedure preceding further interventions. Contraindications to the procedure are relative and include: (1) periodontal disease, (2) inability or unwillingness to undergo perioperative orthodontic care, and (3) difficulty adhering to distraction.

Diagnostic Workup

We strongly recommend a preoperative attended polysomnography (PSG), with attention to airflow limitation. Maxillofacial computed tomography (CT) is necessary for virtual surgical planning (VSP) and assessment of surgical landmarks (premaxilla thickness, nasopalatine nerve position, and distance between central incisors roots). The thickness of the maxilla dictates the length of screws used on the expander. Pre- and posttreatment photos are recommended. It is important to note that one's facial appearance does not change significantly posttreatment.

Specific Risks, Patient Information, and Consent

Patients must be counseled about the goals of treatment. The most significant and reproducible outcome is the subjective decrease in nasal obstruction as measured by the nasal obstruction symptom evaluation (NOSE) scale and the functional component of the Standardized Cosmesis and Health Nasal Outcomes Survey (SCHNOS). For severe OSA, surgical success is approximately 70%, and these patients will continue to receive further interventions either in the form of other surgical procedures or CPAP. For patients with upper airway resistance syndrome (UARS), the reduction in the apnea-hypopnea index (AHI) is significant, but surgical success cannot be defined by the Sher's criteria because pretreatment AHI is usually less than ten events per hour.

Surgical risks include loss of dental vitality, particularly of the central incisors; asymmetric maxillary expansion; inadequate expansion; and persistent paresthesia from the vestibular incision. VSP has significantly reduced these risks. Moreover, the MINI-DOME approach significantly reduces the risk of paresthesia and swelling [16]. Pain is minimal post procedure and could be managed with over-the-counter analgesia. A minority may require narcotics for the first few days postoperatively. The risk of palatal fistula is around 2% and most self-resolve.

Anesthesia and Patient Positioning

Oral intubation with total intravenous anesthesia is preferred to reduce postoperative nausea and vomiting. A flexible reinforced tube is secured to one side of the oral commissure. The patient is turned 180° away from the anesthesia cart. Hypotensive anesthesia is rarely required as only Lefort level 1 osteotomies are performed. If both anterior and posterior maxilla need expansion (posterior for occlusion indications), then the pterygoid junctions are separated.

Equipment

A standard head and neck or maxillofacial set including Bovie electrocautery, Molt periosteal elevators, toe-out retractors, curved Freer elevator, reciprocating saw, piezoelectric saw (optional), several straight osteotomes, and 3–0 and 4–0 chromic sutures. For MINI-DOME, a 0° rigid endoscope and a surgical assistant are required. Patient-specific cutting guides are recommended to reduce the chances of asymmetrical osteotomies, particularly in minimally invasive approaches.

Surgical Steps with Focus on Endoscopic Approach

Prior to surgery, the collaborating orthodontist has designed and sometimes placed the expander with the transpalatal implants. It is crucial that the implants are placed as medially as possible, straddling the midpalatal suture. Additional implants can be placed against the sides of the alveolus bilaterally near the molar region.

In the MINI-DOME approach, needle tip cautery is used to make a 1–1.5 cm incision parallel to the piriform rim at the level of the head of inferior turbinate, and toward the anterior maxilla. This helps with closure at the end of the procedure. Molt periosteal elevator is used initially to obtain a subperiosteal pocket. Once an adequate pocket is developed, 0° endoscope is introduced to visualize the remainder of the inferolateral dissection toward the lateral maxillary buttress. Subperiosteal dissection can be quite limited because with guides, there is not a need to expose the infraorbital nerve and inferiorly to identify the canine eminence (Fig. 6.3). A small malleable blade is fashioned to rest against the lateral buttress to retract the soft tissue away from the bony structures. It is helpful to first cut at the middle of the classic Lefort osteotomy, where the anterior maxillary wall is located. This would allow a natural drainage hole for the irrigation from ultrasonic cutting blades. This allows one less instrument in the nasal cavity (suction tip). After this drainage hole is created, the osteotomy is carried forward past the buttress and then outwards toward the piriform rim. The nasal incisions are closed on each side with 4–0 chromic sutures.

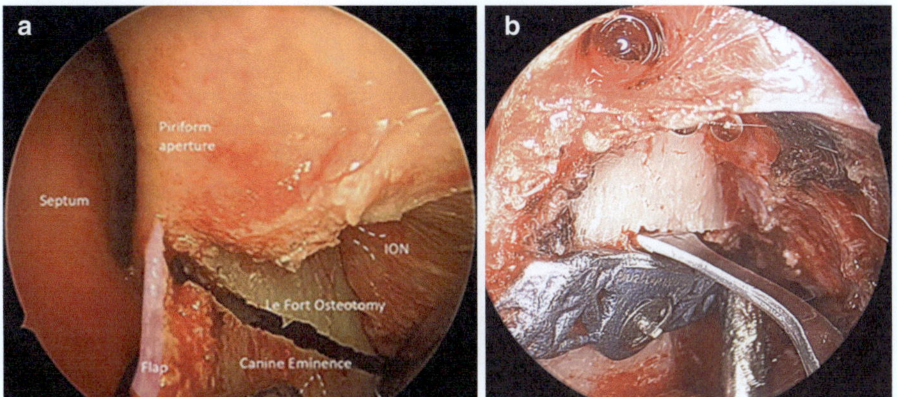

Fig. 6.3 (**a**) Depicts the extent of dissection in a MINI-DOME. The Lefort I osteotomy. *ION* infraorbital nerve. (**b**) A custom made cutting-guide is inserted and secured. The bony cut is made with a piezoelectric saw

The primordial groove of the midpalatal suture is seen inferior to the anterior nasal spine, and between the apices of the maxillary central incisors. A piezoelectric saw, which does not cut the mucosa of the palate across the maxillary alveolus, is used to deepen the groove. Osteotomes are used in sequential fashion to wedge open the midpalatal suture from the groove. A diastema between the central incisors is seen immediately as the suture opens. The expander is then turned to ensure easy and symmetric separation of the maxilla bilaterally, until a 2 mm separation is created. In adults, it is generally advisable to place a cancellous or a bone progenitor bone graft between the separated maxillae and not activate the expansion for about 10–14 days. This will allow improved bony healing, which is not a concern in children. Closure of the vestibular wound is performed by 3–0 chromic sutures.

Complications

Major complications include bone healing issues such as malunion, nonunion, and asymmetric expansion. Minor asymmetric expansion can be corrected with orthodontics. Most bone healing issues self-resolve with completion of distraction. Rarely, they may require a secondary bone graft. V_2 paresthesia is usually temporary and resolves between 1 and 6 months. Nasal sinus and odonotogenic infections have not been reported with DOME. Maxillary central incisors occasionally show signs of decreased perfusion. Loss of central incisors vitality requiring root canal treatment is less than 5%. No loss of dentition is reported with DOME. Patients with thin gingiva, which is common in OSA, likely benefit from presurgical periodontal and bone grafting to prevent the dental complications.

Postoperative Care

Patients can be discharged home the same day. There are no true diet restrictions, though we advise a soft diet for a few days as the bone graft and wounds heal. Limited epistaxis and nasal congestion are expected and are self-resolving and is best addressed by nasal irrigation. Blood and blood clots collect in the maxillary sinus during the procedure.

Patients turn the expander daily at a rate of 0.25 mm. For most patients, 7–12 mm of expansion at the nasal floor is achieved within 4–6 weeks. Orthodontic treatment is then applied to close the diastema, while the expander is left in place to prevent relapse during the bone consolidation period. Typically, the consolidation period is around 3-months for pediatric patients and 6–8 months in adults. The expander does not interfere with dental movement, allowing the restoration of proper occlusion without its removal. Average orthodontic treatment required is 12–18 months. Following orthodontic treatment, the expansion can be maintained passively by a removable retainer.

Outcomes

The early Stanford experience suggests the adult OSA patients with narrow and high-arched palate improve the most with DOME if they also have an acute internal nasal valve angle, narrow nasal floor, no significant septal deviation or turbinate hypertrophy, and TMH recalcitrant to palatopharyngoplasty. For adults with moderate to severe OSA, multilevel or multistage treatments remain the hallmarks of effective surgical treatment. We have performed DOME in conjunction with genioglossus/genioplasty advancements. For patients with both transverse maxillary and maxillary-mandibular hypoplasia, multistage treatment may be required. That is usually in the form of DOME followed by UPPP (uvulopalato-preservation pharyngoplasty), upper airway stimulation, or maxillomandibular advancement (MMA). Post-DOME patients have shown resolution of circumferential collapse of the velum that would otherwise disqualify them from receiving upper airway stimulation.

Hypoglossal Nerve Stimulation (HGNS)

Loss of genioglossus muscle tone and upper airway collapse were first reported by Remmers et al. in the late 1970s [17]. Since then, attempts to stimulate the pharyngeal muscles with transcutaneous, intraoral, and intramuscular electrodes to treat OSA were of limited success [18–20]. However, hypoglossal nerve stimulation has emerged as a viable alternative option to CPAP in treating moderate to severe OSA due to the technological advancement over the last decade [21, 22]. The indications, patient selection process, contraindications, surgical technique, postoperative care, and complications are reviewed.

Indications and Patient Selection Process

All patients being considered for HGNS surgery must undergo a comprehensive sleep medicine history and upper airway evaluation including drug induced sleep endoscopy (DISE). HGNS is still considered a second line procedure after CPAP therapy intolerance or failure in patients with moderate to severe OSA. Additional screening criteria include a body mass index (BMI) of less than or equal 32 kg/m^2, and the absence of concentric velum collapse on DISE. The BMI cutoff has recently been increased to 35 kg/m^2 [23]. It is important to note that these criteria oversimplify the complexity of OSA. The patient's medical comorbidities and skeletal phenotype should factor in the selection process. A history of breast cancer or breast augmentation may present a significant challenge. Moreover, a patient with a narrow, high-arched palate might be at a higher risk of failing the procedure due to the limited space for tongue displacement during stimulation, as well as persistent nasal obstruction.

Contraindications

Contraindications to HGNS can be relative or absolute. Relative contraindications include BMI more than 32 kg/m^2, electromagnetic incompatibility and interference from other implantable medical devices, and incompatibility and interference from diagnostic or therapeutic devices. Absolute contraindications include sleep study showing greater than 25% central or mixed apneas, concentric palatal collapse seen on DISE, inability to operate the therapy, pregnancy, severe anatomical challenges to implantation, severe neurological conditions, and anticipated or ongoing need for magnetic resonance imaging evaluation of the head, cervical spine, or thorax.

Surgical Technique

There are multiple upper airway neurostimulation devices in development. However, there is only one currently approved by the Food and Drug Administration. Therefore, the outlined surgical steps are for the Inspire II Upper Airway Stimulation device (Inspire Medical Systems, Inc., Maple Grove, MN). The outlined steps are meant to provide a high-level overview and do not address the nuances beyond the scope of this chapter. In addition, the senior author has moved away from the original three-incision technique to a contemporary two-incision technique.

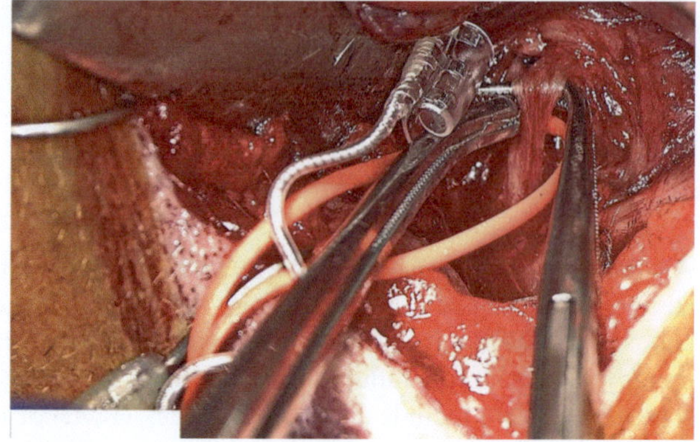

Fig. 6.4 The stimulation cuff electrode is placed around the distal protrusor branches of the hypoglossal nerve

The steps are as follows: after general orotracheal anesthesia, sensing electrodes are placed in the genioglossus muscle and the hyoglossus/styloglossus muscles for intraoperative nerve monitoring. After standard sterile prep and drape, a 4 cm incision is made in the right upper neck parallel to a natural skin crease and carried down to the floor of the submandibular triangle, where the main trunk of the hypoglossal nerve is identified. Nerve monitoring is used to selectively capture the distal tongue protrusor branches and to exclude branches innervating the tongue retractor muscles. The stimulation cuff electrode is placed around the distal protrusor branches and C1 and secured to the digastric tendon (Fig. 6.4). A second incision is made in the right upper chest with the development of a subcutaneous pocket overlying the pectoralis fascia for the pulse generator. The pocket is carefully sized to fit the implantable pulse generator with minimal dead space to minimize seroma formation. The sensing lead is then inserted between the external and the internal oblique intercoastal muscles and secured to a cuff of the external intercoastal muscle. The sensing lead and stimulation lead are each then tunneled into the right upper chest pocket and connected to the implantable pulse generator (IPG), which is secured to the pectoralis fascia. The telemetry unit is then activated, and the implant confirmed with both a good sensing lead waveform and uninhibited tongue protrusion.

Postoperative Care

Postoperative radiographs of the neck and chest are obtained before the patient is discharged to document the baseline position of the device and rule out pneumothorax. Patients can be discharged home the same day, but as they tend to be older, an overnight stay is advisable. They are instructed to avoid strenuous or repetitive activity of the ipsilateral arm for the first 3–4 weeks, although this is more permissive without the former third incision at right lower chest. Device activation is done at approximately the 1-month mark. After patients adjust to the therapy, optimization of stimulation voltage is performed during an attended PSG.

Complications

Serious complications are uncommon in the published literature. Bleeding, infection, and injury to the hypoglossal nerve or marginal mandibular nerve and pneumothorax formation are the main complications. Hardware failure can also be an issue, particularly with detachment of sensing or stimulation leads. Sleep disturbance and aggravation of insomnia are potential side effects of device activation.

Uvulopalato-"Preservation" Pharyngoplasty (UPPP)

Often referred as the workhorse of sleep apnea surgery, uvulopalatopharyngoplasty (UPPP) is performed alone or in conjunction with other surgeries. The procedure traces its origin to the 1950s [24]. Many technique variations have been described with varying degree of tissue sacrifice. Moreover, most of these techniques do not account for the interaction between the vectors of tissue suspension and physiologic muscle function [25, 26]. The indications, patient selection process, contraindications, postoperative care, complication, and outcomes are thoroughly described in the literature. Therefore, the focus in this section is on the senior author's surgical technique that emphasizes tissue preservation and augmentation of airway dilator muscle function.

Surgical Technique

When present, tonsillectomy is performed in the standard fashion. After removal of the tonsils, the following vectors of horizontal mattress sutures are performed. First, the palatopharyngeus muscle is anchored to a fibrous pad at the retromolar trigone and secured to the palatoglossus muscle. Next, the medial palatopharyngeus muscle is sutured toward the levator veli palatini muscle. Finally, the newly approximated medial palatopharyngeus and levator muscles are anchored toward the tensor veli palatini muscle. The first two vectors dilate the soft palate, whereas the last vector advances it. Overall, the vector of suspension augments the function of pharyngeal dilators and allows for maximal tissue preservation reducing postoperative pain and scarring in the long term (Fig. 6.5). The uvula muscle is always preserved. However, there is often long-term negative pressure that results in elongated mucosa. The mucosa can be trimmed slightly, although this is often not necessary and needs to be judiciously performed to prevent velopharyngeal insufficiency or globus sensation.

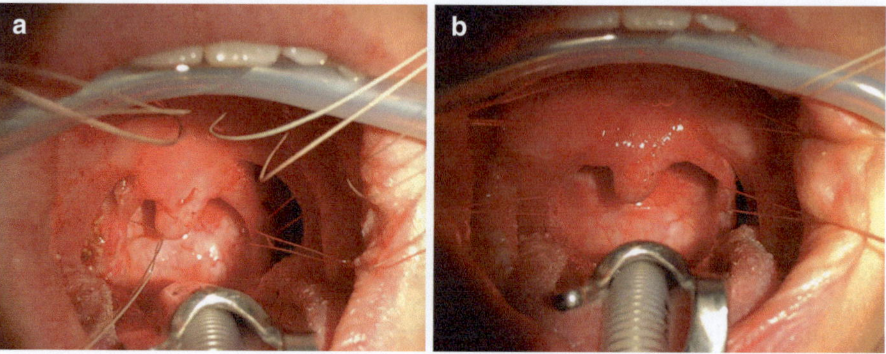

Fig. 6.5 Using 3–0 Vicryl the palatopharyngeus muscle is anchored to a fibrous pad at the retromolar trigone and secured to the palatoglossus muscle. Next, the medial palatopharyngeus muscle is sutured toward the levator veli palatini muscle. Finally, the newly approximated medial palatopharyngeus and levator muscles are anchored toward the tensor veli palatini muscle. (**a**) Depicts presuspension and (**b**) Depicts postsuspension. Note that the uvula and muscles of the pillars are preserved

Postoperative Care

Unlike tonsil surgery for children, the senior author focuses on adequate pain control for the adult patients so that they can eat as regular of a diet as possible. Active swallowing is important to prevent bleeding resulting from tearing of scab tissue as the wounds heal. Antibiotics have been shown to reduce the incidence of bleeding in OSA patients following UPPP [27].

Complications

The most serious complication is bleeding, and this is 5% [28]. Patients can help reduce incidence of bleeding by the postoperative care regimen as described. Surgically, the use of low heat on monopolar cautery and meticulous hemostasis with bipolar cautery are helpful. The less scabs created with accurate dissection in the avascular plane, the less likely for delayed bleeding. Hemostasis should also be checked with anesthesia directed Valsalva maneuver.

Genioglossus Advancement (GGA)

GGA was initially described by Riley and Powell in 1984 as an intervention for base of tongue collapse in a patient who had failed palate surgery [29]. Many variations of the original GGA have since been described, but they all share the common goal of advancing the genial tubercle, genioglossus muscle, and tongue base anteriorly to prevent hypopharyngeal collapse during sleep [30–32]. There are two main types of GGAs: (1) those that incorporate just the genial tubercle without including the inferior border of the mandible—also referred to as genial tubercle advancement—and (2) those that include the inferior border of the mandible and the suprahyoid muscles attached to it is also referred to as genioplasty, mortised genioplasty, and sliding genioplasty with GGA.

Indications and Patient Selection

GGA is most often performed with nasal and palate procedures as a multilevel approach to tongue-base collapse can be identified with DISE, and it is important to differentiate physiologic tongue-base collapse from lingual tonsil hypertrophy.

Planning Considerations

Ideally, the genial tubercle is incorporated in the movement with avoidance of the dental roots and mental nerve on either side. Weakening of the alveolar bone must be avoided, and some degree of bony overlap must be achieved for proper union. When GGA involves advancement of the inferior border of the anterior mandible, it is important to assess the patient's facial proportions and ensure balance is achieved with advancement of the chin. Custom osteotomy cutting guides and fixation plates allows precise movements and adjustments to achieve consistent esthetic and physiologic results.

Operative Technique

An incision is made perpendicular to the lip before angling through the mentalis muscle and toward the inferior border of anterior mandible. This is critical for closure, especially with advancement of the chin. The extent of dissection depends on the osteotomy design, but it is limited laterally by the mental foramina and inferiorly at the border to preserve the attachments of the suprahyoid muscles and the blood supply for the advancement graft.

Once exposure has been obtained, the osteotomy cutting guide is placed, and the saw can be used to mark the planned cut. If a custom plate has been made, the osteotomy guide will also include guides for screw placement. Once fixated, the patient's soft tissue should be redraped, and chin position should be assessed for adequate advancement and appropriate introduction of any planned pitch, roll, or yaw movements (Fig. 6.6). Closure requires reapproximation of the mentalis muscle to

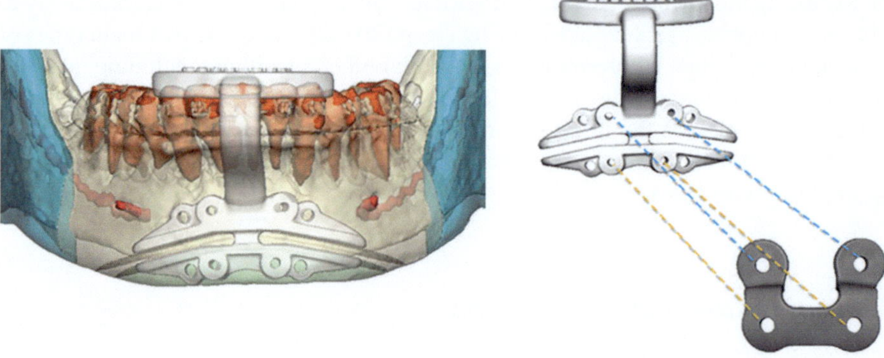

Fig. 6.6 The cutting guide is placed. Note the guides for screw placement. Once the bony cut is made, it is fixated with a custom plate

prevent a witch's chin deformity and the mucosal edges to safeguard against dehiscence and infection. Interrupted sutures should be used here with the knot tied to the lip, as opposed to the gingival side.

Complications

Significant, but uncommon, complications include avulsion of the genioglossus muscle and mandibular fracture. Genioglossus avulsion is a worrisome complication as it carries significant airway risk. Mandibular fractures resulting from GGA can be difficult to repair. If it is on the alveolar side, open reduction with internal fixation is not possible, and hence, maxillomandibular fixation is the only option. If it occurs on the cortical side (inferior to the advancement graft), there is usually inadequate room for plate placement. This does argue for the genioglossus advancement with genioplasty, in one piece, especially for older adults.

Other complications include loss of tooth vitality, paresthesia of the lower lip and chin, and persistent wound dehiscence leading to infection.

Outcomes

The literature on GGA outcomes is limited but demonstrates low complication rates and favorable respiratory and quality-of-life outcomes [33, 34]. Studies have shown that GGA alone confers a 40–50% decrease in AHI and a surgical success rate of greater than 60% in patients with severe OSA [32, 35]. Two key factors have been shown to influence the likelihood of success with GGA: lower preoperative BMI and AHI. Specifically, patients with a BMI less than 30 kg/m^2 experience a surgical success rate of 64% after GGA, whereas those with a BMI greater than 30 kg/m^2 experience a 41% success rate. Similarly, patients with a preoperative AHI of less than 50 events per hour experience a 71% success rate, whereas those with an AHI greater than 50 events per hour experience a 32% success rate. No difference in outcomes has been found between GGA with just the genial tubercle versus GGA including the inferior mandibular border and suprahyoid musculature.

Maxillomandibular Advancement

MMA is a facial skeletal surgery that provides tension and stability of the upper airway muscles implicated in OSA. It has a documented success rate using the universal Sher's criteria OSA of 85–90% [36–39]. The procedure was originally described for OSA by Riley et al., as a 10-mm advancement of the maxilla and mandible for patients who had failed phase I surgery [40]. Despite its impressive impact on the airway, it sometimes resulted in suboptimal esthetic outcomes. The contemporary Stanford MMA is patient specific, with attention to balancing both airway improvement and overall facial balance [41]. In the updated Stanford sleep surgery protocol, there are three main indications to recommend MMA. As with the old protocol, those who have not responded adequately to phase I surgery may be recommended MMA. There are two phenotypes to which we recommend MMA first, which are (1) patients with dentofacial deformity, presenting with any degree of OSA, and (2) patients presenting with both complete concentric collapse of the velum and lateral pharyngeal wall collapse.

Even though VSP is helpful, starting with the correct head position is crucial for planning. The natural head position in a patient with OSA is not healthy. The neck tends to extend forward to compensate for a narrow, obstructive, or collapsible airway. A patient with bimaxillary retrusion may appear to have normal class I facial skeletal position with the forward neck extension. Similarly, a patient with class III malocclusion may have bimaxillary hypoplasia when the head position is not extended and with the neck in neutral position.

Since esthetic results of the midface largely depend on the degree of distortion of the nose and having adequate incisal show (and preferably with a nice smile arc), placement of the maxilla cannot be planned based on bony position alone. A way to allow flexibility while maintaining efficiency of the procedure may be to approach surgery with two plans. One would have more rotation and less advancement, and the other may be less rotation but more advancement. Ultimately, since the surgeon controls the pitch, the two intermediate splints that are designed for these movements allow for optimization of maxillary placement on the table. This combines the best of VSP with concepts borrowed from esthetic orthognathic surgery using the single splint technique [42].

Preoperative Planning

The earliest indications for MMA included severe OSA, morbid obesity, severe mandibular deficiency, and failure of other forms of therapy. Today, appropriate patient selection begins with a thorough history, subjective questionnaires (Epworth Sleepiness Scale and Nasal Obstructive Symptom Evaluation), head and neck physical examination, polysomnography interpretation, and fiberoptic nasopharyngoscopy observation. Moreover, selection criteria for MMA include the use of dynamic examinations, such as drug-induced sleep endoscopy (DISE). MMA is particularly effective when DISE shows lateral pharyngeal wall or concentric velum collapse [43]. Because concentric collapse of the velum is a contraindication for hypoglossal nerve stimulation and lateral pharyngeal wall collapse is difficult to address with soft tissue pharyngeal procedures, MMA can be a first-line recommendation in OSA patients exhibiting these airway collapse patterns (Fig. 6.7) [44].

Maxillomandibular advancement is also performed in OSA patients with dentofacial deformity. However, in patients with Class 1 occlusion, MMA with airway-specific counterclockwise (CCW) rotation can be expeditiously performed with minimal orthodontic decompensation.

The most unique aspect of today's Stanford MMA in preoperative planning is the center of rotation for the maxillomandibular complex (MMC). When counterclockwise rotation is appropriate, the center of rotation is at the maxillary buttress to maximize both airway stability and facial aesthetics (Fig. 6.8). Additionally, the main reference points and movements for planning are (1) advancement from a point at the piriform rim just below level of the inferior turbinate, (2) degree of occlusal plane change dictated by the maxilla, and (3) postoperative position of the pogonion. If patients also exhibit dentofacial deformity, this is certainly addressed, but the general principle of movement, as described here, remains consistent.

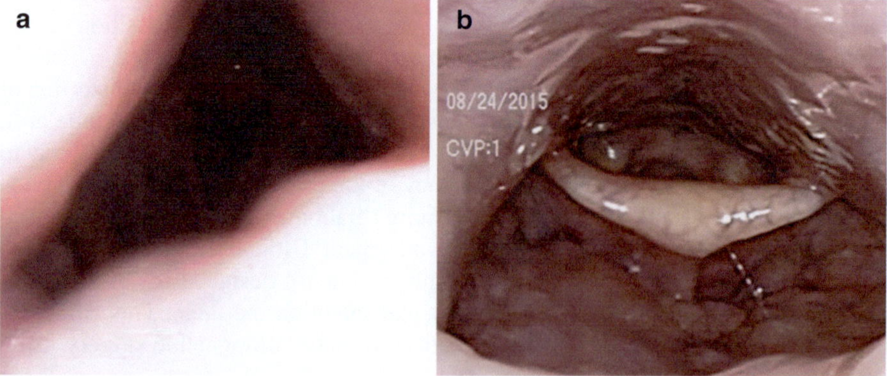

Fig. 6.7 (**a**) Lateral pharyngeal collapse on drug induces sleep endoscopy pre-MMA. (**b**) Stable lateral pharyngeal walls on drug-induced sleep endoscopy post-MMA

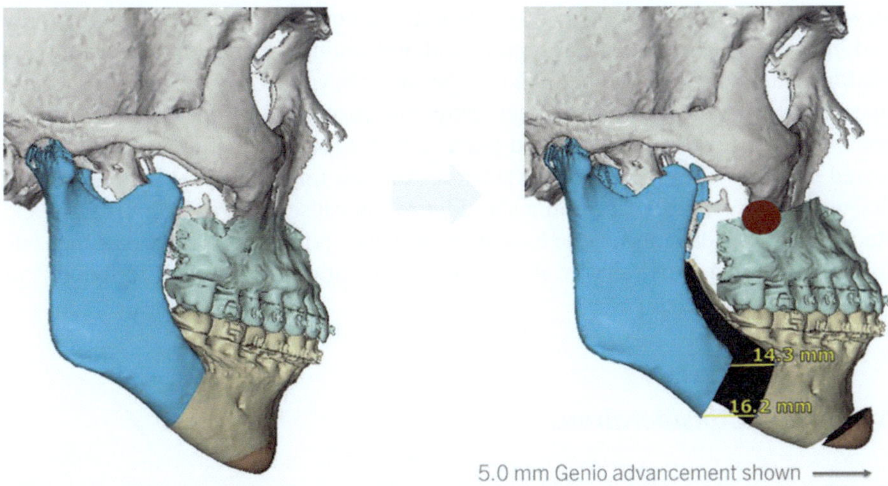

Fig. 6.8 The red dot represents the center of counterclockwise rotation (maxillary buttress). Note the degree of chin advancement

Virtual Surgical Planning

Prior to virtual surgical planning (VSP), Riley and Powell performed what is commonly described in the orthognathic literature as a single-splint technique [42]. This requires extensive experience to control the pitch, roll, and yaw of the MMC and is difficult to reproduce consistently. With VSP, surgical movements are planned, and two intermediate splints are usually produced to provide a clinical outcome that balances bite, beauty, and breathing. Regarding the movement, a differential anterior impaction is performed with the rotation center in line with the buttress. CCW rotation has been described with centers at the anterior nasal spine (ANS) or posterior nasal spine (PNS). The buttress may seem like a peculiar landmark. The rationale is that when the maxilla is rotated in line with the buttress and the level of the first molar is maintained, the CCW rotation brings the entire maxilla posterior to the original piriform rim (Fig. 6.8). From here, an advancement of approximately 3–5 mm anterior to the piriform translates to a final pogonion position approximately 12–18 mm anterior and 2–4 mm superior to its original position. Concurrent orthognathic problems, if present, are corrected during the planning session.

Preparation and Patient Positioning

There are two important nuances to the positioning of the MMA patient compared with the orthognathic patient. Classically, nasal Ring, Adair, and Elwyn (RAE) tubes are used for orthognathic cases. However, OSA patients tend to have longer airways, requiring longer RAE tubes, which are bulkier, distorting nasal anatomy and limiting access to the nasal septum and prohibiting accuracy in performing the piriformplasty. Instead, the authors use the microlaryngoscopy tube (MLT), where there is adequate length and thinner diameters (usually 5 mm). The authors trim back the tube toward the nares and place a 120° reverse metallic attachment, followed in-line with an accordion extension. Another important positioning element is that patients are not placed on a shoulder roll because this overextends the neck. Recall that OSA patients tend to have extended neck position already to compensate for compromised upper airway. A neutral head position is important for control of the occlusal plane change.

Anesthetic Considerations

Total intravenous anesthesia with agents such as propofol and remifentanil is used. Although controlled hypotension with a target mean arterial pressure of 60 mmHg is recommended for orthognathic procedures, many OSA patients undergoing MMA have cardiovascular comorbidities. Keeping the mean arterial pressure this low is both difficult for the anesthesiologist and sometimes contraindicated. The authors still aim for a brief period of controlled hypotension during maxillary downfracture but most often are doing this at a mean arterial pressure of approximately 80 mmHg. Total blood loss is approximately 250–350 mL for the procedure. Mean operative time is approximately 3 h without GGA and 3.5 h with GGA.

Surgical Technique

Approach to general aspects of MMA surgery is not discussed in detail. However, critical steps are highlighted.

At the time of LeFort I osteotomy, a wedge can be created that determines the degree of CCW rotation. An appropriate degree of CCW rotation should not compromise incisor show in the final maxillary position.

The maxilla is never mobilized aggressively with instruments like the Rowe disimpaction forceps (Sklar Surgical Instruments, West Chester, PA). With a wire through the anterior nasal spine area to control the maxilla, lateral forces are applied concurrently to the posterior maxillary wall to mobilize the maxilla.

With large CCW rotations, muscle tension associated with the maxilla and mandible is significant. For this reason, maxillomandibular fixation prior to rigid fixation is performed with the aid of suspension wires. The authors use suspension wires anchored to the alveolus with intermaxillary fixation (IMF) screws and through a hole by the piriform rim above the LeFort osteotomy for the maxilla and to the arch wire for the mandible. Maxillomandibular fixation prior to fixation with the use of 24-gauge wires on dental brackets or the arch bar may debond brackets or shift the arch bar. Minor discrepancy greatly affects accuracy of the final fixation.

The authors do not perform sagittal split osteotomy with instruments like Smith spreaders. Older patients tend to have little bone marrow space. With the need of longer osteotomy (anterior extent to the second premolar) for fixation after large advancements, the use of Smith spreaders leads to poorly controlled fractures. Instead, the authors focus on an accurate horizontal osteotomy taking down the lingula, anterior osteotomy not past the midline of the inferior mandibular border and wedging open the segments with 3 osteotomes in a sequential sandwiched fashion.

For fixation, the authors use two to three bicortical fixation screws, coupled with a long 2.4-mm plate across the osteotomy site. The rigidity allows the patient a rapid return to function. Patients are not kept in a splint, and only guiding elastics are used immediately after surgery. This allows MMA patients to breathe orally in the immediate postoperative period. By the end of the second week postoperatively, patients progress beyond the liquid diet. Minimal use of narcotic pain medications is expected.

Complications

The most serious complication is airway obstruction. The authors do not band the jaws of post-MMA patients tightly nor place them in a splint. By not using a splint postoperatively and only using guiding elastics, patients are able to orally breathe while congested and have additional access to suctioning when needed. If there is a well-supported ENT ward, patients do not need to for observation in the intensive care unit.

Based on a review of more than 370 MMA patients from Stanford, approximately 18.7% underwent functional or esthetic nasal surgery approximately 1.5 years after surgery. This rate has decreased to less than 5% in the recent 120 patients with judicious midfacial contouring and intraoperative septoplasty and inferior turbinate reduction with outfracture [45]. Perioperative considerations and interventions are also critical. In a review comparing OSA patients to dentofacial deformity patients, the morbidity and mortality rates of MMA are higher. Early, late, minor, and major complications were present. The patients with OSA were older, had a higher American Society of Anesthesiologists classification, had a greater number of medical comorbidities, and had a higher body mass index [46].

Clinical Outcomes

Although there are variations on how MMA is performed around the world, it consistently demonstrates high rates of surgical success and moderate rates for cure. The systematic review and meta-analysis published by Holty et al. in 2010 with 22 unique patient populations (627 adults with OSA) report mean Apnea/Hypopnea Index (AHI) decrease from 63.9/h to 9.5/h, with pooled surgical success and cure

(AHI <5/h) rates of 86% and 43.2% [36]. An update to this meta-analysis was performed by Zaghi and colleagues in 2016, which included 518 patients across 45 studies. They reported success and cure rates of 85.5% and 38%, respectively [39]. When compared with continuous positive airway pressure (CPAP), both Riley and Powell, of Stanford, and Vicini of Forli, Italy, independently showed MMA to be as effective based on the AHI and Epworth Sleepiness Scale in evidence level 2 and level 3 studies [47, 48].

MMA compares favorably to CPAP regarding improvement in sleep quality. Although the increase in rapid eye movement sleep is comparable between CPAP and MMA, MMA has shown additional decrease in wakefulness after sleep onset, a measure for sleep disturbance. A patient treated with MMA can restore sleep architecture comparable to a younger, healthy individual [49]. Therefore, MMA leads to significant improvements in neurocognitive performance Moreover, MMA is effective in reducing cardiovascular risk by lowering blood pressure [50].

Conclusions

The updated Stanford sleep surgery protocol aims to provide a roadmap for all practitioners across the continuum of care. At its core, it is about precision in patient-selection, phenotype recognition, and surgical application. With the technological advances described, the principles described can be better adopted and applied in a universal manner. This would then allow optimization of personalized care across all ages, gender, and ethnicity.

References

1. Awad M, Gouveia C, Zaghi S, Camacho M, Liu SY-C. Changing practice: trends in skeletal surgery for obstructive sleep apnea. J Craniomaxillofac Surg. 2019;47(8):1185–9.
2. Liu SY-C, Awad M, Riley R, Capasso R. The role of the revised Stanford protocol in today's precision medicine. Sleep Med Clin. 2019;14(1):99–107.
3. Riley RW, Powell NB, Guilleminault C. Obstructive sleep apnea syndrome: a surgical protocol for dynamic upper airway reconstruction. J Oral Maxillofac Surg. 1993;51(7):742–7; discussion 748.
4. Liu SY-C, Riley RW, Yu MS. Surgical algorithm for obstructive sleep apnea: an update. Clin Exp Otorhinolaryngol. 2020;13(3):215–24.
5. Wang M, Liu SY-C, Zhou B, Li Y, Cui S, Huang Q. Effect of nasal and sinus surgery in patients with and without obstructive sleep apnea. Acta Otolaryngol. 2019;139(5):467–72.
6. Williams R, Patel V, Chen Y-F, Tangbumrungtham N, Thamboo A, Most SP, et al. The upper airway nasal complex: structural contribution to persistent nasal obstruction. Otolaryngol Head Neck Surg. 2019;161(1):171–7.
7. Principato JJ. Upper airway obstruction and craniofacial morphology. Otolaryngol Head Neck Surg. 1991;104(6):881–90.
8. Tsai M-S, Chen H-C, Liu SY-C, Lee L-A, Lin C-Y, Chang G-H, et al. Holistic care for obstructive sleep apnea (OSA) with an emphasis on restoring nasal breathing: a review and perspective. J Chin Med Assoc. 2022;85(6):672–8.

9. Zhao Z, Zheng L, Huang X, Li C, Liu J, Hu Y. Effects of mouth breathing on facial skeletal development in children: a systematic review and meta-analysis. BMC Oral Health. 2021;21(1):108.
10. Kim J-E, Hwang K-J, Kim S-W, Liu SY-C, Kim S-J. Correlation between craniofacial changes and respiratory improvement after nasomaxillary skeletal expansion in pediatric obstructive sleep apnea patients. Sleep Breath. 2022;26(2):585–94.
11. Yoon A, Abdelwahab M, Bockow R, Vakili A, Lovell K, Chang I, et al. Impact of rapid palatal expansion on the size of adenoids and tonsils in children. Sleep Med. 2022;92:96–102.
12. Camacho M, Chang ET, Song SA, Abdullatif J, Zaghi S, Pirelli P, et al. Rapid maxillary expansion for pediatric obstructive sleep apnea: a systematic review and meta-analysis. Laryngoscope. 2017;127(7):1712–9.
13. Liu SY-C, Guilleminault C, Huon L-K, Yoon A. Distraction osteogenesis maxillary expansion (DOME) for adult obstructive sleep apnea patients with high arched palate. Otolaryngol Head Neck Surg. 2017;157(2):345–8.
14. Alyessary AS, Othman SA, Yap AUJ, Radzi Z, Rahman MT. Effects of non-surgical rapid maxillary expansion on nasal structures and breathing: a systematic review. Int Orthod. 2019;17(1):12–9.
15. Fitzpatrick MF, McLean H, Urton AM, Tan A, O'Donnell D, Driver HS. Effect of nasal or oral breathing route on upper airway resistance during sleep. Eur Respir J. 2003;22(5):827–32.
16. Liu SY-C, Ibrahim B, Abdelwahab M, Chou C, Capasso R, Yoon A. A minimally invasive nasal endoscopic approach to distraction osteogenesis maxillary expansion to restore nasal breathing for adults with narrow maxilla. Facial Plast Surg Aesthet Med. 2022;24:417.
17. Remmers JE, deGroot WJ, Sauerland EK, Anch AM. Pathogenesis of upper airway occlusion during sleep. J Appl Physiol. 1978;44(6):931–8.
18. Steier J, Seymour J, Rafferty GF, Jolley CJ, Solomon E, Luo Y, et al. Continuous transcutaneous submental electrical stimulation in obstructive sleep apnea: a feasibility study. Chest. 2011;140(4):998–1007.
19. Randerath WJ, Galetke W, Domanski U, Weitkunat R, Ruhle K-H. Tongue-muscle training by intraoral electrical neurostimulation in patients with obstructive sleep apnea. Sleep. 2004;27(2):254–9.
20. Smith PL, Eisele DW, Podszus T, Penzel T, Grote L, Peter JH, et al. Electrical stimulation of upper airway musculature. Sleep. 1996;19(10 Suppl):S284–7.
21. Kezirian EJ, Boudewyns A, Eisele DW, Schwartz AR, Smith PL, Van de Heyning PH, et al. Electrical stimulation of the hypoglossal nerve in the treatment of obstructive sleep apnea. Sleep Med Rev. 2010;14(5):299–305.
22. Schwartz AR, Bennett ML, Smith PL, De Backer W, Hedner J, Boudewyns A, et al. Therapeutic electrical stimulation of the hypoglossal nerve in obstructive sleep apnea. Arch Otolaryngol Head Neck Surg. 2001;127(10):1216–23.
23. Steffen A, Sommer JU, Hofauer B, Maurer JT, Hasselbacher K, Heiser C. Outcome after one year of upper airway stimulation for obstructive sleep apnea in a multicenter German post-market study. Laryngoscope. 2018;128(2):509–15.
24. Heinberg CJ. A surgical procedure for the relief of snoring. Eye Ear Nose Throat Mon. 1955;34(6):389; passim.
25. Simmons FB, Guilleminault C, Silvestri R. Snoring, and some obstructive sleep apnea, can be cured by oropharyngeal surgery. Arch Otolaryngol. 1983;109(8):503–7.
26. Fujita S, Conway W, Zorick F, Roth T. Surgical correction of anatomic azbnormalities in obstructive sleep apnea syndrome: uvulopalatopharyngoplasty. Otolaryngol Head Neck Surg. 1981;89(6):923–34.
27. Abdelwahab M, Marques S, Previdelli I, Capasso R. Perioperative antibiotic use in sleep surgery: clinical relevance. Otolaryngol Head Neck Surg. 2022;166(5):993–1002.
28. Tami TA, Parker GS, Taylor RE. Post-tonsillectomy bleeding: an evaluation of risk factors. Laryngoscope. 1987;97(11):1307–11.
29. Riley R, Guilleminault C, Powell N, Derman S. Mandibular osteotomy and hyoid bone advancement for obstructive sleep apnea: a case report. Sleep. 1984;7(1):79–82.

30. García Vega JR, de la Plata MM, Galindo N, Navarro M, Díez D, Láncara F. Genioglossus muscle advancement: a modification of the conventional technique. J Craniomaxillofac Surg. 2014;42(3):239–44.
31. Hendler B, Silverstein K, Giannakopoulos H, Costello BJ. Mortised genioplasty in the treatment of obstructive sleep apnea: an historical perspective and modification of design. Sleep Breath. 2001;5(4):173–80.
32. Li KK, Riley RW, Powell NB, Troell RJ. Obstructive sleep apnea surgery: genioglossus advancement revisited. J Oral Maxillofac Surg. 2001;59(10):1181–4; discussion 1185.
33. Song SA, Chang ET, Certal V, Del Do M, Zaghi S, Liu SY, et al. Genial tubercle advancement and genioplasty for obstructive sleep apnea: a systematic review and meta-analysis. Laryngoscope. 2017;127(4):984–92.
34. Kezirian EJ, Goldberg AN. Hypopharyngeal surgery in obstructive sleep apnea: an evidence-based medicine review. Arch Otolaryngol Head Neck Surg. 2006;132(2):206–13.
35. Foltán R, Hoffmannová J, Pretl M, Donev F, Vlk M. Genioglossus advancement and hyoid myotomy in treating obstructive sleep apnoea syndrome—a follow-up study. J Craniomaxillofac Surg. 2007;35(4–5):246–51.
36. Holty J-EC, Guilleminault C. Maxillomandibular advancement for the treatment of obstructive sleep apnea: a systematic review and meta-analysis. Sleep Med Rev. 2010;14(5):287–97.
37. John CR, Gandhi S, Sakharia AR, James TT. Maxillomandibular advancement is a successful treatment for obstructive sleep apnoea: a systematic review and meta-analysis. Int J Oral Maxillofac Surg. 2018;47(12):1561–71.
38. Camacho M, Noller MW, Del Do M, Wei JM, Gouveia CJ, Zaghi S, et al. Long-term results for maxillomandibular advancement to treat obstructive sleep apnea: a meta-analysis. Otolaryngol Head Neck Surg. 2019;160(4):580–93.
39. Zaghi S, Holty J-EC, Certal V, Abdullatif J, Guilleminault C, Powell NB, et al. Maxillomandibular advancement for treatment of obstructive sleep apnea: a meta-analysis. JAMA Otolaryngol Head Neck Surg. 2016;142(1):58–66.
40. Riley RW, Powell NB, Guilleminault C. Maxillary, mandibular, and hyoid advancement for treatment of obstructive sleep apnea: a review of 40 patients. J Oral Maxillofac Surg. 1990;48(1):20–6.
41. Liu SY-C, Awad M, Riley RW. Maxillomandibular advancement: contemporary approach at Stanford. Atlas Oral Maxillofac Surg Clin North Am. 2019;27(1):29–36.
42. Yu C-C, Bergeron L, Lin C-H, Chu Y-M, Chen Y-R. Single-splint technique in orthognathic surgery: intraoperative checkpoints to control facial symmetry. Plast Reconstr Surg. 2009;124(3):879–86.
43. Liu SY-C, Huon L-K, Iwasaki T, Yoon A, Riley R, Powell N, et al. Efficacy of maxillomandibular advancement examined with drug-induced sleep endoscopy and computational fluid dynamics airflow modeling. Otolaryngol Head Neck Surg. 2016;154(1):189–95.
44. Huyett P, Kent DT, D'Agostino MA, Green KK, Soose RJ, Kaffenberger TM, et al. Drug-induced sleep endoscopy and hypoglossal nerve stimulation outcomes: a multicenter cohort study. Laryngoscope. 2021;131(7):1676–82.
45. Liu SY-C, Lee P-J, Awad M, Riley RW, Zaghi S. Corrective nasal surgery after maxillomandibular advancement for obstructive sleep apnea: experience from 379 cases. Otolaryngol Head Neck Surg. 2017;157(1):156–9.
46. Passeri LA, Choi JG, Kaban LB, Lahey ET. Morbidity and mortality rates after maxillomandibular advancement for treatment of obstructive sleep apnea. J Oral Maxillofac Surg. 2016;74(10):2033–43.
47. Riley RW, Powell NB, Guilleminault C. Maxillofacial surgery and nasal CPAP. A comparison of treatment for obstructive sleep apnea syndrome. Chest. 1990;98(6):1421–5.
48. Vicini C, Dallan I, Campanini A, De Vito A, Barbanti F, Giorgiomarrano G, et al. Surgery vs ventilation in adult severe obstructive sleep apnea syndrome. Am J Otolaryngol. 2010;31(1):14–20.

49. Liu SYC, Huon LK, Ruoff C, Riley RW, Strohl KP, Peng Z. Restoration of sleep architecture after maxillomandibular advancement: success beyond the apnea-hypopnea index. Int J Oral Maxillofac Surg. 2017;46(12):1533–8.
50. Boyd SB, Chigurupati R, Cillo JE, Eskes G, Goodday R, Meisami T, et al. Maxillomandibular advancement improves multiple health-related and functional outcomes in patients with obstructive sleep apnea: a multicenter study. J Oral Maxillofac Surg. 2019;77(2):352–70.

Chapter 7
Oral Dysplasia

Lior Aljadeff and Anthony B. Morlandt

Terminology

The term "precancer" was initially introduced in 1805 when a panel of physicians in Europe suggested that some benign disease can progress to invasive malignancy if given enough time [1]. Over time, the terms "precancer," "premalignancy," and "precursor lesion" have become synonymous with oral dysplasia. However, during the 2005 WHO workshop (published in 2007), a panel of experts proposed replacing these terms with the more precise term "oral potentially malignant disorder" (OPMD) [2]. This term is defined as any "clinical presentations that carry a risk of cancer development in the oral cavity, whether in a clinically definable precursors lesion or in clinically normal oral mucosa." [3]. The reasons for this shift were multifold. For one, the phrase "potentially malignant" highlights the fact that not all patients diagnosed with an OPMD will develop an oral malignancy. The new term implies that there is an unknown potential for carcinogenesis, rather than framing it as inevitable given enough time. Additionally, the term "disorder" highlights the fact that patients diagnosed with an OPMD have an increased risk of developing carcinoma anywhere in their mouth over their lifetime. Data show that patients can develop oral squamous cell carcinoma in sites that are separate from the mucosal changes of their OPMD [2]. This reinforces the importance of shifting our view of OPMDs from "precancerous lesions" to disorders that represent a field of molecular mucosal changes in which cancer is more likely to develop [4, 5]. Recently, a newer term, "potentially premalignant oral epithelial lesion (PPOEL)," has emerged in the literature to replace OPMDs. However, the 2020 WHO working group rejected this terminology because the term OPMD is now well-established in the literature since

L. Aljadeff · A. B. Morlandt (✉)
Department of Oral and Maxillofacial Surgery, Section of Oral Oncology, University of Alabama at Birmingham, Birmingham, AL, USA
e-mail: laljadeff@uabmc.edu; amorlandt@uabmc.edu

J. C. Melville et al. (eds.), *Advancements and Innovations in OMFS, ENT, and Facial Plastic Surgery*, https://doi.org/10.1007/978-3-031-32099-6_7

its introduction in 2007, and they felt PPOEL neither added nor changed anything significant [6, 7].

Fundamentally speaking, OPMD is a broad term that encompasses anything that has a risk of progressing to oral cancer, including clinically normal oral mucosa. OPMD includes both strictly clinical conditions (e.g., leukoplakia, erythroplakia, and erythroleukoplakia) and a variety of diagnoses that have well-established clinical and histologic characteristics (e.g., submucous fibrosis, dyskeratosis congentia, smokeless tobacco keratosis, chronic candidiasis lichen planus, discoid lupus erythematosus, syphilitic glossitis, and actinic keratosis). In contrast, dysplasia is a *histological diagnosis* that describes "abnormal growth" at the cellular level, as its name implies. The WHO defines oral epithelial dysplasia (OED) as "a spectrum of architectural and cytological epithelial changes caused by an accumulation of genetic changes, associated with an increased risk of progression to squamous cell carcinoma" [3]. The distinction between these two is important.

OPMDs carry a risk of malignant transformation; however, they may or may not contain histological evidence of the epithelial dysplasia. In fact, although OED is a common finding in erythroplakia and erythroleukoplakia, it is only present in a minority of leukoplakias, despite the malignant potential of many leukoplakic lesions. The presence of dysplasia is important because it has been shown to carry prognostic significance in predicting malignant transformation, even in clinically normal appearing mucosa. Thus, any lesion with dysplasia is, by definition, an OPMD (although the converse is not true). However, OPMDs can progress to oral squamous cell carcinoma (OSCC) without any previous histological evidence of dysplasia. Chaturvedi et al. demonstrated that a substantial proportion of cancers (39.6%) arose from lesions histologically classified as *non*dysplastic [8].

The diagnostic criteria for epithelial dysplasia includes both architectural and cytological epithelial changes that serve as evidence of the cellular misbehavior that is thought to progress to oral squamous cell carcinoma (OSCC). However, although a plethora of grading scales, models, and biomarkers exist, no one has been able to reliably predict *if and when* epithelial dysplasia will traverse the basement membrane and invade the underlying connective tissue to progress to OSCC. This leaves clinicians with a difficult conundrum in the management and surveillance of these historically controversial conditions. Before surgeons can intelligently use the most recent data and technology to personalize treatment plan for a patient with OPMD or OED, they must have a clear understanding of the terminology described above.

Oral Potentially Malignant Disorders

It is outside the scope of this chapter to discuss all OPMDs; however, leukoplakia, erythroplakia, and erythroleuoplakia are the most common, controversial, and confusing OPMDs and are thus included herein.

First, it is important to understand that leukoplakia, erythroplakia, and erythroleukoplakia are *clinical terms* that simply describe a lesion as "white plaque," "red patch," or a predominantly white plaque with red areas, respectively. To be clear, these are not histologic diagnoses. In fact, there is a broad range of conditions that can present as a white plaque in the oral cavity, many of which have well-characterized clinicohistopatholgic findings that allow for a formal diagnosis. These include frictional keratosis, lichen planus, oral candidiasis, and white sponge nevus, to name a few. Thus, the term leukoplakia can first be used as a provisional diagnosis at the time of detection if nothing else on the list of differential diagnoses appears more likely. However, a biopsy is indicated to rule out the many other well-established diagnoses that present as white plaques of the oral cavity in order to establish oral leukoplakia as the diagnosis of exclusion [9, 10]. The same is true for erythroplakia and erythroleukoplakia.

Oral leukoplakia is the most common OPMD with a prevalence of 1–4% [10]. The published malignant transformation rate of oral leukoplakia is highly variable, ranging from 0 to 36%, largely due to differences in geographic region, population risk profiles, definitions, and study design [8]. Iocca et al. recently published the most thorough systematic review and meta-analysis on OPMDs to date, and they calculated a malignant transformation rate of 9.5% with an annual transformation rate of 1.5% [11]. Waldron and Shafer studied 3256 cases of oral leukoplakia and reported that 19.9% had some degree of epithelial dysplasia [12]. Risk factors for malignant transformation of oral leukoplakia include: (1) female patients, (2) non-smokers, (3) longstanding lesions, (4) floor-of-mouth and tongue subsites (5) non-homogeneous leukoplakia, (6) presence of Candida albicans within the lesion, and (7) presence of epithelial dysplasia in the lesion [13]. Proliferative verrucous leukoplakia (PVL) is an aggressive and problematic subtype of leukoplakia that is most common in elderly women with a malignant transformation rate of approximately 50% and an annual malignant transformation rate of 9.3% [11, 14].

In 1911, Vincent Jules Louis Queyrat, a French dermatologist, described a bright-red precancerous lesion of the glans penis, which he termed "erythroplasie," and is known today as Erythroplasia of Queryat [15]. The term was subsequently adapted to "erythroplakia" and used to describe potentially premalignant red patches of the oral cavity that were thought to be analogous to the already well-described potentially premalignant white plaques of the oral cavity, leukoplakia. Years later, the term "erythroplakia" was recognized to be a misnomer because, in contrast to leukoplakia, erythroplakia does not typically form plaques at all but are more erosive or atrophic-appearing lesions that are continuous with or even depressed below the surrounding mucosa [13, 16]. Over the years, the definition of oral erythroplakia has changed; however, the most widely accepted definition today was proposed by Pindborg and colleagues in 1997: "a fiery red patch that cannot be characterized clinically or pathologically as any other definable lesion" [17]. An array of lesions with overlapping clinical appearances have since been described, and terms such as erythroleukoplakia, erosive leukoplakia, leukoerythroplakia, and speckled erythroplakia were coined, which further complicated the literature.

Shafer et al. has shown that 51% of homogenous erythroplakia had evidence of invasive carcinoma at the time of biopsy, and 40% showed carcinoma in situ [18]. Furthermore, Iocca et al. have shown that the rate of malignant transformation of oral erythroplakia, even without any prior evidence of dysplasia, was still as high as 33.1% [11]. Although poorly understood at the molecular level, clinical evidence of erythroplakia represents an ominous disease process that should be managed more aggressively than its more common and benign counterpart, leukoplakia.

Oral Dysplasia: Grading and Classification

In 1957, Slaughter popularized the principle of "field cancerization," which stated that if carcinogens caused clinically detectable premalignant or malignant changes in one part of the oral cavity, there is equal risk of it causing those changes in other parts of the oral cavity that were exposed to those carcinogens as well [19]. This concept helped reconcile the rising number of synchronous and metachronous tumors that were being observed and reported in the literature. Ultimately, it shed light on the existence of subclinical lesions that made the entire oral cavity, especially high-risk sites such as the tongue and the floor of the mouth, susceptible to malignancy. Years later, in 1996, Califano and colleagues published their landmark description of the genetic progression model for head and neck cancer. This model proposed a "genetic pathway to malignancy." They proposed that mutations begin in clinically and histologically normal mucosa and accumulate to cause phenotypic changes at the microscopic and/or clinical level that eventually culminate in the development of dysplasia and cancer [20]. This model lay the foundation for our current understanding of oral epithelial dysplasia as a continuum of cytological and architectural changes in epithelium that may progress to oral squamous cell carcinoma. Califano's model also provided a molecular explanation for the "field cancerization" that Slaughter carefully observed and described [19].

The challenge that continues to plague clinicians, scientists, and ultimately patients is predicting which dysplastic lesions will progress to carcinoma and when. Over the years, many methods have been proposed and tested to predict the progression from dysplasia to carcinoma; the most well-known of which is histological grading.

Smith and Pindborg were the first to describe a classification system for grading epithelial dysplasia of oral mucosa in 1969 [21]. They evaluated 13 histologic features, which were standardized by a set of photographs. After comparing the slides with the photographic standard, each feature was graded as absent, slight, or marked and given a score. The scores were then added to produce an epithelial atypia index (EAI) (which could range from 0 to 75). A score of 10 or less was considered non-dysplastic, a score between 11 and 25 was considered mild dysplasia, a score of 26–45 was considered moderate dysplasia, and a score above 45 was considered severe dysplasia.

Currently, the most widely used grading system for dysplasia is the one first proposed by the WHO in 1997 and revised in 2005 and then again in 2017 [22]. In 1967, the WHO established a Collaborating Center for Oral Precancerous Lesions in Copenhagen, Denmark that set out to characterize and define oral lesions that

Table 7.1 1978 WHO criteria for oral epithelial dysplasia

1. Loss of polarity of basal cells
2. Basaloid appearance in more than one layer of cells
3. An increased nuclear-cytoplasmic ratio
4. Drop-shaped rete pegs
5. Irregular epithelial stratification
6. Increased number of mitotic figures
7. Mitotic figures in the superficial half of the epithelium
8. Cellular polymorphism
9. Nuclear hyperchromatism
10. Enlarged nucleoli
11. Reduction of cellular cohesion
12. Keratinization of single cells or cell groups in the prickle cell layer

Data taken from: WHO (1978). Collaborating Centre for Oral Precancerous Lesions. Definition of leukoplakia and related lesions: an aid to studies on oral precancer. Oral Surg Oral Med Oral Pathol Oral Radiol Endod 46:518–539

should be considered "precancer" and to determine their relative risk of becoming malignant. They published their first report in 1978, which defined 12 characteristics of epithelial dysplasia (Table 7.1), and graded it as mild, moderate, or severe based on whether dysplastic features were restricted to the lower third of epithelium, involved the middle third as well, or went all the way to the upper third, respectively [23]. In 2005, the classification was expanded to five stages based on the level of architectural and cytological alterations that were present. Briefly, these were squamous hyperplasia, mild dysplasia, moderate dysplasia, severe dysplasia and carcinoma in situ (CIS) [2]. In 2017, the WHO dropped the terms "squamous hyperplasia" and "carcinoma in situ" from their classification system (Table 7.2) and made minor changes to the diagnostic criteria [3].

Unfortunately, data have shown that the inter- and even intra-observer reproducibility of this classification system is poor [24–26]. A study by Brothwell et al. showed that when three oral pathologists were asked to simply identify the presence or absence of oral epithelial dysplasia in 64 slides, the inter-observer agreement was only moderate with a kappa score of 0.51 [24]. The intra-observer agreement was extremely variable; one pathologist had a kappa score of only 0.22, which means he had only mild agreement with himself. Other studies have shown equally poor inter- and intra-observer agreement using the WHO classification with one reporting a kappa agreement scores as low as 0.15 between six pathologists reviewing 150 slides [25]. This lack of consistency in the diagnosis and grading of oral epithelial dysplasia significantly confounds the data on the prognostic implications of dysplasia and makes it highly controversial [26].

In 2006, Warnakulasuriya et al. sought to address this problem by proposing a two-tier classification for lesions: low risk (no dysplasia, questionable dysplasia, or mild dysplasia) versus high risk (moderate or severe dysplasia) for undergoing malignant transformation [27]. They felt this would have better reproducibility and clinical utility. Kujan et al. argued that the binary system has superior

Table 7.2 Comparison of the evolving WHO classification for oral epithelial dysplasia

1978 classification	2005 classification	2017 classification
Mild dysplasia	Squamous hyperplasia	Mild dysplasia
	Mild dysplasia	
Moderate dysplasia	Moderate dysplasia	Moderate dysplasia
Severe dysplasia	Severe dysplasia	Severe dysplasia
	Carcinoma in situ	

1978 WHO Classification taken from: WHO (1978). Collaborating Centre for Oral Precancerous Lesions. Definition of leukoplakia and related lesions: an aid to studies on oral precancer. Oral Surg Oral Med Oral Pathol Oral Radiol Endod 46:518–539

2005 WHO Classification taken from: Warnakulasuriya S, Johnson NW, van der Waal I. Nomenclature and classification of potentially malignant disorders of the oral mucosa. J Oral Pathol Med. 2007;36:575–580

2017 WHO Classification taken from: Reibel J, Gale N, Hille J, et al. Oral potentially malignant disorders and oral epithelial dysplasia. In: El-Naggar AK, Chan JKC, Grandis JR, Takata T, Slootweg PPJ, eds. WHO Classification of Head and Neck Tumours. 4th ed. Lyon, France: IARC; 2017: 112–115.

reproducibility and a similar prognostic ability when compared to the three-tier WHO system; however, when they tested this binary system with four architectural and five cytological criteria for dysplasia, they still only demonstrated a moderate inter-observer agreement (κ of 0.5) [28]. Nankivell et al. tested the binary system with four architectural and four cytological features and had a slightly higher inter-observer kappa of 0.59 [29].

Oral Dysplasia: Detection and Diagnosis

As mentioned early, oral epithelial dysplasia is a histological diagnosis and thus requires tissue biopsy. Furthermore, current guidelines suggest that a biopsy is also indicated to make the provisional diagnosis of leukoplakia or erythroplakia a definitive one by excluding other conditions. However, there has a been a strong practical and financial incentive to identify minimally invasive adjunctive tests that can be used to either screen for dysplasia or further characterize lesions with a suspicious clinical appearance. Additionally, they can help guide clinicians in selecting a specific location to obtain their tissue biopsy.

Although it is outside the scope of this chapter to review the ever-evolving landscape of chairside adjuncts developed for oral epithelial dysplasia and OSCC, we will briefly review some important principles about using them and a few of the most common types.

First, it is important to understand that adjuncts are not intended to replace tissue biopsy when a lesion appears frankly invasive or even highly concerning for dysplasia [30]. Second, it is important to understand that there are two main ways to use these technologies: as a screening test or a "case-finding" test [30]. Lingen and colleagues, citing the WHO Public Health Papers from 1968, say that a screening test is defined as a test used for "people who are apparently free from the disease in question in order to sort out those who probably have the disease from those who probably do not. The important factor is that screening involves checking for the presence of disease in a person who is symptom free." Meanwhile, they define a case-finding test as a test that is "applied to a patient who has abnormal signs or symptoms in order to establish a diagnosis and bring the patient to treatment." These distinctly different applications of a technology have significant implications for the test's sensitivity, specificity, positive predictive value, and negative predictive value. Unfortunately, there is a lot of literature that confuses these terms and even uses them interchangeably, which confounds epidemiologic data and emphasizes the importance of critically evaluating the literature supporting an adjunct before incorporating it into a practice [30].

A conventional oral examination with special attention to high-risk subsites has long been the standard of care method to screen for oral cancer and dysplasia. A large meta-analysis done by Downer et al. calculated a sensitivity of 85% and a specificity of 97% [31]. Furthermore, Kerala et al. conducted a randomized controlled trial that was initiated in 1995 and involved over 130,000 individuals randomized into two groups (screening or control) with results presented at 3, 6, and 9 years. At 9 years, although there was no increase in survival observed for the overall population, they found a decreased mortality among males who were using tobacco and alcohol and received oral cancer screening.

Light-based detection systems have been studied as both screening tests and case-finding tests. There are two main categories of light-based detection tests: tests that assess tissue reflectance (e.g., ViziLite Plus and MicroLux DL) and tests that assess tissue autofluorescence (e.g., VELscope). Tissue reflectance was being used as an adjunct in cervical mucosa long before it was used in the oral cavity. In the oral cavity, these tests begin with a 1% acetic acid solution pre-rinse that is thought to remove surface cellular debris and cause mild dehydration of epithelial cells to increase visibility of their nuclei. A blue-white LED light is then applied to the oral mucosa, and normal tissue absorbs it, causing it to appear dark, whereas abnormal tissue reflects it, causing it to appear white. However, there is no data to demonstrate that this technology can identify mucosal abnormalities not already detected by visual examination. Furthermore, there is no data to show it can reliably predict histopathological abnormalities in clinically suspicious lesions identified by visual exam [30].

Tissue autofluorescence is based on the principle that cellular alterations in dysplasia and carcinoma change the concentration of fluorophores in tissue, which affect the way abnormal tissue scatters and absorbs certain wavelengths of light. Tissue autofluorescence technology does not require the use of a pre-rinse. The VELscope uses a blue light (with a wavelength of 400–460 nm) to excite the tissue. Normal oral mucosa emits a pale green autofluoresence when viewed through a narrow-band filter in the handpiece. In contrast, abnormal tissue has less autofluoresence and appears dark in comparison to the bright surrounding normal mucosa. When used as a case-finding test (on suspicious lesions that were detected by visual exam under incandescent light), one study showed a high sensitivity (98%) and high specificity (100%) in discriminating mucosa with histologic evidence of carcinoma or dysplasia from mucosa that is histologically normal [32]. However, the data is mixed with one systematic review reporting sensitives as low as 15.3% and specificities as low as 30% [33]. Furthermore, there is no good evidence to show tissue autofluorescence can reliably identify histopathologically abnormal mucosa that is not detectable by clinical oral exam, which limits its use as a screening test [30].

Another popular adjunct is brush biopsy. This technology is used as a case-finding test and works by allows clinicians to collect exfoliated cells in a clinically suspicious lesion. The cells are then fixed on a histology slide and undergo specialized computer-aided analysis. Because the test evaluates individual cells, its assessment is based solely on cellular atypia. Thus, it cannot evaluate epithelial architecture and cannot differentiate dysplasia from invasive carcinoma. It was introduced in 1999 and marketed as a minimally invasive adjunct that could further characterize innocuous appearing lesions that clinicians would not normally biopsy. If the test resulted as "abnormal" or "positive," clinicians are encouraged to follow up with a formal scalpel biopsy for definitive diagnosis. The data on this has been mixed as well with sensitivities and specificities ranging from 71% to 100% and 32% to 100%, respectively [30]. However, Lingen and colleagues argue that this adjunct may be helpful in patients with multiple lesions throughout the oral cavity who are not willing to undergo scalpel biopsy for all of them.

A third main category of adjuncts is dyes, most commonly toluidine blue, which have a high affinity for nucleic acids and thus presumably stain dysplastic and malignant tissue because of their high DNA content. Toluidine blue has been used for decades in other countries as both a screening test and case-finding test for oral cavity dysplasia and cancer [34]. Surgeons have also used toluidine blue to decide on margins for excision of a lesion [35]. Although a lot of data exist on toluidine blue, there is none that supports its use as a screening test. Overall, its sensitivity and specificity for detecting oral cancer ranges from 78% to 100% and 31% to 100%, respectively [30].

In summary, these adjuncts may have a role in the detection and diagnosis of dysplasia, but only in the hands of informed clinicians who understand their indications and use them appropriately.

Oral Dysplasia: Management (Treatment and Surveillance)

Treating dysplasia before it progresses to oral cancer can be lifesaving; however, there is still no way to accurately predict which dysplastic lesions will progress and when. Furthermore, because dysplasia is a disease that is restricted to the epithelium, there are many different management options including observation, topical therapy (retinoids and vitamin A), cryotherapy, laser vaporization, and surgical excision. Each of these have different levels of morbidity, rely on different amounts of patient compliance, have different costs, and require different expertise and equipment from clinicians. Additionally, unlike oral squamous cell carcinoma, there is no consensus or data-drive guidelines to follow. Thus, the management of dysplasia has become a matter of surgeon preference and a source of significant controversy.

For purposes of this chapter, we will review a few algorithms that help provide a framework for managing patients with oral epithelial dysplasia. In 2015, the University of Liverpool published an algorithm that divides epithelial dysplasia into two main categories: mild or moderate/severe/CIS [36]. This is based on strong data that lesions with a higher degree of dysplasia have a higher tendency to undergo malignant transformation [37]. Specifically, a meta-analysis conducted by Iocca et al. showed that the "the odds of malignant transformation in moderate/severe dysplasia are much higher than mild dysplasia (OR 2.37, 99% CI 1.47–3.79)" [11]. They calculated an annual malignant transformation rate of 1.7% for mild dysplasia and 3.57% for severe dysplasia. Furthermore, Speight has shown that while less than 5% of mild dysplasia will undergo malignant transformation, up to 50% of severe dysplasia will [37]. In the Liverpool algorithm, mild dysplasia gets monitored for 5 years by a specialist and then discharged to their primary care for surveillance, whereas moderate and severe dysplasia gets treated, re-biopsied, or closely observed long term by a specialist. The only exception to this is that mild dysplasia that has a concerning clinical appearance or exists in a patient with significant risk factors gets managed more vigilantly along the moderate/severe dysplasia pathway of the treatment algorithm.

In 2018, Awadallah and colleagues published their own algorithm for managing dysplasia [38]. Similar to the Liverpool algorithm, their algorithm was based on risk stratification; however, they proposed a unique treatment for moderate dysplasia rather than grouping it with severe dysplasia and CIS. Interestingly, they excise severe dysplasia and CIS with 5 mm margins and moderate dysplasia with 2 mm margins and combine excision with laser ablation. Although there is no strong data to support their selection of margins, it reflects their concern that lesions with severe dysplasia and CIS identified on biopsy are more likely to have a focus of Squamous cell carcinoma (SCCa) that may be identified after complete excision. Additionally, the surveillance is different for moderate dysplasia versus severe dysplasia/CIS. The surveillance for severe dysplasia/CIS closely mimics the regimen outlined by the National Comprehensive Cancer Network (NCCN) for head and neck cancer, again, reflecting the concern that severe dysplasia and CIS are most likely to undergo malignant transformation. Meanwhile, mild dysplasia in patients with clinically innocuous lesions and no risk factors undergo "conservative management," whereas higher-risk patient undergo excision with or without laser ablation. The long-term follow-up they propose for mild dysplasia is similar to their follow up for moderate dysplasia.

Ultimately, both the Liverpool and Awadallah algorithms focus on two main modalities of treatment: surgical excision or CO2 laser ablation. The main advantage of surgical excision over CO2 laser ablation is that it provides a specimen for histopathological analysis that may affect treatment (for example, if a focus of carcinoma was found in the specimen). However, laser ablation is often less morbid that surgical excision and can be used in lesions that are not amenable to excision either because of location or distribution.

Oral Dysplasia: Risk of Malignant Transformation

Although there is no way to definitively predict when an OPMD will undergo malignant transformation, some tools exist to stratify patients into risk categories.

Unfortunately, the malignant transformation rate of oral epithelial dysplasia varies widely in the literature, ranging from 0.13% to 36% [39]. This is, in large part, due to significant differences in population risk factors, study design, inclusion criteria, and terminology. As discussed earlier in this chapter, the largest met analysis to date was conducted by Iocca et al., and they calculated an annual malignant transformation rate of 1.7% for mild dysplasia and 3.57% for severe dysplasia [11]. Furthermore, Speight has shown that while less than 5% of mild dysplasia will undergo malignant transformation, up to 50% of severe dysplasia will [37].

In 2018, Speight et al. published an excellent review of risk factors for malignant transformation of oral epithelial dysplasia and proposed an algorithm that incorporates some of the most important clinical risk factors along with histopathologic grading to classify lesions as either high or low risk [4]. According to this algorithm, female gender, nonsmokers, high-risk subsites (tongue and floor of mouth), erythroplakia, nonhomogenous or speckled leukoplakia, PVL (that is persistent, recurrent, or in multiple spots), and severe dysplasia all pose a high risk for malignant transformation. Meanwhile, homogenous leukoplakia that histopathologically demonstrates mild dysplasia is the only lesion that is considered low risk. However, risk stratifying patients must always be balanced against the reality that lesions without any evidence of epithelial dysplasia can still undergo malignant transformation and malignant transformation of high-risk lesions is not inevitable.

This conundrum highlights the urgent need for a data-driven method to distinguish dysplastic lesions that will progress to cancer from those that will not. As the molecular underpinnings of the "hallmarks of cancer" have become better understood, molecular biomarkers of these critical processes have received a lot of attention as potential predictors of malignant transformation [40, 41]. As Speight puts it, "The Holy Grail in terms of risk assessment is to discover a biomarker that can be used in a histologic or chairside test to predict malignant transformation of oral lesions" [4]. Some of the most investigated markers have been p53, S100A7, Ki67, survivin, MMP-9, and p16 [42]. Additionally, there is emerging data that genetic abnormalities such as loss of heterozygosity and aneuploidy, as well as epigenetic changes such as histone modification, post-transcriptional regulation of mRNA, and DNA methylation, are important in progression from dysplasia to carcinoma [4, 25]. However, although many molecular markers and genetic and epigenetic changes have been shown to correlate with oral epithelial dysplasia and tumorigenesis, no single biomarker has been shown to reliably predict malignant transformation [4]. Unfortunately, the literature is full of poorly designed studies with little to no clinical application. A systematic review published by Smith et al. identified 2550 studies published on molecular biomarkers for the malignant transformation of oral dysplasia. However, only 13 of them were longitudinal studies with adequate follow up that met their quality standards [42].

Interestingly, artificial intelligence (AI) has shown some promise as a tool for integrating large amounts of data to estimate risk of malignant transformation [43]. The ability to digitize stained tissue specimens and develop machine learning tools in digital pathology have paved the way to a myriad of AI-based tests in oncology. One such test designed specifically for oral dysplasia is Straticyte, marketed by Proteocyte AI (Toronto, ON). This prognostic test uses digitized immunohisto-chemical stains for a panel of biomarkers, including S100A7, to calculate a quantitative risk of malignant transformation [44]. Many molecular diagnostics are in use developed for breast cancer, prostate cancer, and brain cancer with encouraging preliminary results [43] and are commercially available. Historically, the management of dysplasia has been as diverse and variable as the opinions of all the clinicians treating it; however, this exciting technology may allow standardization of treatment practices and afford new levels of sophistication in the management of dysplasia based on objective assessments of patient-specific histopathological data and molecular signatures. Ultimately, the management of dysplasia deserves increasingly *standardized and customized* practices, to limit the morbidity of unnecessary and costly treatment for those patients whose OPMDs are unlikely to undergo malignant transformation, and discourage watchful waiting for those with aggressive lesions, which may ultimately progress to cancer.

References

1. Baillie S, Simms W. Queries and responses from the medical committee of the society for investigating the nature and cure of cancer. Edinb Med Surg J. 1806;2:382–9.
2. Warnakulasuriya S, Johnson NW, van der Waal I. Nomenclature and classification of potentially malignant disorders of the oral mucosa. J Oral Pathol Med. 2007;36:575–80.
3. Reibel J, Gale N, Hille J, et al. Oral potentially malignant disorders and oral epithelial dysplasia. In: El-Naggar AK, Chan JKC, Grandis JR, Takata T, Slootweg PPJ, editors. WHO classification of head and neck tumours. 4th ed. Lyon: IARC; 2017. p. 112–5.
4. Speight PM, Khurram SA, Kujan O. Oral potentially malignant disorders: risk of progression to malignancy. Oral Surg Oral Med Oral Pathol Oral Radiol. 2018;125(6):612–27.
5. Warnakulasuriya S, Kujan O, Aguirre-Urizar JM, Bagan JV, González-Moles MÁ, Kerr AR, Lodi G, Mello FW, Monteiro L, Ogden GR, Sloan P, Johnson NW. Oral potentially malignant disorders: a consensus report from an international seminar on nomenclature and classification, convened by the WHO Collaborating Centre for Oral Cancer. Oral Dis. 2021;27(8):1862–80.
6. Nikitakis NG. Special focus issue on potentially premalignant oral epithelial lesions: introduction and perspective. Oral Surg Oral Med Oral Pathol Oral Radiol. 2018;125(6):575–6.
7. Van der Waal I. Historical perspective and nomenclature of potentially malignant or potentially premalignant oral epithelial lesions with emphasis on leukoplakia-some suggestions for modifications. Oral Surg Oral Med Oral Pathol Oral Radiol. 2018;125(6):577–81.
8. Chaturvedi AK, Udaltsova N, Engels EA, Katzel JA, Yanik EL, Katki HA, Lingen MW, Silverberg MJ. Oral leukoplakia and risk of progression to oral cancer: a population-based cohort study. J Natl Cancer Inst. 2020;112(10):1047–54.
9. Axell T, Pindborg JJ, Smith CJ, et al. Oral white lesions with special reference to precancerous and tobacco related lesions: conclusions of an international symposium held in Uppsala, Sweden, May 18-21, 1994. J Oral Pathol Med. 1996;25:49–54.

10. Hogewind WFC, van der Kwast WAM, van der Wall I. Oral leukoplakia, with emphasis on malignant transformation. J Craniomaxillofac Surg. 1989;17:128–33.
11. Iocca O, Sollecito TP, Alawi F, Weinstein GS, Newman JG, De Virgilio A, Di Maio P, Spriano G, Pardiñas López S, Shanti RM. Potentially malignant disorders of the oral cavity and oral dysplasia: a systematic review and meta-analysis of malignant transformation rate by subtype. Head Neck. 2020;42(3):539–55.
12. Waldron CA, Shafer WG. Leukoplakia revisited. Cancer. 1975;36:1386–92.
13. Reddi SP, Shafer AT. Oral premalignant lesions: management considerations. Oral Maxillofac Surg Clin North Am. 2006;18:425–33.
14. Abadie WM, Partington EJ, Fowler CB, Schmalbach CE. Optimal management of proliferative verrucous leukoplakia: a systematic review of the literature. Otolaryngol Head Neck Surg. 2015;153:504–11.
15. Goette DK. Review of erythroplasia of queyrat and its treatment. Urology. 1976;8(4):311–5.
16. Cawson RA, Langdon JD, Eveson JW. Ertyroplasia ('ertyroplakia'). In: Cawson RA, editor. Surgical pathology of the mouth and jaws. Oxford: Wright; 1996. p. 180.
17. Pindborg JJ, Reichart PA, Smith CJ, et al. Histological typing of cancer and precancer of the oral mucosa. 2nd ed. Berlin: Springer; 1997.
18. Shafer WG, Waldron CA. Erththroplakia of the oral cavity. Cancer. 1975;36:1021–8.
19. Slaughter DP, Southwick HW, Smejkal W. "Field cancerization" in oral stratified squamous epithelium: clinical implications of multicentric origin. Cancer. 1953;6(5):963–8.
20. Califano J, van der Riet P, Westra W, Nawroz H, Clayman G, Piantadosi S, et al. Genetic progression model for head and neck cancer: implications for field cancerization. Cancer Res. 1996;56:2488–92.
21. Smith C, Pindborg JJ. Histologic grading of oral epithelial atypia by the use of photographic standards. Copenhagen: C. Hamburgers Bogtrykkeri; 1969.
22. Pindborg JJ, Reichart PA, Smith CJ, van der Waal I. World Health Organization: histological typing of cancer and precancer of the oral mucosa. Berlin: Springer; 1997.
23. WHO, Collaborating Centre for Oral Precancerous Lesions. Definition of leukoplakia and related lesions: an aid to studies on oral precancer. Oral Surg Oral Med Oral Pathol Oral Radiol Endod. 1978;46:518–39.
24. Brothwell DJ, Lewis DW, Bradley G, Leong I, Jordan RC, Mock D, Leake JL. Observer agreement in the grading of oral epithelial dysplasia. Community Dent Oral Epidemiol. 2003;31(4):300–5.
25. Ranganathan K, Kavitha L. Oral epithelial dysplasia: classifications and clinical relevance in risk assessment of oral potentially malignant disorders. J Oral Maxillofac Pathol. 2019;23(1):19–27.
26. Abbey LM, Kaugars GE, Gunsolley JC, Burns JC, Page DG, Svirsky JA, Eisenberg E, Krutchkoff DJ, Cushing M. Intraexaminer and interexaminer reliability in the diagnosis of oral epithelial dysplasia. Oral Surg Oral Med Oral Pathol Oral Radiol Endod. 1995;80(2):188–91.
27. Warnakulasuriya S, Reibel J, Bouquot J, Dabelsteen E. Oral epithelial dysplasia classification systems: predictive value, utility, weaknesses and scope for improvement. J Oral Pathol Med. 2008;37:127–33.
28. Kujan O, Oliver RJ, Khattab A, Roberts SA, Thakker N, Sloan P, et al. Evaluation of a new binary system of grading oral epithelial dysplasia for prediction of malignant transformation. Oral Oncol. 2006;42:987–93.
29. Nankivell P, Williams H, Matthews P, Suortamo S, Snead D, McConkey C, et al. The binary oral dysplasia grading system: validity testing and suggested improvement. Oral Surg Oral Med Oral Pathol Oral Radiol. 2013;115:87–94.
30. Lingen MW, Kalmar JR, Karrison T, et al. Critical evaluation of diagnostic aids for the detection of oral cancer. Oral Oncol. 2008;44(1):10–22.
31. Downer MC, Moles DR, Palmer S, Speight PM. A systematic review of test performance in screening for oral cancer and precancer. Oral Oncol. 2004;40(3):264–73.

32. Lane PM, Gilhuly T, Whitehead P, Zeng H, Poh CF, Ng S, et al. Simple device for the direct visualization of oral-cavity tissue fluorescence. J Biomed Opt. 2006;11(2):024006.
33. Rashid A, Warnakulasuriya S. The use of light-based (optical) detection systems as adjuncts in the detection of oral cancer and oral potentially malignant disorders: a systematic review. J Oral Pathol Med. 2015;44(5):307–28.
34. Mashberg A. Final evaluation of tolonium chloride rinse for screening of high-risk patients with asymptomatic squamous carcinoma. J Am Dent Assoc. 1983;106(3):319–23.
35. Portugal LC, Wilson KM, Biddinger PW, et al. The role of toluidine blue in assessing margin status after resection of squamous cell carcinomas of the upper aerodigestive tract. Arch Otolaryngol Head Neck Surg. 1996;122:517–9.
36. Field EA, McCarthy CE, Ho MW, Rajlawat BP, Holt D, Rogers SN, Triantafyllou A, Field JK, Shaw RJ. The management of oral epithelial dysplasia: the Liverpool algorithm. Oral Oncol. 2015;51(10):883–7.
37. Speight PM. Update on oral epithelial dysplasia and progression to cancer. Head Neck Pathol. 2007;1(1):61–6.
38. Awadallah M, Idle M, Patel K, Kademani D. Management update of potentially premalignant oral epithelial lesions. Oral Surg Oral Med Oral Pathol Oral Radiol. 2018;125(6):628–36.
39. Kademani D, Dierks E. Surgical management of oral and mucosal dysplasias: the case for surgical excision. J Oral Maxillofac Surg. 2007;65(2):287–92.
40. Hanahan D, Weinberg RA. Hallmarks of cancer: the next generation. Cell. 2011;144:646–74.
41. Nikitakis N, Pentenero M, Georgaki M, Poh C, et al. Molecular markers associated with development of potentially premalignant oral epithelial lesions: current knowledge and future implications. Oral Surg Oral Med Oral Pathol Oral Radiol Endod. 2008;125:650–69.
42. Smith J, Rattay T, McConkey C, Helliwell T, Mehanna H. Biomarkers in dysplasia of the oral cavity: a systematic review. Oral Oncol. 2009;45:647–53.
43. Bera K, Schalper KA, Rimm DL, Velcheti V, Madabhushi A. Artificial intelligence in digital pathology—new tools for diagnosis and precision oncology. Nat Rev Clin Oncol. 2019;16(11):703–15.
44. Hwang JT, Gu YR, Shen M, Ralhan R, Walfish PG, Pritzker KP, Mock D. Individualized five-year risk assessment for oral premalignant lesion progression to cancer. Oral Surg Oral Med Oral Pathol Oral Radiol. 2017;123(3):374–81.

Chapter 8
Pharyngoesophageal Reconstruction

Ray Y. Wang, Caitlin M. Coviello, Mohammad S. Jafferji, Shawn Groth, and Andrew T. Huang

Introduction

Defects of the pharynx and cervical esophagus represent a significant challenge for reconstructive surgeons due to the unique technical, functional, and outcome considerations involved. Reconstruction following ablative procedures for malignancy is the most common indication and is complicated by the need for expedient recovery to avoid delays in adjuvant therapy and additional technical challenges posted by prior treatment, particularly radiation. While the incidence of most head and neck cancers has decreased in recent years, presumably due to a decrease in tobacco use, an estimated 40,000 patients will be diagnosed annually with cancers of the laryngopharynx or esophagus [1, 2]. Historically, advanced laryngeal and hypopharyngeal cancers were treated with primary total laryngectomy with or without pharyngectomy and/or adjuvant radiation [3]. Published in 1991, the landmark Department of Veteran Affairs Laryngeal Cancer Study Group trial demonstrated that an organ preservation approach with induction chemotherapy followed by radiation could achieve comparable overall survival with laryngeal preservation in 64% of patients [3]. Twelve years later, the RTOG 91-11 trial demonstrated superiority of concurrent chemotherapy with radiation for laryngeal preservation and locoregional control compared to induction chemotherapy and radiation or radiation alone, establishing concurrent chemoradiotherapy as the treatment of choice for

R. Y. Wang · C. M. Coviello · A. T. Huang (✉)
Department of Otolaryngology—Head and Neck Surgery, Baylor College of Medicine, Houston, TX, USA
e-mail: ray.wang@bcm.edu; aitlin.coviello@bcm.edu; andrew.huang@bcm.edu

M. S. Jafferji · S. Groth
Division of Thoracic Surgery, Michael E. DeBakey Department of Surgery, Baylor College of Medicine, Houston, TX, USA
e-mail: mohammad.jafferji@bcm.edu; shawn.groth@bcm.edu

J. C. Melville et al. (eds.), *Advancements and Innovations in OMFS, ENT, and Facial Plastic Surgery*, https://doi.org/10.1007/978-3-031-32099-6_8

organ-sparing treatment of advanced laryngeal and hypopharyngeal cancers [4, 5]. Today, total laryngectomy is typically reserved for patients with very advanced (T4) local disease or in the salvage setting [6, 7]. Similarly, while surgery has historically been the primary curative modality for cancers of the esophagus, preoperative or definitive chemoradiation has been increasingly utilized in patients with locally advanced disease [8].

The choice of technique in pharyngeal reconstruction after surgery for advanced cancers of the larynx and hypopharynx is of particular importance as wound complications—particularly pharyngocutaneous fistula (PCF) – carry considerable morbidity. When they occur in the primary setting, these complications can lead to delays in the initiation of adjuvant treatment, which have been shown to negatively impact survival [9]. Meanwhile, patients undergoing laryngectomy with or without pharyngectomy in the salvage setting have been demonstrated in multiple studies to be at increased risk of PCF and wound complications [7, 10]. In the RTOG 91-11 study, 59% of patients in the concurrent chemoradiation arm developed wound complications postoperatively with 30% developing PCF [11].

Furthermore, other functional outcomes such as the ability to tolerate oral nutrition, gastrostomy-tube dependence, stricture formation, and utilization of tracheoesophageal puncture for phonation are impacted by the reconstructive technique and represent important considerations when approaching these patients.

In this chapter, we review fundamental principles of pharyngeal reconstruction after oncologic treatment and existing literature on the various techniques that have been described with regards to functional outcomes and complications.

Principles of Reconstruction

The pharynx is a funnel-shaped structure that serves dual functions as part of the upper respiratory and gastrointestinal tracts. It is divided into three components—the nasopharynx, which is bounded anteriorly by the choanae and inferiorly at the velum; the oropharynx, which is separated from the oral cavity anteriorly along the circumvallate papillae of the base of tongue to the anterior tonsillar pillars and soft palate and inferiorly by the larynx; and the hypopharynx, which comprises the pyriform sinuses, post-cricoid, and esophageal inlet. A representative endoscopic view of the larynx and pharynx is demonstrated in Fig. 8.1. The pharynx serves as a conduit for air to the lower respiratory tract and for food and liquid bolus transit to the esophagus and stomach. As laryngectomy and pharyngoesophagectomy procedures result in opening of the alimentary tract to the neck and external environment, the goals of reconstruction are focused primarily on re-establishing a safe and functional passageway for the transit of food boluses that is robust enough to survive adjuvant therapy. In the primary setting, this closure must also be robust enough to withstand adjuvant radiation or chemoradiotherapy and heal quickly enough so as to not delay initiation of adjuvant treatment. Ideally, the pharyngeal reconstruction should also allow for a tracheoesophageal puncture to facilitate phonation while preventing leakage of saliva or food into the respiratory tract.

Fig. 8.1 Laryngopharyngeal anatomy. (**a**) Greater cornu of thyroid cartilage, (**b**) Pyriform sinus, (**c**) Post-cricoid, (**d**) Glottic inlet, (**e**) Arytenoid, (**f**) Epiglottis, (**g**) Vallecula

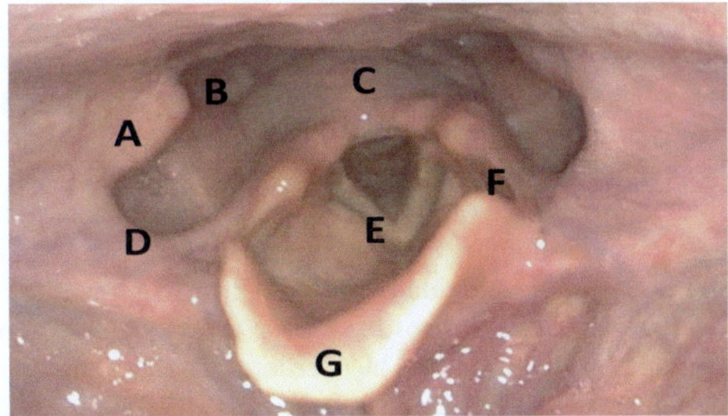

Table 8.1 Reconstructive ladder

Microvascular free tissue transfer
Regional tissue transfer
Local tissue transfer
Tissue expansion
Skin graft
Delayed primary closure
Primary closure
Secondary intention

The concept of the reconstructive ladder (Table 8.1) is well established within the reconstructive literature and describes a spectrum of reconstructive options that may be applied to a particular defect, ranging from healing by secondary intention to microvascular free tissue transfer (MVFTT). Selecting a reconstructive modality is a complex decision that depends on a variety of factors, including the patient's anatomy, anticipated extent of the defect, and medical comorbidities. Depending on the extent of resection, the size of the defect may vary dramatically from small pharyngotomies in mucosa-sparing laryngectomy to total laryngopharyngectomy with total glossectomy or esophagectomy. There have been numerous algorithms described to guide pharyngeal reconstruction, and approaches are highly surgeon and institution-dependent. Ideally, the reconstruction would minimize risk of post-operative pharyngocutaneous fistula and stenosis, allowing for as close to normal function as possible while minimizing donor site morbidity and operative complexity. A variety of techniques ranging from primary closure, skin grafting, local mucosal flap, pedicled flaps, abdominal-based enteric flaps, and microvascular free tissue transfer (MVFTT) have been described.

Primary Closure

While the first laryngectomy performed by Billroth in 1873 involved intentional creation of a pharyngocutaneous fistula above the tracheostoma, pharyngeal defects following resection of laryngeal and hypopharyngeal malignancies have been managed with primary closure in a single stage since the 1890s [12–14]. With the advent of locoregional and MVFTT options and evidence of increased complications rates with primary closure in the salvage setting, primary closure is predominantly utilized in primary laryngectomy cases with limited pharyngeal resection. Primary closure may be utilized in cases of esophageal perforation or partial resection, but total or subtotal esophagectomy defects require additional reconstruction. The exact amount of residual pharyngeal mucosa required to prevent stricture has not been clearly elucidated, although primary closure in patients with as little as 1.5 cm of residual mucosa has been described with functional swallow postoperatively [15]. Other authors have recommended primary closure when at least 3.5 cm of residual mucosa remains, corresponding roughly to a 34Fr bougie catheter [16]. The decision to proceed with primary closure is largely based on surgeon preference and experience as data to delineate candidates for primary closure in both the primary and the salvage setting is lacking [17]. In cases involving significant resection of pharyngeal mucosa, a patch (interposition design) reconstruction sutured to the residual mucosa is often necessary to provide adequate circumference to avoid stricture.

The primary goal of pharyngeal closure is to obtain a water-tight, tension-free closure with care taken to avoid excessive tension resulting in strangulation of the mucosa. Multiple different suture techniques, including Lembert, Cushing, Connell, and Gambee sutures, have been utilized and are shown in Fig. 8.2 [18]. The choice of suture technique varies greatly among surgeons and institutions, and there is little data to suggest superiority of one technique over another, though some studies have suggested that continuous sutures may have lower rates of pharyngocutaneous fistula than interrupted suture [19, 20]. Meticulous technique is imperative as any gaps or tears in the mucosa can lead to a salivary leak and PCF. There is also considerable variation based on institutional and surgeon preference in the orientation of the closure (vertical, horizontal, or "T"-shaped). Due to its orientation, horizontal closure may reduce likelihood of stricture and improve postoperative dysphagia and dysphagia-related quality of life, though this may not be suitable for larger defects [21]. The "T" closure is typically accomplished with a vertical suture line along the medial pyriform mucosa with a horizontal cross-bar at the base of tongue [22]. The "T"-shaped closure has been shown to reduce the incidence of pseudo-diverticula (pseudo-vallecula) separated from the neopharynx by a scar band (pseudoepiglottis); this has been suggested to reduce postoperative dysphagia in some studies although this relationship has not been consistently demonstrated [22–24]. While the trifurcation of the "T"-shaped closure represents a theoretical weak point, which may increase the risk of pharyngocutaneous fistula, there is limited data to support this assertion and retrospective studies have had mixed results [25, 26].

Described by Sofferman et al. in 2000, the mechanical stapling technique has also been advocated as an alternative method to manual suturing techniques, particularly in the international literature [27, 28]. After the trachea has been transected, a linear stapler is clamped and fired across the pyriform sinuses angling superiorly and again at the vallecula aiming inferiorly to separate the larynx from the pharynx [27]. A recent meta-analysis found a lower rate of pharyngocutaneous fistula (13.7%

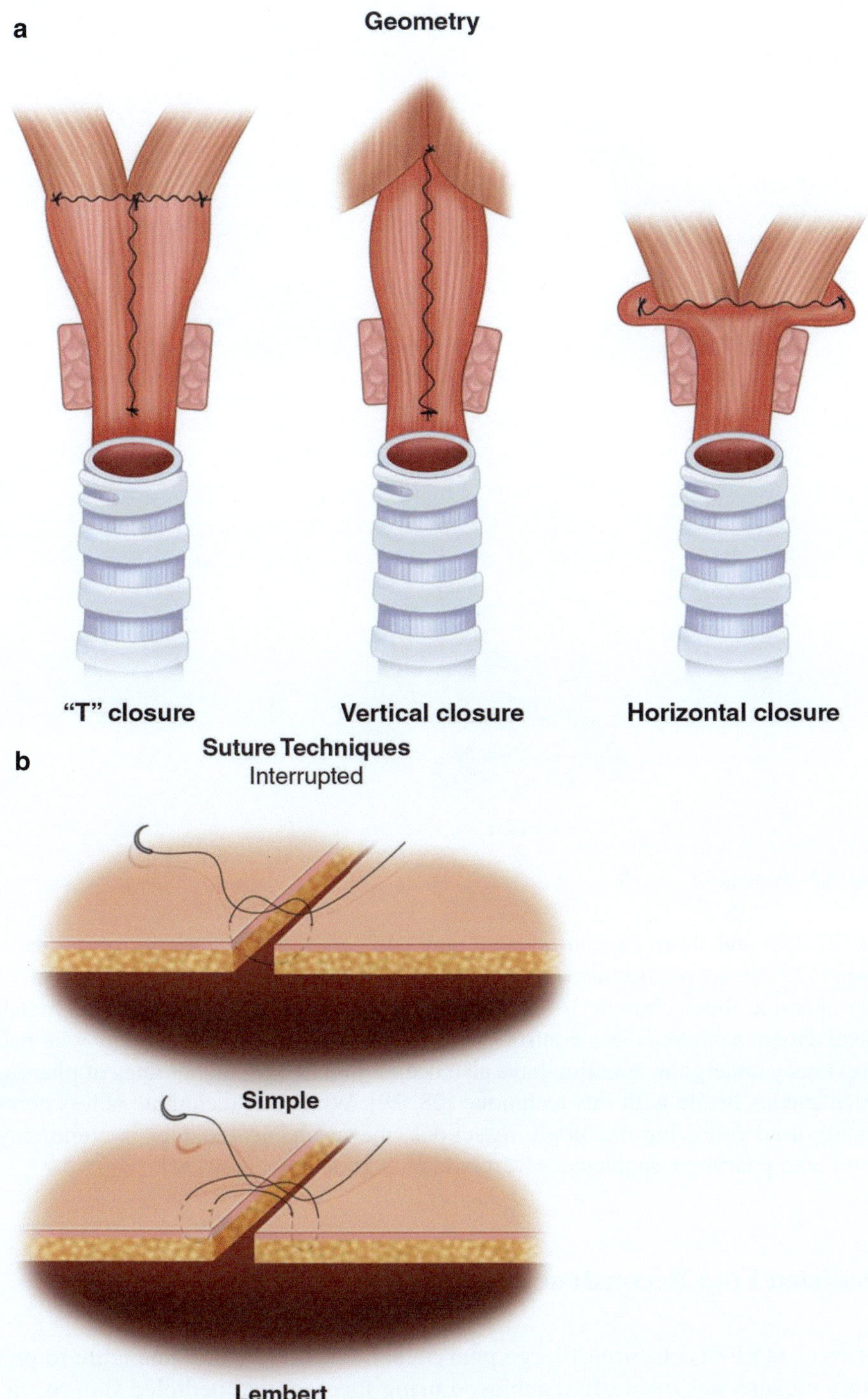

Fig. 8.2 Various suture techniques in the primary repair of pharyngoesophageal deformities. (**a**) Geometry. (**b**) Suture Techniques—Interrupted. (**c**) Suture Techniques—Continuous

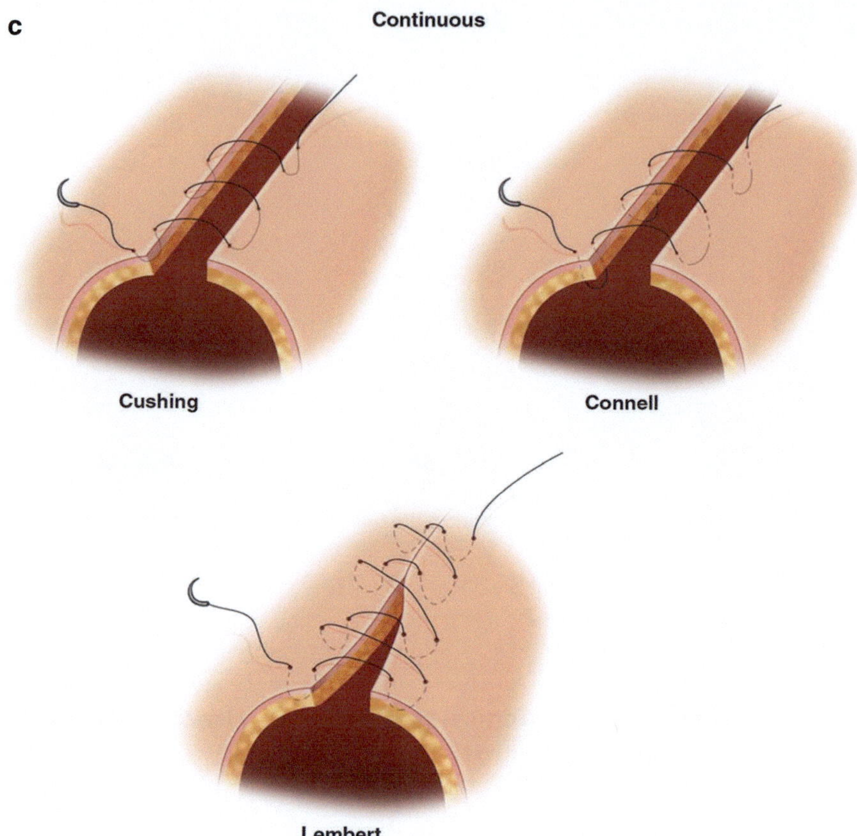

Fig. 8.2 (continued)

vs. 27.2%) and shorter mean hospital stay compared to conventional suture technique [29]. However, because this is a closed technique with limited visualization of the pharynx, this technique is less suitable for tumors with significant pharyngeal involvement as there is less control over the pharyngeal margins. Patients who had previously undergone radiation have also been found to have higher rates of pharyngocutaneous fistula with this technique [28, 29]. While this technique is less commonly used following oncologic resections, the mechanical stapler is commonly used with pharyngoesophageal diverticula with good outcomes [30].

Pedicled Flap Reconstruction

Prior to MVFTT, closure of large pharyngeal deformities not amenable to primary closure was most often achieved using locoregional pedicled flap reconstruction. A variety of different flaps have been reported, with the most frequently cited being the deltopectoral (DP) flap, the internal mammary artery perforator (IMAP) flap, the pectoralis major myofascial (PMMF) and myocutaneous (PMMC) flaps, and the supraclavicular artery island flap (SCAIF) (Table 8.2).

Table 8.2 Locoregional flaps. Blood supply, advantages, and disadvantages

Flap	Blood supply	Reconstructive capability	Advantages	Disadvantages
Deltopectoral	Internal mammary artery and vein, deltoid perforators from thoracoacromial trunk and anterior circumflex vascular bundle	Tubed (circumferential defects)	Safe management of airway and salivary formation	Presence of fistula Donor site morbidity, need for split thickness skin graft (STSG) Distal tip necrosis Two-stage surgery
Internal mammary artery perforator	Internal mammary artery and vein	Onlay/patch Tubed (circumferential defects)	Thin and pliable, minimal tracheostomal obstruction Decreased donor site morbidity when compared to deltopectoral (DP) flap	Small-medium sized defects only May require resection of rib cartilage Can alter breast contour
Pectoralis major Myocutaneous	Thoracoacromial artery and vein	U-shaped (circumferential defects) Onlay/patch	Ease of harvest, single surgeon team Can be used in vessel depleted neck	Flap bulk results in worse speech/ swallowing outcomes Shoulder and arm weakness Chest wall contour asymmetries Can alter breast contour
Pectoralis major myofascial	Thoracoacromial artery and vein	Onlay/patch		
Supraclavicular Artery Island	Supraclavicular artery and vein	Onlay/patch	Thin and pliable Minimal donor site morbidity Can be used to reconstruct anterior neck skin	Small-medium sized defects only Extensive neck dissections may have transverse cervical arteries ligated Anatomic variations in vascular pedicle

Locoregional reconstruction of the pharynx was first reported in 1886, but was not popularized until Wookey introduced the pedicled cervical flap in the 1940s [31]. The Wookey flap was a two-staged reconstruction using a platysmal cervical skin flap tacked to prevertebral fascia. This eventually formed the neopharynx to be closed in a second stage. Salivary contamination, subsequent mediastinitis and great vessel rupture was a frequent occurrence with the Wookey flap, and thus, it has largely been abandoned for the more common locoregional flaps used today [32].

Deltopectoral and Internal Mammary Artery Perforator Flap

The deltopectoral (DP) flap was first reported as a reconstructive option for pharyngeal reconstruction by Bakamjian in 1965 [33]. It was the primary reconstructive method for head and neck defects up until the 1980s, when the pectoralis major flaps and microvascular free tissue transfer became popularized. While it is less frequently used for pharyngeal reconstruction today, it paved the way for current techniques in pharyngeal reconstruction.

The DP flap was initially described as a two-stage perforator flap based on three separate blood supplies: (1) the first to fourth perforators of the internal mammary artery and veins, which are located parasternally; (2) the deltoid perforators arising from the thoracoacromial trunk; and (3) the anterior circumflex vascular bundle that accompanies the deltoid muscle laterally. Given the less reliable nature of the lateral vasculature, the flap is typically harvested based medially on the internal mammary blood supply. A horizontal incision is made below the clavicle and brought inferiorly to the fourth intercostal space. The flap is then elevated deep to the superficial pectoral and deltoid muscle fascia [34]. The flap is tunneled into the defect site, tubed longitudinally, and sutured to the oropharynx superiorly. The esophagus is sutured to the base of the DP flap, thus creating a controlled salivary fistula site. The donor site is closed with a split thickness skin graft (STSG). A second stage for division and inset of the flap and closure of the salivary fistula is performed 4 weeks later. This approach had significant advantages over the Wookey procedure including safe management of the airway and salivary formation. However, the need for multiple-staged surgeries, persistent salivary fistula prior to second stage, donor site morbidity with inability to obtain primary closure, and unreliability of the distal tip of the flap are major drawbacks [32]. Today, the DP flap is utilized less frequently due to the improved versatility and lesser donor site morbidity afforded by the supraclavicular and pectoralis major flaps for similar defects.

The DP flap has most recently been redefined by Yu et al. in 2006 as the internal mammary artery perforator (IMAP) flap and is most commonly described today as such [35]. Basing the pedicle off one arterial supply rather than three as in the DP flap allows for a greater arc of rotation [36]. The internal mammary artery perforator of interest can be found using a Doppler and traced out from the parasternal region. The stronger signal of the second or third IMAP is typically chosen for the vascular bundle. Dissection is similarly carried deep to the muscular fascia, and the flap is tunneled into the defect site in a subcutaneous fashion. Some have reported resecting the associated rib cartilage to allow for better exposure of the vascular bundle. In general, the IMAP flap is thinner, resulting in decreased donor site morbidity compared to the DP flap.

DP and IMAP flaps can be used as onlay flaps or as a tubed flap in cases of circumferential pharyngeal defects [37]. The IMAP flap has also frequently been reported for its use in repair of pharyngocutaneous fistulas and is, therefore, an ideal backup option in case of primary flap failure or complication. Advantages of the IMAP flap include its thin and pliable design, allowing for adequate reconstruction without risk of tracheostomal obstruction [38]. However, the inability to close the donor site primarily in most cases and poor cosmesis that results are significant drawbacks that limit utilization of the IMAP flap.

Pectoralis Major Myofascial and Myocutaneous Flap

The pectoralis major (PM) flap is perhaps the most reported regional flap used in pharyngeal reconstruction and is a workhorse in head and neck reconstruction. It was first described by Ariyan in 1979, where its use was described for various head and neck defects ranging from orbital exenteration to oral cavity and oropharyngeal resections [39].

The pectoralis major flap is based on the thoracoacromial artery, which branches from the axillary artery and then travels under the clavicle for approximately 2–4 cm before coursing obliquely in an inferomedial direction along the pectoralis major muscle. The PM flap is classically harvested through a parasternal incision carried down to the pectoralis fascia. The muscle is then elevated off the chest wall from an inferior to superior direction. The neurovascular bundle can be found on the deep surface of the muscle in the fatty plane separating the pectoralis major and minor muscles. Dissection can then be carried as far wide and proximal as necessary to cover the defect extent. Once defect dimensions are known, the pedicled flap can be released from its attachments, including the humerus. Keeping the vascular pedicle intact, the flap is mobilized and transferred through a subcutaneous tunnel into the neck [34].

The PM flap can be harvested and inset as either a myofascial flap (PMMF) or a myocutaneous flap (PMMC). For pharyngeal reconstruction, the PMMF flap is typically used in an onlay fashion and leaves behind the skin and subcutaneous tissue overlying the pectoralis major. In onlay reconstruction, the pharynx is first closed primarily in a tension-reducing T- or Y-pattern [40]. The PMMF is then sutured to the base of tongue, pharyngeal constrictor muscles, and posterior wall of the trachea to lay external to the primary pharyngeal closure and serve as a vascularized wound bed to assist in pharyngeal healing. Retrospective series have shown mixed results with regards to PCF formation in PMMF flap onlay compared to primary closure alone. Some have shown a decreased PCF formation, whereas others have shown a similar rate of PCF formation but decreased size and severity of fistula formation [7, 40–43].

The PMMC flap was initially described by Fabian in 1984 and later simplified by Spriano et al. in 2001 [44, 45]. It is most commonly used as an anterior patch graft when a posterior mucosal pharyngeal strip is left. If a circumferential pharyngeal defect exists, the PMMC flap can be partially tubed and either sutured directly to prevertebral fascia or with an STSG overlying the prevertebral fascia. In these situations, the PMMC flap serves as the anterior and lateral walls of the neopharynx, and the prevertebral fascia/STSG serves as the posterior wall. The PMMC flap in theory can be completely tubed and was historically done prior to the advent of free flaps; however, given their high incidence in pharyngeal stricture, it is infrequently performed [46].

The PM flap has several major advantages, including relative ease to harvest, decreased time in the operating room, and only requiring a single surgeon team. These are particularly advantageous in the patient with multiple comorbidities that may not be able to withstand longer periods of time under general anesthesia. Additionally, in patients with an irradiated neck, microvascular reconstruction may be challenging due to the vessel depletion.

Multiple studies have evaluated rates of pharyngocutaneous fistula after salvage laryngectomy with primary closure, pedicled flap reconstruction (primarily with pectoralis major flaps), or MVFTT (predominantly RFFF and anterolateral thigh free flap (ALT)) [7, 40, 42, 47–52]. Most studies have demonstrated elevated risk of PCF with primary closure, with rates ranging from 9% to 57%, though with conflicting findings regarding the comparison between pedicled flap and MVFTT reconstruction [7, 42, 49, 52]. In a promising early series published in 2009, Patel et al. found that overlay with PMMF after laryngectomy reduced the rate of PCF to 0% in both the primary and salvage setting [42]. A subsequent meta-analysis demonstrated a 22% decreased risk of fistula with PMMF compared to primary closure alone [53]. While data regarding radiation history and other complications was not reported, this study nonetheless suggested a role for routine prophylactic PMMF in the salve setting to reduce the rate of PCF.

While PM flaps have many advantages, its major disadvantage is the bulk that comes from the pectoralis major muscle. Even with denervation and subsequent muscle atrophy, tissue bulk can often tether the tongue and limit its mobility. This can lead to poor functional outcomes, including difficulty with articulation, speech, and swallowing. This tissue bulk can often impede tracheoesophageal speech through impairment of the vibratory quality of the neopharynx [17]. In comparison to patients undergoing primary closure, Deschler et al. showed patients with PM flap reconstruction had a functional voice with similar intensity, pitch, and range; however, the PM flap group was found to have poorer intelligibility, communicative effectiveness, pitch and loudness usage, and fluency compared to those who underwent primary closure [54]. In addition to these functional disadvantages, the PM flaps are associated with donor site morbidity, including shoulder and arm weakness and chest wall contour asymmetries [17]. Given these disadvantages, the PM flaps are traditionally reserved as a backup reconstructive option in the event that initial reconstructive attempts fail.

Supraclavicular Artery Island Flap

The supraclavicular artery island flap (SCAIF) has gained popularity for pharyngeal locoregional reconstruction in recent years. The flap is based on the supraclavicular artery and vein, which branches off the transverse cervical vessels approximately 3–4 cm from their origin off the subclavian vessels. The supraclavicular vascular bundle can be found in a triangle composed of the posterior edge of the sternocleidomastoid muscle (SCM), the external jugular vein, and the medial aspect of the clavicle The incision is started lateral through the distal part of the flap superior to the deltoid muscle. Dissection is performed in a subfascial plane elevating from lateral to medial. The pedicle can sometimes be identified in the medial third of the flap, but may not always be able to be visualized. Once the medial limit of dissection is met, the overlying skin is superficially incised down to subcutaneous tissue on the superior side of the flap and subfascial on the inferior side of the flap to create a tunnel. The flap is then pulled through the tunnel to reconstruct the pharyngeal defect [55]. If one side of the neck is at risk for great vessel exposure due to prior surgery or radiotherapy, it is recommended to harvest the SCAIF from the affected side, as the proximal soft tissue pedicle can provide vessel coverage in addition to pharyngeal closure. Otherwise, it is recommended to use the patient's nondominant side to minimize donor site morbidity [56].

Emerick et al. reported a large case series in 2014 demonstrating the utility of this flap and popularized its use in pharyngeal reconstruction [56]. The SCAIF can be used as an adipofascial flap to reinforce primary pharyngeal closure in an onlay fashion or as a fasciocutaneous flap to serve as a patch graft in a partial pharyngeal defect. Reconstruction with a tubed SCAIF for circumferential pharyngeal defects has been reported, though this is infrequently performed due to limitation in flap width that can be harvested [57–59].

A major benefit of the SCAIF is its ability to reconstruct anterior neck skin (Fig. 8.3). This is particularly useful in cases of salvage laryngectomy where reduced skin elasticity after radiation can make primary closure challenging. It is also helpful in tracheostomy-dependent patients, where excision of stromal tissue leaves a cutaneous defect. The SCAIF tissue is an excellent thickness match for this area of the neck, especially in comparison to PM flaps. The SCAIF has very minimal donor site morbidity. Similar to other locoregional reconstructive options, the SCAIF can be quickly harvested and can be performed by a single surgeon team [56].

The SCAIF can only be used in selected patient populations. Those undergoing extensive neck dissections may have their transverse cervical vasculature ligated, which removes the SCAIF as a reconstructive option. Additionally, some have experienced variable success due to anatomical variations in the vascular pedicle. This can be potentially be avoided through the use of Doppler to trace out the vessels prior to flap harvest [56].

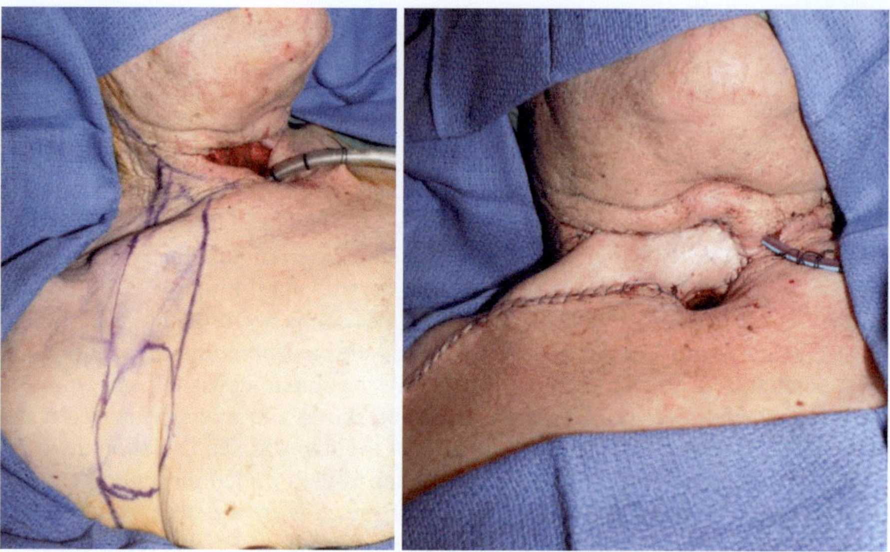

Fig. 8.3 Supraclavicular artery island flap (SCAIF) reconstruction of the anterior neck following laryngectomy

Microvascular Free Tissue Transfer (MVFTT)

Visceral flaps such as jejunal flaps were originally described in pedicled fashion for esophageal reconstruction and have been utilized as free flaps in animal models since as early as 1959 [60]. Over the past several decades, MVFTT has emerged as a popular modality for reconstruction of complex defects throughout the head and neck [61]. With recent advances in surgical technique and postoperative care, head and neck MVFTT has become increasingly reliable with failure rates ranging from 0 to 3.8% in recent series [62, 63]. A variety of donor sites have been described in the literature for pharyngoesophageal reconstruction since the 1980s (Table 8.3) and offer a range of options to fit each patient's defect. Fasciocutaneous thigh-based and forearm-based free flaps were the first described for pharyngoesophageal reconstruction and remain among the most popular options to this day. Careful consideration of patient factors (comorbidities, body habitus, prior surgery, prior radiation history, etc.), the anticipated defect, and donor site morbidity are mandatory for successful MVFTT reconstruction.

Forearm Free Flaps

Originally described by Yang et al. in 1981, the radial forearm free flap (RFFF) has emerged as a workhorse flap in head and neck reconstruction [64, 65]. Relative ease of harvest, long pedicle length, and thin, pliable tissue make it a versatile option for

Table 8.3 Free flaps utilized in laryngopharyngeal reconstruction

Upper extremity
Radial forearm free flap (RFFF)
Ulnar forearm free flap (UFFF)
Lateral arm free flap
Lower extremity
Anterolateral thigh free flap (ALT)
Anteromedial thigh free flap (AMT)
Profunda artery perforator flap (PAP)
Medial sural artery perforator flap (MSAP)
Tensor fascia Lata free flap (TFL)
Subscapular system
Parascapular free flap
Latissimus Dorsi free flap
Head and neck
Temporoparietal fascia free flap
Abdominal
Jejunal free flap
Gastro-omental free flap

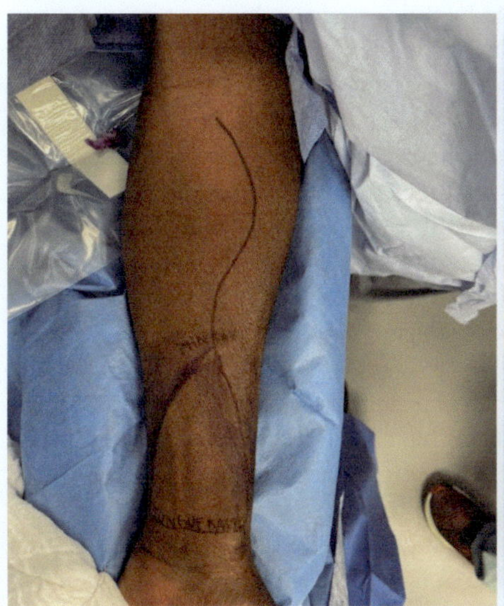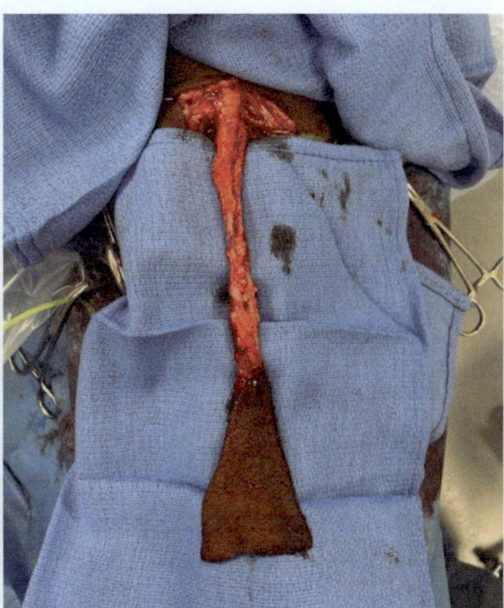

Fig. 8.4 "Shield" design of radial forearm free flap

a variety of defects. The radial forearm free flap is based on the radial artery as it courses toward the wrist with deep venous drainage coming from venae comitantes associated with the radial artery, but can also be designed to include superficial accessory drainage from the cephalic vein. The skin paddle is typically centered over the radial artery and may be designed in a shield pattern to account for the greater circumference at the base of tongue compared to the esophagus (Fig. 8.4). A preoperative Allen's test, either by clinical examination or by duplex sonography, should be performed to ensure adequate perfusion to the hand through an intact palmar arch will be maintained after sacrifice of the radial artery. The flap is typically harvested from the nondominant hand to minimize functional deficits after surgery. In most cases, the donor site defect cannot be closed primarily and requires either skin grafting or local flap closure. Typically the wrist is kept in a splint for several weeks to prevent shearing of the skin graft from the underlying tendons and musculature. Donor site morbidity is typically minor, but can include decreased grip strength and range of motion, hypesthesia from injury to the superficial branch of the radial nerve, and poor cosmesis [66]. Flexor carpi radialis tendon exposure can develop due to failure of the overlying skin graft from shearing and if left untreated can result in impaired mobility of the wrist [67]. The exposed tendon may be covered with a skin graft, local flap, or biologic dressing to facilitate healing [66].

Described as an alternative to the radial forearm free flap in the 1980s, the ulnar artery perforator free flap (UAPFF) serves as another option for reconstructions requiring thin, pliable tissue [68]. The UAPFF is a thin flap with the additional benefit of allowing chimeric design with multiple independent skin paddles based on individual perforators. The perforators can be identified using preoperative Doppler assessment when planning for chimeric designs. The skin of the medial forearm also tends to be less hirsute than that of the lateral forearm, which can be an advantage in oral cavity reconstruction (particularly after glossectomy), though this is less critical in pharyngeal reconstruction. However, given concerns that sacrificing the ulnar artery would compromise blood flow to the hand and the risk of injury to the ulnar nerve during pedicle dissection, the ulnar forearm free flap has been less popular than the radial forearm [69]. Furthermore, the pedicle tends to be slightly shorter than that of the radial forearm with smaller-caliber vessels, particularly in the ulnar vena comitantes [69]. In patients in whom a radial forearm flap is not an option or a more complex chimeric design is desired for multilayered or through-and-through defects (e.g., for reconstruction of tracheoesophageal fistulae), the UAPFF serves as a useful alternative to the RFFF [70].

Since Harii et al. first utilized the RFFF in pharyngoesophageal reconstruction as a tubed flap in 1985, a variety of modifications have been described to address additional reconstructive concerns [61, 71]. For example, subcutaneous fat and fascia may be harvested around the vascular pedicle to provide additional bulk and protection at the anastomosis, or an additional skin paddle can be designed to serve as an external monitor paddle [72, 73]. The medial or lateral antebrachial cutaneous nerve can also be harvested with the UAPFF or RFFF to create a sensate flap [74]. Because of the pliability of the tissue, the forearm flaps can be folded to reconstruct the pharyngeal defect and skin simultaneously [75]. This technique can also be applied to reconstruct the tracheal and esophageal walls in patients who develop tracheoesophageal fistulae (TEF) after tracheoesophageal puncture [76]. The RFFF is much less bulky than the pedicled pectoralis flap or most other free flaps, making it a good option in overweight and obese patients. This decreased bulk also facilitates recovery of swallowing function postoperatively and restoration of speech with tracheoesophageal puncture [77–79]. However, this may come at the cost of increased risk of postoperative pharyngocutaneous fistulae relative to other reconstructive options [79]. Early studies with RFFF demonstrated rates of PCF ranging from 17% to 25% with higher rates of fistula and anastomotic stricture with tubed RFFF, particularly when compared to jejunal free flaps [79–81]. While direct comparisons with patients undergoing primary closure or pedicled flaps were not available in these studies, these rates of complications are comparable to those described with the PMMF.

Anterolateral Thigh Free Flap (ALT)

Along with the RFFF, the ALT free flap has been established as one of the primary options for soft tissue reconstruction of the head and neck. First described as a fasciocutaneous flap based on perforators from the descending branch of the circumflex femoral artery by Song et al. in 1984, the ALT can also be harvested as a myocutaneous, adipofascial, or even osteocutaneous flap by including muscular perforators to the vastus lateralis muscle or femur cortex [82]. With the possibility of multiple skin paddles based on individual perforators and including vastus lateralis muscle supplied by perforators from the distal pedicle, the ALT has great versatility to fit a variety of complex defects (Fig. 8.5). The pedicle tends to be quite long with large vessel caliber [82]. If desired, it can also be harvested with the lateral femoral cutaneous nerve to create a sensate flap. Donor site morbidity tends to be minimal, although the long incision along the lateral thigh can be unsightly. Primary closure of the donor site can often be achieved after harvest of wide fasciocutaneous components (up to approximately 10 cm depending on skin laxity). The bulk of the flap can be a limitation in some cases, as the flap can be quite thick in obese patients. The perforator anatomy of the ALT free flap can also be somewhat variable; in some cases, perforators from the lateral circumflex femoral artery may be absent, necessitating conversion to the anteromedial thigh (AMT) flap based on a medial

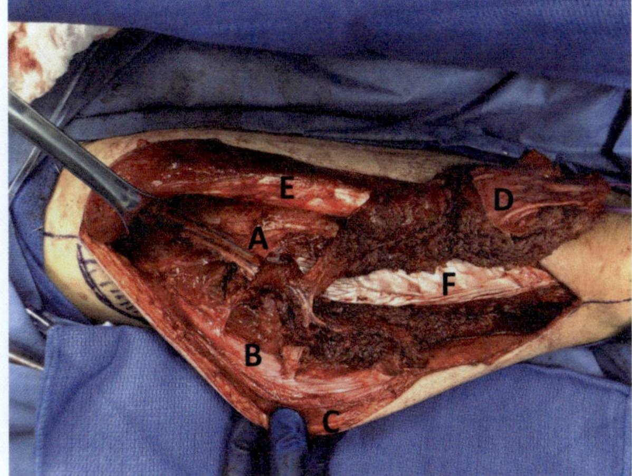

Fig. 8.5 Anterolateral thigh free flap with pedicled vastus lateralis muscle flap. (**a**) Pedicle, (**b**) Skin perforators, (**c**) Skin paddle, (**d**) Vastus lateralis, (**e**) Rectus femoris, (**f**) Vastus intermedius

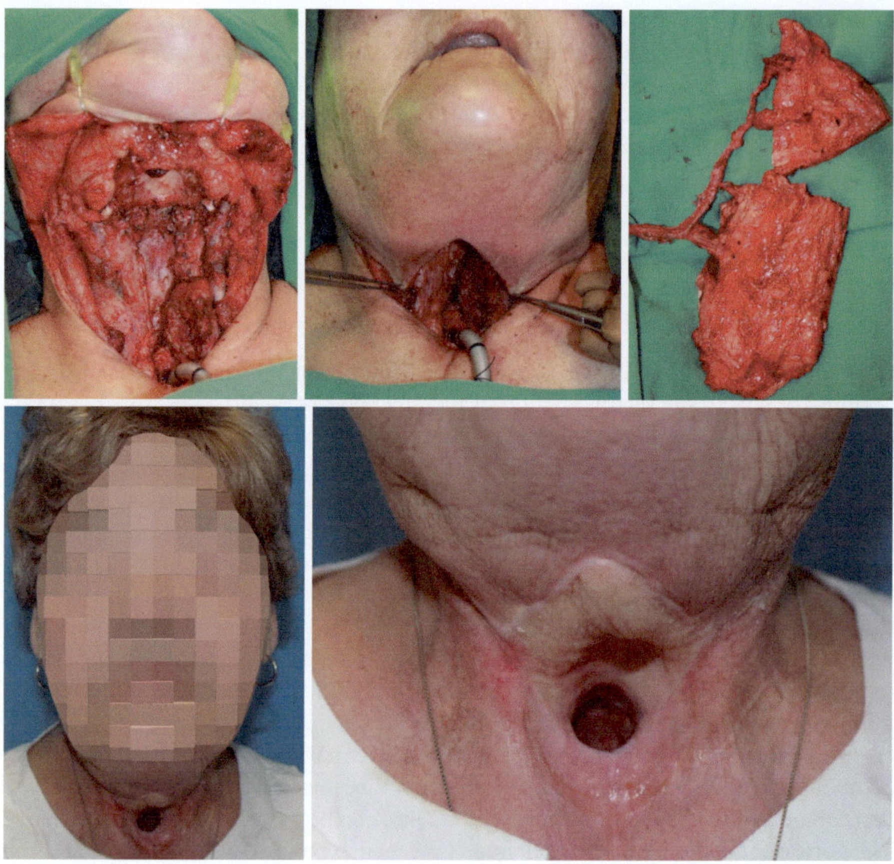

Fig. 8.6 Chimeric anterolateral thigh free flap (ALT) microvascular free tissue transfer (MVFTT) reconstruction of a total laryngopharyngectomy requiring anterior neck soft tissue reconstruction

descending branch [83]. Evaluation of perforator anatomy using the Doppler can be helpful for planning purposes, particularly when very large skin paddles or chimeric designs are desired. Because much of the flap can be raised without committing to specific dimensions on the skin paddle, flap harvest can start earlier in the case before the final defect size is known, allowing for greater efficiency.

As with the RFFF, the ALT can be used both as an interpositional or patch design and as a tubed graft after total pharyngectomy. In cases where skin resection is required or there is insufficient skin laxity for closure, as is often the case in salvage cases after prior radiation, an additional skin paddle can be harvested in a chimeric fashion to resurface the skin and serve as a monitor paddle (Fig. 8.6) [51]. Alternatively, when a radical or modified radical neck dissection is performed with resection of the sternocleidomastoid muscle, a vastus lateralis muscle flap based off perforators from the distal pedicle can also be used with a skin graft to provide skin coverage (Fig. 8.3). To bolster the pharyngeal repair, the fascia can be wrapped around the flap and secured to the prevertebral fascia to create a two-layer closure of the pharynx [51]. Because of its greater size and bulk, the ALT also serves as a good option when total glossectomy is performed with laryngopharyngectomy as it can fill the floor of mouth defect and close the pharyngeal defect with a single paddle.

The ALT free flap is favored by many surgeons for pharyngeal reconstruction due to the additional flexibility afforded by the flap to perform multilayered reconstruction using fascia and muscle, which is not possible with other flaps. Yu et al. described a series of patients constructed using a multilayered closure with the ALT for both partial and circumferential defects using fascia to reinforce suture lines with a fistula rate of 9%, including 10% among patients in the salvage setting [51]. Similarly, Chen et al. found that closure utilizing multilayer closure with fascial underlay significantly decreased rates of PCF (3% vs. 20%) when compared to single-layer closure.

Because most studies comparing the impact of reconstructive techniques were small, underpowered retrospective series, larger multicenter studies were designed to further elucidate the efficacy of various reconstructive modalities in preventing PCF. Patel et al. described a multicenter retrospective study of 359 patients and found that the rate of PCF was highest in the primary closure cohort (34%) [69]. There were lower rates of fistula with pectoralis muscle onlay flap (15%) than with free flap (25%), though this difference was not statistically significant. Of note, the majority of free flaps performed in this cohort were RFFF, which may have contributed to the higher rate of PCF. In 2019, the Microvascular Committee of the American Academy of Otolaryngology-Head & Neck Surgery published a separate large, multicenter retrospective review of 486 patients who underwent salvage laryngectomy or laryngopharyngectomy [69]. As with the Patel study, this study demonstrated significant reduction in the rate of PCF with vascularized tissue compared to primary closure, although it did not find any significant difference in the rate of fistula among reconstructions with or without augmentation with muscle. Ultimately, these large retrospective studies were unable to distinctly identify a superior reconstructive approach, though both clearly demonstrated the importance of vascularized tissue augmentation compared to primary closure alone in the post-radiation setting.

Enteric Conduit Options for Pharyngoesophageal Replacement

Gastric Conduit

Enteric conduits are generally utilized in the setting of pharyngectomies requiring concurrent esophagectomy beyond the cervical esophagus. In these deformities, either the length of required soft tissue replacement is too long for regional flap or MVFTT reconstruction (e.g., deformity of the pharynx to the stomach in total esophagectomy) or the reconstructive suture line is intrathoracic, precluding a safe soft tissue anastomosis as any breakdown could lead to mediastinitis. While there are several enteric donor tissues for pharygnoesophageal reconstruction, the tubularized gastric conduit is considered the preferred method for esophageal replacement given its ease of construction and requirement of only a single pharyngeal anastomosis (Fig. 8.7), [84, 85]. The stomach is a well-vascularized organ, which is supplied by the left gastric artery that arises from the celiac axis, the right gastric artery that arises from the proper hepatic artery, the left gastroepiploic artery arising from the splenic artery, the right gastroepiploic artery arising from the gastroduodenal artery, and short gastric vessels arising from the distal splenic artery [86]. For a tubularized gastric conduit, the vascular supply is exclusively the right gastroepiploic artery [87]. Consequently, this vessel must be identified and preserved at all costs during conduit construction and intraoperative factors associated with hypoperfusion should be mitigated.

Preoperatively, because anastomotic complications are a significant source of morbidity after pharyngoesophectomy, it is prudent to optimize medical comorbidities associated with such complications, including cigarette use, malnutrition, obesity, chronic obstructive pulmonary disease, corticosteroid use, renal insufficiency, hypertension, and heart failure preoperatively [88–91].

Following transthoracic mobilization of the esophagus and mediastinal lymphadenectomy, the operation proceeds with transabdominal construction of the conduit, which can be performed via a traditional "open" approach or minimally invasive techniques. During the gastric mobilization, a strict "no touch" technique should be used to minimize trauma to the microvascular blood supply of the eventual gastric conduit. Conduit preparation is begun by taking down the gastrohepatic

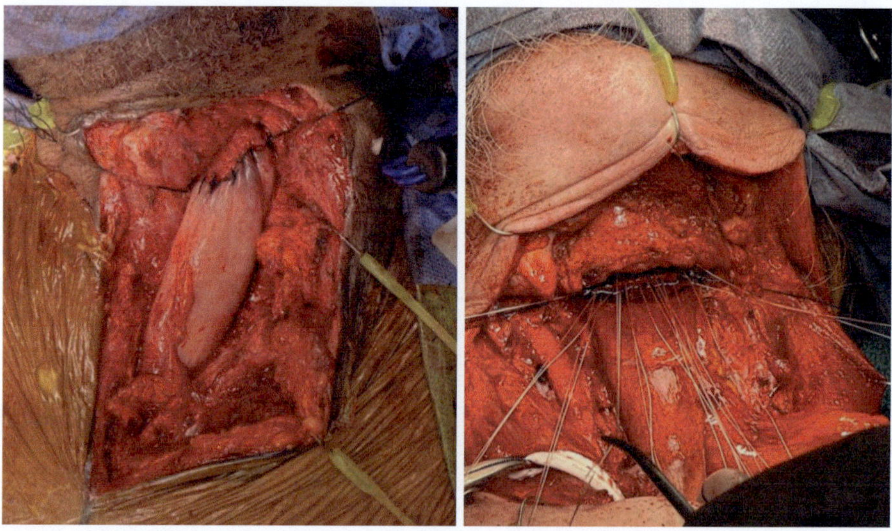

Fig. 8.7 Gastric pull up reconstruction of total laryngopharyngectomy and esophagectomy defect

ligament and continuing to the base of the right crus. The left gastric artery and vein are skeletonized and divided. At the greater curvature, after identifying the course of the right gastroepiploic artery, the greater omentum is separated from the transverse mesocolon, and the short gastric vessels are taken down all of the way to the angle of His. Any remaining retrogastric attachments are also taken down. Because the stomach is tethered by the hilum of the liver rather than the lateral attachments of the duodenum, a former Kocher maneuver has little value. However, it is important to take down all retrogastric and antropyloric attachments, and, for those patients who have undergone cholecystectomy, adhesions to the gallbladder fossa, as these can impair mobility of the gastric conduit. The esophagus is circumferentially mobilized into the mediastinum until the transabdominal dissection plane communicates with the transthoracic dissection plane. During the thoracic phase of the operation, the distal esophagus is looped with a Penrose drain to assure that esophagus has been fully mobilized. If desired, a gastric emptying procedure and feeding jejunostomy tube may be placed.

Though anastomotic complications are similar, because of its greater reach, (likely) improved conduit emptying, and superior functional outcomes, a gastric tube is preferred over the whole stomach as a gastric conduit [92]. Because of the location of microvascular anastomotic branches between the left gastric and right gastroepiploic vessels, the preferred width of the conduit is approximately 4 cm [87]. While preserving one to two branches of the right gastric artery along the lesser curve, conduit construction begins with a linear stapler approximately 5 cm cephalad to the pylorus and continues along a line parallel to the greater curvature. A key technical maneuver is to provide simultaneous cephalad (at the apex of the fundus) and caudal retraction (on the body of the stomach), in order to create a long, straight conduit, without spiraling.

Anastomotic complications are a significant source of morbidity and mortality after pharyngoesophagectomy. A meta-analysis of mainly retrospective reviews and case series of laryngopharyngectomies followed by gastric pull up from 1990 to 2014 found the risk of anastomotic leak to range from 0 to 23% [85]. Most were successfully treated with nonoperative management including NPO status, nutritional support, antibiotics, and drainage. For larger leaks, soft tissue coverage over a salivary bypass tube may be required [93]. Gastric conduit necrosis, which is a feared complication, has been reported in up to 5% of patients, is a significant risk for perioperative mortality, and may require resection and diversion if there is significant conduit loss [94]. As a consequence of ischemia, tension, and healed leaks, anastomotic strictures occur in approximately 5–10% of patients; dilatation is the primary method of treatment [95].

Given the significant source of morbidity and mortality associated with anastomotic complications, investigators have explored methods to mitigate this risk. Several have investigated gastric ischemic preconditioning by embolization of, or laparoscopic ligation of, the left gastric artery typically at least a week before esophagectomy. However, strong evidence supporting this technique is lacking, and it has not gained widespread acceptance [96]. However, there are certain populations (yet to be clarified) where preconditioning may have specific value, such as current or recent smokers. To improve blood flow to the tip of the gastric tube, others have explored the use of a supercharged anastomoses to the transverse cervical artery and to the external jugular vein, anterior jugular vein, or internal jugular vein [97]. Further studies are needed to determine when microvascular anastomoses have added value.

An alternative to the standard isoperistaltic gastric tube is a reversed gastric tube based on the left gastroepiploic pedicle. It has the advantages of greater length compared with an isoperistaltic gastric tube and, like an isoperistatic tube, only requires a single anastomosis. Its long staple line and tenuous blood supply are distinct disadvantages. To enhance blood flow, investigators have explored use of a supercharged graft with promising results [98]. However, this technique has not gained widespread acceptance, and an isoperistatic tube remains the first conduit of choice.

Colonic Interposition

Despite the stomach being the most popular choice for esophageal replacement, the colon has reliably been used as a conduit since the early 1900s [99]. The stomach may not be a suitable conduit either because it does not have the appropriate length, there is prior gastric surgery such as weight loss operations, or underlying gastric pathology. The colon interposition is an appropriate alternative conduit that can reliably reach the pharynx. It has advantages of its length, resistance to bile and acid reflux, and its robust vascular supply [100]. The colon is also a good option in cases of surgical salvage of a failed gastric conduit. Careful preoperative evaluation of the entire colon is needed to determine if the colon is a suitable replacement option.

A CT scan with arterial enhancement is helpful for assessing the colonic vasculature or colonic pathology. Patients with underlying cardiovascular disease may have calcification or stenosis of the superior and inferior mesenteric arteries and the colic vessels and may influence whether a left or right interposition or alternative conduit is used [101]. To exclude underlying pathology, all patients 45 years of age and older, younger patients with known colon pathology, and those with a family history of colon cancer should have a colonoscopy within the proceeding 5 years.

The blood supply for an ascending colon graft originates off the superior mesenteric artery (SMA) and the ileocolic artery, whereas the blood supply for a descending colon graft originates from the inferior mesenteric artery (IMA) and the ascending branch of the left colic. In addition, the Marginal Artery of Drummond forms a variable and important anastomotic connection between the SMA and IMA [101]. The right colon has a more variable vascular anatomy. As a result, the descending colon graft is generally preferred for most patients. It is also important to note that anatomic variations of the middle colic artery include complete absence in up to 25% of patients with presence of an accessory middle colic artery in 10% [102].

During graft harvest, the colon should be fully mobilized off its peritoneal and retroperitoneal attachments to allow splaying of its mesentery and assessment of the vascular arcades. Transillumination is done to identify the blood supply. Prior to vascular division, the vessels are temporarily clamped, and a handheld Doppler is used to assure adequate flow to the tip of the planned conduit and to the colocolostomy. It is important to preserve the distal vascular arcades during the mesenteric dissection. Both left and right interpositions are typically prepared in an isoperistaltic fashion, which has been shown to improve functional outcomes and minimize the risk of spasms [103, 104]. There is typically ample length to perform a handsewn anastomosis to as high as the base of the tongue. If the anastomosis is under tension, additional length can be achieved by further dividing the mesentery while preserving the blood supply to the graft, although most colonic conduits can reach the pharynx without additional lengthening maneuvers [105]. In the rare instance that the arterial flow or the venous drainage of the tip of the conduit is impaired, a supercharged microvascular arterial and/or venous anastomosis can be performed (Fig. 8.8), [106, 107].

It is preferable to construct the distal anastomosis of the colon interposition to the stomach, even if the amount of stomach remaining is limited. When a total gastrectomy has been performed, anecdotally, colon interpositions function better when the anastomosis is constructed on the duodenum rather than a roux limb of jejunum. A key technical point of all esophageal replacement grafts is for the graft to lie as straight as possible in order to facilitate conduit emptying and thus improve functional outcomes. Conduit emptying is mainly passive relying on gravity. Redundancy of the conduit can lead to dysphagia and aspiration [103]. After gently pulling down the redundancy in the graft from the abdomen, it is recommended to tack the interposition graft to the hiatus to minimize tension with permanent braided suture.

Though colon interposition has been a reliable conduit for esophageal replacement after pharyngoesophagectomy, it has a longer operative time and requires

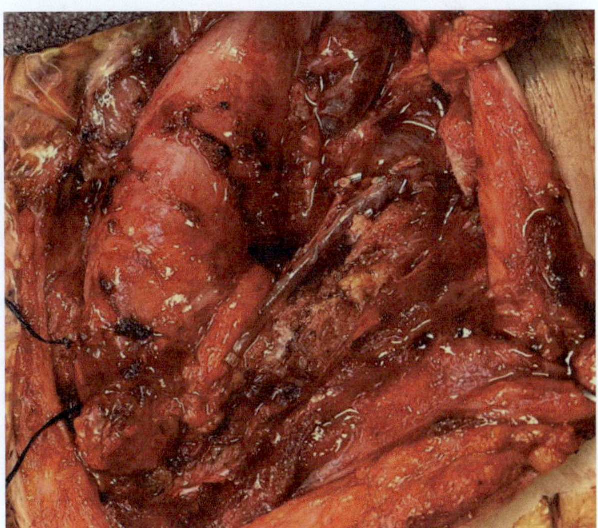

Fig. 8.8 Supercharged colon interposition graft reconstruction of a total esophagectomy defect

more (three rather than one) anastomoses as compared with the gastric pull up [108]. Postoperative mortality has been reported to be as high as 5–17% but is typically less than 5% in high volume centers [109–111]. Published anastomotic leak rates vary widely from 0 to 50%, but larger studies from high volume centers suggest a rate of approximately 10%. Graft necrosis represents the most serious surgical complication, occurring in less than 2.4% of patients in experienced centers but is the most common cause of reoperation and a significant cause of mortality [112, 113].

Functional outcomes after colon interposition are excellent and may be better than a gastric conduit due to a lower risk of reflux and dysphagia [114]. The majority of patients (75–100%) after colon interposition are able to resume oral intake, and more than half resume a normal diet. In one prospective study looking at the long-term functional outcomes in a selected group of long-term survivors who underwent colonic interposition, 89% of patient reported no dysphagia, 84% reported no regurgitation or reflux, and 91% were able to consume three or more meals daily [115]. Quality of life metrics 21 months and 10 years after interposition were at normal values. Of note, 11% had required surgical revision for symptoms related to redundancy, highlighting the importance of minimizing this technical complication during the index operation.

Supercharged Jejunal Interposition

Another alternative to a tubularized gastric conduit is a pedicled jejunal graft and a microvascular ("supercharged") anastomosis. The jejunum has been used for decades as a conduit, and supercharging allows for a generous length of jejunum to be utilized for high neck anastomoses [116]. As compared with a colon interposition graft, advantages of a supercharged jejunal conduit are its more reliable vascular supply. It also offers a similar size to the native esophagus, is generally free of intrinsic disease, is less prone to redundancy, and maintains peristalsis, which may improve functional outcomes [117]. However, it tends to be more at risk for marginal ulceration and requires a trained microvascular surgeon to construct the supercharged microvascular anastomosis, which increases the operative time [118].

Harvest of a supercharged jejunal conduit starts with identifying a segment of jejunum 20 cm to 30 cm from the ligament of Treitz. The vascular supply should be carefully assessed. The first jejunal branch off the SMA is preserved while the second branch is divided and clamped and used for the eventual microanastomosis. The third branch can be ligated to allow for appropriate length, and the fourth branch should be preserved to its SMA supply [119]. Like other conduit options, transillumination and Doppler ultrasonography is important to assure an intact vascular arcade. Once fully mobilized, the conduit should be exteriorized and brought to the desired location at the neck to determine if there is adequate length for a tension-free anastomosis. If there is not adequate length, one option is to divide some of the mesentery between the jejunal branches while preserving the arcades. An indicator flap is fashioned by dividing a short segment of the most superior portion of the jejunum (but remains connected to the mesentery). Typically, a left partial first rib resection and hemimanubriectomy with resection of the head of the clavicle is performed at the neck to allow space for the conduit and its mesentery. Arterial and venous microvascular anastomoses from the second jejunal branch to the chest (internal mammary artery) or neck (most commonly the transverse cervical artery) are performed. The end-to-end pharyngo-jejunal anastomosis is typically hand-sewn. The distal end of the jejunum is then anastomosed to the posterior stomach, or it can be connected in a Roux-en-Y formation [120].

Several small studies have looked at outcomes following supercharged jejunal interposition and found low rates of mortality, anastomotic leak, and graft loss. The largest series (60 patients) noted a 30-day mortality of 5% [118]. The anastomotic leak rate was 32%. However, half of those leaks were of minimal clinical significance, identified by contrast study alone and were managed with simple drainage. Conduit loss was reported in 8.3% of cases contributing to the majority of the 31% of reoperations. In this series, functional outcomes were favorable with 83% able to return to an oral diet. Interestingly, postoperative manometry of some of these patients with successful reconstruction revealed intact jejunal peristalsis, which is thought to aid in passage of food boluses. However, in those undergoing total larnygopharyngectomy and tracheoesophageal puncture, peristalsis may interfere with speech production. Long-term functional outcome were good with 80% of patients having no dysphagia and 78% able to maintain a total oral diet for nutrition [121].

Route of Conduit

Enteric conduits can be passed from the abdomen to the neck via one of four routes. The most common and preferred route is the *posterior mediastinal* position or the orthotopic esophageal location. This provides the shortest path and forms the most natural lie for a gastric, colon or jejunal conduit [122]. However, in cases where the posterior mediastinum is hostile (i.e., after esophageal exclusion), an alternative route is needed.

The *substernal* route is the most common option when the posterior mediastinum is not available. The conduit sits between the sternum and the anterior pericardium. Typically, the graft can be tunneled in the substernal space without performing a full sternotomy. Care must be taken for patients who have had a prior median sternotomy, especially those that have undergone coronary artery bypass grafting due to the risk of iatrogenic injury during sternal re-entry [123]. Typically, performance of a left hemimanubriectomy and resection of the left sternoclavicular joint to avoid impingement on the conduit should be performed.

A large Japanese retrospective analysis of gastric conduits undergoing retrosternal versus posterior mediastinal review found a lower leak rate 11.7% versus 13.8% in the posterior mediastinal group but a higher rate of surgical site infection (14.9% vs. 8.4%). In addition, the risk of pneumonias were higher in the posterior mediastinal route (13.7% vs. 12.2%) [124, 125]. No difference in morbidity was seen. Other studies have also demonstrated an increased leak rate when using the substernal route.

The *intra-pleural* route, which involves passage of the conduit through the left pleural space anterior or posterior to the pulmonary hilum, is a rarely used alternative to a substernal pull up that requires a longer length of conduit as compared with the posterior mediastinum or substernal route [124]. A *subcutaneous* route is also seldom used, but when other spaces are not available, a subcutaneous tunnel above the sternum with the conduit exiting the abdomen via a subxyphoid ventral hernia can be created and connected to the subcutaneous neck where the pharyngeal anastomosis is performed. The conduit again will require a longer length and comes with a poorer cosmetic outcome.

Postoperative Considerations

Voice Rehabilitation

Loss of the ability to phonate is a debilitating consequence of total laryngectomy. Since early attempts to develop an artificial larynx for phonation in the late nineteenth century, numerous advances have been made in vocal rehabilitation after laryngectomy in both available prostheses and devices, and in techniques that can be utilized to optimize communication [126]. Today, the primary modalities utilized by patients for phonation are the electrolarynx, tracheoesophageal (TE) speech, and esophageal speech. Understanding of these options is important for the reconstructive surgeon as the techniques used in pharyngeal reconstruction can impact patients' ability to communicate postoperatively.

Electrolarynx

Replacing older mechanical devices, the electrolarynx is a battery-powered device that vibrates the tissues of the oral cavity and pharynx to produce speech either through direct contact in the neck or a plastic tube that is placed in the oral cavity. Because it is easy to use and can be utilized by virtually all patients who have undergone laryngectomy, the electrolarynx is often the first option offered to patients after surgery. Further, it does not preclude use of esophageal or tracheoesophageal (TE) speech and serves as a useful backup. Although some patients may be unable to use the device directly on the neck if there is excessively thick tissue, most are typically able to use it intraorally. Despite its versatility, the electrolarynx does have some drawbacks. While newer models do allow pitch modulation to allow for more natural-sounding speech, the electrolarynx has a mechanical sound quality and allows limited intonation due to its fixed fundamental frequency which may limit intelligibility. As with other forms of alaryngeal speech, a fair amount of time and practice is required to achieve maximum intelligibility. Most models also require the user to hold the device during phonation, although some newer devices have hands-free functionality. While the electrolarynx is typically readily available to patients in the United States, access may be more difficult in other settings. Nonetheless, the electrolarynx is an excellent option for most patients and with proper training can serve as an effective means of verbal communication after laryngectomy.

Esophageal Speech

Because it relies on the vibration of the patient's pharyngoesophageal tissues to generate sound and does not require any additional prostheses or equipment, esophageal speech is the oldest form of alaryngeal speech. With esophageal speech, air is ingested and forcefully passed back through the pharyngoesophageal segment, generating vibrations which serve as the foundation of the voice. Unlike with the electrolarynx, the voice quality with esophageal speech more closely approximates that of normal laryngeal speech [127]. Furthermore, it does not require the user to use any prostheses or devices, allowing for hands-free speech. While esophageal speech only relies on the patient's normal remaining anatomy for generation of voice, it requires a significant amount of training and expertise to generate reliable speech. Even with practice, speech intelligibility tends to be inferior to that with TE speech and is limited in duration due to the need to expel air from the gastrointestinal tract rather the lungs. Esophageal speech is a good option in motivated patients who are unwilling or unable to undergo tracheoesophageal puncture (TEP) and have access to speech pathologists who are knowledgeable with the technique.

Tracheoesophageal Puncture (TEP)

In the appropriate patient, TE speech is the gold standard in alaryngeal speech as it produces a voice more similar to native laryngeal speech than either the electrolarynx or esophageal speech. TE speech allows for greater clarity, maximum intensity, and phonatory duration than esophageal speech and a much more natural quality than electrolarynx. These advantages allow TE speakers to enjoy improved voice-related quality of life than those using either electrolarynx or esophageal speech [128].

To facilitate TE speech, a tracheoesophageal puncture is performed, generating a controlled fistula between the trachea and the neopharynx or esophagus through which a prosthesis with a one-way valve is placed. This valve allows for direction of air into the pharyngoesophageal segment with occlusion of the tracheostoma while preventing aspiration of food or secretions. TEP can be performed primarily at the time of laryngectomy or at a later time. There is concern regarding the risk of postoperative complications with primary TEP as a prior analysis of the National Surgical Quality Improvement Program (NSQIP) database demonstrated increased overall wound complication rate, though the rates of surgical site infection and return to the operating room did not differ [129]. Patients requiring complex reconstruction with MVFTT or bowel transposition may not be candidates for primary TEP, though some of these patients may be eligible after sufficient time has passed for wound healing. It is the author's preference to wait at least 3 months after reconstruction before placing TEP. A retrospective series by Gitomer et al. found that in patients undergoing MVFTT for pharyngeal reconstruction, those undergoing secondary TEP had higher utilization rates that those who underwent primary TEP [130]. The method of reconstruction of the pharynx may also affect speech outcomes, as patients with muscle augmentation—primarily from the pectoralis flaps—have been shown to have worse speech and swallowing outcomes [52].

While TE speech is an excellent modality for voice rehabilitation after laryngotomy, a high level of cognitive function and dexterity is required to use and maintain the prosthesis. Furthermore, most patients will require exchange of their prosthesis at least a few times a year if not more frequently, adding greater complexity and expense to their care [131]. While surgical complications from the TEP are uncommon, issues that interfere with patients' ability to produce TE speech are more common [131]. These can include spasms or stenosis of the pharynx, stenosis of the stoma, prosthesis malfunction, and enlargement of the TEP site. The latter complication may be particularly problematic as leakage through the TEP can result in increased risk of pneumonia [132]. Enlarging TEP sites can usually be managed with conservative measures such as placement of larger prostheses, though a small proportion of patients will require closure of the fistula [132]. These defects often arise in radiated patients and can be challenging to manage due to the need for robust tissue to repair the defect without excessive bulk, which would obstruct the pharynx or tracheostoma; techniques using folded or double-paddled forearm free flaps have been described to manage these complex defects [70, 133].

Swallowing Outcomes

Patients with advanced laryngeal and pharyngeal cancers often suffer from significant dysphagia, which results from either their malignancy or adverse effects from treatment. For example, subsequent analysis of RTOG 91-11—which excluded patients with very advanced T4 disease—demonstrated that 27% of patients were gastrostomy dependent prior to treatment due to severe laryngeal dysfunction [134]. Patients undergoing concurrent chemoradiation suffer high rates of severe toxicity; 77% of patients in the concurrent chemoradiation arm of RTOG 91-11 suffered from grade 3 or 4 adverse effects during treatment with 35% experience severe pharyngeal or esophageal toxicity [4]. Retrospective analysis of functional outcomes following concurrent chemoradiation in RTOG 91-11, 97-03, and 99-14 demonstrated high rates of severe late toxicity (43%) with older age, advanced T stage, and laryngeal/hypopharyngeal primaries identified as independent risk factors on multivariate analysis [134]. While patients who undergo laryngectomy are no longer at risk of aspiration, restoration of functional swallow can be a challenge, particularly in the salvage setting. Furthermore, while much has been published in the literature regarding the impact of reconstructive techniques of development of pharyngocutaneous fistula, the data describing functional outcomes are relatively sparse.

Postoperative dysphagia following total laryngectomy is quite common with up to 72–87% of patients reporting dysphagia after surgery, which may be related to alterations in contractility of the residual pharynx and dysfunction from prior treatment [135]. Similarly, rates of gastrostomy tube dependence vary with retrospective series report rates of up to 57% after salvage total laryngectomy [49, 50, 81, 136]. Worley et al. found patients who had advanced disease (pT4 or pN2+) or underwent re-irradiation to be at high risk of long-term gastrostomy dependence [135]. Comparison of gastrostomy tube rates among different reconstructive options is challenging as operative technique varies greatly among surgeons and institutions, and numerous factors unrelated to the reconstruction influence the need for gastrostomy [137]. Nonetheless, many patients are able to regain some degree of swallowing function. Hutcheson et al. reported a series of 23 patients undergoing salvage laryngectomy for laryngopharyngeal dysfunction and found that all patients tolerated oral intake with only 17% of patients requiring supplemental enteral nutrition postoperatively despite 74% being gastrostomy dependent prior to surgery.

Strictures occur relatively frequently after laryngectomy, with rates ranging from 13% to 50% [138]. Strictures are particularly common in tubed flaps (up to 50%), likely due to the circumferential repair at the esophageal anastomosis [81, 137]. Sweeny et al. found that patients undergoing primary closure had lower rates of stricture than those who underwent RFFF reconstruction, with similar rates of stricture regardless of prior radiation [138]. In their series, they also found that patients who required only a single dilation had better dietary outcomes than those who required serial dilations [138]. Yu et al. published a series of 114 patients who underwent reconstruction with ALT free flaps and reported a much lower stricture rate (6%) including only a 9% stricture rate in patients with circumferential defects [51]. In their series, a vertical incision was carried along the anterior esophageal wall to increase the diameter of the anastomosis, which has contributed to their lower stricture rate.

References

1. SEER*Explorer: an interactive website for SEER cancer statistics [Internet]. Surveillance Research Program, N.C.I.C.S.A.f.h.s.c.g.
2. Siegel RL, et al. Cancer statistics, 2022. CA Cancer J Clin. 2022;72(1):7–33.
3. Wolf GT, et al. Induction chemotherapy plus radiation compared with surgery plus radiation in patients with advanced laryngeal cancer. N Engl J Med. 1991;324(24):1685–90.

4. Forastiere AA, et al. Concurrent chemotherapy and radiotherapy for organ preservation in advanced laryngeal cancer. N Engl J Med. 2003;349(22):2091–8.

5. Forastiere AA, et al. Long-term results of RTOG 91-11: a comparison of three nonsurgical treatment strategies to preserve the larynx in patients with locally advanced larynx cancer. J Clin Oncol. 2013;31(7):845–52.

6. Rosenthal DI, et al. Long-term outcomes after surgical or nonsurgical initial therapy for patients with T4 squamous cell carcinoma of the larynx: a 3-decade survey. Cancer. 2015;121(10):1608–19.

7. Patel UA, et al. Impact of pharyngeal closure technique on fistula after salvage laryngectomy. JAMA Otolaryngol Head Neck Surg. 2013;139(11):1156–62.

8. Shah MA, et al. Treatment of locally advanced esophageal carcinoma: ASCO guideline. J Clin Oncol. 2020;38(23):2677–94.

9. Graboyes EM, et al. Effect of time to initiation of postoperative radiation therapy on survival in surgically managed head and neck cancer. Cancer. 2017;123(24):4841–50.

10. Ganly I, et al. Postoperative complications of salvage total laryngectomy. Cancer. 2005;103(10):2073–81.

11. Weber RS, et al. Outcome of salvage total laryngectomy following organ preservation therapy: the radiation therapy oncology group trial 91-11. Arch Otolaryngol Head Neck Surg. 2003;129(1):44–9.

12. Kierzek A, et al. The first polish total laryngectomies. Contemp Oncol (Pozn). 2013;17(6):473–6.

13. Ceachir O, Hainarosie R, Zainea V. Total laryngectomy—past, present, future. Maedica. 2014;9(2):210–6.

14. Matev B, et al. Losing one's voice to save One's life: a brief history of laryngectomy. Cureus. 2020;12(6):e8804.

15. Hui Y, et al. Primary closure of pharyngeal remnant after total laryngectomy and partial pharyngectomy: how much residual mucosa is sufficient? Laryngoscope. 1996;106(4):490–4.

16. Ragbir M, Brown JS, Mehanna H. Reconstructive considerations in head and neck surgical oncology: United Kingdom National Multidisciplinary Guidelines. J Laryngol Otol. 2016;130(S2):S191–7.

17. Yeh DH, Sahovaler A, Fung K. Reconstruction after salvage laryngectomy. Oral Oncol. 2017;75:22–7.

18. Chotipanich A. Total laryngectomy: a review of surgical techniques. Cureus. 2021;13(9):e18181.

19. Avci H, Karabulut B. Is it important which suturing technique used for pharyngeal mucosal closure in total laryngectomy? Modified continuous Connell suture may decrease pharyngocutaneous fistula. Ear Nose Throat J. 2020;99(10):664–70.

20. Haksever M, et al. Modified continuous mucosal Connell suture for the pharyngeal closure after total laryngectomy: zipper suture. Clin Exp Otorhinolaryngol. 2015;8(3):281–8.

21. Thrasyvoulou G, et al. Horizontal (vs. vertical) closure of the neo-pharynx is associated with superior postoperative swallowing after total laryngectomy. Ear Nose Throat J. 2018;97(4–5):E31–5.

22. Davis RK, et al. The anatomy and complications of "T" versus vertical closure of the hypopharynx after laryngectomy. Laryngoscope. 1982;92(1):16–22.

23. van der Kamp MF, Rinkel RNPM, Eerenstein SEJ. The influence of closure technique in total laryngectomy on the development of a pseudo-diverticulum and dysphagia. Eur Arch Otorhinolaryngol. 2017;274(4):1967–73.

24. Maclean J, et al. Impact of a laryngectomy and surgical closure technique on swallow biomechanics and dysphagia severity. Otolaryngol Head Neck Surg. 2011;144(1):21–8.

25. Walton B, et al. Post-laryngectomy stricture and pharyngocutaneous fistula: review of techniques in primary pharyngeal reconstruction in laryngectomy. Clin Otolaryngol. 2018;43(1):109–16.

26. Deniz M, Ciftci Z, Gultekin E. Pharyngoesophageal suturing technique may decrease the incidence of pharyngocutaneous fistula following total laryngectomy. Surg Res Pract. 2015;2015:363640.

27. Sofferman RA, Voronetsky I. Use of the linear stapler for pharyngoesophageal closure after total laryngectomy. Laryngoscope. 2000;110(8):1406–9.
28. Sansa-Perna A, et al. Pharyngeal closure after a total laryngectomy: mechanical versus manual technique. J Laryngol Otol. 2020;134(7):626–31.
29. Lee Y-C, et al. Stapler closure versus manual closure in total laryngectomy for laryngeal cancer: a systematic review and meta-analysis. Clin Otolaryngol. 2021;46(4):692–8.
30. Smith SR, Genden EM, Urken ML. Endoscopic stapling technique for the treatment of Zenker diverticulum vs standard open-neck technique: a direct comparison and charge analysis. Arch Otolaryngol Head Neck Surg. 2002;128(2):141–4.
31. Wookey H. The surgical treatment of carcinoma of the hypopharynx and the oesophagus. Br J Surg. 1948;35(139):249–66.
32. Patel RS, et al. Circumferential pharyngeal reconstruction: history, critical analysis of techniques, and current therapeutic recommendations. Head Neck. 2010;32(1):109–20.
33. Bakamjian VY, Long M, Rigg B. Experience with the medially based deltopectoral flap in reconstructuve surgery of the head and neck. Br J Plast Surg. 1971;24(2):174–83.
34. Andrews BT, et al. Deltopectoral flap revisited in the microvascular era: a single-institution 10-year experience. Ann Otol Rhinol Laryngol. 2006;115(1):35–40.
35. Yu P, Roblin P, Chevray P. Internal mammary artery perforator (IMAP) flap for tracheostoma reconstruction. Head Neck. 2006;28(8):723–9.
36. Ibrahim A, et al. The deltopectoral flap revisited: the internal mammary artery perforator flap. J Craniofac Surg. 2016;27(2):e189–92.
37. Shayan R, Syme DY, Grinsell D. The IMAP flap for pharygoesophageal reconstruction following stricture release. J Plast Reconstr Aesthet Surg. 2012;65(6):810–3.
38. Mirghani H, et al. Pharyngotracheal fistula closure using the internal mammary artery perforator Island flap. Laryngoscope. 2014;124(5):1106–11.
39. Ariyan S. The pectoralis major myocutaneous flap. A versatile flap for reconstruction in the head and neck. Plast Reconstr Surg. 1979;63(1):73–81.
40. Burke MS, et al. Pectoralis major myocutaneous flap for reconstruction of circumferential pharyngeal defects. Ann Plast Surg. 2013;71(6):649–51.
41. Righini C, et al. The pectoralis myofascial flap in pharyngolaryngeal surgery after radiotherapy. Eur Arch Otorhinolaryngol. 2005;262(5):357–61.
42. Patel UA, Keni SP. Pectoralis myofascial flap during salvage laryngectomy prevents pharyngocutaneous fistula. Otolaryngol Head Neck Surg. 2009;141(2):190–5.
43. Comert E, et al. Pectoralis major myofascial flap in salvage laryngectomy. J Laryngol Otol. 2014;128(8):714–9.
44. Fabian RL. Reconstruction of the laryngopharynx and cervical esophagus. Laryngoscope. 1984;94(10):1334–50.
45. Spriano G, Piantanida R, Pellini R. Hypopharyngeal reconstruction using pectoralis major myocutaneous flap and pre-vertebral fascia. Laryngoscope. 2001;111(3):544–7.
46. Richmon JD, Brumund KT. Reconstruction of the hypopharynx: current trends. Curr Opin Otolaryngol Head Neck Surg. 2007;15(4):208–12.
47. Teknos TN, et al. Free tissue reconstruction of the hypopharynx after organ preservation therapy: analysis of wound complications. Laryngoscope. 2001;111(7):1192–6.
48. Disa JJ, et al. Microvascular reconstruction of the hypopharynx: defect classification, treatment algorithm, and functional outcome based on 165 consecutive cases. Plast Reconstr Surg. 2003;111(2):652–60. discussion 661–3.
49. Sandulache VC, et al. Salvage total laryngectomy after external-beam radiotherapy: a 20-year experience. Head Neck. 2016;38(Suppl 1(Suppl 1)):E1962–8.
50. Chen DW, et al. Free flap inset techniques in salvage Laryngopharyngectomy repair: impact on fistula formation and function. Laryngoscope. 2021;131(3):E875–81.
51. Yu P, et al. Pharyngoesophageal reconstruction with the anterolateral thigh flap after total laryngopharyngectomy. Cancer. 2010;116(7):1718–24.
52. Microvascular Committee of the American Academy of Otolaryngology-Head & Neck Surgery. Salvage laryngectomy and laryngopharyngectomy: multicenter review of outcomes associated with a reconstructive approach. Head Neck. 2019;41(1):16–29.

53. Guimarães AV, et al. Efficacy of pectoralis major muscle flap for pharyngocutaneous fistula prevention in salvage total laryngectomy: a systematic review. Head Neck. 2016;38(S1):E2317–21.

54. Deschler DG, et al. Quantitative and qualitative analysis of tracheoesophageal voice after pectoralis major flap reconstruction of the neopharynx. Otolaryngol Head Neck Surg. 1998;118(6):771–6.

55. Pallua N, Magnus Noah E. The tunneled supraclavicular Island flap: an optimized technique for head and neck reconstruction. Plast Reconstr Surg. 2000;105(3):842–51. discussion 852–4.

56. Emerick KS, Herr MA, Deschler DG. Supraclavicular flap reconstruction following total laryngectomy. Laryngoscope. 2014;124(8):1777–82.

57. Makiese O, et al. Huge proliferating trichilemmal tumors of the scalp: report of six cases. Plast Reconstr Surg. 2010;126(1):18e–9e.

58. Liu PH, Chiu ES. Supraclavicular artery flap: a new option for pharyngeal reconstruction. Ann Plast Surg. 2009;62(5):497–501.

59. Taylor R, Sionis S, Varley I. Spiralised supraclavicular artery Island flap for total pharyngeal reconstruction: a technical note. Br J Oral Maxillofac Surg. 2021;59(2):242–3.

60. Seidenberg B, et al. Immediate reconstruction of the cervical esophagus by a revascularized isolated jejunal segment. Ann Surg. 1959;149(2):162–71.

61. Nagel TH, Hayden RE. Advantages and limitations of free and pedicled flaps in reconstruction of pharyngoesophageal defects. Curr Opin Otolaryngol Head Neck Surg. 2014;22(5):407–13.

62. Corbitt C, et al. Free flap failure in head and neck reconstruction. Head Neck. 2014;36(10):1440–5.

63. Ligh CA, et al. An analysis of early oncologic head and neck free flap reoperations from the 2005-2012 ACS-NSQIP dataset. J Plast Surg Hand Surg. 2016;50(2):85–92.

64. Yang GF, et al. Forearm free skin flap transplantation: a report of 56 cases. 1981. Br J Plast Surg. 1997;50(3):162–5.

65. Megerle K, Sauerbier M, Germann G. The evolution of the pedicled radial forearm flap. Hand. 2010;5(1):37–42.

66. Foissac R, et al. Coverage of tendon exposure after radial forearm free flap by the dorsoulnar artery perforator flap. Otolaryngol Head Neck Surg. 2017;156(5):822–7.

67. Hartwig S, et al. Treatment of wound healing disorders of radial forearm free flap donor sites using cold atmospheric plasma: a proof of concept. J Oral Maxillofac Surg. 2017;75(2):429–35.

68. Lovie MJ, Duncan GM, Glasson DW. The ulnar artery forearm free flap. Br J Plast Surg. 1984;37(4):486–92.

69. Huang JJ, et al. Anatomical basis and clinical application of the ulnar forearm free flap for head and neck reconstruction. Laryngoscope. 2012;122(12):2670–6.

70. Huang AT, Day TA. Double paddle ulnar perforator free flap in reconstruction of through-and-through and fistulous defects of the head and neck. Laryngoscope. 2017;127(6):1302–5.

71. Harii K, et al. Pharyngoesophageal reconstruction using a fabricated forearm free flap. Plast Reconstr Surg. 1985;75(4):463–76.

72. Urken ML, et al. A modified design of the buried radial forearm free flap for use in oral cavity and pharyngeal reconstruction. Arch Otolaryngol Head Neck Surg. 1994;120(11):1233–9.

73. Pellini R, et al. External monitor for buried free flaps in head and neck reconstructions. Acta Otorhinolaryngol Ital. 2006;26(1):1–6.

74. Kuriakose MA, et al. Sensate radial forearm free flaps in tongue reconstruction. Arch Otolaryngol Head Neck Surg. 2001;127(12):1463–6.

75. Ahmed A, et al. Use of double skin paddle for pharyngoesophageal reconstruction using tubed radial forearm free flap. Br J Oral Maxillofac Surg. 2014;52(7):661–3.

76. Machado RA, Moubayed SP, Urken ML. Repair of pharyngoesophageal stenosis and a tracheoesophageal fistula using a dual-paddled radial forearm free flap: flap design and surgical technique. Laryngoscope. 2017;127(9):2081–4.

77. Sinclair CF, et al. Primary versus delayed tracheoesophageal puncture for laryngopharyngectomy with free flap reconstruction. Laryngoscope. 2011;121(7):1436–40.
78. Kelly KE, Anthony JP, Singer M. Pharyngoesophageal reconstruction using the radial forearm fasciocutaneous free flap: preliminary results. Otolaryngol Head Neck Surg. 1994;111(1):16–24.
79. Azizzadeh B, et al. Radial forearm free flap pharyngoesophageal reconstruction. Laryngoscope. 2001;111(5):807–10.
80. Cho BC, et al. Pharyngoesophageal reconstruction with a tubed free radial forearm flap. J Reconstr Microsurg. 1998;14(8):535–40.
81. Withrow KP, et al. Free tissue transfer to manage salvage laryngectomy defects after organ preservation failure. Laryngoscope. 2007;117(5):781–4.
82. Song YG, Chen GZ, Song YL. The free thigh flap: a new free flap concept based on the septocutaneous artery. Br J Plast Surg. 1984;37(2):149–59.
83. Park CW, Miles BA. The expanding role of the anterolateral thigh free flap in head and neck reconstruction. Curr Opin Otolaryngol Head Neck Surg. 2011;19(4):263–8.
84. Marmuse JP, Guedon C, Koka VN. Gastric tube transposition for cancer of the hypopharynx and cervical oesophagus. J Laryngol Otol. 1994;108(1):33–7.
85. Butskiy O, Anderson DW, Prisman E. Management algorithm for failed gastric pull up reconstruction of laryngopharyngectomy defects: case report and review of the literature. J Otolaryngol Head Neck Surg. 2016;45(1):41.
86. Tsai WS, Levy RM, Luketich JD. Technique of minimally invasive Ivor Lewis esophagectomy. Oper Tech Thorac Cardiovasc Surg. 2009;14(3):176–92.
87. Liebermann-Meffert DM, Meier R, Siewert JR. Vascular anatomy of the gastric tube used for esophageal reconstruction. Ann Thorac Surg. 1992;54(6):1110–5.
88. Jiang H, et al. Risk factors for anastomotic complications after radical McKeown esophagectomy. Ann Thorac Surg. 2021;112(3):944–51.
89. Hagens ERC, et al. Risk factors and consequences of anastomotic leakage after esophagectomy for cancer. Ann Thorac Surg. 2021;112(1):255–63.
90. Van Daele E, et al. Risk factors and consequences of anastomotic leakage after Ivor Lewis oesophagectomy†. Interact Cardiovasc Thorac Surg. 2016;22(1):32–7.
91. Kassis ES, et al. Predictors of anastomotic leak after esophagectomy: an analysis of the society of thoracic surgeons general thoracic database. Ann Thorac Surg. 2013;96(6):1919–26.
92. Zhang W, et al. Gastric-tube versus whole-stomach esophagectomy for esophageal cancer: a systematic review and meta-analysis. PLoS One. 2017;12(3):e0173416.
93. Yu P, et al. Comparison of clinical and functional outcomes and hospital costs following pharyngoesophageal reconstruction with the anterolateral thigh free flap versus the jejunal flap. Plast Reconstr Surg. 2006;117(3):968–74.
94. Kamiyama R, et al. A clinical study of pharyngolaryngectomy with total esophagectomy: postoperative complications, countermeasures, and prognoses. Otolaryngol Head Neck Surg. 2015;153(3):392–9.
95. Triboulet JP, et al. Surgical management of carcinoma of the hypopharynx and cervical esophagus: analysis of 209 cases. Arch Surg. 2001;136(10):1164–70.
96. Heger P, et al. Gastric preconditioning in advance of esophageal resection-systematic review and meta-analysis. J Gastrointest Surg. 2017;21(9):1523–32.
97. Takeda FR, et al. Supercharged cervical anastomosis for esophagectomy and gastric pull-up. J Thorac Cardiovasc Surg. 2021;162(3):688–697.e3.
98. Huang PM, et al. Supercharged reversed gastric tube technique: a microvascular anastomosis procedure for pharyngo-oesophageal reconstruction after total laryngopharyngo-oesophagectomy. Eur J Cardiothorac Surg. 2013;44(2):258–62.
99. Thomas P, et al. Colon interposition for esophageal replacement: current indications and long-term function. Ann Thorac Surg. 1997;64(3):757–64.
100. DeMeester TR, et al. Indications, surgical technique, and long-term functional results of colon interposition or bypass. Ann Surg. 1988;208(4):460–74.

101. Sakorafas GH, Zouros E, Peros G. Applied vascular anatomy of the colon and rectum: clinical implications for the surgical oncologist. Surg Oncol. 2006;15(4):243–55.
102. Lees W. Colonic replacement after pharyngolaryngectomy. Br J Surg. 1967;54(6):541–7.
103. Bakshi A, Sugarbaker DJ, Burt BM. Alternative conduits for esophageal replacement. Ann Cardiothorac Surg. 2017;6(2):137–43.
104. Rice T. Colon replacement. In: Pearson F, Deslauriers J, Ginsberg R, editors. Esophageal surgery. New York: Churchill Livingstone; 1995. p. 761–74.
105. Mansour KA, Bryan FC, Carlson GW. Bowel interposition for esophageal replacement: twenty-five-year experience. Ann Thorac Surg. 1997;64(3):752–6.
106. Shirakawa Y, et al. Colonic interposition and supercharge for esophageal reconstruction. Langenbeck's Arch Surg. 2006;391(1):19–23.
107. Saeki H, et al. Esophageal replacement by colon interposition with microvascular surgery for patients with thoracic esophageal cancer: the utility of superdrainage. Dis Esophagus. 2013;26(1):50–6.
108. Davis PA, Law S, Wong J. Colonic interposition after esophagectomy for cancer. Arch Surg. 2003;138(3):303–8.
109. Kesler KA, et al. "Supercharged" isoperistaltic colon interposition for long-segment esophageal reconstruction. Ann Thorac Surg. 2013;95(4):1162–8. discussion 1168–9.
110. Ninomiya I, et al. Feasibility of esophageal reconstruction using a pedicled jejunum with intrathoracic esophagojejunostomy in the upper mediastinum for esophageal cancer. Gen Thorac Cardiovasc Surg. 2014;62(10):627–34.
111. Popovici Z. A new philosophy in esophageal reconstruction with colon. Thirty-years experience. Dis Esophagus. 2003;16(4):323–7.
112. Reslinger V, et al. Esophageal reconstruction by colon interposition after esophagectomy for cancer analysis of current indications, operative outcomes, and long-term survival. J Surg Oncol. 2016;113(2):159–64.
113. Knezević JD, et al. Colon interposition in the treatment of esophageal caustic strictures: 40 years of experience. Dis Esophagus. 2007;20(6):530–4.
114. Cerfolio RJ, et al. Esophageal replacement by colon interposition. Ann Thorac Surg. 1995;59(6):1382–4.
115. Greene CL, et al. Long-term quality of life and alimentary satisfaction after esophagectomy with colon interposition. Ann Thorac Surg. 2014;98(5):1713–9. discussion 1719–20.
116. Longmire WP Jr, Ravitch MM. A new method for constructing an artificial esophagus. Ann Surg. 1946;123:819–35.
117. Gaur P, Blackmon SH. Jejunal graft conduits after esophagectomy. J Thorac Dis. 2014;6(Suppl 3(Suppl 3)):S333–40.
118. Blackmon SH, et al. Supercharged pedicled jejunal interposition for esophageal replacement: a 10-year experience. Ann Thorac Surg. 2012;94(4):1104–11; discussion 1111–3.
119. Swisher SG, Hofstetter WL, Miller MJ. The supercharged microvascular jejunal interposition. Semin Thorac Cardiovasc Surg. 2007;19(1):56–65.
120. Rice D, Yu P. Use of supercharged Jejunal flap for esophageal reconstruction. Oper Tech Thorac Cardiovasc Surg. 2010;15:243–57.
121. Poh M, et al. Technical challenges of total esophageal reconstruction using a supercharged jejunal flap. Ann Surg. 2011;253(6):1122–9.
122. DeMeester SR. Colonic interposition for benign disease. Oper Tech Thorac Cardiovasc Surg. 2006;11(3):232–49.
123. Zheng YZ, et al. Comparison between different reconstruction routes in esophageal squamous cell carcinoma. World J Gastroenterol. 2012;18(39):5616–21.
124. de Delva PE, et al. Surgical management of failed colon interposition. Eur J Cardiothorac Surg. 2008;34(2):432–7; discussion 437.
125. Motoyama S, et al. Surgical outcome of colon interposition by the posterior mediastinal route for thoracic esophageal cancer. Ann Thorac Surg. 2007;83(4):1273–8.

126. Lorenz KJ. Rehabilitation after total laryngectomy-a tribute to the pioneers of voice restoration in the last two centuries. Front Med. 2017;4:81.
127. Robbins J. Acoustic differentiation of laryngeal, esophageal, and tracheoesophageal speech. J Speech Hear Res. 1984;27(4):577–85.
128. Moukarbel RV, et al. Voice-related quality of life (V-RQOL) outcomes in laryngectomees. Head Neck. 2011;33(1):31–6.
129. Panwar A, et al. Impact of primary tracheoesophageal puncture on outcomes after total laryngectomy. Otolaryngol Head Neck Surg. 2018;158(1):103–9.
130. Gitomer SA, et al. Influence of timing, radiation, and reconstruction on complications and speech outcomes with tracheoesophageal puncture. Head Neck. 2016;38(12):1765–71.
131. Lewin JS, et al. Device life of the tracheoesophageal voice prosthesis revisited. JAMA Otolaryngol Head Neck Surg. 2017;143(1):65–71.
132. Hutcheson KA, et al. Outcomes and adverse events of enlarged tracheoesophageal puncture after total laryngectomy. Laryngoscope. 2011;121(7):1455–61.
133. Dewey EH, et al. Reconstruction of expanding tracheoesophageal fistulae in post-radiation therapy patients who undergo total laryngectomy with a bipaddled radial forearm free flap: report of 8 cases. Head Neck. 2016;38(S1):E172–8.
134. Machtay M, et al. Factors associated with severe late toxicity after concurrent chemoradiation for locally advanced head and neck cancer: an RTOG analysis. J Clin Oncol. 2008;26(21):3582–9.
135. Worley ML, et al. Factors associated with gastrostomy tube dependence following salvage total laryngectomy with microvascular free tissue transfer. Head Neck. 2019;41(4):865–70.
136. Chen WF, et al. Outcomes of anterolateral thigh flap reconstruction for salvage laryngopharyngectomy for hypopharyngeal cancer after concurrent chemoradiotherapy. PLoS One. 2013;8(1):e53985.
137. Hanasono MM, et al. Closure of laryngectomy defects in the age of chemoradiation therapy. Head Neck. 2012;34(4):580–8.
138. Sweeny L, et al. Incidence and outcomes of stricture formation postlaryngectomy. Otolaryngol Head Neck Surg. 2012;146(3):395–402.

Chapter 9
Trends in Microvascular Surgery

Andrew Beech and Justine Moe

Introduction

The field of microvascular surgery has evolved in the past 150 years. In 1896, American surgeon John Murphy performed the first vascular anastomosis for repair of a severed femoral artery following a gunshot wound to the lower extremity [1]. In 1902, Alexis Carrel described a triangulation of vessel technique for the end-to-end arteriovenous anastomosis and is credited by many as the father of vascular surgery [2]. In 1957, Seidenberg et al. performed the first free tissue transfer, the autotransplantation of a segment of jejunum for reconstruction of a pharyngolaryngectomy defect [3]. Jacobson and Suarez first described use of the operative microscope for small vessel anastomosis in 1960 and coined the term "microsurgery" [4]. Subsequently, microvascular surgical techniques were utilized for digital transplantation and the first toe-to-thumb transplantation in the 1960s [2] and the first omental flap for scalp reconstruction in 1972 by McLean and Buncke [5]. Musculocutaneous free flaps were popularized in the 1970s, and osteocutaneous free flaps were developed in the 1970s and 1980s, including the description of the fibula free flap for mandibular reconstruction by Hidalgo in 1989 [6].

Advances in the understanding of vascular anatomy, microsurgical technique, preoperative imaging, and flap monitoring have led to an evolution in the predictability of free tissue transfer reconstruction [7]. At present, anastomotic and free flap success rates range from 90% to 99%, with a shift in focus from flap survival to optimizing the restoration of function and esthetics and minimizing donor site morbidity. Customizable reconstructive options are possible through the emergence of

A. Beech · J. Moe (✉)
Department of Oral and Maxillofacial Surgery, University of Michigan, Ann Arbor, MI, USA

Department of Oral and Maxillofacial Surgery, Thomas Jefferson University, Philadelphia, PA, USA
e-mail: andrew.beech@jefferson.edu; jusmoe@med.umich.edu

J. C. Melville et al. (eds.), *Advancements and Innovations in OMFS, ENT, and Facial Plastic Surgery*, https://doi.org/10.1007/978-3-031-32099-6_9

supermicrosurgery, perforator flaps, and free-style flaps to optimize reconstructive outcomes. In this chapter, we describe the current technologic innovations at the disposal of the microvascular reconstructive surgeon for preoperative planning for flap harvest, intraoperative microanastomosis and flap assessment, and postoperative flap monitoring.

Preoperative Donor Site Assessment

The preoperative characterization of donor site vascular anatomy is critical to ensure safe harvest of the reconstructive flap. Preoperative imaging modalities for vascular anatomy are particularly important for the assessment of vascular anatomy prior to fibula free flap harvest which blood supply to the distal lower extremity can be compromised following harvest in the setting of aberrant vascular anatomy or severe peripheral vascular disease. Additionally, advances in imaging modalities over the last 30 years have allowed for detailed preoperative evaluation of cutaneous perforator localization as an adjunct to intraoperative identification (Fig. 9.1), and perforasome assessment which has utility in the assessment of perforator flaps.

Surgeons in the early 1990's relied upon handheld Doppler ultrasound for perforator localization; however, this technique was found to have a high false-positive rate and was less reliable when perforators were traveling transversely though fascial planes [8]. Modern imaging modalities including computed tomography angiography (CTA) and color Doppler ultrasonography are more accurate than the handheld Doppler in perforator localization. Additional techniques for preoperative perforator localization include thermography and indocyanine green angiography (ICGA). ICGA is discussed in the following section.

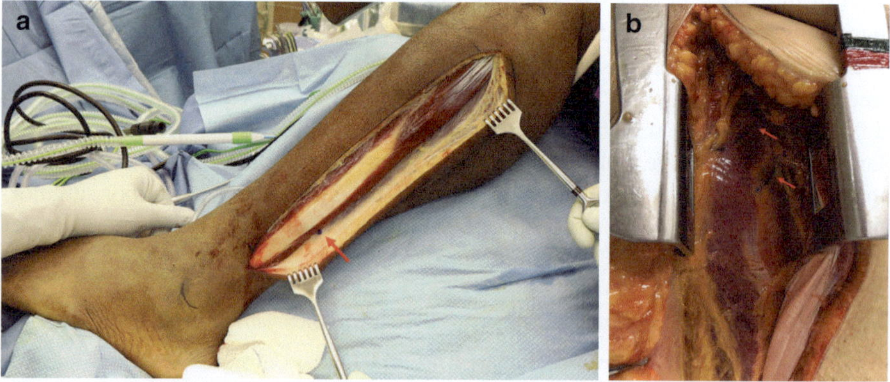

Fig. 9.1 (**a**) Intraoperative identification of septocutaneous perforators during fibula free flap harvest. (**b**) Intraoperative identification of musculocutaneous perforators during anterolateral thigh free flap harvest

Computer Tomography Angiography (CTA)

CTA imaging allows for the acquisition of more than 1000 slices over single bolus dose of IV contrast and uses multidetector and reformatting software to generate a three-dimensional (3D) volumetric analysis. CTA provides detailed information regarding vessel mapping and allows for evaluation of vessel size, course, and relationship to adjacent structures. Preoperative CTA is the standard of care for assessing vascular anatomy prior to fibula free flap (Fig. 9.2). Additionally, CTA is highly accurate in identifying perforators as small as 0.3 mm, with over 95% sensitivity and 95% accuracy [9].

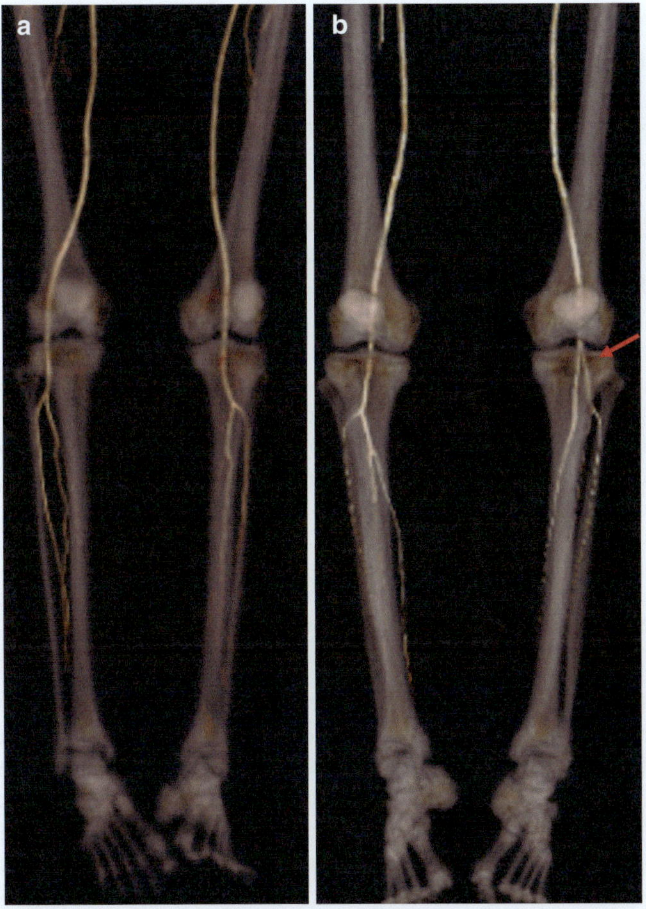

Fig. 9.2 (a) Computed tomography angiography (CTA) showing two vessel runoff on the left lower extremity with a diminutive anterior tibial artery. (b) CTA showing bilateral three vessel runoff with the left lower extremity exhibiting a high takeoff of the tibioperoneal trunk

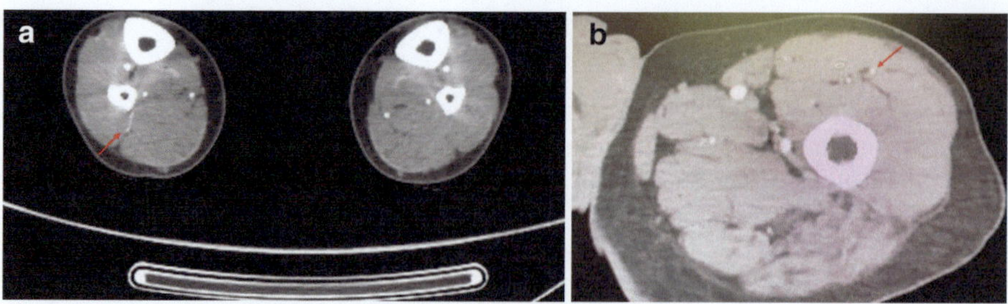

Fig. 9.3 (**a**) Cutaneous perforator of the peroneal artery identified on CTA for fibula free flap harvest. (**b**) Cutaneous perforator of the descending branch of lateral circumflex femoral artery on computed tomography angiography (CTA) for anterolateral thigh free flap harvest

CTA data can be used to map cutaneous perforators for a multitude of flap types (Fig. 9.3) [10, 11]. A prospective study of 60 patients undergoing fibula free flap reconstruction described a technique of cutaneous perforator mapping on CTA and integration with computer-assisted surgical design, in which the position of the patient-specific cutting guide was based on the localization of the cutaneous perforator and planned skin paddle [12]. In comparison to perforators identified intraoperatively, CTA perforator identification had a 96.2% accuracy with a median precision of localization of 0.3 mm, a positive predictive value (PPV) of 99.29%, and a negative predictive value of 90.00% [12]. In the preoperative planning of deep inferior epigastric perforator (DIEP) flaps, perforator localization on CTA as compared to Doppler ultrasound was associated with decreased surgical times, decreased complications including flap partial or total failure, and led to a cost savings of $3000 USD per patient [13]. Limitations to use of CTA include the need for IV contrast and ionizing radiation and the lack of vessel flow dynamics.

Magnetic Resonance Angiography (MRA)

Gadolinium contrast-enhanced MRA imaging has been employed for preoperative donor site evaluation and precludes the need for ionizing radiation and produces detailed 3D images for assessment of vessel course, size, and branching pattern [14]. MRA has a 100% specificity but decreased sensitivity (91%) in perforator detection, providing detailed visualization of septocutaneous perforators greater than 1 mm in diameter but less accurate when evaluating perforators less than 1 mm as compared to CTA [15]. An additional limitation to the utility of MRA is the length of time required for image acquisition, which may be anxiety-provoking in patients who suffer from claustrophobia and can result in poor-quality images in patients who are unable lie still.

Color Duplex Ultrasound (CDU)

CDU is a noninvasive and portable imaging modality for evaluation of pedicle vascular anatomy, perforator size and course, and vessel flow dynamics (Fig. 9.4). CDU combines Brightness-mode ultrasound and Doppler signal measurements to provide real time a visualization of vessels and quantification of the blood flow velocity. This can be done using either a 5 or 13 MHz linear array Doppler probe. In addition to providing an assessment of vascular anatomy and perforator localization, a quantitative assessment of peripheral arterial disease can be given through ankle brachial indices (ABI), toe brachial indices (TBI), and arterial duplex measurements (Fig. 9.5).

A prospective CDU exam of 38 patients prior to fibula free flap detected vascular anomalies in 2.6% and severe peripheral arterial disease in 7.9% of patients, leading to an altered flap selection [16]. Additionally, cutaneous perforator mapping was found to be 100% sensitive and specific in correlation to peroneal perforators identified intraoperatively [16]. The efficacy of CDU has been described in the localization of perforators for the anterolateral thigh (ALT) free flap, allowing selection of the thigh with the largest vessels and shortest intramuscular course in order to reduce the difficulty of dissection [17].

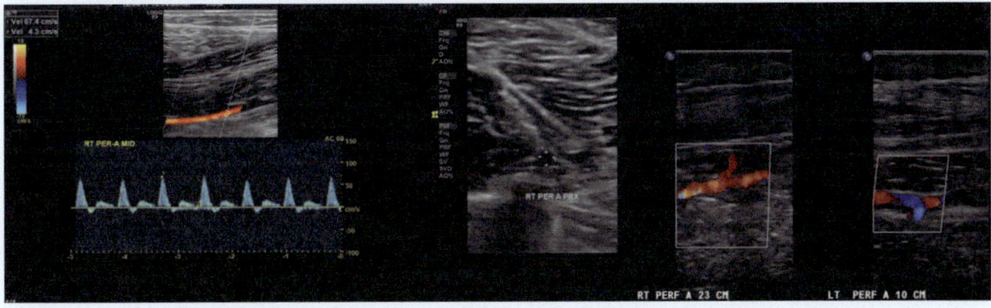

Fig. 9.4 Right peroneal artery identification, flow, and perforator identified on color duplex ultrasound (CDU)

Lower Exrtemity Arterial Duplex

R PSV (cm/s)		R EDV (cm/s)		L PSV (cm/s)		L EDV (cm/s)	
EIA Dst	136	EIA Dst	20	EIA Dst	151	EIA Dst	30
CFA prx	116	CFA prx	16	CFA prx	86	CFA prx	3
CFA dist	66	CFA dst	9	CFA dst	55	CFA dst	4
Profunda	56	Profunda	10	Profunda	50	Profunda	6
SAF prx	71	SFA prx	5	SFA prx	83	SFA prx	8
SFA mid	80	SFA mid	8	SFA mid	85	SFA mid	3
SFA dst	70	SFA dst	2	SFA dst	60	SFA dst	3
Pop prx	63	Pop prx	6	Pop prx	53	Pop prx	4
Pop dst	67	Pop dst	5	Pop dst	55	Pop dst	8
Post Tib Prx	75	Post Tib Prx	5	Post Tib Prx	119	Post Tib Prx	3
PTA Dst	90	PTA Dst	5	Post Tib Dst	70	Post Tib Dst	6
Peroneal	46	Peroneal	3	Peroneal	50	Peroneal	6
Pero A Dst	46	Pero A Dst	2	Pero A Dst	48	Pero A Dst	2
Ant Tib	59	Ant Tib	3	Ant Tib	49	Ant Tib	3
ATA Dst	72	ATA Dst	2	ATA Dst	48	ATA Dst	4

History/Presentation

The patient presents today for pre-op evaluation.

The patient has had a previous DVU study of the same type on 12/7/2017.

Today's ABI results: Right ABI: 1.17 Left ABI: 1.19; Right TBI: 0.91 Left TBI: 0.84.

Fig. 9.5 Assessment of peripheral arterial disease on color duplex ultrasound (CDU) using arterial duplex measurements, ankle brachial indices, and toe brachial indices

Although CDU is most commonly used preoperatively, CDU also has applicability in the intraoperative and postoperative settings. Intraoperatively, CDU can be utilized for perforator mapping of propeller flaps and by utilizing flow velocity to determine the optimal side of rotation [18]. Postoperatively, CDU can also be used to assess perforator patency, to identify the presence of a thrombosis, and to trend flow velocity in a flap with a questionable status [18]. Limitations of CDU include a significant inter-provider variability depending on the experience level of the examiner.

Thermography

Infrared thermography (IRT) is a noninvasive imaging modality that has more recently been investigated as a promising technology for preoperative flap assessment, intraoperative perfusion evaluation, and postoperative flap monitoring, although this technology is not new. Infrared (IR) radiation was described by Sir William Herschel in 1800, and the first IR camera was developed in 1929 by Kalman Tihanyi [19]. IRT cameras detect emitted IR radiation and provide a heat map. Cutaneous temperature depends on vascularization with IR radiation skin emission reflecting local vascularity, which can be modulated by changes in cardiac output [20]. As such, IRT provides a rapid, continuous, and real-time assessment of skin paddle perfusion through the indirect measurement of the skin temperature. The flow of blood in a vessel emits an infrared signal, which can be used to localized perforators that are visualized as "hot spots." Professional IRT cameras can elucidate temperature differences as subtle as $0.04°C$ [20].

Handheld IRT devices have been shown to be as effective as the conventional handheld Doppler ultrasound in the localization of cutaneous perforators of the abdomen, thigh, and sacrum. A study assessing cutaneous perforators of the abdomen, sacrum, and bilateral anterolateral thighs in 20 volunteers reported that 97% of "hotspots" identified by IRT were confirmed with handheld Doppler [21]. A smartphone IRT imaging camera has been found to be effective in thermographic identification of cutaneous perforator hot spots, with resolution slightly inferior to the larger and expensive handheld IRT devices [22]. The smartphone IRT has the potential to serve as a less expensive and more readily accessible alternative, with a cost of approximately 1% that of a professional IRT camera [22].

Dynamic infrared thermography (DIRT) is a technique in which a cold challenge is administered to a skin area of interest, and patterns of flow through perforating vessels and surrounding skin areas are qualitatively assessed during rewarming [20, 23]. DIRT has shown utility in evaluating the speed at which hotspots appear following a cold challenge with findings correlating to volume changes on CDU when used in the preoperative planning for deep inferior epigastric perforator (DIEP) and superficial inferior epigastric artery (SIEA) flaps [23]. A study of 25 subjects planned for DIEP flap found that the location of hotspots using DIRT matched the position of the dominant perforators identified on handheld Doppler and CTA [24].

DIRT has been shown to identify perforators larger than 1 mm when compared to CTA [25]. Additionally, DIRT allows for a qualitative assessment of the pattern of rewarming between interperforator zones to identify the better perfused regions, allowing for improved skin paddle planning [25]. While IRT obviates the need for radiation and contrast exposure necessitated with CTA, the use of IRT for perforator localization has several limitations including the inability to distinguish vessel morphology or perforator caliber, origin, or path after penetrating the deep fascia [20].

Intraoperative Techniques

Advances in Microvascular Anastomotic Technique

The success of free tissue transfer is dependent on the patency of the arterial and venous anastomoses and directly correlates to the quality of the anastomoses. Since first described in the early 1900s, the simple interrupted suture technique remains the primary modality of microvascular anastomosis (Fig. 9.6). The evolution of microsurgical techniques has included refinements in microscope systems and in the microsurgical armamentarium such as fine suture and instrumentation (Fig. 9.7). Currently used innovations including anastomotic coupler systems address the importance of decreasing operative time while maintaining high anastomotic patency rates.

Anastomotic Coupler Systems

In 1900, Payr described a nonsuture method of anastomosis utilizing magnesium tubes to couple vessels; however, success rates were compromised by significant tissue necrosis secondary to strong electrochemical forces generated by the

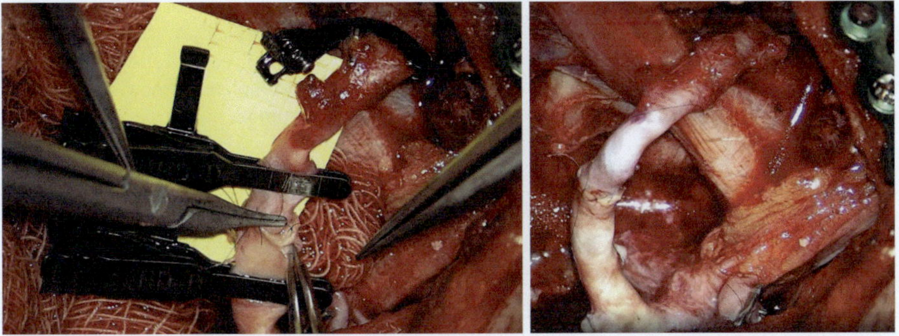

Fig. 9.6 Hand-sewn arterial anastomosis employing the interrupted suture technique

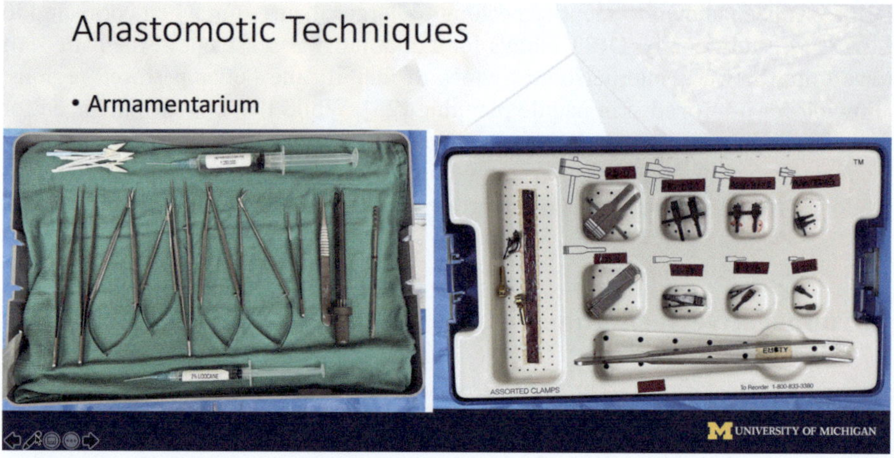

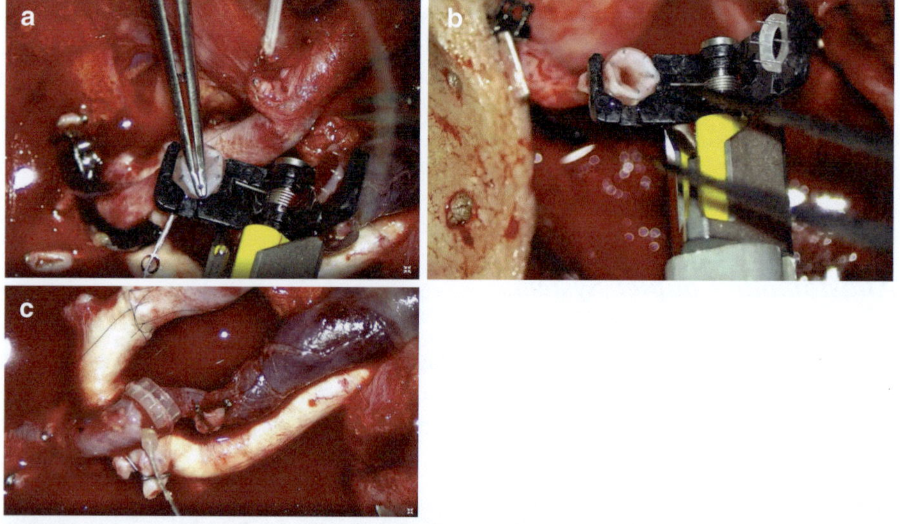

Fig. 9.7 Amamentariam for microvascular surgery

Fig. 9.8 Venous anastomosis using the coupler system. (**a**) Eversion of vessel wall onto interlocking pins. (**b**) Positioning of vessel end on polyethylene ring. (**c**) Completed venous anastomosis using the coupler system with the connected implantable Doppler probe

magnesium [26]. In 1986, Ostrup and Berggren introduced the Unilink Microvascular Anastomotic System, which served as the basis for design for currently used coupler systems (Fig. 9.8) [27]. The Unilink system consisted of two rings composed of high-density polyethylene and six interlocking pins allowing for 90° eversion of the vessel wall for intima to intima contact without the introduction of foreign material [27]. Since its introduction, multiple studies have showed venous couplers decrease operative time while maintaining low rates of venous thrombosis [28–30].

The use of arterial coupler systems has not been widely adopted by microvascular surgeons to the same degree as venous couplers. Early reports from the 1990s reported a high incidence of arterial thrombosis with use of arterial couplers, attributed to the fact that arterial walls are much thicker, less elastic, and more subject to radiation-induced fibrosis and atherosclerosis [31–33]. A greater difficulty in the arterial wall eversion is suggested to result in intimal tears or a greater incidence of obstruction of the arterial lumen with a resultant decrease in laminar blood flow and predisposing to thrombosis. A recent systematic review found a 92.1% success rate of arterial couplers as determined by arterial anastomosis patency and flap viability and up to 3.2% rate of arterial thrombosis [34]. Additionally, a 12.8% (range 0–50%) rate of troubleshooting was reported secondary to a multitude of reasons including: traumatic injury or intimal tear during instrumentation, a need to abort the coupler due to small arterial diameter (<1.5 mm), challenges everting thick arterial vessel walls, and challenges managing vessel wall and coupler luminal diameter discrepancies [34]. Despite the increased risk of significant complications, arterial couplers are associated with a reduction in the time for arterial anastomosis and operating time as compared to the hand-sewn technique; however, technical challenges and inexperience in arterial coupling can limit the advantage of time gained using the coupler device [34].

Case selection for applying the arterial coupler is of utmost importance, with its use only considered for select cases in which: a coupler size of greater than 2.0 mm can be used, vessel size mismatch is limited to 1:1.5, there is a low wall thickness to lumen ratio, and arteries are devoid of severe fibrosis or atherosclerotic plaques [34]. Additional techniques have been described to mitigate complications, including: meticulous adventitiectomy, dilation to upsize vessels 1.5 mm in diameter, and slit arteriotomy when upsizing vessels less than 1.5 mm in diameter [34]. While artery-specific coupler systems are available, coupler systems used for venous anastomosis are FDA-approved for arterial anastomosis as well [35].

Advances in the Operative Microscope

The evolution of the operative microscope over the past century has revolutionized operations in head and neck surgery, plastic surgery, ophthalmic, neurosurgery, and dentistry. The microscope was first introduced into the operating room in 1921 by Carl Olof Nylen, an otolaryngologist at the University Clinic of Stockholm [2]. In 1922, Gunnar Holmgren developed the binocular microscope attached with a light source, which provided the added benefit of stereopsis [2]. In 1961, Jacobson developed the first double binocular microscope, named the diploscope, which allowed for improved surgical assistance [36].

Contemporary operative microscopes allow for autofocusing with automation, improved portability, and coaxial designs for improved maneuverability (Fig. 9.9). Optical carriers and binocular tubes allow for positioning of the microscope in orientations which maintains operator efficiency and comfort. Modern innovations

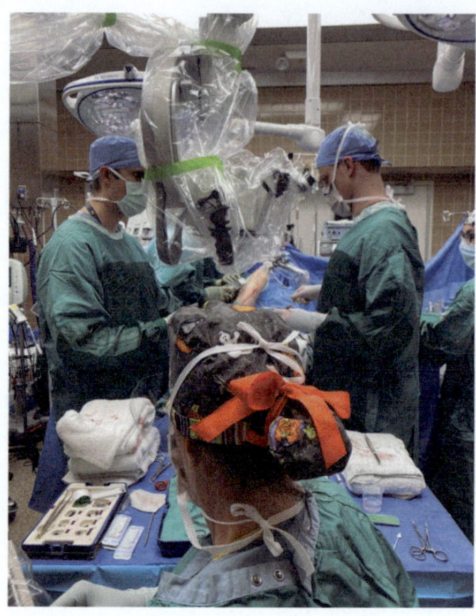

Fig. 9.9 Use of binocular operative microscope for microvascular anastomosis

have allowed for additional capabilities including intraoperative fluorescence systems and neuronavigation software integration [37]. Despite these innovations, the operative microscope still holds a relatively large footprint, making it cumbersome to position intraoperatively. Depending on the unit, the operative field of view can be restricting and can place the surgeon in nonergonomic positions, which can contribute to operator fatigue. New technologies including the exoscope and robotic microscope have been developed to address these challenges.

Exoscope

The exoscope is an extracorporeal video telescope operating system introduced in the last decade. A three-dimensional (3D) camera held by a supporting arm projects a magnified, high definition (HD), 4 K video of the surgical field onto an HD monitor, and operators view the monitor using polarized 3D glasses. This "heads up" display has become increasingly popular as it potentially allows for a more ergonomic position for the surgeon, along with better visualization for team members in the operatory [38]. The exoscope allows for a magnification power of 8–30 times, a depth of field between 7 and 44 mm, and a focal distance of 20–50 cm. The camera is controlled with a sterilely draped joystick, allowing for the operator to zoom, focus, and adjust the position of the camera with minimal change in position.

Several exoscopes are currently on the market [39, 40] and have been shown to provide equivalent outcomes as compared to a standard operative microscope when used for microvascular surgery [41, 42]. The first microvascular free flap anastomosis using the exoscope was described in 2017 using a DIEP flap for breast reconstruction [43]. A simulation noninferiority trial reported that the exoscope was noninferior to the operating microscope with good focusing of the surgical field with high image quality and strong luminance but found that the exoscopic microvascular anastomosis was more time consuming [42]. A case-control pilot study of 22 microvascular free flaps performed using an exoscope and 27 free flaps performed with an operative microscope found no difference in operative time, ischemia time, or microsurgical complications between groups, with operator reported favorable ergonomics, excellent image quality, and ease of equipment manipulation using the exoscope [41].

Potential benefits of the exoscope include versatility of camera positioning to allow for improved comfort of the operator and assistant, a large working length to allow for freedom of movement for hands and instrumentation, and the same view of the operative field for operators and observers, which allows for a more immersive experience not provided with a typical two-dimensional conventional scope screen [42]. A potential disadvantage of the exoscope includes a decrease in resolution at higher magnifications, which has been variably reported [38, 41].

Robotic Microscope

A robotic operative microscope has only been very recently commercially available (Fig. 9.10) [44]. It consists of a high-resolution 3D camera on a robotic arm articulating along six axes. The 3D HD images are transmitted to a head-mounted display (HMD) worn by the operator and an HD external display. The HMD has a weight of approximately 0.5 kg and consists of two micro-displays with adjustable interpupillary distance. A foot pedal is used to unlock a control menu with which the operator interacts through the HMD using motion detection. This allows the surgeon to change the camera position, angle, magnification, and focus without changing body position. The currently available system enables a magnification factor ranging from 2.7 to 30.1 times and a field of view range from 5.8 by 4.3 mm to 64.5 by 48.4 mm with full optical zoom. Additional functionality allows the operator to save multiple views and camera positions and can return to a previously saved view

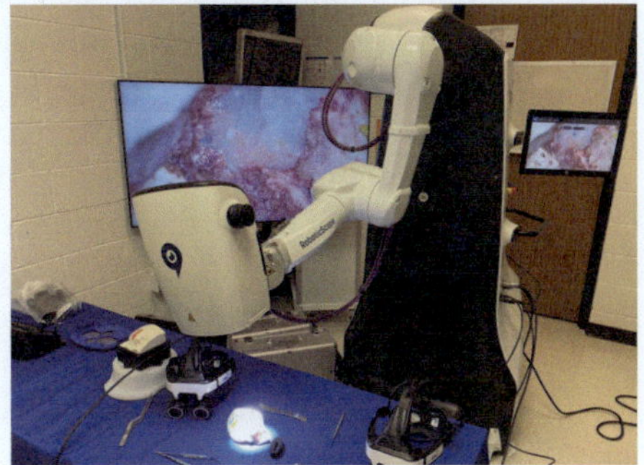

Fig. 9.10 The robotic microscope with head-mounted display and HD external display

through the control menu display [45]. The utility of this emerging technology for microvascular surgery remains to be shown through clinical studies.

Intraoperative Flap Assessment

The patency of the arterial and venous anastomoses is vital for flap survival, with early flap failure commonly related to technical error in performing the vascular anastomoses. Clinical patency tests including vessel filling, flap color and bleeding, and the strip or milk test continue to be the traditional method for assessing anastomotic patency. Adjunct tools including implantable Doppler probe systems (discussed in the next section) allow confirmation of vessel patency. Indocyanine green angiography allows evaluation of flap perfusion and vessel patency.

Indocyanine Green Angiography

Indocyanine green angiography (ICGA) is an imaging technique that allows for real-time evaluation of blood flow and is an invaluable tool for the microvascular reconstructive surgeon. First FDA approved for clinical use in 1955, indocyanine green (ICG) is an amphiphilic contrast agent consisting of a near infrared (NIR) tricarbocyanine florescent dye [46, 47]. Once administered intravenously, the anions bind to plasma proteins [47]. Clinically approved ICGA systems operate in the "NIR-1" window (700–900 nm) with an excitation wavelength of 740–800 nm and emission wavelength of 800–860 nm [48]. The high contrast, which is the manifestation of a high signal to noise ratio (SNR), allows for detailed visualization of blood vessels because the high-pass filter removes the light from the light source, while the low-pass filter allows for emitted light to be received by the sensor [49]. While there is no consensus about the optimal intravenous dose, a systematic review found the most commonly administered total dose of ICG was 12.5 mg, although maximal doses of 1–3 mg/kg have been reported [50]. ICG is hepatically metabolized and excreted through the kidneys with a half-life of 3–5 min, allowing for safe repeat administration. ICGA has been utilized in the evaluation of flap perfusion and selection of dominant perforators with greater utility in performing perforator flaps (Fig. 9.11). ICGA is also useful in assessing microvascular anastomosis patency and for postoperative flap monitoring.

ICGA is helpful in the assessment of flap perfusion, particularly in the setting of questionable physical exam findings. A study of 88 adipo- or fasciocutaneous free flaps performed with intraoperative ICGA reported a sensitivity of 100% and specificity of 98.8% [51]. Microscope-integrated ICGA can be used for early detection of anastomotic problems. A prospective study of 50 patients undergoing free microvascular transfer found that delays in transit time through the arterial and venous anastomoses identified using ICGA correlated with arterial or venous occlusion or

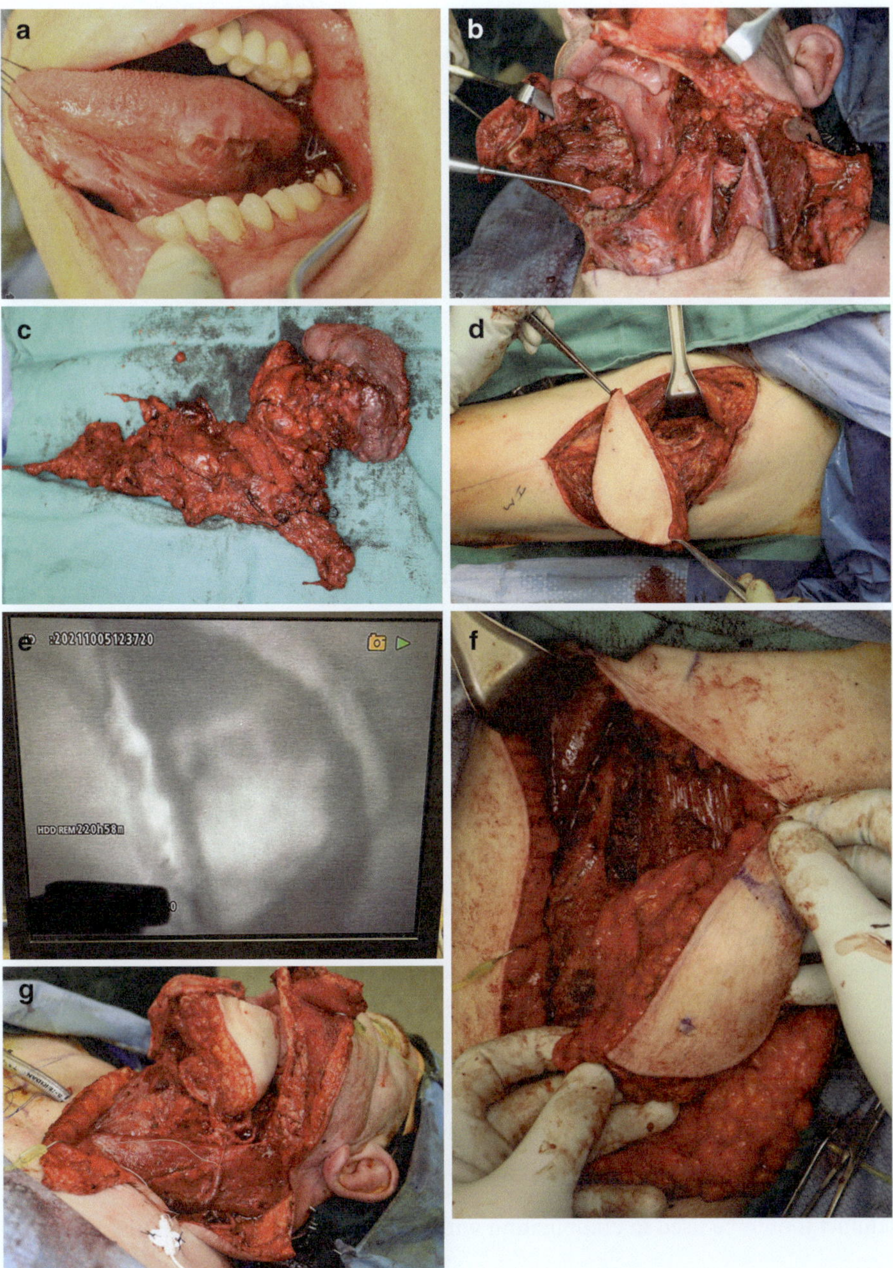

Fig. 9.11 (**a**) 72 year old male with a squamous cell carcinoma of the left ventrolateral tongue. (**b**) Ablative defect following mandibulotomy, subtotal glossectomy, resection of left lateral pharyngeal wall, left soft palate and bilateral neck dissection. (**c**) Tumor and neck dissection specimen. (**d**) Harvest of anterolateral thigh (ALT) free flap. (**e**) Intraoperative indocyanine green angiography demonstrating poor perfusion of the proximal flap. (**f**) Planned flap modification to excise poorly perfused portion of skin paddle. (**g**) Inset of ALT flap. (**h**) Immediate postoperative reconstruction. (**i**) Postoperative reconstruction at 3 months demonstrating a viable flap

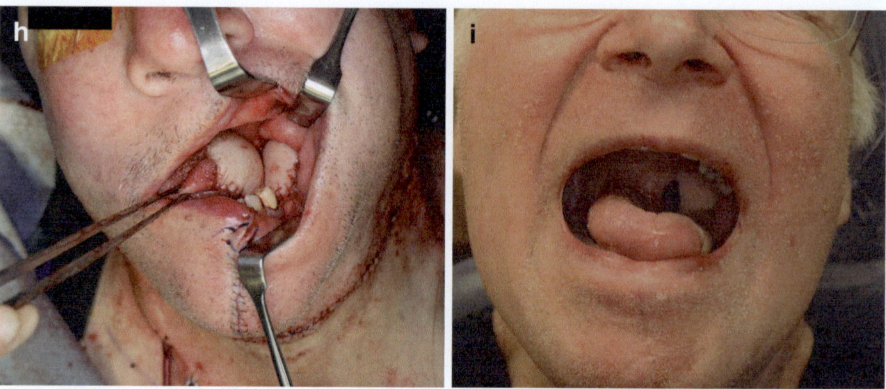

Fig. 9.11 (continued)

alterations in blood flow, potentially predisposing toward postoperative flap failure [52].

ICGA has variable value in perforator assessment. A retrospective comparative study of 28 patients who had undergone ALT flap found that ICGA was reliable in intraoperatively identifying the dominant perforator and found the use of ICGA resulted in a decrease in operator time and an increase in distal flap survival [53]. A prospective study of 12 patients undergoing ALT perforator flap found that in comparison to handheld Doppler CDU, ICGA was superior in identifying perforator anatomy with 100% sensitivity and 100% PPV [54]. Conversely, a study of 50 patients undergoing free flap reconstruction found the PPV and sensitivity of ICGA, multidetector-row computed tomography (MDCT), and Doppler flowmetry were 84% and 76%, 100% and 70%, and 80% and 100%, respectively, in the preoperative evaluation of flap perforator anatomy [55]. In this study, MDCT was less accurate in flaps with a thickness less than 8 mm, and ICGA was less reliable in flaps with a thickness greater than 20 mm, suggesting the mode of examination should be determined based on the characteristics of the flap [55].

ICGA is likely better utilized to assess flap perfusion than mapping perforators. Limitations of ICGA include providing information on arterial perfusion limited to a depth less than 1 cm, issues with both underestimation and overestimation of perfusion, and being subject to dynamic changes affected by patient temperature, cardiac output, volume status, blood pressure, volume support, and the local microvascular environment [47]. Additionally, protocols for optimal dosing and timing of contrast administration are not standardized. As such, ICGA should be considered as an adjunct tool to be used in combination with additional examination modalities.

Postoperative Flap Monitoring

The greatest risk to free flap vitality is a thrombotic occlusion of the vein or artery. Over 95% of these events occur within the first 72 h postoperatively. Early detection of pedicle thrombosis is essential for successful thrombectomy and salvage. The gold standard for free flap monitoring remains frequent intermittent clinical examination and is associated with low false-negative and low false-positive rates. Clinical examination includes an assessment of flap color, capillary refill, warmth, turgor, and bleeding on pinprick (Fig. 9.12). However, clinical monitoring can be labor intensive and subjective, dependent on the experience of the examiner. Additionally, clinical exam alone has a low salvage rate of approximately 63%, potentially as a result of subclinical changes in flap perfusion occurring significantly earlier than clinically evident manifestations of congestion or ischemia [56].

External handheld Doppler systems can supplement the clinical examination and are effective when assessing changes in arterial patency but are less sensitive when assessing venous flow. These devices are useful in monitoring an external skin paddle but less helpful for buried flaps. Additionally, reliance on external Doppler signal can delay identification of venous insufficiency, as the arterial signal can be present in the setting of completed venous occlusion for up to 6 h. The use of the implantable venous Doppler is now widely used for postoperative flap monitoring. Additional postoperative monitoring methods include tissue spectroscopy, intravenous fluorescein, thermography, transcutaneous laser Doppler, photoplethysmography, and transcutaneous PO_2 monitoring.

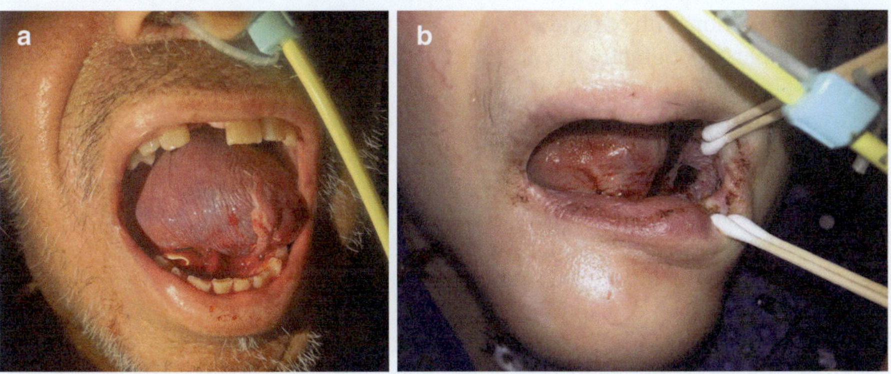

Fig. 9.12 (**a**) Clinical signs of a viable flap. (**b**) Clinical signs of venous congestion

Implantable Doppler Probe Systems

In response to challenges in monitoring buried and intraoral free flaps, Hartley and Cole described the 20-MHz unidirectional ultrasound Doppler probe in 1974 [57]. In 1988, Swartz et al. described a 1.0 mm Doppler probe with a 20 Hz ultrasonic probe applied to a silicone cuff which could be wrapped around the vessel of interest [58]. This allowed for continuous, real-time monitoring of vessel blood flow through both audible and visual monitor display. More recently, Doppler probes integral to the anastomotic coupler system have been developed [59], avoiding the additional step of applying the separate monitoring cuff around the anastomosis and improving operating time.

Multiple studies have shown improved detection of ischemia when using the implantable Doppler probe, particularly when monitoring buried flaps. A retrospective study comparing 259 microvascular free flaps monitored with implantable Doppler and 289 flaps monitored by clinical means across a wide spectrum of surgical subspecialties found improved overall success rates in the implantable Doppler group (96% vs. 89%) with the greatest benefit of the device seen in head and neck procedures (95% vs. 84%) and improved salvage rates in the implantable Doppler group (95% vs. 40%) [60]. A study of 1142 free flaps for head and neck reconstruction using the implantable Doppler reported a 12% detection rate of incipient failures in the operating room leading to immediate revision prior to closure and reported an overall flap survival rate of 98% [61]. While the implantable Doppler has a high sensitivity (87% to 100%) and specificity (99%) for detecting loss of flap perfusion, it suffers from a variable false positive rate (<1% to 88%), which potentially leads to a high proportion of subsequent negative surgical explorations [62, 63]. Corroboration with clinical exam and the use of a second assessment tool such as color duplex sonography to confirm the implantable Doppler findings has been described [63].

Arterial vessel monitoring has been described with fewer false-positive results but with greater false-negative rates, and both arterial and venous monitoring are routinely done postoperatively based on surgeon preference [64]. A systematic review of 763 flaps with implantable Doppler probes on 527 arteries and 388 veins found a 74% reduction in risk of false positives and 63% reduction in risk of signal loss with arterial monitoring, and no difference in sensitivity, specificity, false negative rate, salvage rate, or flap failure rate between venous and arterial implantable Doppler probes; however, the clinical significance of these findings is not ascertained due to study limitations [65].

Tissue Spectroscopy (Visible Light and Near Infrared)

Tissue spectroscopy is a noninvasive, continuous method of monitoring of flap perfusion and can further be subclassified as either visible light spectroscopy or near infrared spectroscopy. Visible light spectroscopy (VLS) uses shallow penetrating visible light (475–625 nm) to measure tissue hemoglobin saturation at the capillary level [66]. Decreases in tissue oxygen saturation suggest arterial inflow compromise related to an isolated arterial thrombosis or a venous thrombosis impeding arterial inflow. Additionally, total hemoglobin concentration is measured to quantify venous drainage, providing an indirect measure of blood volume within the flap. Increased total hemoglobin concentration suggests venous drainage compromise. A prospective controlled study comparing VLS and clinical examination with intermittent Doppler in the postoperative monitoring of free flaps found that VLS was able to detect compromised flap perfusion prior to changes in physical exam or handheld Doppler, resulting a 100% successful flap salvage in cases of compromised flap perfusion [67]. Limitations of VLS technology include the need for an external skin paddle larger than 2 cm, which precludes its use with buried flaps and the inability of the probe to adhere to mucosal surfaces, limiting its use in oral reconstructions. Additionally, instability in SpO_2 values during the first 8 h following arterial anastomosis potentially secondary to mild ischemia-reperfusion injury with free flap transfer can obfuscate potential vascular compromise of the flap [67].

Near-infrared spectroscopy (NIRS) monitors changes in tissue perfusion and oxygenation status based on the differential scattering and absorption of infrared light by tissue chromophores contained in hemoglobin, allowing for real-time measurement of oxygenated, deoxygenated, and total hemoglobin concentrations and detection of altered tissue hemodynamics and potential flap compromise [68]. Postoperative NIRS monitoring allows for earlier detection of subclinical vascular compromise resulting in lower flap loss rates and improved salvage rates as compared to clinical assessment with handheld Doppler [69]. A recent systematic review found that in comparison to free flaps with vascular compromise monitored clinically, flaps monitored with NIRS had a significantly higher salvage rate (89% vs. 50%), a lower rate of partial loss (15% vs. 80%), and an earlier detection of vascular compromise of approximately 82 min [68].

VLS confers several advantages over NIRS. The absorption of visible light by hemoglobin is 100 times that of infrared light, allowing for more sensitive evaluation of variation in tissue oxygenation. Additionally, the smaller VLS probe, as narrow as 6 mm, allows for easier adaptation to tissue surfaces for monitoring as compared to the larger NIRS probe. Conversely, NIRS can monitor to greater depth as compared to VLS, up to 30 mm, which may be useful for evaluating some buried flaps [70].

Conclusion

The field of microsurgery has significantly evolved over the past century. Advances in preoperative imaging have allowed for more sensitive assessment of donor site vessel anatomy and perforator planning. Venous coupler systems decrease operative time while maintaining low rates of venous thrombosis. Implantable Doppler probe systems allow for improved flap monitoring, resulting in earlier detection of microvascular thrombosis and flap compromise. Multiple technologies are available to the microvascular reconstructive surgeon to optimize the preoperative assessment, intraoperative microvascular anastomosis, and postoperative monitoring of free flaps; however, these should be considered as adjunctive tools to supplement rather than replace clinical judgment and excellent surgical technique. These advances have allowed for improved flap predictability and a shift toward custom personalized reconstructions with the goal of providing improved functional and esthetic outcomes in microvascular reconstruction.

References

1. Friedman SG. The end-to-end anastomosis of John B. Murphy. J Vasc Surg. 2015;62(2):515–7.
2. Moritz WR, Raman S, Pessin S, Martin C, Li X, Westman A, Sacks JM. The history and innovations of blood vessel anastomosis. Bioengineering (Basel). 2022;9(2):75.
3. Seidenberg B, Rosenak SS, Hurwitt ES, Som ML. Immediate reconstruction of the cervical esophagus by a revascularized isolated jejunal segment. Ann Surg. 1959;149(2):162–71.
4. Jacobson JH II, Suarez EL. Microsurgery in anastomosis of small vessels. Surg Forum. 1960;11:243–5.
5. McLean DH, Buncke HJ Jr. Autotransplant of omentum to a large scalp defect, with microsurgical revascularization. Plast Reconstr Surg. 1972;49(3):268–74.
6. Hidalgo DA. Fibula free flap: a new method of mandible reconstruction. Plast Reconstr Surg. 1989;84(1):71–9.
7. Tamai S. History of microsurgery—from the beginning until the end of the 1970s. Microsurgery. 1993;14(1):6–13.
8. Giunta RE, et al. The value of preoperative Doppler sonography for planning free perforator flaps. Plast Reconstr Surg. 2000;105(7):2381–6.
9. Garvey PB, Chang EI, Selber JC, Skoracki RJ, Madewell JE, Liu J, Yu P, Hanasono MM. A prospective study of preoperative computed tomographic angiographic mapping of free fibula osteocutaneous flaps for head and neck reconstruction. Plast Reconstr Surg. 2012;130(4):541e–9e.
10. Rozen WM, et al. The accuracy of computed tomographic angiography for mapping the perforators of the DIEA: a cadaveric study. Plast Reconstr Surg. 2008;122(2):363–9.
11. Battaglia S, et al. Osteomyocutaneous fibular flap harvesting: computer-assisted planning of perforator vessels using computed tomographic angiography scan and cutting guide. J Craniomaxillofac Surg. 2017;45(10):1681–6.
12. Ettinger KS, Morris JM, Alexander AE, Nathan JM, Arce K. Accuracy and precision of the computed tomographic angiography perforator localization technique for virtual surgical planning of composite Osteocutaneous fibular free flaps in head and neck reconstruction. J Oral Maxillofac Surg. 2022;S0278-2391(22):00238–5.
13. Smit JM, et al. Preoperative CT angiography reduces surgery time in perforator flap reconstruction. J Plast Reconstr Aesthet Surg. 2009;62(9):1112–7.
14. Nassar AH, et al. Comparison of various modalities utilized for preoperative planning in microsurgical reconstructive surgery. J Reconstr Microsurg. 2021;38:170. https://doi.org/10.1055/s-0041-1736316.
15. Rodkin B, et al. A review of visualized preoperative imaging with a focus on surgical procedures of the breast. Gland Surg. 2019;8(S4):S301–9.
16. Futran ND, Stack BC Jr, Zaccardi MJ. Preoperative color flow Doppler imaging for fibula free tissue transfers. Ann Vasc Surg. 1998;12(5):445–50.
17. Dorfman D, Pu LLQ. The value of color duplex imaging for planning and performing a free anterolateral thigh perforator flap. Ann Plast Surg. 2014;72(Supplement 1):S6–8.

18. Cho M-J, et al. The role of duplex ultrasound in microsurgical reconstruction: review and technical considerations. J Reconstr Microsurg. 2020;36(07):514–21.
19. John HE, Niumsawatt V, Rozen WM, Whitaker IS. Clinical applications of dynamic infrared thermography in plastic surgery: a systematic review. Gland Surg. 2016;5(2):122–32.
20. Muntean MV, et al. Dynamic infrared mapping of cutaneous perforators. J Xiangya Med. 2018;3:16. https://doi.org/10.21037/jxym.2018.04.05. Accessed 23 Jan 2022.
21. Sheena Y, Jennison T, Hardwicke JT, Titley OG. Detection of perforators using thermal imaging. Plast Reconstr Surg. 2013;132(6):1603–10.
22. Hardwicke JT, et al. Detection of perforators using smartphone thermal imaging. Plast Reconstr Surg. 2016;137(1):39–41.
23. de Weerd L, et al. The value of dynamic infrared thermography (DIRT) in perforator selection and planning of free DIEP flaps. Ann Plast Surg. 2009;63(3):274–9. https://doi.org/10.1097/sap.0b013e318190321e.
24. Weum S, et al. Evaluation of dynamic infrared thermography as an alternative to CT angiography for perforator mapping in breast reconstruction: a clinical study. BMC Med Imaging. 2016;16(1):43.
25. Chubb DP, Taylor GI, Ashton MW. True and 'choke' anastomoses between perforator angiosomes: part II. Dynamic thermographic identification. Plast Reconstr Surg. 2013;132(6):1457–64.
26. Leveen HH. Nonsuture method for vascular anastomosis utilizing the Murphy button principle. Arch Surg (1920). 1949;58(4):504–10. https://doi.org/10.1001/archsurg.1949.01240030512010.
27. Ostrup LT, Berggren A. The UNILINK instrument system for fast and safe microvascular anastomosis. Ann Plast Surg. 1986;17(6):521–5.
28. Nakatsuka T, Harii K, Asato H, Takushima A, Ebihara S, Kimata Y, Yamada A, Ueda K, Ichioka S. Analytic review of 2372 free flap transfers for head and neck reconstruction following cancer resection. J Reconstr Microsurg. 2003;19(06):363–8.
29. Grewal A, Erovic B, Struman N, et al. The utility of the microvascular anastomotic coupler in free tissue transfer. Can J Plast Surg. 2012;20(02):98.
30. Shindo M, Costantino P, Nalbone V, Rice D, Sinha U. Use of a mechanical microvascular anastomotic device in head and neck free tissue transfer. Arch Otolaryngol Head Neck Surg. 1996;122(5):529–32.
31. Spector JA, et al. Routine use of microvascular coupling device for arterial anastomosis in breast reconstruction. Ann Plast Surg. 2006;56(4):365–8.
32. Shindo ML, et al. Use of a mechanical microvascular anastomotic device in head and neck free tissue transfer. Arch Otolaryngol Head Neck Surg. 1996;122(5):529–32.
33. DeLacure MD, et al. Clinical experience with a microvascular anastomotic device in head and neck reconstruction. Am J Surg. 1995;170(5):521–3.
34. Pafitanis G, et al. Microvascular anastomotic arterial coupling: a systematic review. J Plast Reconstr Aesthet Surg. 2021;74(6):1286–302.
35. GEM Synovis MCA. Microvascular anastomotic coupler. https://www.synovismicro.com/html/products/gem_microvascular_anastomotic_coupler.html.
36. Rickard RF, Hudson DA. A history of vascular and microvascular surgery. Ann Plast Surg. 2014;73(4):465–72.
37. Liczbik O, et al. From magnifying glass to operative microscopy—the historical and modern role of the microscope in microsurgery. Pol J Pathol. 2019;70(1):14–20.
38. De Virgilio A, et al. Free flap microvascular anastomosis in head and neck reconstruction using a 4K three-dimensional exoscope system (VITOM 3D). Int J Oral Maxillofac Surg. 2020;49(9):1169–73.
39. Karl Storz-Endoskope. VITOM® 3D—3D visualization for microsurgery and open surgery. https://www.karlstorz.com/de/en/microscopy.htm.
40. Olympus. ORBEYE™ exoscope. https://medical.olympusamerica.com/products/orbeye.
41. Ahmad FI, et al. Application of the ORBEYE three-dimensional exoscope for microsurgical procedures. Microsurgery. 2019;40(4):468–72.

42. Pafitanis G, et al. The exoscope versus operating microscope in microvascular surgery: a simulation non-inferiority trial. Arch Plast Surg. 2020;47(03):242–9.
43. Piatkowski AA, Keuter XHA, Schols RM, van der Hulst RRWJ. Potential of performing a microvascular free flap reconstruction using solely a 3D exoscope instead of a conventional microscope. J Plast Reconstr Aesthet Surg. 2018;71:1664–78.
44. BHS Technologies. The RoboticScope®. https://www.bhs-technologies.com/the-robotic-scope-change-of-perspective/.
45. Boehm F, et al. Performance of microvascular anastomosis with a new robotic visualization system: proof of concept. J Robot Surg. 2021;16(3):705–13.
46. Pruimboom T, et al. Optimizing Indocyanine green fluorescence angiography in reconstructive flap surgery: a systematic review and ex vivo experiments. Surg Innov. 2019;27(1):103–19.
47. Ott P. Hepatic elimination of Indocyanine green with special reference to distribution kinetics and the influence of plasma protein binding. Pharmacol Toxicol. 1998;83:1–48.
48. Starosolski Z, et al. Indocyanine green fluorescence in second near-infrared (NIR-II) window. PloS One. 2017;12(11):e0187563.
49. Alander JT, et al. A review of Indocyanine green fluorescent imaging in surgery. Int J Biomed Imaging. 2012;2012:1.
50. Li K, et al. Application of indocyanine green in flap surgery: a systematic review. J Reconstr Microsurg. 2017;34(02):077–86.
51. Bigdeli AK, Thomas B, Falkner F, Gazyakan E, Hirche C, Kneser U. The impact of Indocyanine-green fluorescence angiography on intraoperative decision-making and postoperative outcome in free flap surgery. J Reconstr Microsurg. 2020;36(8):556–66.
52. Holm C, Mayr M, Höfter E, Dornseifer U, Ninkovic M. Assessment of the patency of microvascular anastomoses using microscope-integrated near-infrared angiography: a preliminary study. Microsurgery. 2009;29(07):509–14.
53. La Padula S, et al. Intraoperative use of Indocyanine green angiography for selecting the more reliable perforator of the anterolateral thigh flap: a comparison study. Microsurgery. 2018;38(7):738–44. https://doi.org/10.1002/micr.30326.
54. Ritschl LM, et al. Comparison between different perforator imaging modalities for the anterolateral thigh perforator flap transfer: a prospective study. J Reconstr Microsurg. 2020;36(09):686–93. https://doi.org/10.1055/s-0040-1714425.
55. Onoda S, et al. Preoperative identification of perforator vessels by combining MDCT, Doppler flowmetry, and ICG fluorescent angiography. Microsurgery. 2013;33(4):265–9.
56. Chubb D, et al. The efficacy of clinical assessment in the postoperative monitoring of free flaps: a review of 1140 consecutive cases. Plast Reconstr Surg. 2010;125(4):1157–66. https://doi.org/10.1097/prs.0b013e3181d0ac95. Accessed 12 Nov 2021.
57. Hartley CJ, Cole JS. A single-crystal ultrasonic catheter-tip velocity probe. Med Instrum. 1974;8(4):241–3.
58. Swartz WM, Jones NF, Cherup L, Klein A. Direct monitoring of microvascular anastomoses with the 20-MHz ultrasonic Doppler probe: an experimental and clinical study. Plast Reconstr Surg. 1988;81(2):149–61. https://doi.org/10.1097/00006534-198802000-00001.
59. GEM Synovis MCA. Flow coupler device and system. https://www.synovismicro.com/html/products/gem_flow_coupler_device_and_system.html.
60. Schmulder A, et al. Eight-year experience of the cook-swartz Doppler in free-flap operations: microsurgical and reexploration results with regard to a wide spectrum of surgeries. Microsurgery. 2011;31(1):1–6. https://doi.org/10.1002/micr.20816. Accessed 13 May 2022.
61. Wax MK. The role of the implantable Doppler probe in free flap surgery. Laryngoscope. 2014;124(S1):S1–S12.
62. Chang EI, et al. Deciphering the sensitivity and specificity of the implantable Doppler probe in free flap monitoring. Plast Reconstr Surg. 2016;137(3):971–6.
63. Rosenberg JJ, et al. Monitoring buried free flaps: limitations of the implantable Doppler and use of color duplex sonography as a confirmatory test. Plast Reconstr Surg. 2006;118(1):109–13.

64. Karinja SJ, Lee BT. Advances in flap monitoring and impact of enhanced recovery protocols. J Surg Oncol. 2018;118(5):758–67. https://doi.org/10.1002/jso.25179. Epub 2018 Aug 21.
65. Klifto KM, Milek D, Gurno CF, Seal SM, Hultman CS, Rosson GD, Cooney DS. Comparison of arterial and venous implantable Doppler postoperative monitoring of free flaps: systematic review and meta-analysis of diagnostic test accuracy. Microsurgery. 2020;40(4):501–11. https://doi.org/10.1002/micr.30564. Epub 2020 Feb 7.
66. Fox PM, Zeidler K, Carey J, Lee GK. White light spectroscopy for free flap monitoring. Microsurgery. 2012;33(3):198–202.
67. Mericli AF, et al. A prospective clinical trial comparing visible light spectroscopy to handheld Doppler for postoperative free tissue transfer monitoring. Plast Reconstr Surg. 2017;140(3):604–13.
68. Newton E, et al. Outcomes of free flap reconstructions with near-infrared spectroscopy (NIRS) monitoring: a systematic review. Microsurgery. 2020;40(2):268–75.
69. Koolen PGL, et al. Does increased experience with tissue oximetry monitoring in microsurgical breast reconstruction Lead to decreased flap loss? The learning effect. Plast Reconstr Surg. 2016;137(4):1093–101.
70. Lindelauf AAMA, et al. Near-infrared spectroscopy (NIRS) versus hyperspectral imaging (HSI) to detect flap failure in reconstructive surgery: a systematic review. Life (Basel). 2022;12(1):65.

Chapter 10
Use of Three-Dimensional Technology for Virtual Surgical Planning in Oral and Maxillofacial Surgery

Salah Al Din Al Azri ⓘD, Yohaann Ali Ghosh ⓘD, and Jonathan Shum

Introduction

The use of virtual surgical planning has had a significant impact on oral and maxillofacial surgery. Virtual planning has been utilized since 1980 and has now been implemented into all aspects of osseous surgery and reconstructions of the face. The success of these virtually planned cases depends on each step of the workflow process: patient workup, quality of the image modality, data acquisition, virtual planning, and surgical execution. Each component of the process should be thorough and meticulous in order to minimize the possibility of error during the surgical execution. The overwhelming utility of virtual surgical planning and the ability to create guides and implants to translate virtual reconstructions into reality have led to increased efficiency, reduce costs, and ultimately improve surgical outcomes.

S. A. D. Al Azri (✉)
Maxillofacial Oncology and Microvascular Reconstructive Surgery, Houston, TX, USA

Department of Oral and Maxillofacial Surgery, The University of Texas Health Science Center at Houston, Houston, TX, USA
e-mail: salah.al.din.alazri@uth.tmc.edu

Y. A. Ghosh
School of Medicine and Dentistry, Griffith University, Gold Coast, Australia

Integrated Prosthetics and Reconstruction, Department of Head and Neck Surgery, Chris O'Brien Lifehouse, Sydney, NSW, Australia
e-mail: yohaann.ghosh@lh.org.au

J. Shum
Maxillofacial Oncology and Microvascular Reconstructive Surgery, Houston, TX, USA

Department of Oral and Maxillofacial Surgery, The University of Texas Health Science Center at Houston, Houston, TX, USA

The University of Texas Health Science Center at Houston, Houston, TX, USA
e-mail: jonathan.shum@uth.tmc.edu

J. C. Melville et al. (eds.), *Advancements and Innovations in OMFS, ENT, and Facial Plastic Surgery*, https://doi.org/10.1007/978-3-031-32099-6_10

These processes and applications are outlined in this chapter to provide an overview of the advancements that allow for accurate maxillofacial reconstructions.

Imaging Modality Hard Tissue Considerations

The initial step of virtual surgical planning necessitates obtaining the appropriate images that are processed, used for planning sessions and construction of the appropriate surgical guides and hardware. Different imaging modalities have different spatial and contrast resolution. Spatial resolution is the ability for an image modality to differentiate between two separate objects in a radiographic image, whereas contrast resolution is the ability to differentiate image intensities between two areas (i.e., fat stranding vs. normal adipose tissue) [1] (Fig. 10.1).

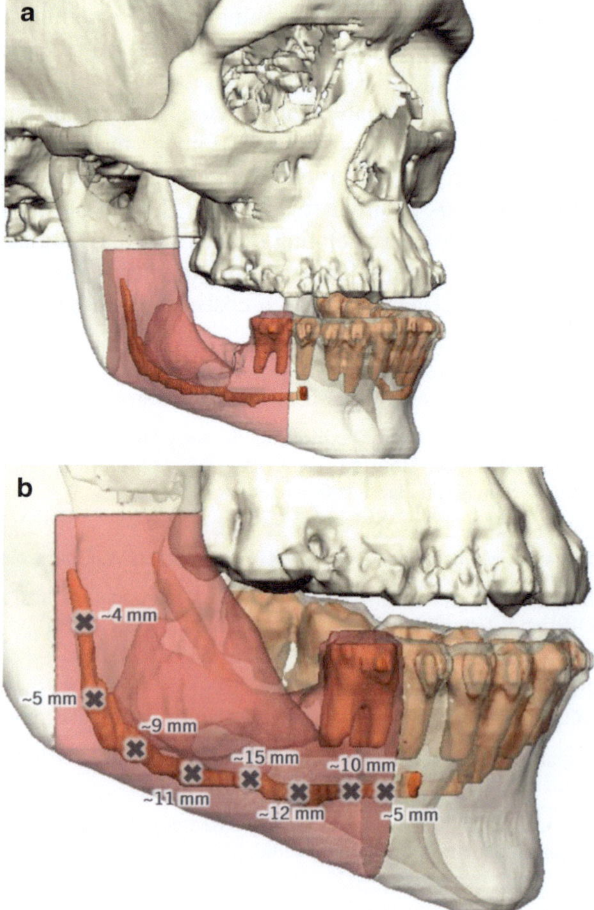

Fig. 10.1 (**a**) Inferior alveolar nerve location within the mandible rendered from computed tomography (CT) scan. (**b**) Depth determined in millimeters from mandible buccal cortex. *(Courtesy of KLS Martin group)*

Computed tomography (CT) scans and Cone Beam CT (CBCT) both have good spatial resolution, whereas Magnetic Resonance Imaging (MRI) has higher contrast resolution. MRI is superior to computed tomography in determining soft tissue alterations; however, its ability to provide high-resolution images of bone can be limited [2]. For this reason, CT scans are widely used in oral and maxillofacial surgery cases since they often involve hard tissue interventions. CBCT offers high spatial resolution with less radiation exposure compared to CT scans but has poor contrast resolution [3]. The disadvantage of the previous imaging modalities is the inability to capture very fine details of teeth structures such as the ridges and grooves which might be necessary when constructing, for example, occlusal splints for orthognathic surgery or dental implant surgical guides. 3-dimensional (3D) intraoral laser scanning (IOS) is used to provide the fine details necessary to facilitate procedures when meticulous details are necessary. IOS creates images that are stored as stereolithography file (STL) then undergoes Digital Imaging and Communications in Medicine (DICOM) encapsulation. This process produces a reliable 3D image that can be used to create an accurate virtual representation of an object, that is, dentition and gingiva. The high accuracy of virtual surgical planning (VSP) design and translation through cutting guides and hardware have been thoroughly studied and established in the literature [4–7]. In addition, this method to plan surgery has been shown to reduce operative time and minimize complications in all its applications [8–11].

Imaging Modalities—Soft Tissue Considerations

VSP for maxillofacial bony reconstruction is often done in conjunction with imaging of related soft tissue structures to obtain adequate coverage of the ablative defect. With respect to soft tissue reconstruction, head and neck surgeons predominantly choose between two approaches: pedicled flaps and free flaps. The fibula and radial forearm regions are among the most common osteomusculocutaneous free flap donor sites to be harvested with a skin island [12]. Adequate perfusion of the tissue is necessary for these flaps to be viable. Indeed, perfusion to the donor region should be assessed preoperatively, with methods depending on the chosen site. For example, CT-angiography can be used to confirm the presence of three-vessel runoff in the lower leg for fibula free flaps. Upon visualizing the perforators from the peroneal artery, fibula osteotomies can be planned to obtain a long pedicle and reliable cutaneous portion [13].

Additionally, the anterolateral thigh (ALT) is the workhorse fasciocutaneous flap for when soft tissue bulk is needed. Emerging technologies such as handheld thermal imaging provide a novel intraoperative modality for perforator identification, negating the need for conventional Doppler imaging [14]. Such devices supplement the surgical armamentarium, providing greater confidence in the design and perfusion of the skin paddle.

Data Acquisition

Appropriate use of the previously discussed imaging modalities is pertinent to a successful virtual surgical plan when using custom devices. Any anatomical inaccuracies made during data acquisition can compromise the final surgical outcome.

Most procedures in oral and maxillofacial surgery involving bony reconstruction require CT imaging. An image slice thickness of 1 mm is an acceptable compromise between high resolution and minimal radiation exposure for the patient [15].

To facilitate virtual modeling and editing between various software and various clinical applications, CT data is stored in a DICOM format. Conversion of this format to a 3D object file for use in VSP requires virtual stacking of each radiographic section. Proprietary software such as *Materialize Mimics* (Materialize, Leuven, Belgium) can be used to build a virtual model. If required, the model can be 3D printed at this stage. However, where editing, rendering, and analysis of the virtual model is required, computer-assisted design (CAD) software should be employed. Such commercially available software includes *Geomagic® Freeform® PLUS* (3D Systems, Rock Hill, SC, USA) and *Proplan* (Materialize, Leuven, Belgium). The ultimate purpose of these software is to finalize the surgical plan and export the model into additional programs for fabrication of cutting guides or other operative hardware.

Optical scanning is another technology that has proven to be high-yield with regards to data acquisition for VSP in maxillofacial procedures involving dentition. Occlusion-driven, reverse VSP provides the optimal workflow for preprosthetic considerations. For example, the Chris O'Brien Lifehouse Cancer Center digital workflow for mandible reconstruction begins with the optical scanning of an ideal denture wax-up positioned onto a 3D printed model of the reconstructed bone [16]. This data is superimposed with scans of the existing teeth, denture wax-up, planned reconstruction, dental implants, and native bone using CAD software such as 3ds Max® (Autodesk®, San Rafael, California). This model can then be 3D printed for preoperative bending of an off-the-shelf titanium fixation plate if needed. Alternatively, the data obtained from the virtual surgery workflow can be used to fabricate customized hardware [17]. Registration of the fixation plate and any necessary screws can again be done using optical scanning and superimposition onto the virtual plan.

Applications

Orthognathic

Virtual surgical planning (VSP) has revolutionized orthognathic surgery planning. It provides precise and predictable movements of the maxillofacial skeleton compared to conventional surgical planning (CSP), which is attributed to numerous opportunities for error and inaccuracies [18]. Combining different imaging modalities and intraoral laser scanning (IOS) for virtual surgical planning has replaced the traditional orthognathic workup and need for dental impressions, and face bow measurements with the added benefit of reduced inaccuracies and costs [6, 18]. Jones and colleagues [6] found that the use of patient-specific cutting guides and implants constructed with VSP provide more accurate maxillary repositioning during bimaxillary surgery than the use of an interim splint constructed by traditional methods. Resnick and colleagues [19] further examined operative time and cost of bimaxillary surgeries of 43 patients to show that operative time and costs were significantly higher in all the patients with conventional orthognathic workup compared with VSP surgeries. These findings are significant because prolonged operative time is closely correlated with increased postoperative complications [20]. VSP has made orthognathic surgeries more accurate and efficient when compared to conventional surgical planning [21, 22]. A standard orthognathic VSP workflow is outlined in Fig. 10.2.

Pathology and Reconstruction

Oncologic resection and reconstruction of maxillofacial defects has seen an immense benefit from 3D technology such as VSP. Throughout the digital workflow, 3D technology provides the ability to accurately visualize the pathology and more confidently plan the required osteotomies (Fig. 10.3). Particularly, with respect to areas of the midface, where direct visualization of some pathologies can be hard to obtain, that is, within the paranasal sinuses and nasal cavity. Using existing imaging techniques, patient-specific cutting guide designs can be optimized to prevent inadvertent injury to vital structures, such as at the skull base while maintaining safe oncologic margins.

Additionally, immediate intraoperative feedback can be achieved through the integration of both live 3D navigation and VSP together. Osteotomies made using these modalities in anatomical models have been more accurate in distance, pitch, and roll [23].

Clinically, the margins for surgical resection of lesions can be difficult to discern, such as in osteoradionecrosis (ORN). In these patients, dosimetry-guided VSP has emerged as a new technique that can be used to plan optimal osteotomies, with the goal of obtaining healthy native bone margins. By superimposing previously delivered radiotherapy dosimetry data onto the corresponding virtual mandible, Jenkins and colleagues [24] have been able to use *IPS®* planning software (KLS Martin IPS Service UK Ltd) to integrate a radiation "heat-map" of the affected mandible with CT data to redefine the necessary margins. This additional planning stage is important where the mandible has received >60Gy of radiation, placing the native bone at higher risk of ORN [25].

The recent adoption of Titanium Milling and Selective Laser Melting (SLM) manufacturing techniques in high-volume surgical centers has heralded a shift from

Data Collection

1. Obtain intraoral and extraoral photographs with a standardized background (white or blue wall)
2. Fabricate stone or digital models (intraoral scans) in reproducible centric occlusion
3. Deliver data to processing center for rendering (digital upload or physical media)
4. Often stone casts are sent with digital scans as a reference mark to the final occlusion
5. Though optional, casts are particular helpful in segmental surgical planning

Pre-Planning

1. Stone models are superimposed with CT images to check for inaccuracies
2. Once verified, scans are imported into digital cephalometric program such as Dolphin
3. Cephalometric points and planned osteotomies are imported into the digitized facial skeleton
4. Coordinate planning session with surgeon, engineer, and possibly orthodontist

Planning Session (Digital Model Surgery)

1. First, assess for maxillary cant and maxillary dental and facial midline (refer to clinical photos)
2. Le Fort osteotomy is virtually placed based on anatomical landmarks (i.e. canine apices)
3. If required, interdental maxillary osteotomies can be placed at this time
4. Cephalometric measurements are placed in the lateral view (SNA, SNB, maxillary depth, etc.)
5. Determine vertical position of maxilla based on clinical photos
6. Once the maxilla is in ideal position, the mandible can be placed into class I canine occlusion
7. The type of mandible osteotomy (SSO vs. VRO) should be made known to all planning members
8. A genioplasty can be virtually executed at this point, if necessary

Manufacturing Considerations

1. Osteotomy guides are typically based on occlusal surfaces for stability
2. Occlusal splints are fabricated to guide the final position of the osteotomy segments
3. Stereolithic models allow evaluation of critical landmarks (i.e. neurovascular bundle)

Fig. 10.2 Orthognathic surgery workflow. *SNA* Sella Nasion A, *SNB* Sella Nasion B, *SSO* sagittal split osteotomy, *VRO* vertical ramus osteotomy. *(Reproduced with permission from Hua, Jack et al. "Virtual Surgical Planning in Oral and Maxillofacial Surgery." Oral and maxillofacial surgery clinics of North America vol. 31,4 (2019): 519–530. doi:10.1016/j.coms.2019.07.01)*

off-the-shelf fixation plates to personalized patient-specific plates. As a result of VSP, titanium plates can be purpose-built for specific cases, taking care to avoid any vital structures detected on imaging. Milled mandibular plates are manufactured from a titanium alloy block, for which a computer-assisted design (CAD) is generated using a digital contour of the reconstructed virtual mandible. Conversely, SLM

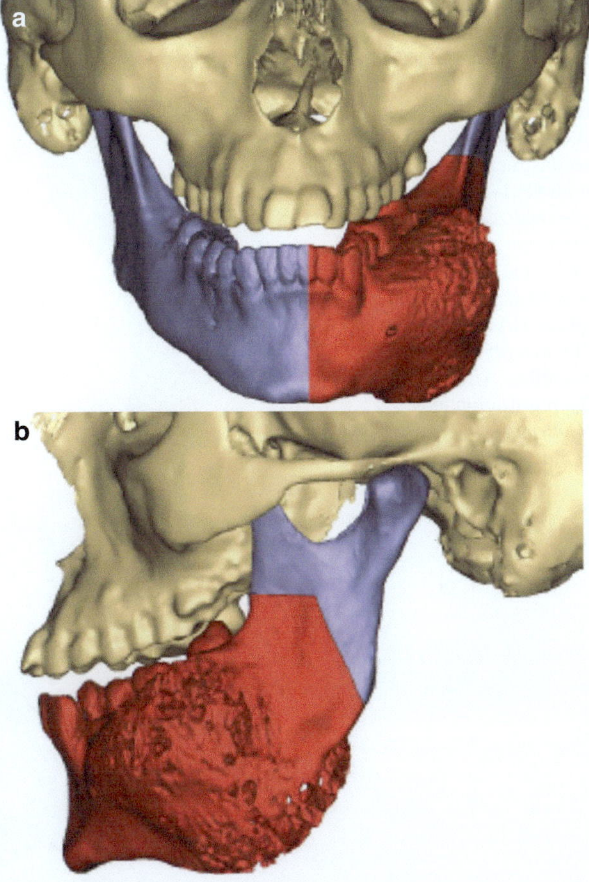

Fig. 10.3 Resection margins are determined during virtual surgical planning. Three-dimensional (3D) objects are created from computed tomography (CT) and cone beam scan images. (**a**) 3D reconstructed coronal view of myxoma in the left mandible. Area of resection highlighted in red. (**b**) 3D reconstructed Sagittal view of myxoma in the left mandible. Area of resection highlighted in red. *(Courtesy of DePuy Synthes/Materialise)*

manufacturing of personalized plates involves a type of 3D printing where titanium particles are melted and fused together in the desired fashion. Because of their exact manufacturing technique, personalized plates may provide a better biomechanical outcome compared to conventional plates that undergo material deformation during bending [26]. Personalized plates also allow for further modifications to be made. Smith and colleagues [27] have introduced an additional tab to their SLM plates that wraps around the lateral mandibular segment for additional fixation (Fig. 10.4). When planned correctly, the temporary fixation holes of each cutting guide can also be repurposed for subsequent parts of the reconstruction such as permanent fixation and dental implant placement, taking care to avoid any vital neurovascular structures. Additionally, adequate occlusion for oral rehabilitation can be obtained through using VSP for precise implant placement, preventing buccal or lingual rotation of the implant and osseous flap [28].

A relatively novel application of this technology has been the 3D printing of single-unit titanium plates for vascularized maxillary reconstruction (Fig. 10.5). The University of Texas Health Sciences Center at Houston (UTHealth) were the

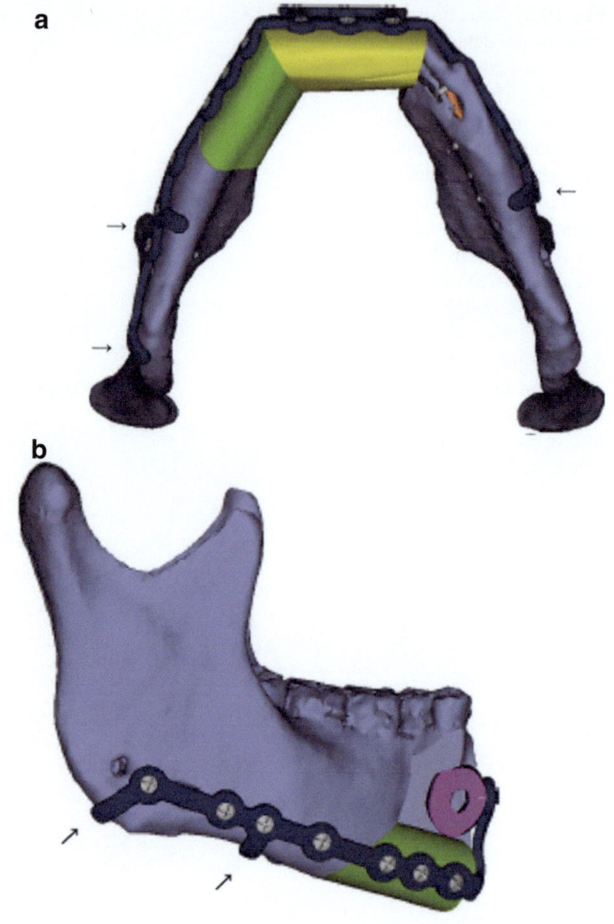

Fig. 10.4 Virtually constructed three-dimensional (3D) printed bone plate with added registration tables. (**a**) Axial view of 3D reconstructed mandible with fibula segments and personalized plate. Fibula segments are highlighted in green and yellow. Arrows denote the registration tables. (**b**) Lateral view of 3D reconstructed mandible. Arrows denote the registration tabs. (*Courtesy of DePuy Synthes/Materialise*)

first reported surgical team to use a customized single-unit system for this purpose (Synthes PSI TRUMATCH CMF Solutions; Depuy Synthes CMF, West Chester, PA) [29]. The primary goal of using VSP in maxillary cases is to preoperatively design a specific plate for the neomaxilla that maximizes contact with the thickest portion of the remaining healthy midface bone. This enables engagement of an optimal bilateral zygomaticomaxillary buttress (Fig. 10.6). The secondary goal of these custom plates is to minimize the plate profile, thus preventing extrusion out of the soft tissue. Ultimately, customized plates designed with VSP provide a comprehensive and efficient approach to maxillary reconstruction.

Using VSP has also facilitated accurate localization and reconstruction of soft tissue structures within bone (Fig. 10.7).

For the maxillofacial cancer patient, oral health-related quality of life can be negatively impacted by problems related to chewing, esthetics, and speech that arise

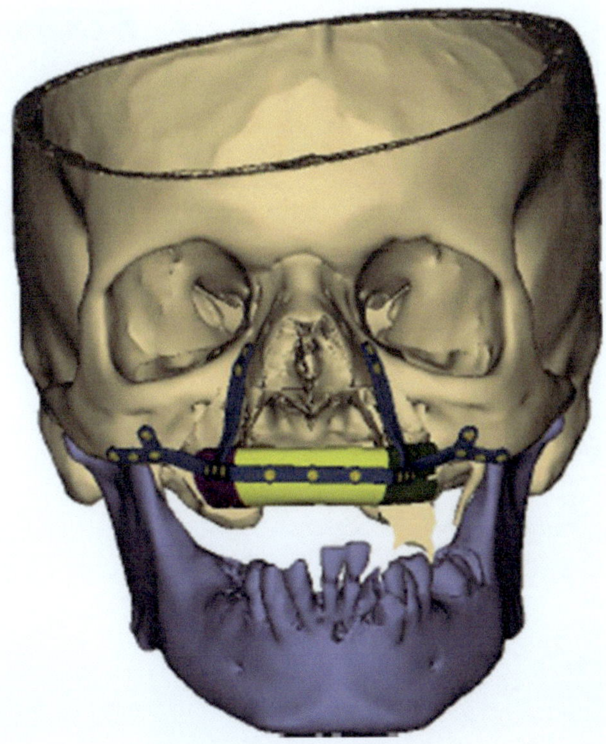

Fig. 10.5 Virtually constructed three-dimensional (3D) printing single unit titanium plate for vascularized maxillary reconstruction. Coronal view of personalized hardware. Fibula segments are highlighted in purple, yellow, and green. *(Courtesy of DePuy Synthes/Materialise)*

from missing teeth. Therefore, the paradigm of occlusion-driven planning for implant reconstruction and prosthetics has dominated head and neck surgery in recent years. For example, following the virtual design of a neomandible using fibular reconstruction, the occlusion can be superimposed to be coincident with the opposing arch. This will guide the placement of dental implants to support a fixed or removable prosthesis.

Although the fibula remains the workhorse flap for reconstructing composite maxillofacial defects, alternative approaches continue to be developed. In 2017, Gellrich and colleagues [30] were the first to describe a novel patient-specific titanium framework implant system used for the oral rehabilitation of patients with severe alveolar atrophy or resected maxilla. Using the aforementioned SLM technology, a patient-specific titanium scaffold and implant construct is engineered following digital prosthetic assessment and planning. To obtain this virtual plan, the surgeon must obtain a stereolithographic (STL) file of the future denture using an optical scanner before digitally fusing that data with the patients' CT scans and planning the reconstruction starting at the occlusion [30]. These processes can be done in-house if needed, using a planning tool such as *iPlan*® (Brainlab®, Feldkirchen, Germany) and a computer-aided design software such as *Geomagic*®

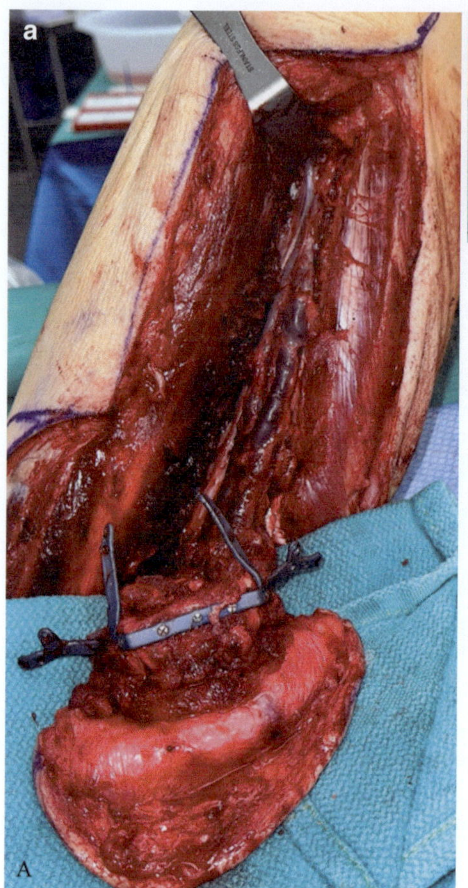
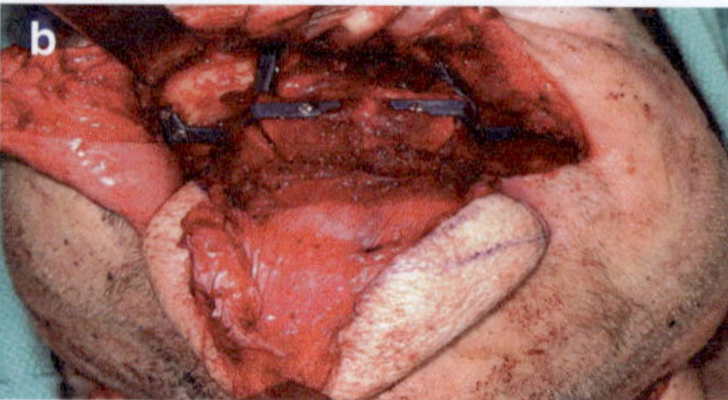

Fig. 10.6 The three-dimensional (3D) printed single unit maxillary plate fixed to the fibula segments. (**a**) After harvest/prior to inset to the maxilla. (**b**) Maxillary construct with custom plate, installed into recipient site, after inset

Freeform® PLUS (3D Systems, Rock Hill, SC, USA). By using this workflow, Spalthoff and colleagues [31] demonstrated that the dental rehabilitation of patients using the novel implant system was comparable to conventional rehabilitation without digital planning. Therefore, computerized planning of these prosthetics and reverse engineering of the implant scaffold provides a promising alternative to conventional soft and hard tissue reconstruction following ablative surgery.

However, development of the plan and manufacturing of guides necessitates extra time. Most centers do not have the resources to complete a full workflow in-house and must outsource this to an external collaborator. Despite being criticized for potentially delaying surgery, incorporating the VSP workflow has not been shown to compromise oncologic outcome and has shown a statistically significant reduction in operating time between 30 and 90 mins including free flap reconstruction [32].

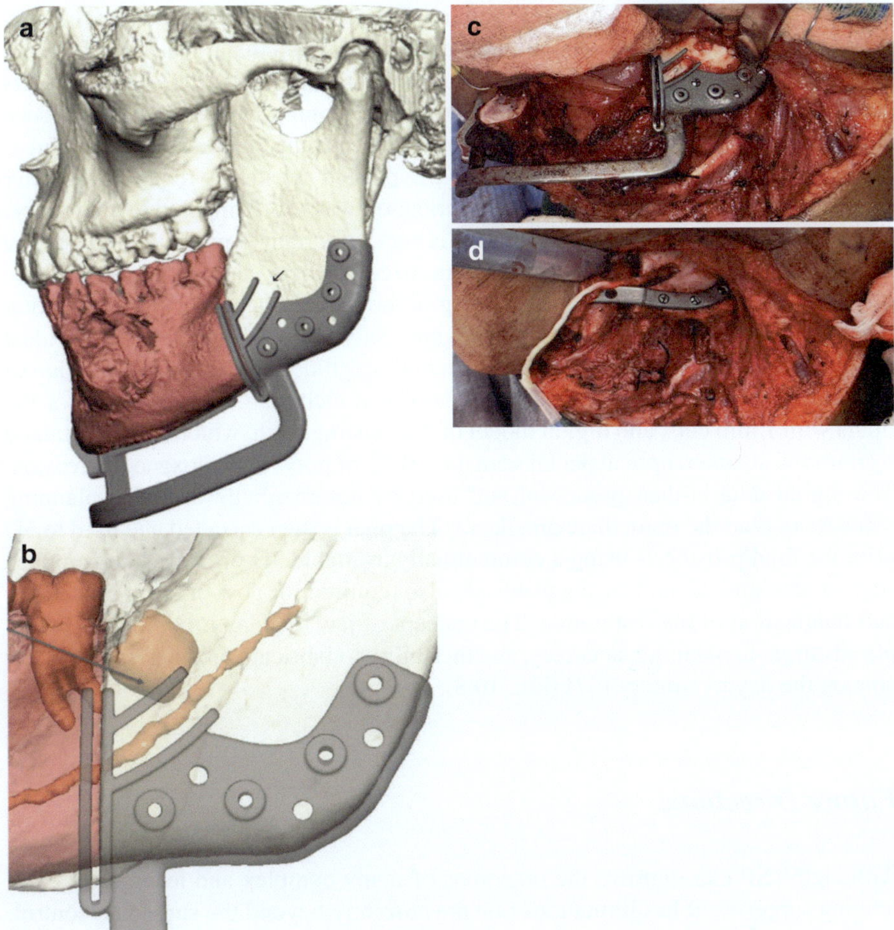

Fig. 10.7 (**a**) Integration of cutting slots in the cutting guide to assist in lateral corticotomy window and localize the inferior alveolar nerve. *(Courtesy of KLS Martin Group)*. Arrow denotes groove for the location of the inferior alveolar nerve. (**b**) Close up of the cutting guide and osteotomy window. (**c**) Inferior alveolar nerve lateralization as assisted by the integrated slots in the cutting guide followed by (**d**). Reconstruction with nerve graft

Jaw in a Day

Placement of osseointegrated dental implants primarily in vascularized free flap was first described in 1989 by Urken et al. [33]. The immediate placement of dental implants into the neomandible, while it is still at the donor site, has the advantage of access to ensure accurate placement of the dental implant, adequate assessment of ridge thickness and height, and less stages involved as compared to implant placement after bone and soft-tissue healing, which ultimately means earlier dental rehabilitation [34]. These dental implants were restored traditionally in collaboration with dental laboratories, which resulted in unavoidable delays and patient dissatisfaction. Hutchison and Dawood first performed immediate loading of dental implants placed in reconstructed microvascular scapula flap in 2007 [35]. This has further evolved to in-house creation of 3D printed dental prosthesis, which has been described and popularized recently with the advent of point-of-care three-dimensional (3D) printing. The in-house 3D printed prosthesis required a shorter time to be constructed, and the cost of fabrication was less compared to laboratory-fabricated prostheses [36]. Case selection is very important to predict the soft-tissue needs for composite defects. VSP revolutionized osteocutaneous vascularized free flap planning in terms of ideal positioning in the maxillofacial skeleton and taking into account the occlusal relationships which subsequently can be used for ideal position of dental implants using the same cutting guides. The digital data required for planning immediate dental implants on fibula include: CBCT, CT scan of the fibula with 1 mm cuts, and digital model of the existing teeth, which can be obtained by intraoral scanner, optical dental scan, or CBCT of polyvinyl siloxane impression. The digital data is then processed and used by commercially available planning software to plan the immediate prosthesis. The plan is then executed and used to 3D print the final prosthesis using a commercially available 3D printer. Other supplies such as alcohol bath and curing ovens are also required for post-printing processing and finalization of the restoration. The concept of jaw in a day is combining multiple advances in planning, accuracy, and the ability to fabricate prosthesis to be available on the day of surgery [37] (Fig. 10.8).

Future Directions

Although VSP can improve the outcomes of many complex and technically challenging surgeries, it has limitations that are currently beyond the surgeons' control. Barriers to the effective use of VSP are associated with the inherent delays associated with current manufacturing capabilities and human error. On average, the authors' experience with the turnover between VSP planning session to delivery of implant/guides can range between 7 and 14 days for pre-bent and milled hardware, whereas 3D-printed plates and laser-sintered hardware can be produced in 14–17 days. These limitations are due to the logistics involved in the processing, quality control, and transportation of the prostheses. Several options are available to reduce the turnaround time, through the use of in office or institutional 3D printers and resources. Surgeons have become their own engineer to design and facilitate the planning process and create acrylic guides; we are still limited by the ability to print or mill implants and hardware. Data sets can be created faster and forwarded to manufacturing sites to create the implants and hardware. Virtual surgical planning will continue to improve, and methods to acquire and process patient data will become more refined. Meticulous attention to each step is necessary to ensure a positive outcome. Future trends will likely include widespread availability of 3D printing and manufacturing technology and an increasing number of surgeons taking on the role of the engineer.

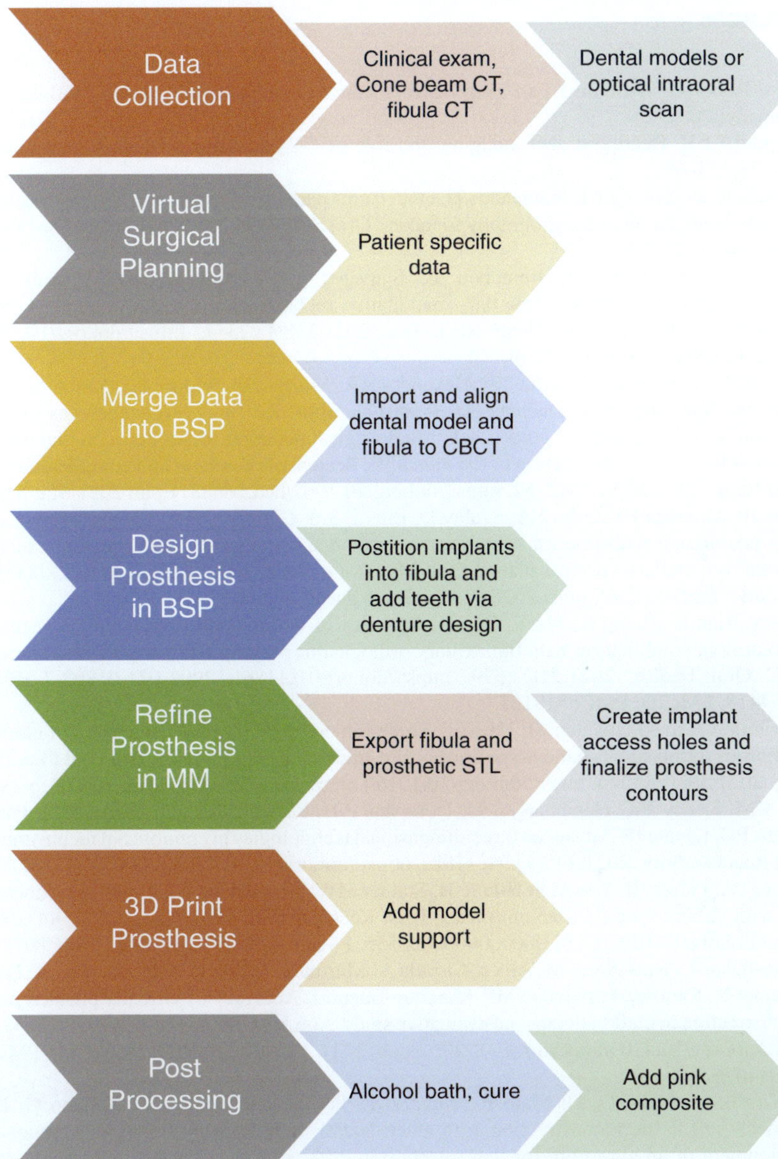

Fig. 10.8 Example of Jaw in A day workflow *(Reproduced with permission from Williams, Fayette C et al. "Immediate Teeth in Fibulas: Planning and Digital Workflow with Point-of-Care 3D Printing." Journal of oral and maxillofacial surgery: official journal of the American Association of Oral and Maxillofacial Surgeons vol. 78,8 (2020): 1320–1327. doi:10.1016/j.joms.2020.04.006)*

References

1. Allisy-Roberts P, Williams J. Farr's physics for medical imaging. New York, NY: W.B. Saunders Company; 2007.
2. Wippold FJ II. Head and neck imaging: the role of CT and MRI. J Magn Reson Imaging. 2007;25:453–65.
3. Pauwels R, Beinsberger J, Stamatakis H, et al. Com- parison of spatial and contrast resolution for cone-beam computed tomography scanners. Oral Surg Oral Med Oral Pathol Oral Radiol. 2012;114(1):127–35.
4. Bartier S, Mazzaschi O, Benichou L, Sauvaget E. Computer-assisted versus traditional technique in fibular free-flap mandibular reconstruction: a CT symmetry study. Eur Ann Otorhinolaryngol Head Neck Dis. 2021;138(1):23–7. https://doi.org/10.1016/j.anorl.2020.06.011; Epub 2020 Jun 30.
5. May MM, Howe BM, O'Byrne TJ, Alexander AE, Morris JM, Moore EJ, Kasperbauer JL, Janus JR, Van Abel KM, Dickens HJ, Price DL. Short and long-term outcomes of three-dimensional printed surgical guides and virtual surgical planning versus conventional methods for fibula free flap reconstruction of the mandible: decreased nonunion and complication rates. Head Neck. 2021;43(8):2342–52. https://doi.org/10.1002/hed.26688; Epub 2021 Mar 31.
6. Jones JP, Amarista FJ, Jeske NA, Szalay D, Ellis E 3rd. Comparison of the accuracy of maxillary positioning with interim splints versus patient-specific guides and plates in executing a virtual bimaxillary surgical plan. J Oral Maxillofac Surg. 2022;S0278-2391(22):00007–6. https://doi.org/10.1016/j.joms.2022.01.006; Epub ahead of print.
7. Ying X, Tian K, Zhang K, Ma X, Guo H. Accuracy of virtual surgical planning in segmental osteotomy in combination with bimaxillary orthognathic surgery with surgery first approach. BMC Oral Health. 2021;21(1):529. https://doi.org/10.1186/s12903-021-01892-7. PMID: 34654418; PMCID: PMC8518167.
8. Rengarajoo J, Syed Husman SI, Hariri F. Three-dimensional surgical contouring of craniofacial fibrous dysplasia via patient-specific cutting guides and depth screws. Br J Oral Maxillofac Surg. 2021;59(7):843–4. https://doi.org/10.1016/j.bjoms.2020.09.028; Epub 2020 Sep 28.
9. Day KM, Kelley PK, Harshbarger RJ, Dorafshar AH, Kumar AR, Steinbacher DM, Patel P, Combs PD, Levine JP. Advanced three-dimensional technologies in craniofacial reconstruction. Plast Reconstr Surg. 2021;148(1):94e–108e. https://doi.org/10.1097/PRS.0000000000008212.
10. Palines PA, Ferrer JR, Yoo A, St Hilaire H, Stalder MW. Simplifying bony midface reconstruction with patient-specific titanium plates. Plast Reconstr Surg Glob Open. 2021;9(4):e3555. https://doi.org/10.1097/GOX.0000000000003555. PMID: 33912374; PMCID: PMC8078310.
11. Rubio-Palau J, Ayats-Soler M, Albert-Cazalla A, Martìnez-Padilla I, Prieto-Gundin A, Prieto-Peronnet N, Ramìrez-Fernández MP, Mareque-Bueno J. Accuracy of virtually planned maxillary distraction in cleft patients—an evaluative study. Ann Maxillofac Surg. 2021;11(1):49–57. https://doi.org/10.4103/ams.ams_331_20; Epub 2021 Feb 18. PMID: 34522654; PMCID: PMC8407633.
12. De Virgilio A, Iocca O, Di Maio P, Malvezzi L, Pellini R, Mercante G, Spriano G. Head and neck soft tissue reconstruction with anterolateral thigh flaps with various components: development of an algorithm for flap selection in different clinical scenarios. Microsurgery. 2019;39(7):590–7.
13. Liu K, Zhang W, Wang Y, Xiang DW, Shi HB, Liu QL. Fibula osteal flap with proximal peroneal perforator skin paddle for composite oromandibular reconstruction: a case report. Medicine (Baltimore). 2020;99(50):e23590.
14. Pereira N, Valenzuela D, Mangelsdorff G, Kufeke M, Roa R. Detection of perforators for free flap planning using smartphone thermal imaging: a concordance study with computed tomographic angiography in 120 perforators. Plast Reconstr Surg. 2018;141(3):787–92.
15. Rajati M, Pezeshki Rad M, Irani S, Khorsandi MT, Motasaddi ZM. Accuracy of high-resolution computed tomography in locating facial nerve injury sites in temporal bone trauma. Eur Arch Otorhinolaryngol. 2014;271(8):2185–9.

16. Cheng K, Leinkram D, Howes D, Clark J. Incorporating 'off-the-shelf' reconstruction plates into the digital plan for mandible reconstruction. Int J Clin Oncol Cancer Ther. 2021;1(1):1–4.
17. Garrido-Martínez P, Quispe-López N, Montesdeoca-García N, Esparza-Gómez G, Cebrián-Carretero JL. Maxillary reconstruction with subperiosteal implants in a cancer patient: a one-year follow-up. J Clin Exp Dent. 2022;14(3):e293.
18. Zhang N, Liu S, Hu Z, et al. Accuracy of virtual Sur- gical planning in two-jaw orthognathic surgery: com- parison of planned and actual results. Oral Surg Oral Med Oral Pathol Oral Radiol. 2016;122(2):143–51.
19. Resnick CM, Inverso G, Wrzosek M, et al. Is there a difference in cost between standard and virtual surgical planning for orthognathic surgery? J Oral Maxillofac Surg. 2016;74(9):1827–33.
20. Cheng H, Chen BP, Soleas IM, et al. Prolonged oper- ative duration increases risk of surgical site infec- tions: a systematic review. Surg Infect (Larchmt). 2017;18(6):722–35.
21. Tondin GM, Leal MOCD, Costa ST, Grillo R, Jodas CRP, Teixeira RG. Evaluation of the accuracy of virtual planning in bimaxillary orthognathic surgery: systematic review. Br J Oral Maxillofac Surg. 2021;S0266-4356(21):00343. https://doi.org/10.1016/j.bjoms.2021.09.010; Epub ahead of print. PMID: 35120785.
22. Chen Z, Mo S, Fan X, You Y, Ye G, Zhou N. A meta-analysis and systematic review comparing the effectiveness of traditional and virtual surgical planning for orthognàthic surgery: based on randomized clinical trials. J Oral Maxillofac Surg. 2021;79(2):471.e1–471.e19. https://doi.org/10.1016/j.joms.2020.09.005. Epub 2020 Sep 9. PMID: 33031773.
23. Bernstein JM, Daly MJ, Chan H, Qiu J, Goldstein D, Muhanna N, de Almeida JR, Irish JC. Accuracy and reproducibility of virtual cutting guides and 3D-navigation for osteotomies of the mandible and maxilla. PloS One. 2017;12(3):e0173111.
24. Jenkins GW, Iqbal S, West N, Ellabban I, Kennedy MP, Adams JR. Dosimetry-guided virtual surgical planning in the reconstruction of mandibular osteoradionecrosis. Br J Oral Maxillofac Surg. 2021;59(8):947–51.
25. Lee IJ, Koom WS, Lee CG, Kim YB, Yoo SW, Keum KC, Kim GE, Choi EC, Cha IH. Risk factors and dose–effect relationship for mandibular osteoradionecrosis in oral and oropharyngeal cancer patients. Int J Radiat Oncol Biol Phys. 2009;75(4):1084–91.
26. Gutwald R, Jaeger R, Lambers FM. Customized mandibular reconstruction plates improve mechanical performance in a mandibular reconstruction model. Comput Methods Biomech Biomed Engin. 2017;20(4):426–35.
27. Smith MH, Schrag CH, Chandarana SP, Cobb JG, Matthews TW, Mckenzie CD, Matthews JL. Novel plate design to improve mandibular and maxillary reconstruction with the Osteocutaneous fibula flap. Plast Reconstr Surg Glob Open. 2019;7(1):e2094.
28. Anolik RA, Nelson JA, Rosen EB, Disa J, Matros E, Allen RJ Jr. Immediate dental implant placement in the oncologic setting: a conceptual framework. Plast Reconstr Surg Glob Open. 2021;9(9):e3671.
29. Melville JC, Manis CS, Shum JW, Alsuwied D. Single-unit 3D-printed titanium reconstruction plate for maxillary reconstruction: the evolution of surgical reconstruction for maxillary defects—a case report and review of current techniques. J Oral Maxillofac Surg. 2019;77(4):874–e1.
30. Gellrich NC, Zimmerer RM, Spalthoff S, Jehn P, Pott PC, Rana M, Rahlf B. A customised digitally engineered solution for fixed dental rehabilitation in severe bone deficiency: a new innovative line extension in implant dentistry. J Craniomaxillofac Surg. 2017;45(10):1632–8.
31. Spalthoff S, Borrmann M, Jehn P, Rahlf B, Gellrich NC, Korn P. Comparison of conventional and digital workflow for dental rehabilitation with a novel patient-specific framework implant system: an experimental dataset evaluation. Int J Implant Dent. 2022;8(1):1–8.
32. Barry CP, MacDhabheid C, Tobin K, Stassen LF, Lennon P, Toner M, O'Regan E, Clark JR. 'Out of house' virtual surgical planning for mandible reconstruction after cancer resection: is it oncologically safe? Int J Oral Maxillofac Surg. 2021;50(8):999–1002.
33. Urken ML, Buchbinder D, Weinberg H, et al. Primary placement of osseointegrated implants in microvascular mandibular reconstruction. Otolaryngol Head Neck Surg. 1989;101:56.

34. Rosen EB, Ahmed ZU, Habib AA, Huryn JM, Randazzo JD, Cracchiolo JR, Matros E, Nelson J, Allen RJ Jr. Interim implant-supported resection prosthesis following fibula free flap reconstruction of the arch with immediate implants: a novel approach for the oncologic patient. Int J Periodontics Restorative Dent. 2020;40(6):861–7. https://doi.org/10.11607/prd.4675. PMID: 33151192; PMCID: PMC8383382.
35. Hutchison IL, Dawood A, Tanner S. Immediate implant supported bridgework simultaneous with jaw reconstruction for a patient with mandibular osteosarcoma. Br Dent J. 2009;206(3):143–6. https://doi.org/10.1038/sj.bdj.2009.57. PMID: 19218947.
36. Patel A, Harrison P, Cheng A, Bray B, Bell RB. Fibular reconstruction of the maxilla and mandible with immediate implant-supported prosthetic rehabilitation: jaw in a day. Oral Maxillofac Surg Clin North Am. 2019;31(3):369–86. https://doi.org/10.1016/j.coms.2019.03.002. Epub 2019 Jun 1. PMID: 31164268.
37. Williams FC, et al. Immediate teeth in fibulas: planning and digital workflow with point-of-care 3D printing. J Oral Maxillofac Surg. 2020;78(8):1320–7.

Chapter 11
Advancing Immediate Dental Rehabilitation in Free Tissue Transfer Utilizing Point-of-Care Digital Workflows and 3D Printing

Daniel Hammer, Marilyn Andersen, Justin Odette, Raymond P. Shupak, Michael Andersen, Fayette C. Williams, and Roderick Y. Kim

Introduction

Maxillofacial reconstructive surgery poses a unique set of challenges to the surgeon. A defect in this region often results from pathology or trauma, and the resulting defect affects both form and function with potential changes to speech, nutrition, swallow function, and esthetics. Maxillofacial defects also have a significant effect on the patients' psychosocial well-being. Therefore, oral and dental rehabilitation is

D. Hammer (✉)
Department of Oral and Maxillofacial Surgery, Naval Medical Center San Diego, San Diego, CA, USA
e-mail: daniel.a.hammer.mil@health.mil

M. Andersen
Department of Oral and Maxillofacial Surgery, Naval Hospital Twentynine Palms, Twentynine Palms, CA, USA
e-mail: marilyn.a.andersen.mil@health.mil

J. Odette
Dental Department, USS Theodore Roosevelt (CVN 71), San Diego, CA, USA
e-mail: justin.r.odette.mil@health.mil

R. P. Shupak
Division of Oral and Maxillofacial Surgery, Geisinger Medical Center, Danville, PA, USA
e-mail: rshupak@geisinger.edu

M. Andersen
Department of Hospital Dentistry, Naval Medical Center San Diego, San Diego, CA, USA
e-mail: michael.r.andersen.mil@health.mil

F. C. Williams · R. Y. Kim
Department of Oral and Maxillofacial Surgery, John Peter Smith Hospital, Fort Worth, TX, USA
e-mail: FWilliam@jpshealth.org; RKim01@jpshealth.org

© The Author(s), under exclusive license to Springer Nature Switzerland AG 2023
J. C. Melville et al. (eds.), *Advancements and Innovations in OMFS, ENT, and Facial Plastic Surgery*, https://doi.org/10.1007/978-3-031-32099-6_11

imperative to fully restore the patient and should not be ignored and completed as soon as predictably possible. Unfortunately, current data suggest that most patients undergoing jaw reconstruction following pathologic resection do not receive immediate implants or an immediate prosthesis at the time of initial surgery [1].

The advantages of immediate dental rehabilitation (dental implants and temporary prosthesis at time of primary reconstruction) include a decrease in the number of surgeries and expedited return to form and function. These advantages can improve the patients' psychosocial and overall well-being. Potential obstacles to immediate dental rehabilitation include the learning curve to optimally virtual plan the reconstruction, gaining familiarity with the complexities of 3D manufacturing, financial reimbursement, and finally, collaborating with a suitable restorative provider capable of delivering a final restoration. Since comprehensive maxillofacial reconstruction incorporates dental rehabilitation, strong consideration should be given to immediate dental rehabilitation when feasible.

Immediate Dental Implant Placement in Osseous Free Flaps

Immediate dental implant placement into osseous free flaps is well documented and has a high success rate [2–4]. The accuracy and success rates have further increased with the incorporation of virtual surgical planning (VSP) [5]. Some of the challenges previously faced by immediate implant placement and dental prosthesis delivery can be simplified by computer-aided design and computer-aided manufacturing (CAD/CAM) technologies [6].

The implant positions should be determined at the time of planning the osseous free flap. This allows for the fabrication of patient-specific cutting guides, which incorporate additional features allowing for guided implant placement. Properly positioned implants are imperative for dental rehabilitation, especially in the immediate setting. This minor shift in protocol greatly increases the likelihood of providing a sound foundation for delivery of an immediate prosthesis. With the use of this protocol, the authors have maintained a high implant success rate in reconstructing defects resultant to both benign and malignant disease and trauma. With the advent and application of CAD/CAM technologies, immediate dental rehabilitation has become predictable and safe.

History of Immediate Dental Rehabilitation in Osseous Free Flaps

Immediate dental rehabilitation with microvascular free tissue reconstruction was first completed by Dr. Iain Hutchison and Dr. Andrew Dawood in 2007 to reconstruct a mandibular continuity defect secondary to ballistic trauma. Previously, dental rehabilitation in free tissue transfer was completed in a staged manner either by using prelaminated flaps 6 weeks after dental implant placement or by placing the dental implants in the osseous free flap transorally after initial healing. Dr. Hutchinson and Dr. Dawood's surgery involved placement of dental implants into a scapula with an immediate provisional prosthesis being delivered before leaving the operating room [7, 8]. Since its inception, immediate dental rehabilitation in free tissue transfer has gained popularity and predictability and has extended its application to a wide variety of clinical situations [9–13].

Expanded Applications of Immediate Dental Rehabilitation in Free Tissue Transfer

Initially, immediate dental rehabilitation was only recommended for secondary trauma reconstruction or reconstruction of defects secondary to benign disease. It was believed that these reconstructions in the setting of malignancy would lead to increased complication rate, especially when the patient required adjuvant radiation treatment. In the authors' experience, postoperative radiation has not been associated with decreased rates of implant integration, further supported by emerging literature [10–13]. When implants are placed immediately during fibula reconstruction, adjuvant radiation therapy does not begin for another 4–6 weeks. After radiation begins, there are several more weeks before radiation doses reach significant biologic levels. Since most of the implant integration is complete before the higher doses of radiation accumulate, the integration rate of implants in fibulas prior to radiation is higher than implants placed after radiation [14, 15].

Furthermore, it is commonly believed that the reconstruction of a composite defect with an osteocutaneous flap is a contraindication to immediate dental rehabilitation with concerns of an inability to achieve a watertight closure and possible decreased skin paddle survival. Our experience has shown that skin paddles can be successfully used with immediate rehabilitation when designed properly. In fact, to perform a successful vestibular reconstruction, the skin paddle is integral. When implants are placed at the suture line between the skin paddle and native mucosa, a near watertight closure can be obtained. This results in a more favorable soft tissue interface leading to less tissue mobility, resulting in improved implant health compared to native non-keratinized oral mucosa. The major disadvantage of utilizing a skin paddle is the potential need for secondary debulking procedures.

Until recently, one of the major challenges to immediate dental rehabilitation of a patient with a malignancy was the prolonged time needed to design and fabricate the temporary dental prosthesis, which could be 6 or more weeks. It was simply not acceptable to delay extirpation of the patient's tumor to offer immediate dental rehabilitation. By leveraging emerging technologies, the temporary dental prosthesis can now be fabricated and ready for delivery within 24 h of the planning the free flap reconstruction. This timeline is possible by utilizing open-source design software and in-house 3D printing (additive resin printing) or polymethylmethacrylate (PMMA) milling. Both technologies have revolutionized the ability to provide a patient-customized rehabilitation within the time constraints of treating malignant tumors [16].

Advantages of using 3D printing (additive resin printing) include rapid manufacturing time and low cost of equipment and consumable resins. The advantages of milled pre-polymerized PMMA, such as polychromatic esthetics, flexural strength, and resistance to the accumulation of biofilms, far surpass those of current 3D-printed resins. However, PMMA mills are more costly compared to resin printers.

The in-house digital workflow used to create the prosthesis provides a high-quality prosthesis in significantly less time and at less cost than using commercially available dental labs [17].

Preoperative Digital Workflow: Data Gathering to Temporary Prosthesis Design

The immediate dental rehabilitation digital workflow can be performed in any office or clinic setting with the appropriate hardware and software. Preoperative imaging includes a maxillofacial CT or cone beam CT (CBCT) and CT angiography of the bilateral lower extremities for evaluation of vessel presence and patency and implant planning. The lower extremity imaging must have a slice thickness of 1 mm or less, and only patient-specific data should be used for virtual surgical planning (VSP). It is important that in the maxillofacial CT or CBCT is obtained with the teeth slightly apart in open occlusion to allow more accurate merging of the preoperative dentition with the CT data. Intraoral scans or stone models can be sent to an appropriate surgical VSP engineer according to the preference of the surgeon.

During the VSP session, the resection and the bony reconstruction are planned as dictated by the pathology and defect, followed by virtual placement of implants. Virtual implant and abutment STL files are brought into the planning environment and adjusted according to standard implant principles. We prefer to have implants emerging from the anterior surface of the fibula as it will position the skin paddle in an orientation to reconstruct the vestibule. However, in cases where this is not possible, implants can also emerge from the posterior surface of the fibula to allow for appropriate flap geometry. The implant guide is digitally built with the fibula osteotomy guide. It is important to note that the drill offset should be built into the guide based on the fully guided implant system that is used (Figs. 11.1 and 11.2).

When planning dental implant placement within the fibula, there should be approximately 15–18 mm of restorative space from the platform of the implant to the opposing occlusal surface. In our experience, the implants themselves should be no less than 7 mm apart from each other (external edge to external edge of adjacent platform) to ensure cleansability of the prosthesis and at least 3 mm from fibular

Simulated Postoperative Anatomy

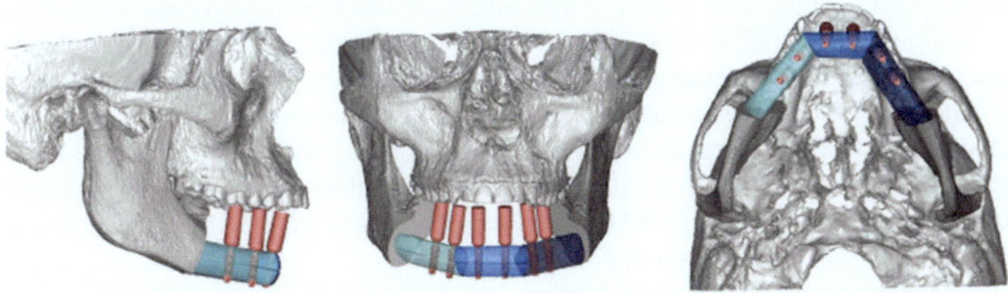

Fig. 11.1 Finalized VSP of an immediate mandibular reconstruction. Note the restorative space (15–18 mm) needed for prosthesis restoration. Here the fibula segments are shown at the inferior border; however, the fibula should be placed to allow for proper implant emergence. This often positions the fibula above the level of the inferior boarder

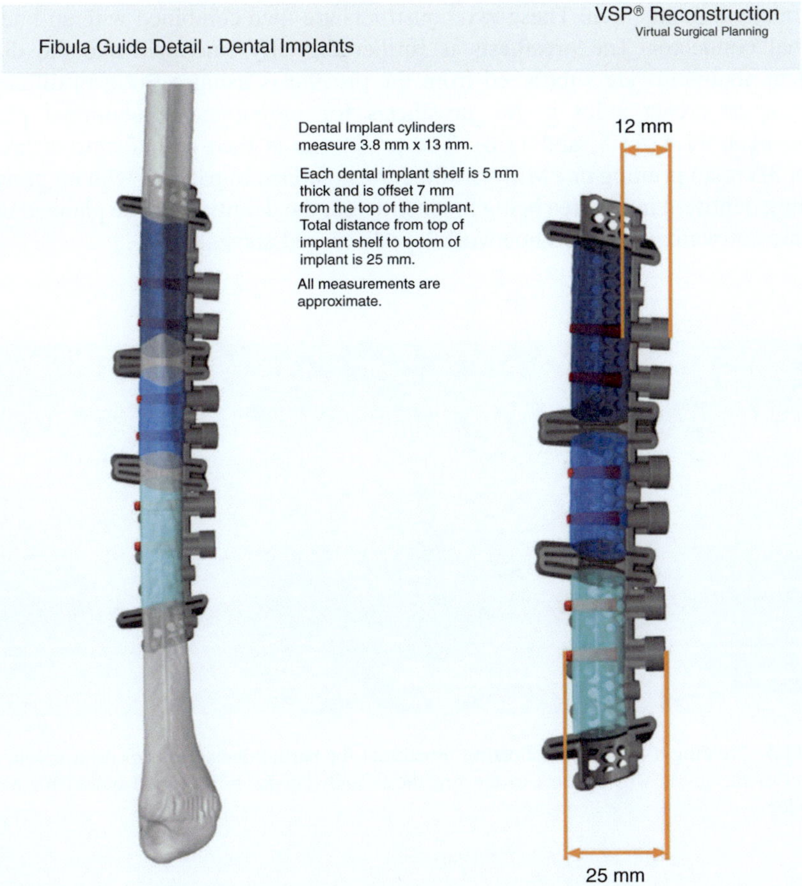

Fig. 11.2 Fibula cut guide with merged guided implant sleeves. Note the implant guide sleeve offset that corresponds to the offset on the guided implant drill length

osteotomies to maintain the integrity of the bony junction. Implant depths should be planned for the platforms to be 1–2 mm subcrestal due to expected crestal bone loss.

Following the VSP session, STL files of the fibula reconstruction with implants are requested from the engineer. This ensures that the shells are accurately overlaid (fibula/implant/existing teeth) in the 3D work environment. This step is critical to ensure that the planning session and implant positioning will align with the in-house fabricated prosthesis. Then the digital in-house workflow is followed, as previously described [15]. The patient's STL files are then imported to the 3D printer software for temporary prosthesis fabrication.

For partial arch dental rehabilitation in a patient with existing dentition in the region that will be removed, the temporary prosthesis design is cloned from the patient's existing dentition. The STL data is recorded from the intraoral scan and modified within the software. A base is created with the close model feature. This creates an identical copy of the patient's dentition. After this step, a tooth-borne guide is created digitally on teeth within the non-resected portion of the patient's contralateral dental arch. These two constructs are then combined with an interpositional connector. The prosthesis is further digitally smoothed and the digital implant abutments are subtracted from the prosthesis using a Boolean difference function to create holes in the prosthesis for intraoperative abutment pickup (Figs. 11.3, 11.4, 11.5, and 11.6). The prosthesis is then manufactured through either 3D resin printing or PMMA milling throughputs. In patients with no previous existing dentition in the area being reconstructed, the dentition can be planned using denture software using the same workflow discussed above.

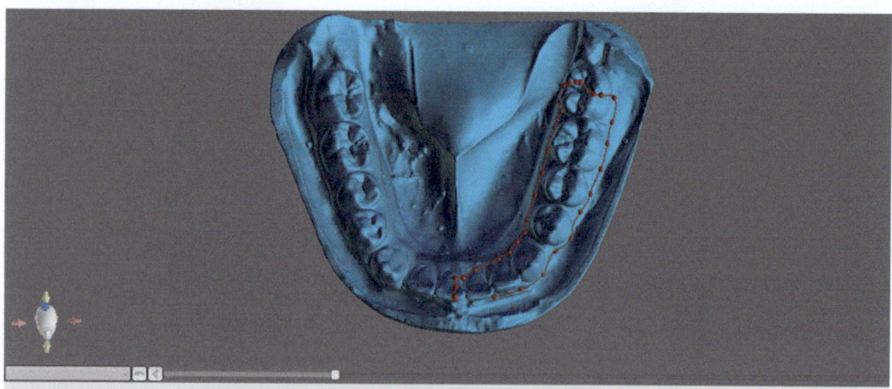

Fig. 11.3 Creating a tooth-borne floating prosthesis for partial dental arch reconstruction. This portion of the guide will connect to the prosthesis and register to a printed model for pickup in the leg

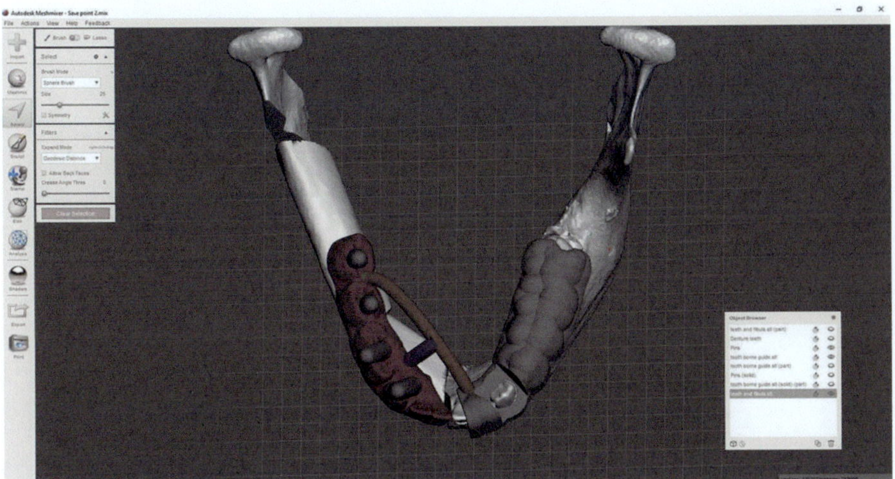

Fig. 11.4 The tooth-borne floating prosthesis joined with the dental prosthesis

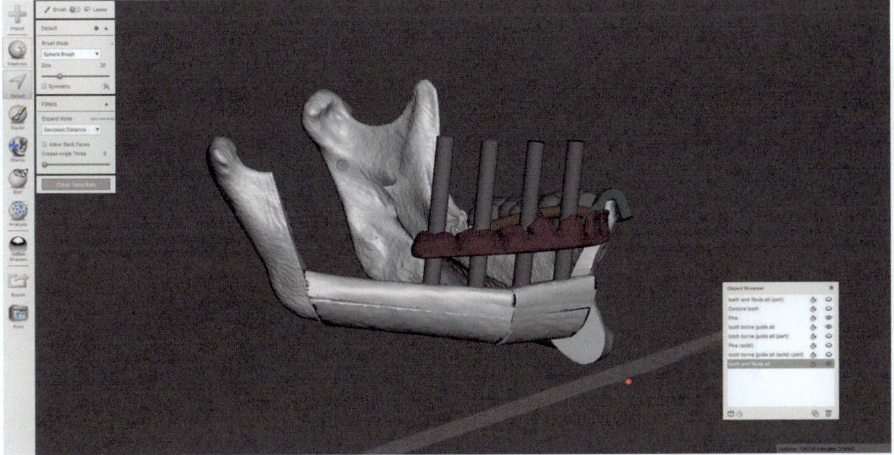

Fig. 11.5 Lateral view of the virtual prosthesis and floating guide. Note the highwater design required for soft tissue skin paddle inset and cleansability

For full-arch dental rehabilitation, the entire maxillary or mandibular arch is duplicated if the patient has reasonable preoperative dentition. Again, the data is taken from an intraoral scan, preoperative CBCT data, or digitization of physical stone models in articulation. If the patient does not have adequate dentition, then a virtual denture is made through a denture module in the software. The prosthesis is then smoothed and refined digitally. The digital implant abutments are again

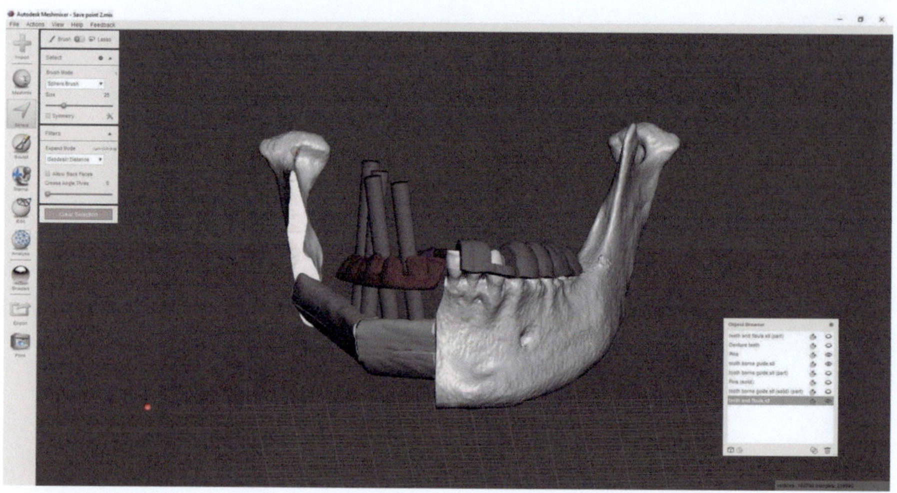

Fig. 11.6 The virtual implant abutments are digitally subtracted from the prosthesis using a Boolean difference function for intraoperative pickup. Note the inferior border offset to achieve the proper interocclusal restorative space

Fig. 11.7 Full-arch prosthesis pickup with contralateral arch 3D model prior to flap ischemia

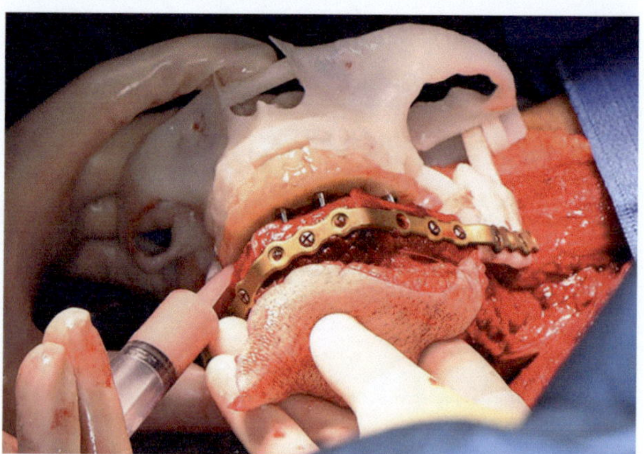

subtracted from the prosthesis with a Boolean difference function for purposes of intraoperative pickup impression (Figs. 11.7, 11.8, 11.9, and 11.10). The prosthesis is then 3D printed using biocompatible crown and bridge resin available from multiple manufacturers or milled PMMA as described above.

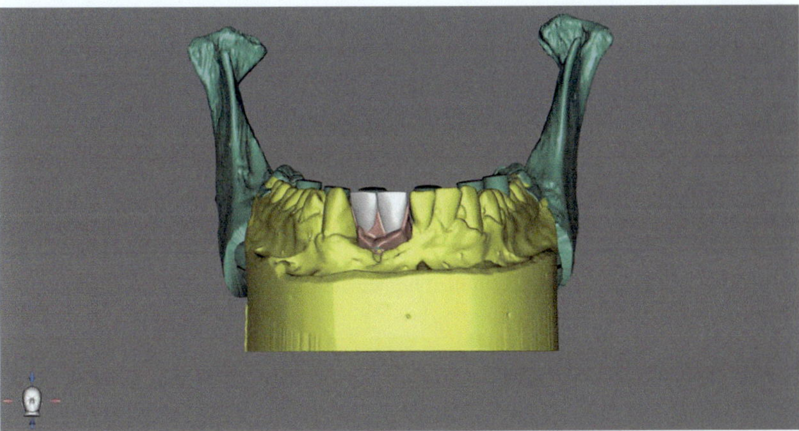

Fig. 11.8 Complete dental arch reconstruction using a combination of the patient's existing dentition and digitally created teeth

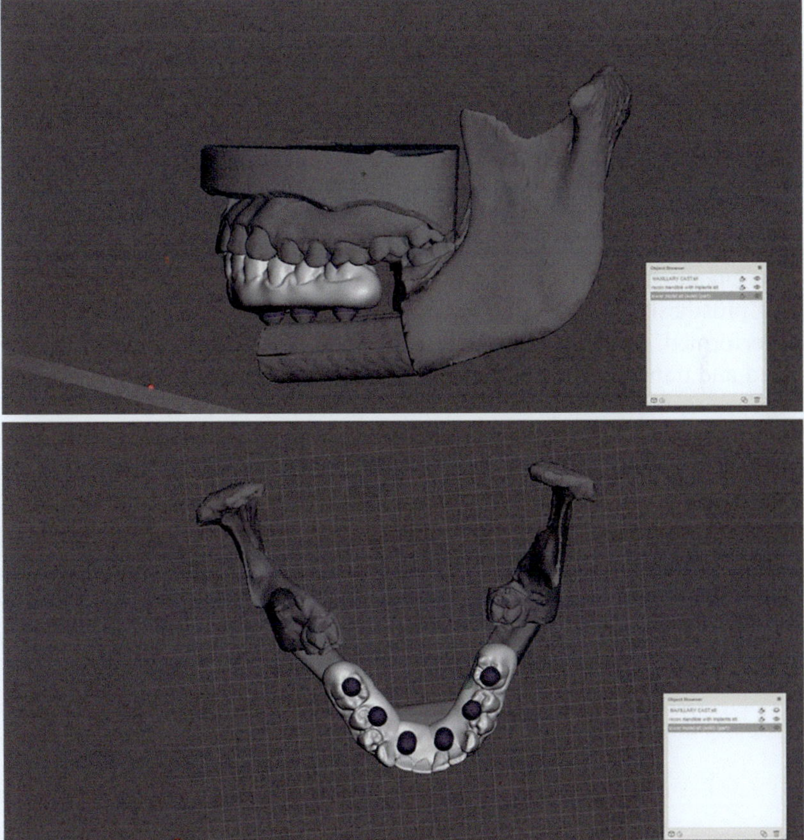

Fig. 11.9 Full-arch reconstruction. The second molars were left until time of pickup. This provides a stable occlusal stop to confirm the correct vertical dimension of occlusion (VDO). The second molars will be removed before final inset of the prosthesis

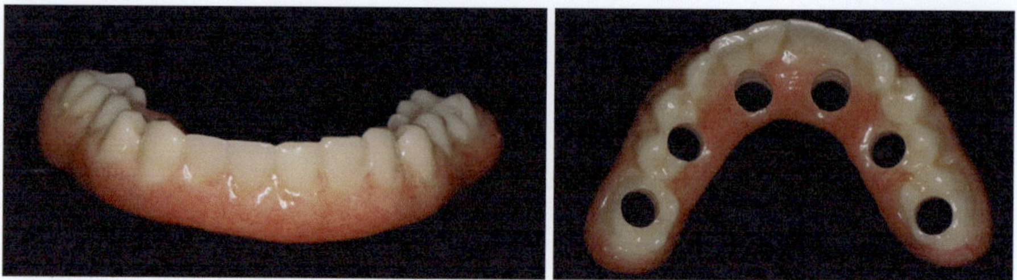

Fig. 11.10 Poly(methyl methacrylate) milled immediate full-arch prosthesis

Intraoperative Technique

A defect model, fibula cutting guide, mandible or maxilla cutting guide, and custom reconstruction plate are requested from the vendor used for the initial VSP panning session. A preoperative fit check on the defect model is performed to ensure correct positioning of implants and prosthesis. The defect model should have predictive holes to attach the plate and fibula construct. Intraoperatively, it is imperative that the resection and fibula cutting guides are placed at the surgical sites according to the preoperative plan. The fibula cutting guide is then secured, predictive holes are drilled, and then the guided dental implants are placed. Following these steps, the closing osteotomies are created with a surgical saw.

The fibula segments are then fit into the defect model and secured to the custom plate. Straight multiunit abutments are placed on the implants and torqued to manufacturer's specifications. Temporary copings are then placed on the multiunit abutments in preparation for attachment of the prosthesis. The tooth-borne guided "floating prosthesis" is placed on the printed STL defect model. A pickup impression is performed, and the prosthesis is removed and converted. At that time, the flap is divided and transferred to the head and neck. In cases where the full dental arch is being reconstructed, the prosthesis can be picked up utilizing a 3D-printed skull model with hinged opposing and vertical dimension of occlusion (VDO) stops (Fig. 11.11). Alternatively, the prosthesis can also be picked up intraorally. While this can be more difficult due to the constraints of operating with limited space within the intraoral surgical field, the occlusion is more accurate and requires minimal final adjustment.

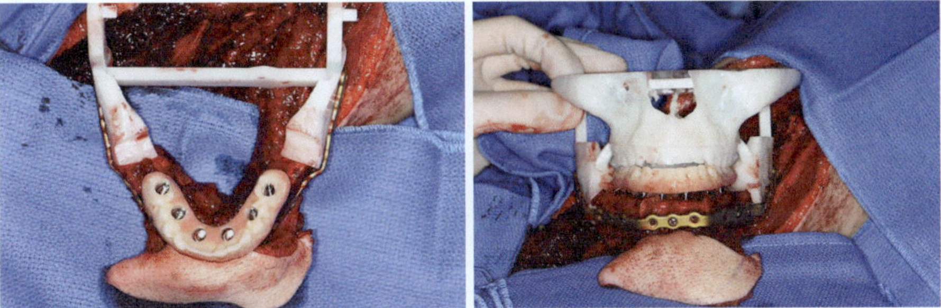

Fig. 11.11 Full-arch pickup performed at the donor site. A hinged model is used to provide opposing dentition

Postoperative Digital Workflow: Naval Medical Center Rapid Restorative Protocol

At the time of surgery, the pre-manufactured prosthesis is converted to a fixed conversion dental prosthesis by fixating multiunit abutment temporary cylinders to the dental prosthesis with autocure acrylic. After the prosthesis is disinfected and taken to the dental laboratory for completion of the conversion, a check-cast of the multiunit abutment analog positions is poured in low-expansion type IV die stone. The intaglio contours of the prosthesis are rounded, hygienically contoured, and polished. In addition, multiunit abutment impression scan bodies are attached to the conversion prosthesis and scanned in the desktop scanner that provides surface scan data of the cameo and intaglio surfaces of the prosthesis and its relationship to the multiunit abutment platforms (Fig. 11.12).

After an appropriate amount of time has elapsed as deemed by the surgeon for restorative recall, maxillomandibular relationship records are made with an intraoral scanner after any additional occlusal adjustments are required (Fig. 11.13). The conversion prosthesis is then removed and the soft tissue is inspected for areas of concern. Corresponding areas of the intaglio surface of the prosthesis are adjusted and polished as appropriate, all multiunit abutments are re-torqued to manufacturer's specifications, and the conversion prosthesis is reinserted intraorally and analyzed for passivity to the multiunit abutments. A PVS wash of the intaglio of the conversion prosthesis or final impression using splinted impression copings and custom tray can also be made to capture the respective soft tissue if indicated. Pre-manufactured verification jigs made from the surgical check cast are then luted intraorally using autocure acrylic to verify passivity of the final master cast. The conversion prosthesis is then disinfected and taken to the dental laboratory, and a final master cast is poured in a low-expansion type IV die stone using the verified passive conversion prosthesis or splinted impression copings with multiunit analogs. The conversion prosthesis is then scanned on a desktop scanner individually and attached to the master cast that captures the cameo and intaglio surfaces and its relationship to the verified master cast (Fig. 11.14).

Fig. 11.12 The scanned STL file of the temporary prosthesis to use for fabrication of the final prosthesis

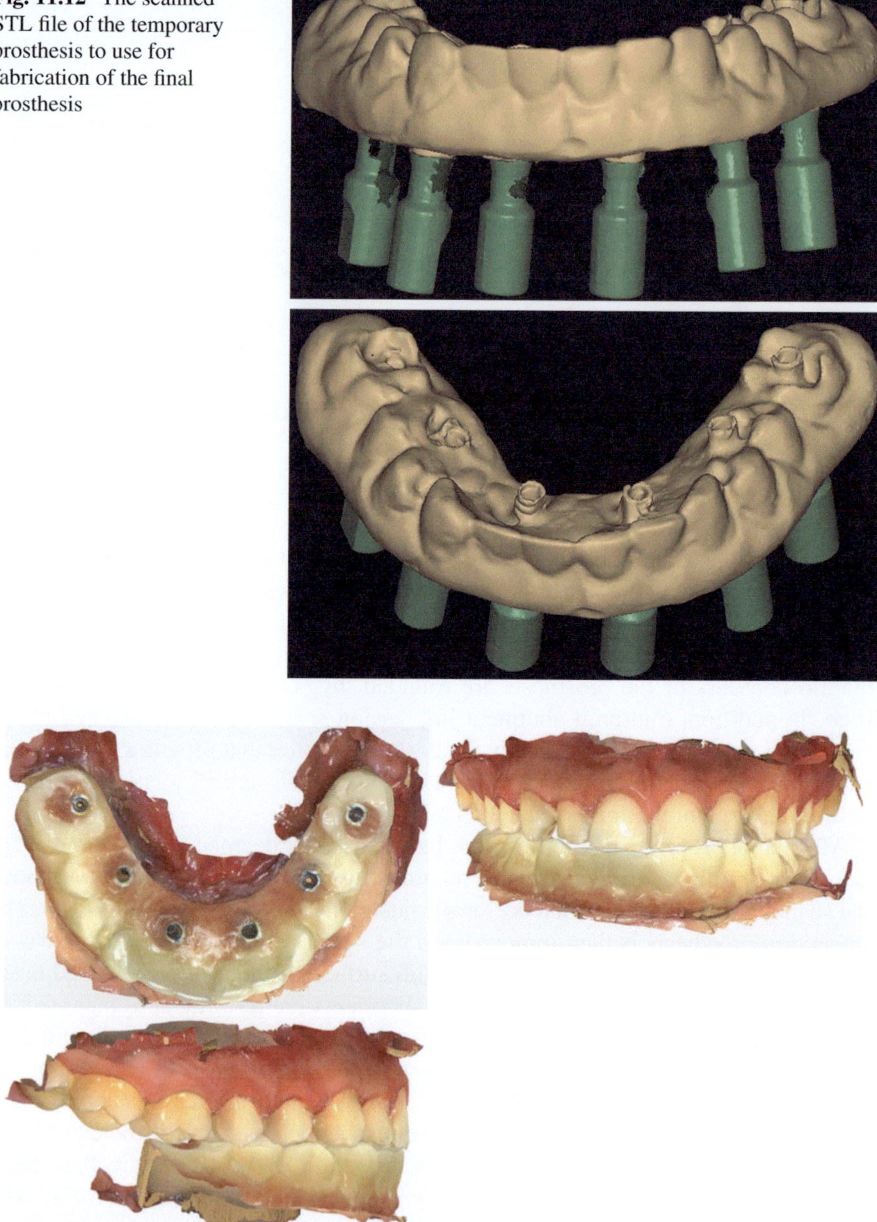

Fig. 11.13 Maxillomandibular relationship records of the conversion prosthesis and opposing dentition made with an intraoral scanner

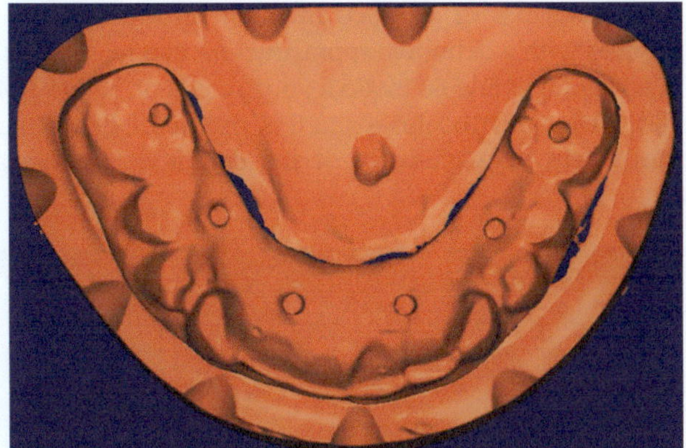

Fig. 11.14 Desktop scan of the conversion prosthesis indexed to the verified master cast

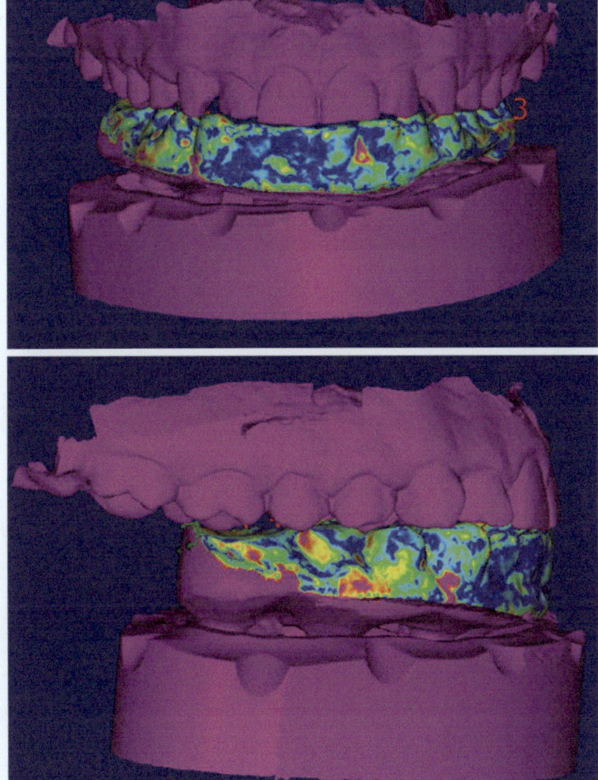

Fig. 11.15 The master cast is then registered to the opposing dentition in the restorative maxillomandibular relationship using the conversion prosthesis as the constant fiduciary surface

These STL models can then be registered within the CAD software for an accurate relationship to each other, and all files are sent to the dental laboratory for manufacture of a definitive prosthesis along with the verified stone master cast for verification of the metal framework milling accuracy (Fig. 11.15). The prosthesis design consists of a milled titanium substructure enhanced by vertical retention grooves with a definitive suprastructure that replicates the presurgical anatomy and occlusion if available made from zirconia or milled PMMA. A 2 mm bilayer pressure form matrix occlusal guard is also fabricated to the prosthesis and delivered to the patient upon delivery of the definitive prosthesis (Figs. 11.16 and 11.17).

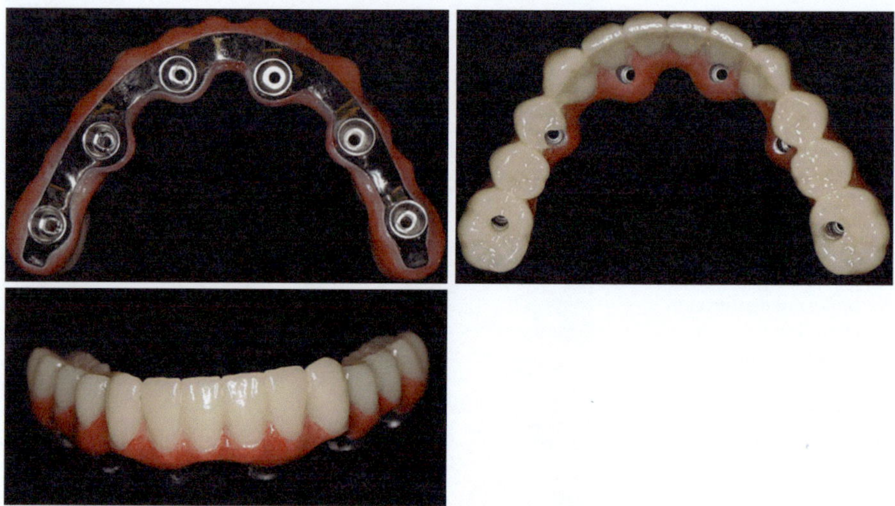

Fig. 11.16 Final prosthesis

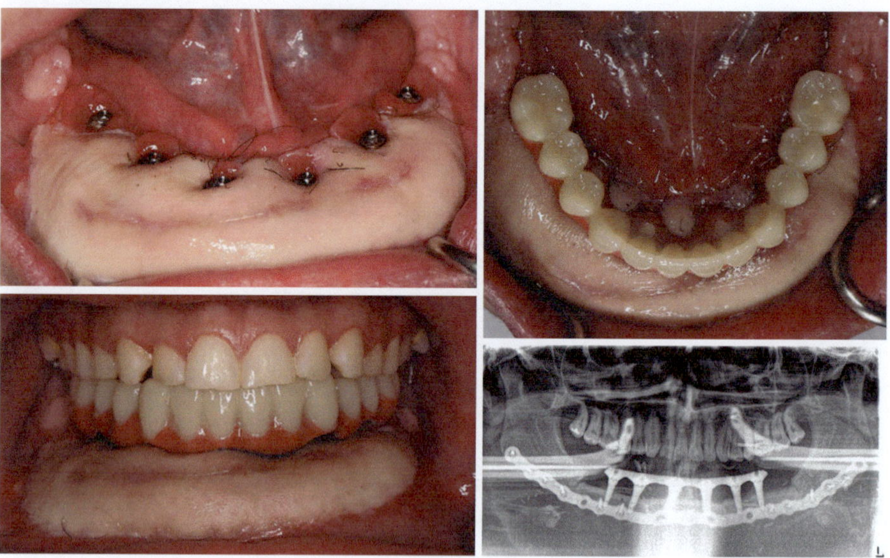

Fig. 11.17 Delivery of prosthesis 14 weeks postoperatively

Homecare instructions are reinforced, and the recall regimen is customized per patient requirements. This protocol has enabled delivery of a final dental prosthesis in less than 4 months postoperatively.

Future Directions

Currently, we strive to complete dental rehabilitation with final prosthesis delivery within 4 months of surgery. The final prostheses can be delivered following implant integration torque testing. With the use of digital workflow and in-house 3D printing, rapid design and fabrication can be achieved even in the time constraints of malignancy. As technology continues to advance, the workflow will continue to simplify and improve accuracy. Thus, patients will benefit from early return to function as immediate maxillofacial reconstruction becomes common practice.

References

1. Cordeiro PG, Disa JJ, Hidalgo DA, Hu QY. Reconstruction of the mandible with osseous free flaps: a 10-year experience with 150 consecutive patients. Plast Reconstr Surg. 1999;104(5):1314–20.
2. Li B, Byun S, Kim S, Lee J. The clinical outcome of dental implants placed through skin flaps. Head Neck. 2014;151(6):945–51.
3. Nooh N. Dental implant survival in irradiated oral cancer patients: a systematic review of the literature. Int J Oral Maxillofac Implants. 2013;28:1233–42.
4. Ch'ng S, Skoracki RJ, Selber JC, et al. Osseointegrated implant based dental rehabilitation in head and neck reconstruction patients. Head Neck. 2016;38:E321–E32.
5. Wei FC, Santamaria E, Chang YM, et al. Mandibular reconstruction with fibular osteoseptocutaneous free flap and simultaneous placement of osseointegrated dental implants. J Craniofac Surg. 1997;8:512–21.
6. Hirsch D, Garfein E, Christianswn A, et al. Use of computer-aided design and computer-aided manufacturing to produce orthognathically ideal surgical outcomes: a paradigm shift in head and neck reconstruction. J Oral Maxillofac Surg. 2009;67:2115–22.
7. Hutchison I. Saving faces: a facial surgeon's craft (Video); pc.tedcdn.com/talk/stream/2010G/Blank/IainHutchison_2010G-1500k.mp4. Accessed 14 Nov 2021.
8. Hutchison I, Dawood A. Maxillofacial treatments; www.dawoodandtanner.co.uk/maxillofacial.
9. Sclaroff A, Haughhey B, Gay WD, Paniello R. Immediate mandibular reconstruction and placement of dental implants: at the time of ablative surgery. Oral Surg Oral Med Oral Pathol. 1994;78:711–7.
10. Qaisi M, Kolodney H, Swedenburg G, Chandran R, Caloss R. Fibula jaw in a day: state of the art in maxillofacial reconstruction. J Oral Maxillofac Surg. 2016;74:1284.e1–1284.e15.
11. Anolik R, Nelson J, Rosen E, et al. Immediate dental implant placement in the oncologic setting: a conceptual framework. Plast Reconstr Surg Glob Open. 2021;9(9):e3671.
12. Sandoval M, Rosen E, Robert A, et al. Immediate dental implants in fibula free flaps to reconstruct the mandible: a pilot study of the short-term effects on radiotherapy for patients with head and neck cancer. Clin Implant Dent Relat Res. 2019;22:91–5.
13. Landes CA, Kovacs AF. Comparison of early telescope loading of non-submerged ITI implants in irradiated and non-irradiated oral cancer subjects. Clin Oral Implants Res. 2006;17:367–74.

14. Jackson R, Price D, Arce K, Moore E. Evaluation of clinical outcomes of osseointegrated dental implantation of fibula free flaps for mandibular reconstruction. JAMA Facial Plast Surg. 2016;18(3):201–6.
15. Ch'ng S, Skoracki R, Selber J, Yu P, et al. Osseointegrated implant-based dental rehabilitation in head and neck reconstruction patients. Head Neck. 2016;38:21–7.
16. Allen R, Shenaq D, Rosen E, et al. Immediate dental implantation in oncologic jaw reconstruction: workflow optimization to decrease time to full dental rehabilitation. Plast Reconstr Surg Glob Open. 2019;7:1–4.
17. Williams FC, Hammer DA, Wentland TR, Kim RY. Immediate teeth in fibulas: planning and digital workflow with point-of-care 3D printing. J Oral Maxillofac Surg. 2020;78(8):1320–7.

Chapter 12
Microvascular Free Tissue Transfer in Osteoradionecrosis and Medication-Related Osteonecrosis of the Jaws

Arshad Kaleem, Neel Patel, Joseph Geiger, and Ramzey Tursun

Introduction

Osteoradionecrosis of the jaws (ORN) and medication-related osteonecrosis f the jaws (MRONJ) are two disease processes that pose unique challenges and require specific considerations in regard to management. These conditions can be managed by way of nonsurgical (medical) management, more conservative surgical measures, or in cases of advanced disease and aggressive surgical intervention such as resection and reconstruction using a variety of techniques.

The first section of this chapter will focus on management of patients with ORN. This is a much feared complication after radiation therapy in head and neck cancer, with an incidence ranging from 2 to 37% [1]. There appears to be a

A. Kaleem
Division of Oral and Maxillofacial Surgery, DeWitt Daughtry Family Department of Surgery, Section of Head and Neck Surgical Oncology and Microvascular Reconstructive Surgery, Miller School of Medicine/Jackson Health System, University of Miami, Miami, FL, USA

N. Patel (✉)
Division of Oral and Maxillofacial Surgery, DeWitt Daughtry Family Department of Surgery, Head and Neck Surgical Oncology and Microvascular Reconstructive Surgery, Miller School of Medicine/Jackson Health System, University of Miami, Miami, FL, USA

J. Geiger
Oral and Maxillofacial Surgery, DeWitt Daughtry Family Department of Surgery, Miller School of Medicine/Jackson Health System, University of Miami, Miami, FL, USA
e-mail: joseph.geigeriii@jhsmiami.org

R. Tursun
Division of Oral and Maxillofacial Surgery, DeWitt Daughtry Family Department of Surgery, Head and Neck Surgical Oncology and Microvascular Reconstructive Surgery Fellowship, Miller School of Medicine/Jackson Health System, University of Miami, Miami, FL, USA

© The Author(s), under exclusive license to Springer Nature Switzerland AG 2023
J. C. Melville et al. (eds.), *Advancements and Innovations in OMFS, ENT, and Facial Plastic Surgery*, https://doi.org/10.1007/978-3-031-32099-6_12

correlation between the development of ORN and the amount of radiation, with 60 Gy being the threshold after which the risk of development of ORN significantly increases, particularly in the mandible [2]. There is also an incremental increased risk of complications from ORN associated with greater time from radiation therapy, owing to the continued effect on tissues over time [3]. The most severe cases of ORN are most often managed surgically with aggressive resection and free flap reconstruction in order to reconstruct the resultant defects. Effective management strategies must be employed to successfully treat these patients and involves considerations in all phases of treatment. A thorough preoperative clinical and radiographic examination must be done, appropriate biopsies done for accurate diagnosis, and risk stratification for potential complications. Intraoperatively, challenges can present during dissection of the severely fibrosed neck, as well as handling and preparation of radiated vessels for reperfusion of flaps. Postoperatively complication rates are higher due to wound healing issues and the continued effect of radiation.

The second focus of this chapter examines the management of advanced MRONJ with resection and free flap reconstruction and the challenges encountered during this process. MRONJ was first reported in 2003 by Marx in 36 patients and is defined as non-healing bone in craniofacial complex that persists for more than 8 weeks in a person who has received a systemic drug known to cause ONJ with no history of radiation to the jaws [4, 5]. These medications include anti-resorptive and anti-angiogenic medications such as bisphosphonates and RANK ligand inhibitors. Similar to ORN, special considerations exist in these patients in the preoperative, intraoperative, and postoperative phases of treatment. Challenges in accurate disease process delineation, healing issues due to immunosuppression, and the overall health of the metastatic cancer patient all serve as issues that must be considered.

The goals of resection and reconstruction in ORN and MRONJ patients are threefold: (1) curative, which involves resection of diseased bone and soft tissue; (2) restoration of form and function, in terms of articulation, mastication, and swallowing; and (3) esthetic, to obtain a cosmetically acceptable result [6]. In this chapter, the authors will discuss some of the issues that present in management of these patients, as well as ways in which to mitigate these problems and avoid potential pitfalls that can be encountered.

Osteoradionecrosis

Management of patients with ORN can be very difficult, with reconstruction of the hard and soft tissues of the facial skeleton after resection in these patients presenting some interesting challenges for the reconstructive surgeon. Historically, options have included reconstruction plates, pedicled soft tissue flaps, secondary reconstruction with non-vascularized bone grafts, and more recently, the use of microvascular free tissue transfer. Though it is been a time-honored approach, reconstruction of these defects using non-vascularized tissue has been shown to result in inconsistent success rates, varying from 20% to 91%, with complication rates approaching as high as 81%, secondary to issues such as decreased tissue bed vascularity leading to poor healing and increased rates of infection [7, 8]. The use of pedicled flaps to bring vascularized tissue to the region has helped to alleviate some of these issues; however in cases of composite bone and soft tissue defects necessitates a multi-stage surgical approach. The advent of composite free tissue transfer in reconstruction of these defects has served to overcome this and provides a means by which surgeons can reconstruct these defects in a single-stage surgery (Fig. 12.1). This proves particularly useful in cases of very advanced disease due to high dose radiation, where treatment often involves extensive resection of both hard and soft tissues, leaving very large composite defects (Figs. 12.2, 12.3, and 12.4). With the advancement of virtual surgical planning, surgeons are now able to provide accurate and predictable results in these complex cases with custom hardware and less operating time (Figs. 12.5, 12.6, and 12.7). Though free flap reconstruction has revolutionized the management of ORN, it is not without its risks and difficulties and has been shown to be associated with increased rates of complications, including flap failure rates anywhere from 1.4% to 24% [9–14]. Patients who present with this complication from radiation therapy display a variety of both anatomic and

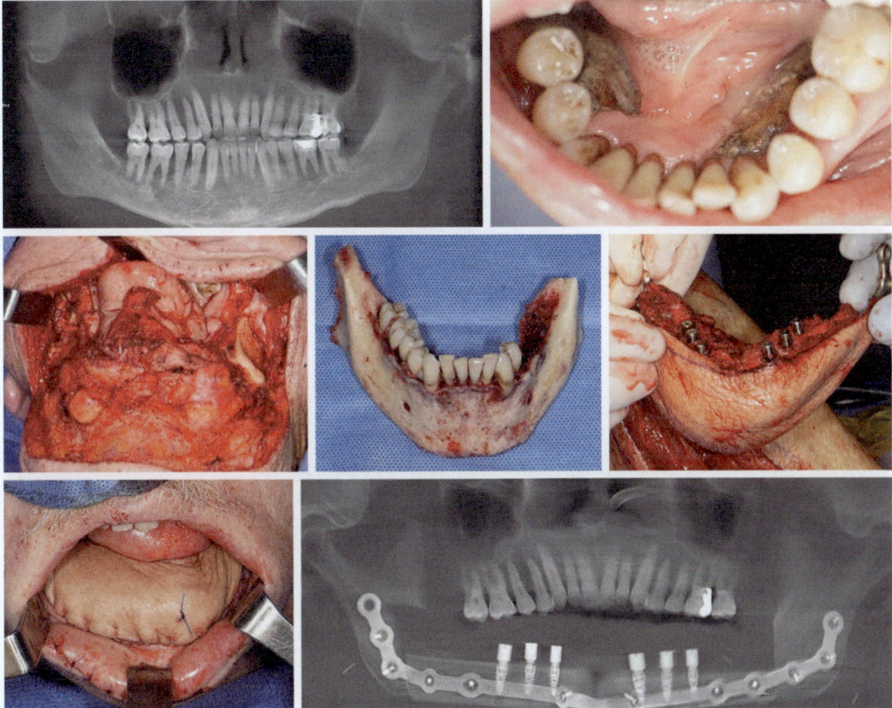

Fig. 12.1 Patient presented with ORN of the mandible bilaterally and was treated with en bloc segmental resection and free fibula flap (FFF) reconstruction with immediate dental implant placement

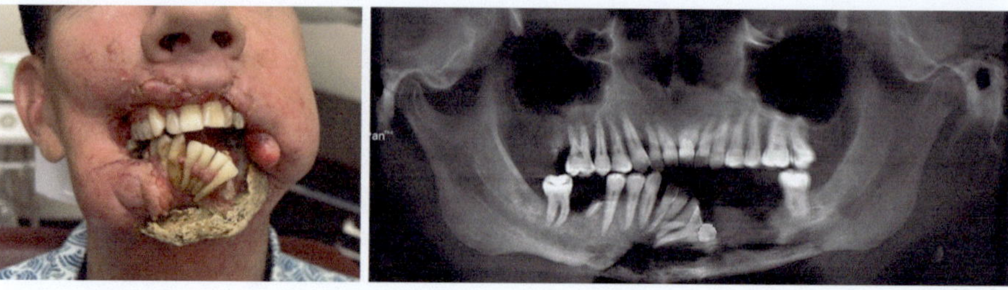

Fig. 12.2 A patient demonstrating extremely advanced ORN of the mandible with necrosis of the soft tissues of the face

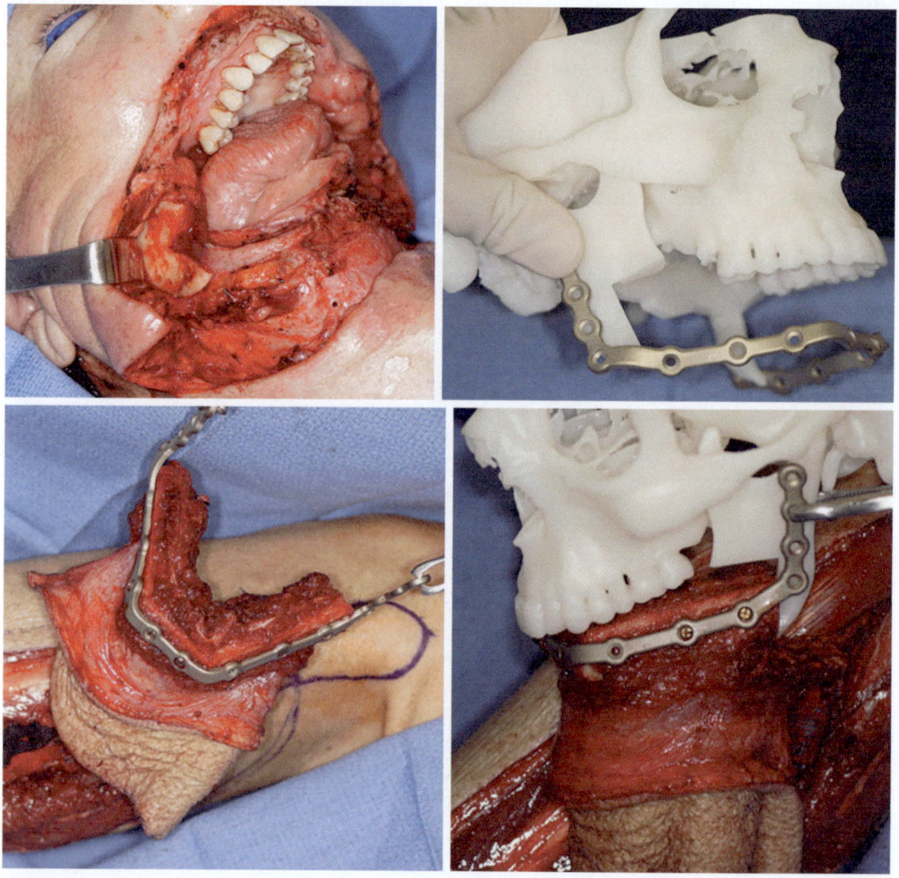

Fig. 12.3 Extensive resection of hard and soft tissues of the facial complex in the advanced ORN patient, with double flap reconstruction using a fibula free flap (FFF) and an anterolateral thigh flap (ALT)

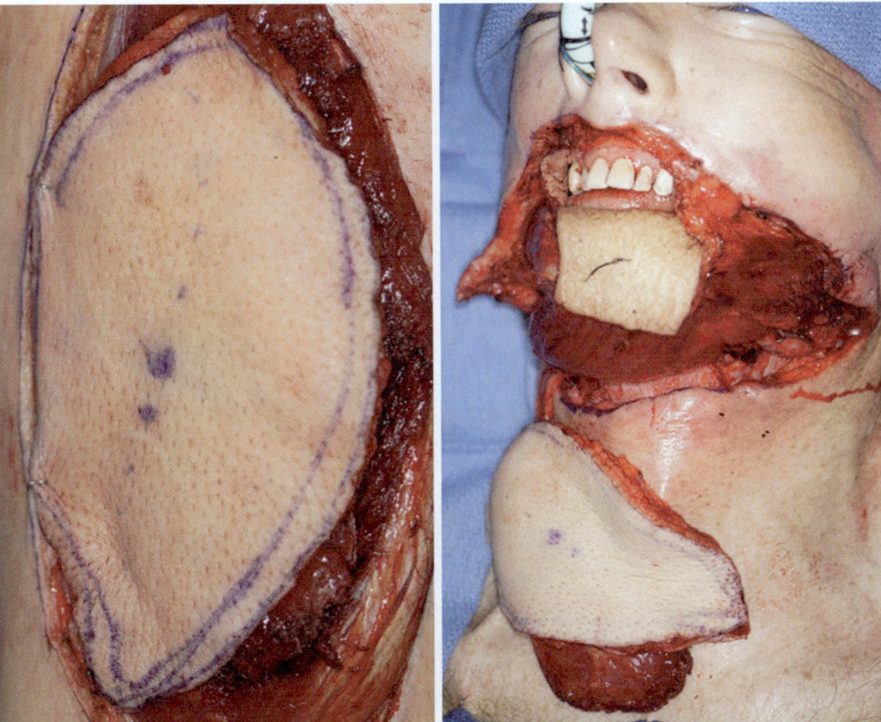

Fig. 12.3 (continued)

physiologic changes that can not only produce intraoperative challenges but can also result in early and late complications postoperatively after free flap surgery.

Vasculature

One of the primary necessities for free tissue transfer procedures is the availability of blood vessels of adequate quality and caliber for microvascular anastomosis to re-vascularize the transplanted tissues. This requires not only the presence of relatively healthy vasculature in the region immediately adjacent to the defect to be reconstructed but also hinges on meticulous and careful dissection and preparation of the vessels to ensure optimal anastomosis. In the case of reconstruction of the facial bones, this usually entails the use of vessels within the neck for this purpose. In patients who have been treated with radiation therapy for malignant disease, unfortunately this often results in the cervical tissues receiving large amounts of radiation, resulting in significant changes in tissue quality that should be taken into consideration. The effects of radiation on vessels have been documented via the use of electron microscopic evaluation and can include such things as direct endothelial

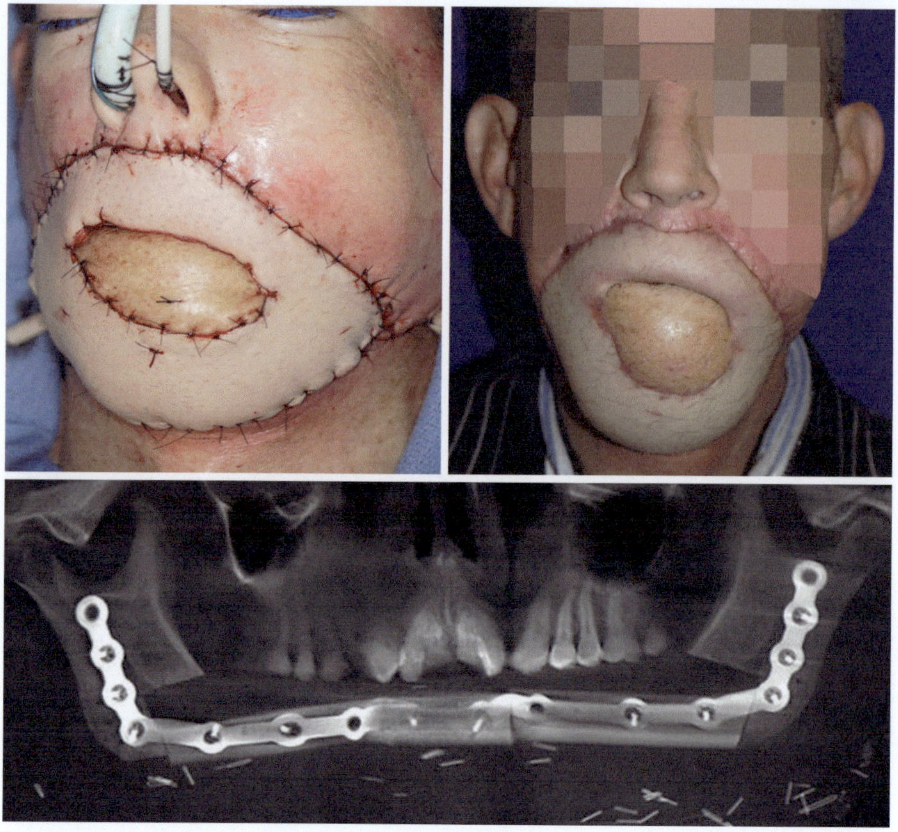

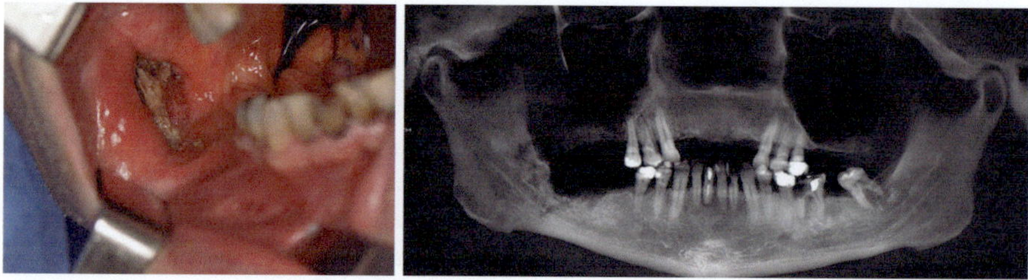

Fig. 12.4 The skin paddle of the FFF is seen here being used to reconstruct the lower lip soft tissues and the ALT to reconstruct the upper lip and remaining facial soft tissues. Below the cone beam CT (CBCT) demonstrates excellent positioning of the FFF for mandibular reconstruction

Fig. 12.5 Patient with ORN of the right mandible

damage, decreased endothelial regeneration, increased fibrin and platelet deposition with formation of plaques and calcifications, increased intramural and subluminal fibrosis, and intimal dehiscence and fragility, in both arteries and veins (Fig. 12.8) [15]. Direct damage to vessels renders them friable and thus easily damaged during

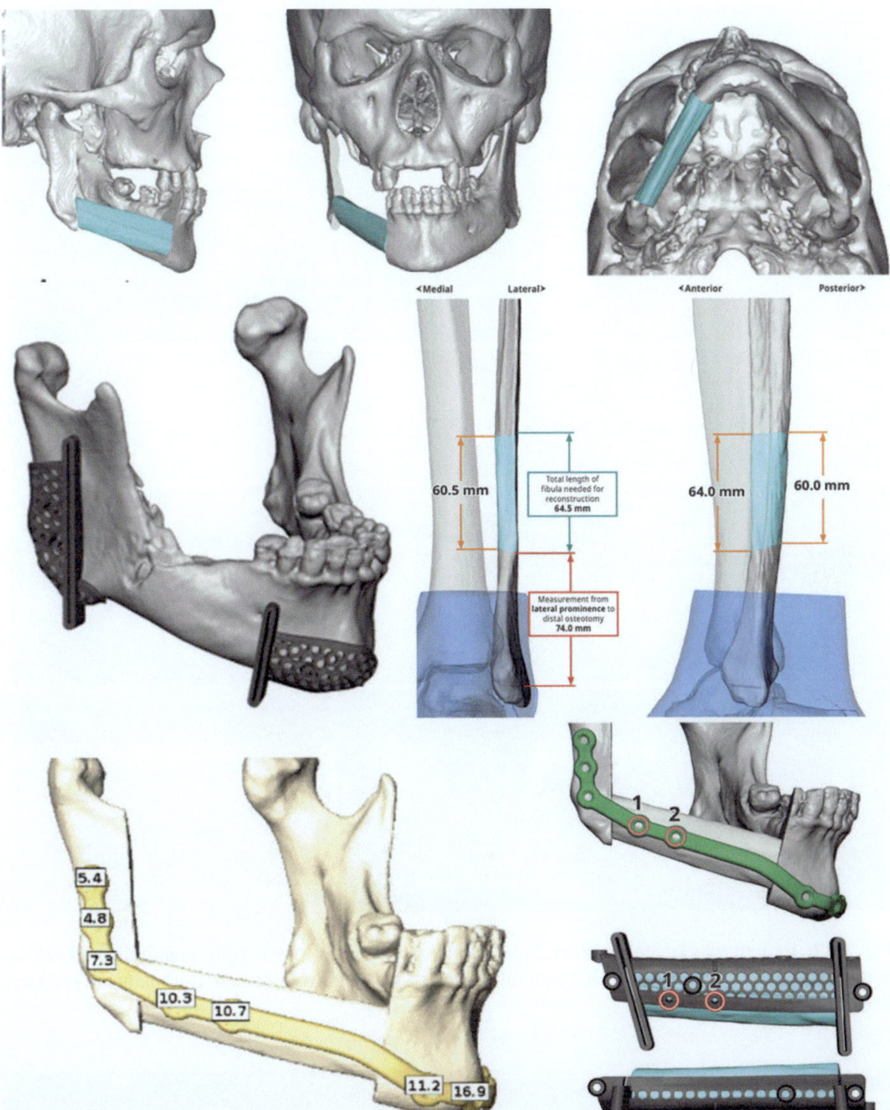

Fig. 12.6 VSP provides predictable and accurate postoperative results with custom hardware

dissection and handling, increased deposition of clot-producing elements leading to increased rates of thrombosis, and damage to the intimal layer leading to increased risk of dissection Fand subsequent anastomotic failure. Extreme care must be taken during both dissection and handling of irradiated vessels in preparation for microvascular anastomosis. Complete vessel preparation should be performed prior to division of the flap pedicle, in the event that the vessels appear compromised during preparation and a second set of vessels needs to be sought out, as this minimizes the

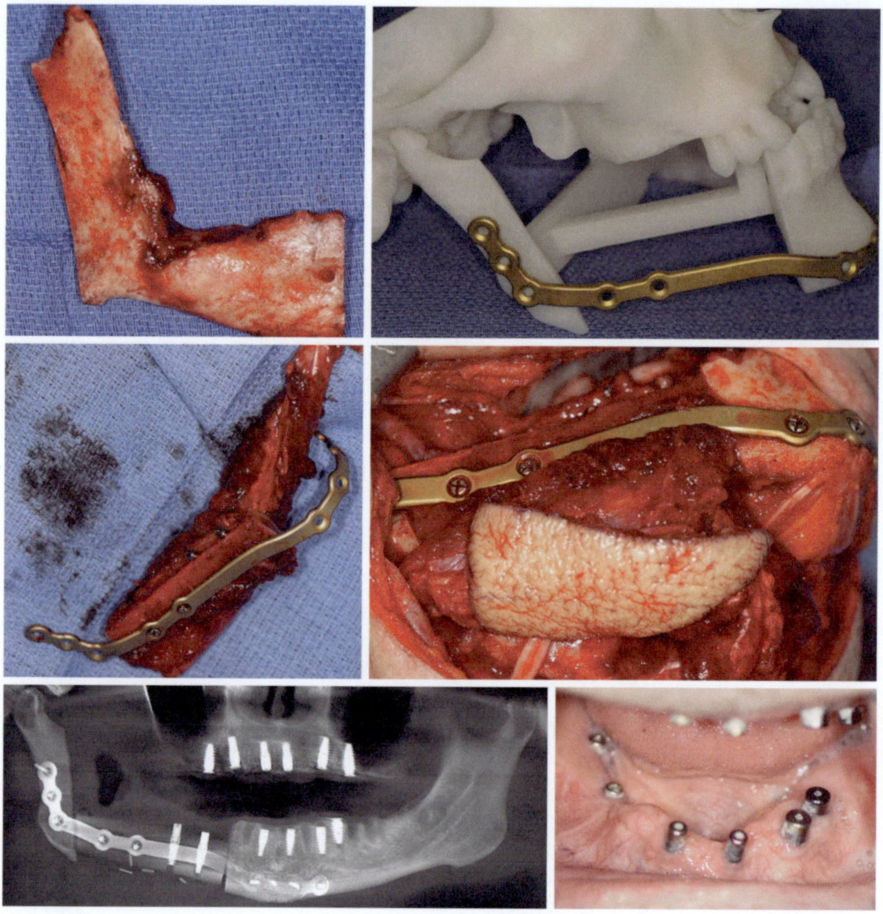

Fig. 12.7 Patient was treated with en bloc segmental resection of the right mandible, and reconstruction with free fibula flap (FFF), and rehabilitated with endosseous dental implants in preparation to receive teeth

Fig. 12.8 Radiated vessel under microscope demonstrating fibrotic walls and damaged endothelium

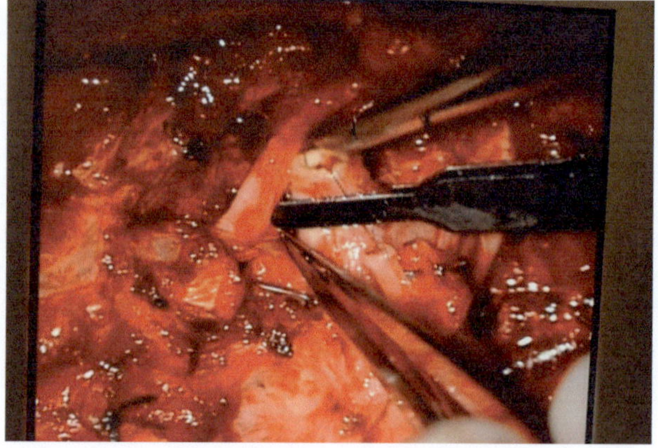

ischemia time for the flap. While microvascular anastomosis in these cases can be challenging, some techniques can be utilized to mitigate some problems that can arise. Avoiding the use of double microvascular clamps can help minimize vessel trauma, and avoiding excessive stretching and dilation can help decrease the risk of damage. In regard to venous anastomosis, most often done using coupler devices, vessel fragility must be taken into account when placing vessel edges on the stainless steel pins of the coupler. In most cases, it is usually ideal to use the largest coupler possible for anastomosis to provide the largest lumen possible for blood flow, and given the relative elasticity of veins, this is often quite easy to do. However, in irradiated veins, given the friability of the vessel walls, one must be cognizant of this, and thus a slightly smaller coupler may be preferable to reduce the risk of tearing the vessel walls. In terms of preparation and anastomosis of the arterial system, several potential issues must be taken into account, with the majority of arterial anastomoses being performed using suture techniques. The "PCA technique" [16] combines three different techniques for vessel anastomosis (i.e., "posterior wall first," "continuous interrupted," and "airborne" [17]) and provides an excellent method for radiated vessel anastomosis (Fig. 12.9). Performing posterior wall anastomosis first eliminates the need to turn the micro-clamps over at any point during anastomosis, thus decreasing twisting and risk of vessel trauma. Furthermore, the combination of the continuous interrupted and airborne suture technique allows for visibility of the lumen throughout the anastomosis process, decreasing the risk of "backwalling." By using this technique, the surgeon avoids tightening and tying each subsequent suture and leaves that until the end, at which time is done in an interrupted fashion. In doing so, the surgeon can ensure to maintain complete visualization of the intima with every passing of the suture needle, whereas if knots are tied along the way, one loses more and more view of the intima as anastomosis proceeds, increasing the risk of intimal damage. The anastomosis is performed in an "in" to "out" direction to minimize the risk of intimal separation.

Poor healing at the anastomotic line with potential breakdown at that level can be a concern, and thus reinforcement at that site can often be performed. When passing the suture needle, the surgeon can include a small cuff of adventitia on either side of the anastomosis to provide an additional bolstering effect while taking care to avoid having the adventitia fold into the site of the anastomosis. During vessel isolation and preparation, surgeons will often use either monopolar or bipolar electrocautery, not only to clear the vessels from the adjacent tissues but also to ligate branches from the vessels. With the increased risk of thrombosis in irradiated vessels, surgeons should minimize the use of monopolar cautery whenever possible and should resort to gentle blunt dissection. Furthermore, even the use of bipolar cautery in ligation of branches carries with it the risk of retrograde thrombosis, and thus ties or clips should be used whenever possible. Surgeons should always maintain a low threshold to refresh vessel margins whenever there is doubt of the quality at the site of anastomosis while always taking into account residual vessel length when doing so to ensure good reach and a tension-free anastomosis. Finally, the option of using vessels outside of the zone of radiation is also possible; however this is contingent on having an adequate pedicle length and good vessel caliber match.

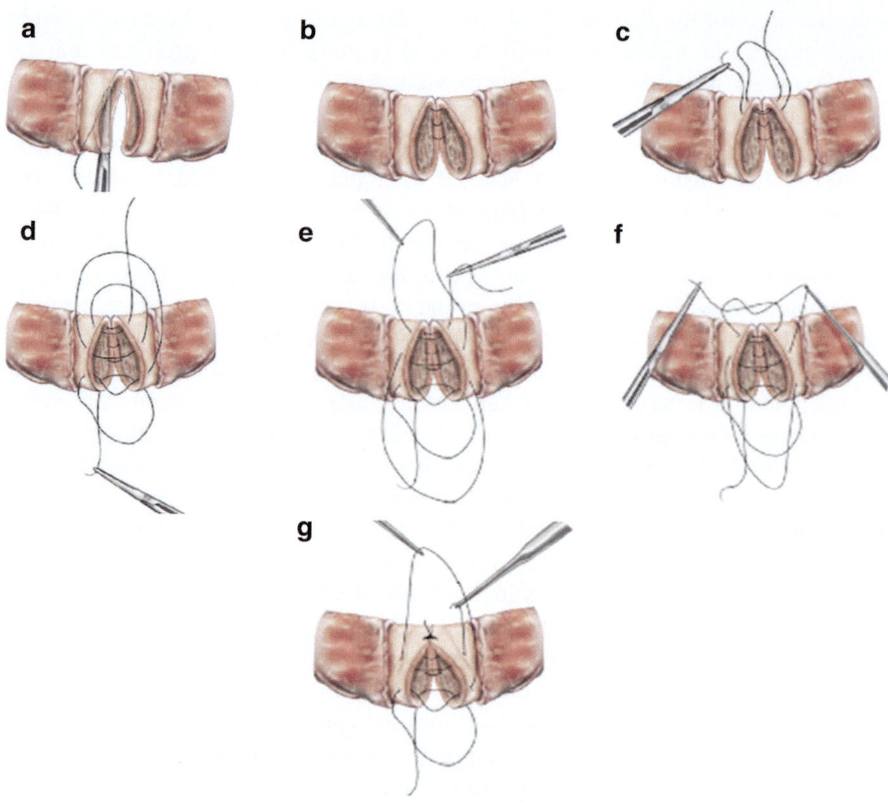

Fig. 12.9 PCA technique begins with suturing of the posterior wall first (**a**, **b**), the sutures are continuously passed without tying (**c**, **d**), and then finally each suture is tied separately with the airborne technique, tying the tail with the opposing loop, and this is continued until the end (**e–g**), such that one ends up with all interrupted tied sutures. (*Cigna E, Cirunga C, Bistoni G, Spalvieri C, Tortorelli G, Scuderi N. Microsurgical anastomosis with the "PCA" technique. J Plastic Recon & Aesth Surg. 2008; 61:762–766 (with permission)*))

In unilaterally radiated necks, using vessels in the contralateral non-irradiated neck is often used by surgeons [18]. One can also use vessels that are outside of the neck such as the superficial temporal system, or vessels lower in the neck such as ones from the thyrocervical system, or even the internal mammary system (Fig. 12.10) and employ techniques such as vein grafts whenever needed. In regard to preoperative assessment of vessels, some surgeons will obtain a CT angiogram of the neck to evaluate vessels ahead of time. However, caution should still be employed even if vessels of apparent adequate caliber and quality are seen on imaging, as sometimes these vessels may demonstrate poor flow or wall lesions under microscopic examination intraoperatively. Given all of this, the surgeon should always keep in mind that the goal is to obtain the best result *possible* for the patient. In very rare instances where appropriate vessels cannot be found, the surgeon may have to consider the option of abandoning a free flap procedure in favor of a local or regional flap reconstruction.

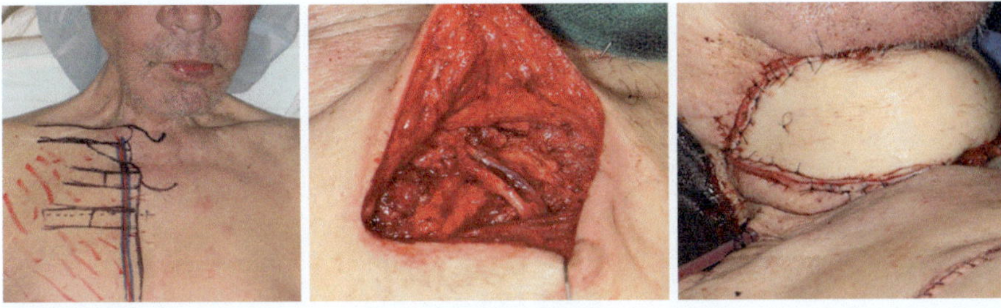

Fig. 12.10 Use of the internal mammary system in head and neck reconstruction

Fig. 12.11 Extensive fibrosis and scarring in the neck of a radiated patient

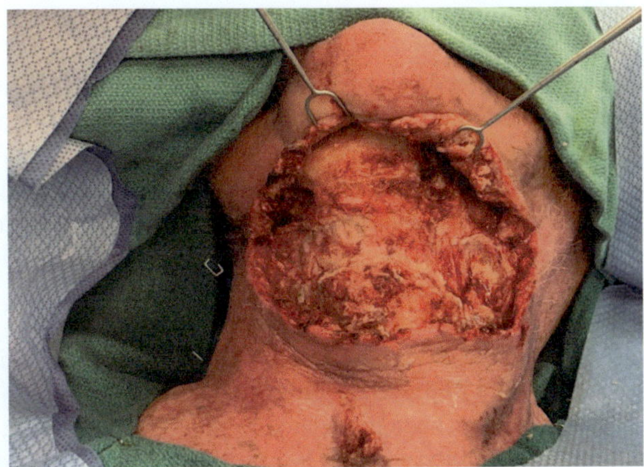

Tissue Quality and Healing

The effects of radiation therapy on tissue beds are well known and can be very apparent in radiated patients. These effects include ionization events, production of free radicals that cause damage to vital cellular components, and cell death [19]. Tissue planes are often obliterated by the fibroblastic response resulting in excessive amounts of collagen deposition leading to extensive fibrosis and scarring (Fig. 12.11). Dissection in these cases should never be underestimated and should be done with care, as normal anatomic relationships are often skewed or non-existent. In patients who have undergone previous neck dissection, this becomes even more challenging, as tissues are often scarred together without the presence of the fibrofatty layer, and structures can be more superficial than expected. Previous neck dissection itself has also been demonstrated to have a strong correlation with free flap loss and microvascular revisions [20]. Moreover, though the effects of radiation begin immediately after exposure, the clinical and histological changes can continue for weeks, months, and even years after treatment. This can result in late complications due to continued changes in both soft and hard tissue even years after resection and reconstruction, thus presenting as soft tissue wound breakdowns and appearance of osteolytic/necrotic changes at the bony resection margins with

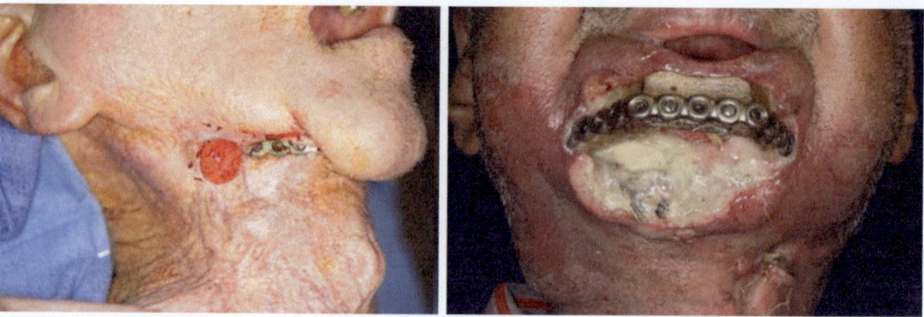

Fig. 12.12 Extraoral hardware exposure (left) and severe hard and soft tissue necrosis (right) in previously reconstructed ORN patients

subsequent related complications such as infections, fistulae, and malunions with or without fracture. To this point, Wang et al. found that increasing time elapsed from radiotherapy was significantly and negatively correlated with quality-of-life scores in regard to speech and recreation, as a result of these complications [21]. Hardware failure can often be associated either by way of exposure either intraorally or via skin breakdown and exposure extraorally (Fig. 12.12) or by virtue of necrosis of the fixated bone segments with subsequent loss of stability. Studies have shown rates of local wound complications such as infection, hardware failure, wound breakdown, and fistula formation can be approximately 40–57%, thus representing about half of patients who will present with some local wound healing issue [22, 23]. One of the methods that has been postulated to potentially result in reduction of complications and increasing success rates has been the use of hyperbaric oxygen therapy (HBO) in this cohort of patients, primarily in the preoperative setting. Given its ability to produce reactive oxygen species that aid in osteoclast differentiation, as well as neovascularization, fibroblast proliferation, and stem cell production, it can result in improved bone turnover and soft tissue healing. A study by Nolen et al. [24] looked at a cohort of 39 patients who had received HBO prior to resection and free flap reconstruction and examined rates of local wound complications, including free flap failure as compared to those patients who did not receive preoperative HBO. They concluded that there was no difference in complication rates between the two groups, and even cited those patients who had a history of failed HBO therapy demonstrated an increased rate of postoperative infection, which is consistent with other studies. A possible reason for this is that this may represent a group of patients where HBO-resistant ORN is more recalcitrant [25].

Extent of Disease

Another concern is the progression of ORN to the remaining bony segments after resection and reconstruction, resulting in local complications. A study by Suh et al. [26] reported the incidence of recurrent or progressive ORN after resection and free flap reconstruction as high as 25% in the mandible, with 70% occurring in the unresected, previously unaffected, proximal segment. This can present an additional echelon of complication if the continued ORN occurs in a bony segment that has already been dentally rehabilitated, as now the surgeon and dentist must address the potential loss and replacement of dental implants and a new prosthesis, adding not only the need for additional surgical procedures but also supplementary expense for the patient. Unfortunately, progression of necrosis and tissue damage is difficult to account for and predict. Preoperative assessment via clinical examination and imaging provides the best tool to assess the extent of disease and should be carefully evaluated to ensure adequate resection margins. Moreover, it is extremely crucial that recurrent malignant disease is ruled out preoperatively with biopsies if indicated, as it has been reported that up to as much as 3.4% of ORN resection specimens demonstrate the presence of malignancy upon postoperative histopathological examination [27]. Some surgeons may opt to minimize the extent of surgery by performing a more conservative resection, for example, to retain the proximal segment (if uninvolved) to avoid a disarticulation mandibular defect to reconstruct and to maintain the patient's natural joint articulation, given some studies that have shown increased rates of complications and patient morbidity after total condylectomy and reconstruction [28]. Others may choose to limit the amount of resection to maximize the dental rehabilitation for the patient by being conservative on the amount of dentate segment they resect. While these approaches can provide some benefit, they must be weighed with the possibility of progression of the osteoradionecrosis within those unresected nearby segments of the bone. Intraoperatively surgeons will often resect to "bleeding bone," which frequently indicates healthy tissue; however given the progressive nature of this disease process, this does not guarantee long-term success. Moreover, it is difficult to assess for bleeding from the proximal segment, in particular the condylar region, as this is dense cortical bone with little to no marrow space. Additionally, decreased blood supply to the proximal segment due to compromise of the inferior alveolar vessels and stripping of periosteum during hardware fixation can contribute to hypovascularity and necrotic changes in the future. Given these findings, many surgeons have become more aggressive with their resection margins and have a lower threshold to resect the proximal segment of the mandible, especially if the ORN extends to the angle or into the ramus and have noted that postoperative function is grossly unaffected with a good composite free flap reconstruction. A recent study by Tang et al. [29] looked at 48 patients who underwent fibula flap reconstruction of the mandibular condyle and assessed both changes in the neo-condylar position and function and concluded that despite slight changes in fibula condyle positioning, patient's postoperative function was intact. Additionally, the free osseous flap can be used in combination with a joint prosthesis in order to reconstruct the condylar segment (Fig. 12.13). Moreover, with all the advances in dental implants and prosthetics, it is certainly acceptable to maintain at least a 1 cm margin from obviously involved necrotic bone during resection and even be slightly more aggressive in resecting more of the ORN-adjacent dentate segments of the jaws if questionable. It is much easier dealing with a slightly larger defect on the front end, rather than having to navigate

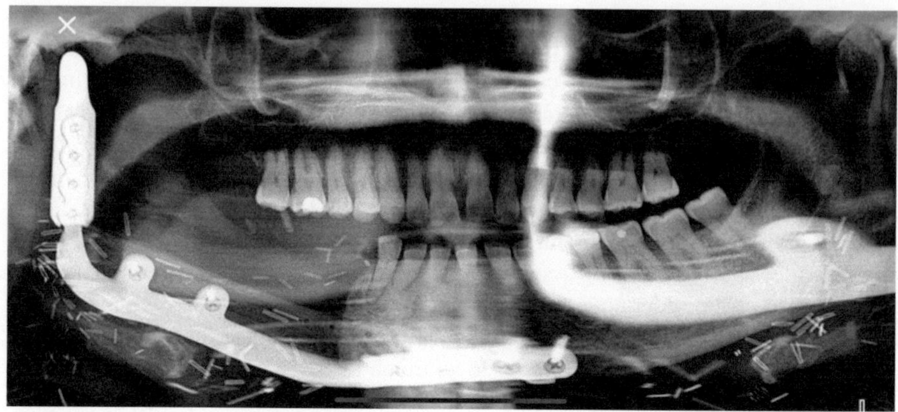

Fig. 12.13 Use of condylar prosthesis in conjunction with free fibula flap in reconstruction of ORN patient

necrotic bone that has already been dentally rehabilitated later on. As resection margins in ORN remain a topic to be elucidated, the concept of tetracycline bone fluorescence has been studied in this cohort of patients. This method has been shown to potentially be helpful in guiding resection margin delineation [30], given that tetracycline is only absorbed by viable bone, to help in determining where necrotic bone ends. Other studies have used near-infrared fluorescence using intravenously administered indocyanine green dye, with subsequent margin evaluation with a portable infrared imaging device [31]. Though these techniques may have some usefulness in this regard, more studies need to be done to determine their reliability.

Perioperative Management

Perioperative management planning is also crucial in patients with ORN undergoing extensive resection and free flap reconstruction procedures. Airway management strategy is important to determine preoperatively, as patients who have received radiation therapy can demonstrate extensive scarring in the oropharynx, hypopharynx, and larynx, predisposing them to potential airway complications. Tracheostomy represents a safe and reliable method to provide a secure airway in these patients and should be discussed with patients in the preoperative phase. Whether it is going to be a planned procedure to be done at the beginning or end of the surgery, or to at least discuss the possibility with the patient in the event that it must be done in an emergent fashion, if the anesthesia team has difficulties during the induction and endotracheal intubation process, given the sometimes extensive airway contracture that can be seen in these patients. Additionally, patients who are being treated with radiation for malignancy often inherently have issues with malnutrition, whether from the cancer diagnosis itself causing weight loss or as a result of dysphagia and odynophagia from the radiation therapy itself. A plan for both preoperative nutritional assessment and optimization and the route of postoperative nourishment should be planned ahead of time. Not only can this have an effect on the overall health of the patient but also has been shown to affect rates of microvascular free tissue transfer success, as low prealbumin levels have been demonstrated as a risk factor for free flap failure [32]. Percutaneous endoscopic gastrostomy (PEG) tubes may be useful in these patients and can either be placed preoperatively for improvement of nutritional status before surgery or at time of surgery to optimize postoperative feeding. If patients have been on medical treatment for their ORN (i.e., pentoxifylline-tocopherol or PENTO protocol, as well as antibiotics), these should not be interrupted until the day of surgery and can be continued postoperatively if indicated.

Medication-Related Osteonecrosis of the Jaws

MRONJ represents an enigma within the medical field that has been proven to be a difficult disease entity to manage (Figs. 12.14, 12.15, 12.16, and 12.17). There has been a long-standing debate on conservative versus more aggressive management strategies, with a consensus yet to be reached. However, despite the lack of high-quality evidence in regard to optimal treatment, the majority of practitioners favor a more conservative approach when possible. When nonsurgical therapy fails or when the disease process presents at a more advanced stage, then conservative surgical options such as local debridement, sequestrectomy, and softening sharp bony edges with the goal of promoting overlying soft tissue healing are favored [33, 34]. More extensive surgical procedures are generally reserved for patients with more advanced disease (stages II and III) and for those patients who have failed previous conservative therapy with or without progression of disease. Patients who present with stage II and III disease managed with conservative measures have historically only shown resolution in about 50% of cases, owing to either a refractory disease process or continued progression of disease [35, 36]. Some authors have stated that more aggressive surgery, such as en bloc segmental resection and free flap reconstruction, is inappropriate because of the patient's poor overall condition, as well as the diminished life expectancy in the case of some metastatic cancer patients [37]. However, radical segmental surgical resection of involved necrotic bone with reconstruction using microvascular free tissue transfer has shown excellent rates of disease eradication, good functional and esthetic results, and improved quality of life, with some authors reporting as high as 100% success rates [38]. Good success rates notwithstanding, free flap reconstruction in these patients can present with a few challenges.

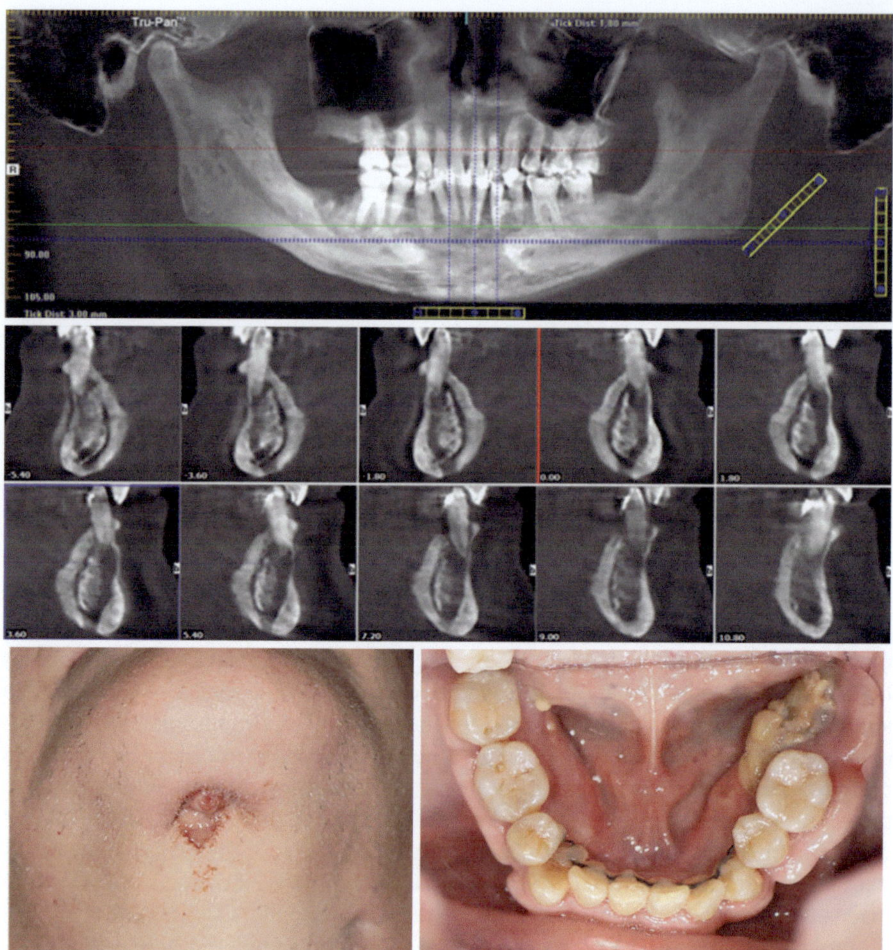

Fig. 12.14 Severe case of MRONJ of the mandible with draining fistula

Malignancy

Reconstruction of these defects using free tissue transfer represents an excellent surgical option in advanced or refractory cases and can be accomplished in several fashions. The use of soft tissue-only flaps can be employed in combination with reconstruction plates to span and stabilize the jaw, leaving a bony discontinuity, with the possibility of returning for secondary non-vascularized bone grafting [39]. This would allow for a more expedited procedure, which is helpful in patients with significant comorbidities and in whom a shorter surgical intervention is desired. Despite this advantage, patients who desire bony reconstruction would necessitate a second surgery, with a second general anesthetic and the associated risks. Furthermore, the risk of hardware failure (such as plate fracture, exposure,

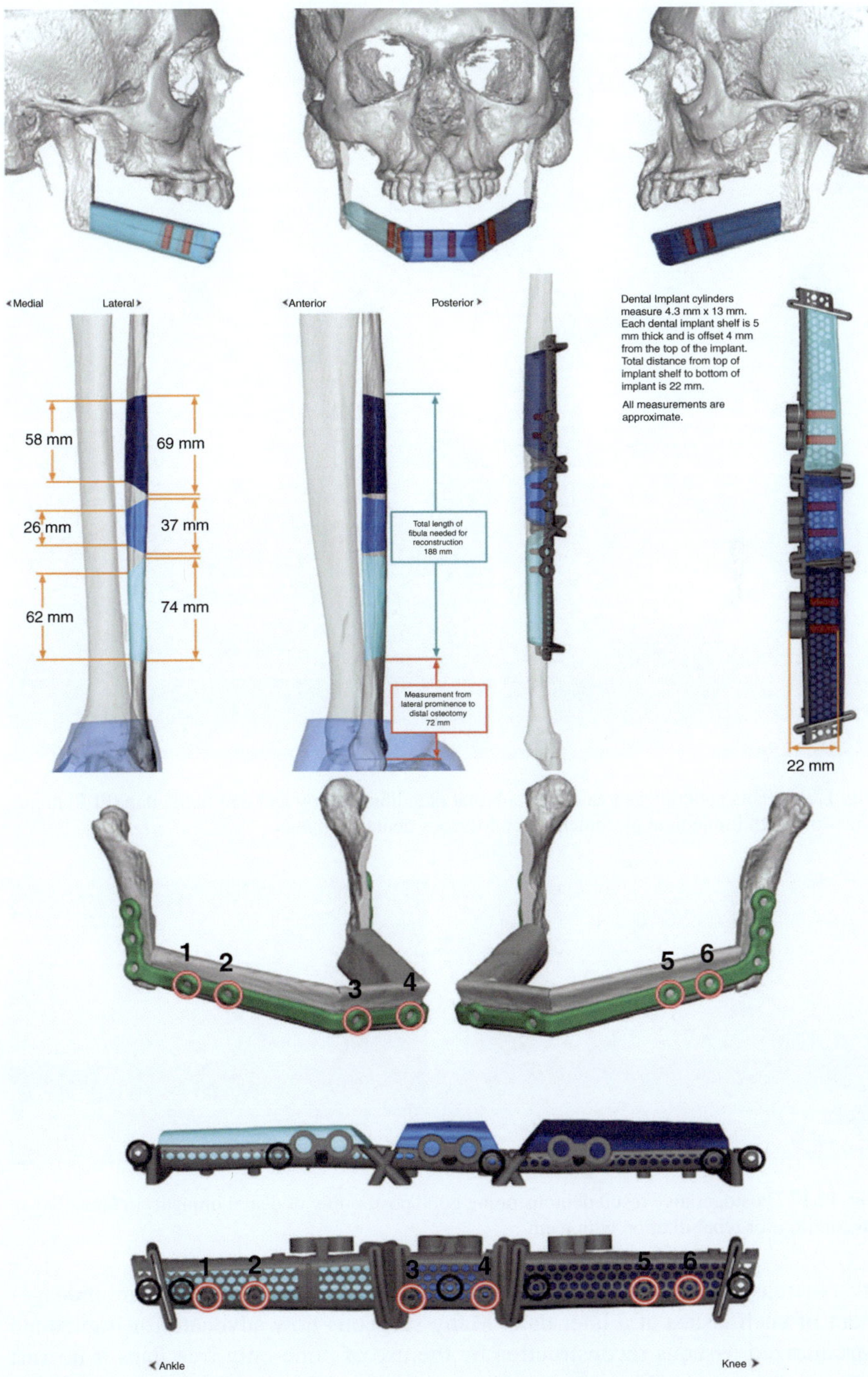

Fig. 12.15 VSP planning allows for a fully guided surgical platform for complex cases, including accurate placement of endosseous dental implants for optimal rehabilitation

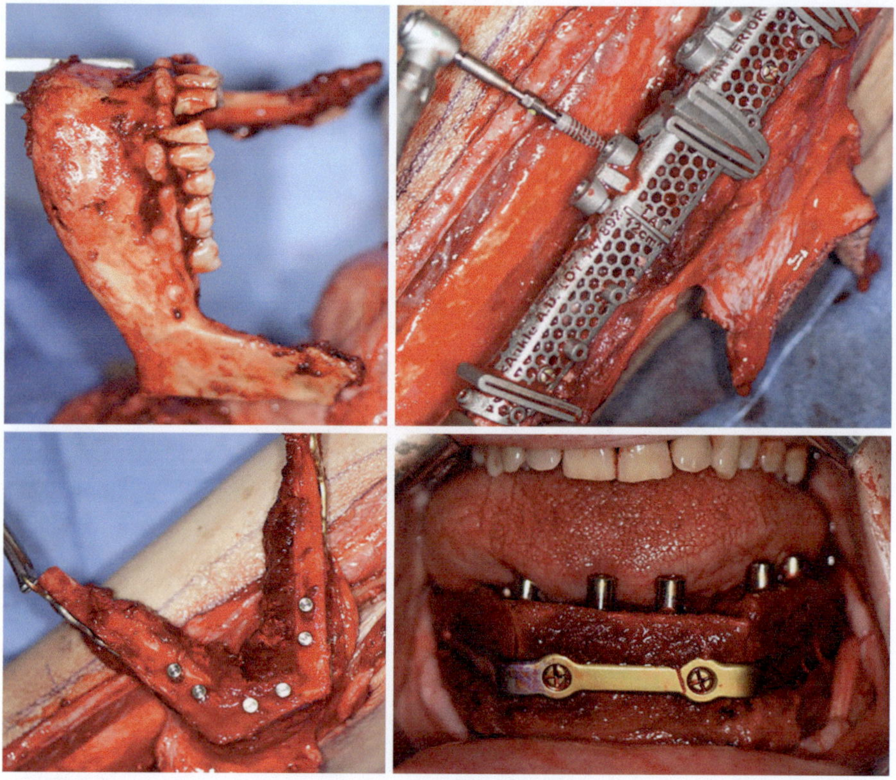

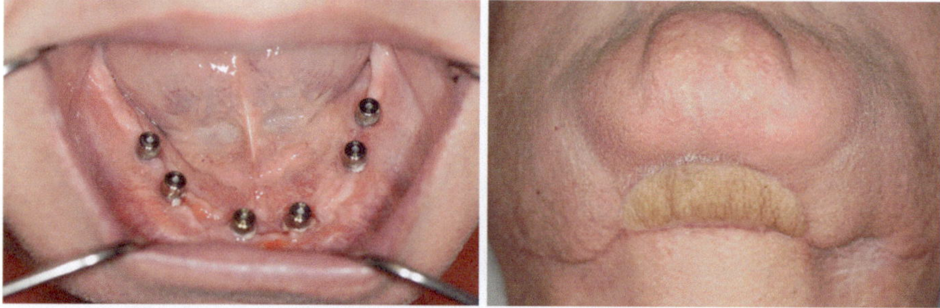

Fig. 12.16 This patient was treated via subtotal mandibulectomy and free fibula flap (FFF) reconstruction, with immediate placement of endosseous dental implants

Fig. 12.17 Postoperative result demonstrating good positioning of dental implants in fibula flap in preparation for rehabilitation with teeth

etc.) increases in this cohort of patients and thus may eventually require management of such issues at a later date. Many surgeons now advocate for immediate vascularized osseous reconstruction by the use of bone-only free flaps if no soft tissue defect exists (Fig. 12.18) or composite free flaps. While this presents an

Fig. 12.18 Patient with advanced MRONJ of the mandible, en bloc segmental resection, and reconstruction was performed with bone-only fibula free flap (FFF). Note remaining aspects of mandible show sclerotic effect of anti-resorptive medications

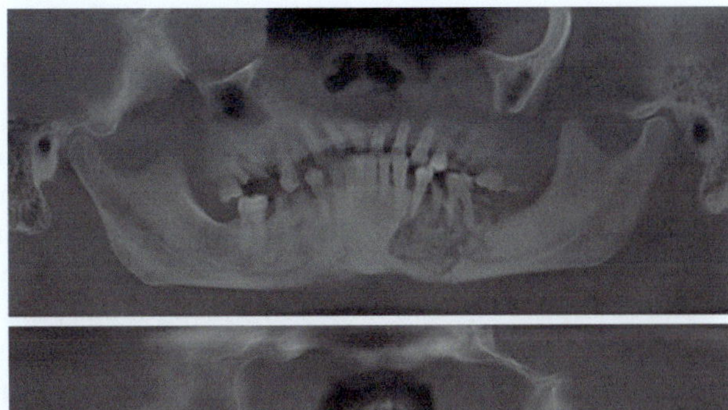

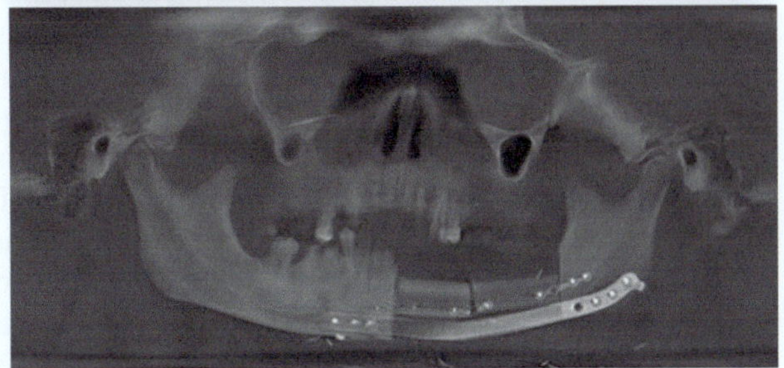

attractive option as patients would obtain complete reconstruction in a one-stage surgical procedure, there exist some concerns nonetheless. Many patients who are on these anti-resorptive and anti-angiogenic agents are those who have metastatic malignant disease involving the bone, for example, patients with multiple myeloma. MRONJ can also occur in patients who are receiving these medications for osteoporosis; however the rate of this disease process in cancer patients is about ten times higher in cancer patients than in osteoporotic patients [40]. There exists the theoretical possibility of transferring a malignant process from the donor bone within the flap to the jaws in metastatic cancer patients [41], though there have been no such reports in the literature. In cases where this is a concern, preoperative full body imaging using positron emission tomography (PET) and/or nuclear bone scans have been considered to rule out malignant lesions in the donor bone; however the sensitivity of these imaging techniques may not be adequate to detect micrometastatic lesions. The fibula represents a rare site for metastatic disease or lesions in multiple myeloma [42, 43], whereas the ilium and the scapula are more common sites of disease in these groups [44, 45]. As such, the fibula free flap may represent a better choice of bone flap for reconstruction of MRONJ defects in cases where malignant cell transfer is a concern. It is also very important, as with ORN, to preoperatively rule out the presence of malignant disease within the area of jaw osteonecrosis, as small deposits of malignancy can be difficult to detect in a background of necrotic bone. In a multicenter review, Carlson et al. [46] showed the presence of microscopic foci of malignancy in 5.3% of biopsy and resection specimens previously diagnosed as MRONJ, and thus a thorough evaluation of involved bone should be employed to ensure the absence of malignant disease.

Healing

Postoperative free flap healing with bony union also presents as a concern in patients with MRONJ, given that many of these patients are immunocompromised, either due to concomitant use of steroids, chemotherapy regimens, or simply by virtue of having advanced stage cancer in itself. Furthermore, some authors state that the risk of nonunion is higher in this cohort of patients given the systemic nature of delivery of anti-resorptive and anti-angiogenic medications such that both the recipient bone and the donor bone likely demonstrate generalized uptake of these agents and thus may have issues with adequate bone turnover and thus bony healing. However despite this claim, reports in the literature do not support this postulation, as the incidence of poor healing and nonunion of bony segments after osseous reconstruction in MRONJ is only about 5–6.5%, with the rate of resultant fistula formation only at about 10% [47]. The concept of a "drug holiday," namely, stopping the offending anti-resorptive and anti-angiogenic medications about 6–9 months prior to undergoing resection and free flap reconstruction, has been suggested; however definitive evidence that this helps in increasing the incidence of healing and decreasing complication rates is still not available and, as such, is not widely practiced. Additionally, given the higher risk of postoperative complications secondary to patients' immunocompromised status, discussion with the patients' oncologist regarding optimal chemotherapy and immunosuppressive regimens is encouraged, though the overall patient condition should always be taken into account and should not be compromised. The role of HBO in MRONJ has not yet been fully elucidated; however it has been studied in the context of more conservative treatment such as medical management and localized surgical interventions such as debridement and sequestrectomy. In a randomized control trial, Frieberger et al. [48] assessed the use of HBO as an adjunct to conservative surgical procedures and antibiotic therapy and concluded that HBO did play a role as part of multimodal therapy in severe cases. However no studies have yet been done to evaluate its role as an adjunct to more extensive surgical procedures such as large resections and free vascularized flap reconstruction. In addition to bony healing, the quality of the overlying and adjacent soft tissues should be taken into consideration, as bisphosphonates have been shown to have a negative effect on oral mucosal healing [49], which could precipitate wound breakdown, plate and bone exposure, and infection. As such, osteotomies should ideally be placed in areas where the vascular supply is robust, such as areas of muscle attachment, and they should be at least 1 cm away from any tooth [50].

Extent of Disease

Postoperative progression of disease is always a cause for concern in these patients, primarily within the jaw bones, given the fact that these medications can remain within these bones for years and even decades. However, an interesting case report by Pautke et al. [51] described the occurrence of MRONJ not within the jaw bones, but within the transplanted free iliac bone flap postoperatively. They reported that intraoperatively the bone appeared vital; however postoperative serial imaging lacked the evidence of bone remodeling at the margins, and biopsies were taken. Histopathology of the biopsied iliac bone revealed the typical signs of MRONJ including bone necrosis, bacterial colonization by actinomyces, and hypervascular tissue surrounding the necrotic bone (Fig. 12.19). It is not possible, however, to deduce whether the process occurred de novo within the iliac bone or was a direct extension from the adjacent mandibular bone, and one single case report by no means can provide a reliable data set upon which to make any viable conclusions. There have also been further reports on the occurrence of MRONJ postoperatively in the contralateral jaw bone and thus can complicate the postoperative course as well [52, 53]. Similar to ORN, the extent of necessary resection in cases of MRONJ can also be difficult to accurately assess, despite excellent clinical and radiographic examination preoperatively. Most commonly surgeons will use one or a

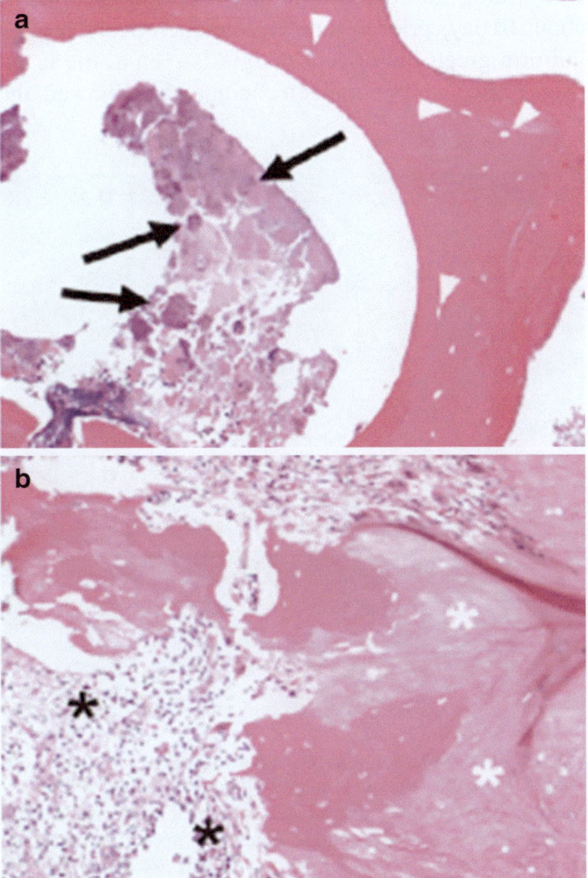

Fig. 12.19 Histology of MRONJ in iliac bone free flap with typical hallmarks. Necrotic bone with no osteocytes (black arrows), bacterial colonization with actinomyces (white arrows), and necrotic bone surrounded by hypervascular tissue (black asterisks) and new trabecular bone (white asterisks). (*Pautke C, Otto S, Reu S, Kolk A. Bisphosphonate related osteonecrosis of the jaw—Manifestation in a microvascular iliac bone flap. Oral Oncology. 2011:47;425–429 (with permission)*)

combination of imaging modalities such as panoramic films, cone beam computerized tomography (CBCT), medical-grade computerized tomography (CT), and magnetic resonance imaging (MRI) to assess the extent of disease prior to surgery. Moreover, intraoperative assessment of bone margin quality is also performed, with resection to apparent healthy bleeding bone, in correlation with preoperative radiographic findings to maximize the chances of obtaining a clear surgical margin. Despite these efforts, occasionally resection margins appear inadequate on postoperative histopathological examination, imposing a risk of persistent and/or recurrent disease, and possible treatment failure, sometimes within 3–6 months [54, 55]. As such, it is always prudent to err on the side of caution, and if an area adjacent to obvious MRONJ-afflicted bone is questionable, surgeons should consider extending the resection to those regions, to decrease the risk of unresected disease. A linear margin of at least 1 cm beyond visible involved bone on imaging should be planned to achieve good, negative margins [56]. As with ORN, the concept of tetracycline bone labeling has also been investigated in patients with MRONJ, to help delineate necrotic versus viable bone. Pautke et al. [57] reported their experience in a pilot study using fluorescence-guided resection, with administration of tetracycline for about 10 days prior to surgery. Intraoperatively, resection is performed until a clean, uniform green fluorescent margin is seen at the level of the residual bone margin (Fig. 12.20), and with this technique, they showed about an 85% success rate [58].

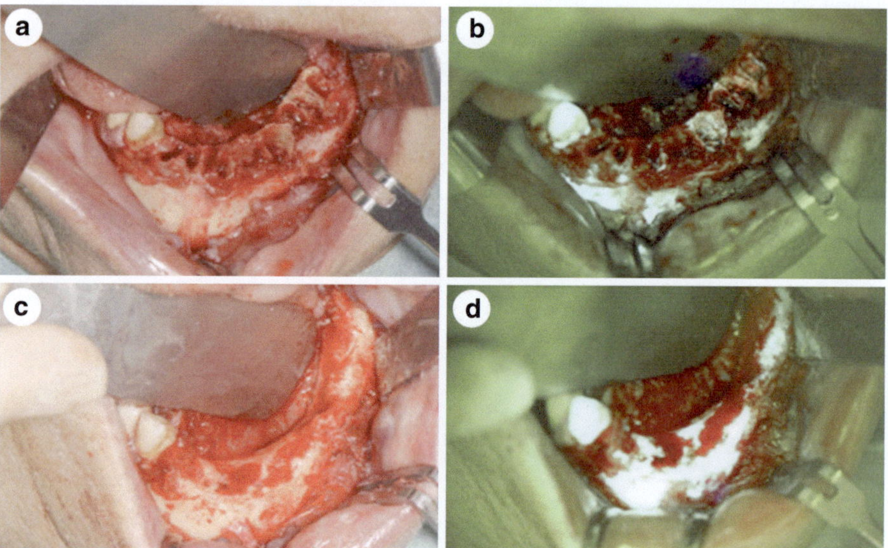

Fig. 12.20 Fluorescence-guided bone resection performed after 10-day doxycycline treatment. Extent of necrosis evident clinically (**a**) and delineated by fluorescence (**b**). After resection, healthy bleeding bone seen (**c**), and a clean margin of viable fluorescent bone seen (**d**). (*Pautko C, Bauer F, Otto S. Fluorescence-guided bone resection in bisphosphonate-related osteonecrosis of the jaws: first clinical results of a prospective pilot study. J Oral Maxillofac Surg. 2011;69:84–91 (with permission)*)

Studies have also shown that even one single intravenous dose of doxycycline about 1 h prior to surgery can provide clinically evident uptake and fluorescence that can prove to be useful in determining resection margins [59]. The concept of autofluorescence has also been investigated, namely, the use of a fluorescence lamp without tetracycline labeling, and has proven to potentially have some value; however no studies currently exist comparing this to tetracycline-labeled fluorescence [59].

Conclusion

Both ORN and MRONJ represent disease entities that can be difficult to manage, with some controversies among surgeons. Segmental resection with free vascularized flap reconstruction has proven to be a very successful treatment option in cases of advanced and refractory disease. Several considerations, however, must be taken into account in this cohort of patients, which can affect overall treatment results and will challenge the surgeon. Accurate diagnosis and disease delineation, intraoperative surgical considerations, and postoperative wound healing issues, disease progression, and compromise of the overall health of these patients can all lead to potential complications that must be dealt with and overcome. Nevertheless, advances in techniques, methodology, and technology have continued to provide the tools to help mitigate some of these challenges.

References

1. Nabil S, Samman N. Risk factors for osteoradionecrosis after head and neck radiation: a systematic review. Oral Surg Oral Med Oral Pathol Oral Radiol. 2012;113:54–69.
2. Studer G, Bredell M, Studer S, Huber G, Glanzmann C. Risk profile for osteoradionecrosis of the mandible in the IMRT era. Strahlenther Onkol. 2016;192:32–9.
3. Cannady SB. Free flap reconstruction for osteoradionecrosis of the jaws—outcomes and predictive factors for success. Head Neck. 2011;33(3):424–8.
4. Aldhalaan NA. Medication-related osteonecrosis of the jaw: a review. Cureus. 2020;12(2):e6944.
5. Marx RE. Pamidronate (Aredia) and Zoledronate (Zometa) induced avascular necrosis of the jaws: a growing epidemic. J Oral Maxillofac Surg. 2003;61(9):1115–7.
6. Chrcanovic BR, Reher P, Sousa AA. Osteoradionecrosis of the jaws—a current overview—Part 2: dental management and therapeutic options for treatment. J Oral Maxillofac Surg. 2010;14:81–95.
7. Foster RD, Anthony JP, Sharma A. Vascularized bone flaps versus nonvascularized bone grafts for mandibular reconstruction: an outcome analysis of primary bony union and endosseous implant success. Head Neck. 1999;21:66.
8. Pogrel MA, Podlesh S, Anthony JP. A comparison of vascularized and nonvascularized bone grafts for reconstruction of mandibular continuity defects. J Oral Maxillofac Surg. 1997;55:1200.
9. Kaleem A, Tursun R, Amailuk P. Free flap surgery in osteoradionecrosis of the head and neck. Front Oral Maxillofac Med. 2021;3:13–6.
10. Deutsch M, Kroll SS, Ainsle N. Influence of radiation on late complications in patients with free fibular flaps for mandibular reconstruction. Ann Plast Surg. 1999;42:662–4.

11. Pohlenz P, Blessmann M, Heiland M. Postoperative complications in 202 cases of microvascular head and neck reconstruction. J Craniomaxillofac Surg. 2007;35:311–5.
12. Singh B, Cordeiro PG, Santamaria E. Factors associated with complications in microvascular reconstruction of head and neck defects. Plast Reconstr Surg. 1999;103:403–11.
13. Lee M, Chin RY, Eslick GD. Outcomes of microvascular free flap reconstruction for mandibular osteoradionecrosis: a systematic review. J Craniomaxillofac Surg. 2015;43:2026–33.
14. Mijiti A, Kuerbantayi N, Zhang ZQ. Influence of preoperative radiotherapy on head and neck free-flap reconstruction: systematic review and meta-analysis. Head Neck. 2020;42:2165–80.
15. De Wilde R, Boeckx W, Van Der Schueren E. A scanning electronic microscopic study of microvascular anastomoses on irradiated vessels: short-term effects of irradiation. Microsurgery. 1983;4:193.
16. Cigna E, Cirunga C, Bistoni G, Spalvieri C, Tortorelli G, Scuderi N. Microsurgical anastomosis with the "PCA" technique. J Plast Reconstr Aesthet Surg. 2008;61:762–6.
17. Chen HC, Mardini S, Tsai FC. "Airborne" suture tying technique for the microvascular anastomosis. Plast Reconstr Surg. 2004;113:1225–8.
18. Ang E, Black C, Irish J, Brown DH, Gullane P, O'Sullivan B, Neligan PC. Reconstructive options in the treatment of osteoradionecrosis of the craniomaxillofacial skeleton. Br J Plast Surg. 2003;56:92–9.
19. Stone HB, Coleman CN, Anscher MS. Effects of radiation on normal tissue: consequences and mechanisms. Lancet Oncol. 2003;4:529–36.
20. Hanasono MM, Barnea Y, Skoracki RJ. Microvascular surgery in the previously operated and irradiated neck. Microsurgery. 2009;29(1):1–7.
21. Wang L. Quality of life in osteoradionecrosis patients after mandible primary reconstruction with free fibula flap. Oral Surg Oral Med Oral Pathol Oral Radiol Endod. 2009;108(2):162–8.
22. O'Connella JE, Browna JS, Rogersa SN. Outcomes of microvascular composite reconstruction formandibular osteoradionecrosis. Br J Oral Maxillofac Surg. 2021;59:1031–5.
23. Benatar MJ, Dassonville O, Chamorey E, Poissonnet G, Etaiche M, Pierre CS. Impact of preoperative radiotherapy on head and neck reconstruction: a report on 429 cases. J Plast Reconstr Aesthet Surg. 2013;66:478–82.
24. Nolen D, Cannady SB, Wax MK. Comparison of complications in free flap reconstruction for osteoradionecrosis in patients with or without hyperbaric oxygen therapy. Head Neck. 2014;36:1701–4.
25. Gal T, Yueh B, Futran N. Influence of prior hyperbaric oxygen therapy in complications following microvascular reconstruction for advanced osteoradionecrosis. Arch Otolaryngol Head Neck Surg. 2003;129:72–6.
26. Suh JD, Blackwell KE, Sercarz JA, Cohen M. Disease relapse after segmental resection and free flap reconstruction for mandibular osteoradionecrosis. Otolaryngol Head Neck Surg. 2010;142:586–91.
27. Marwan H, Green MJ, Tursun R, Marx RE. Recurrent malignancy in osteoradionecrosis specimen. J Oral Maxillofac Surg. 2016;74(11):2132–316.
28. Mercuri LG. Considering total temporomandibular joint replacement. Cranio. 1999;17:44–8.
29. Tang Q, Lil Y. Association between condylar position changes and functional outcomes after condylar reconstruction by free fibular flap. Clin Oral Investig. 2021;25:95–103.
30. Pautke C, Bauer F, Bissinger O. Tetracycline bone fluorescence: a valuable marker for osteonecrosis characterization and therapy. J Oral Maxillofac Surg. 2010;68:125–9.
31. Schilling C, Ahmed N, Jayaram R. Intraoperative assessment of osteoradionecrosis (ORN) affected tissue by near infrared (NIR) fluorescence imaging. Br J Oral Maxillofac Surg. 2015;53:e114.
32. Shum J, Markiewicz MR, Park E, Bui T, Lubek J, Bell RB, Dierks EJ. Low prealbumin level is a risk factor for microvascular free flap failure. J Oral Maxillofac Surg. 2014;72:169–77.
33. Klingelhoffer C, Zeman F, Meier J, Reichert TE, Ettl T. Evaluation of surgical outcome and influencing risk factors in patients with medication-related osteonecrosis of the jaws. J Craniomaxillofac Surg. 2016;44(10):1694–9.

34. Migliorati CA, Casiglia J, Epstein J, Jacobson PL. Managing the care of patients with bisphosphonate-associated osteonecrosis: an American academy of oral medicine position paper. J Am Dent Assoc. 2005;136(12):1658–68.
35. Montebugnoli L, Felicetti L, Gissi DB, Pizzigallo A. Biphosphonate-associated osteonecrosis can be controlled by nonsurgical management. Oral Surg Oral Med Oral Pathol Oral Radiol Endod. 2007;104(4):473–7.
36. van denWyngaert T, Claeys T, Huizing MT, Vermorken JB. Initial experience with conservative treatment in cancer patients with osteonecrosis of the jaw (ONJ) and predictors of outcome. Ann Oncol. 2009;20(2):331–6.
37. Lazarovici TS, Yahalom R, Taicher S, Elad S, Hardan I, Yarom N. Bisphosphonate-related osteonecrosis of the jaws: a single-center study of 101 patients. J Oral Maxillofac Surg. 2009;67:850–5.
38. Caldroney S, Ghazali N, Dyalram D, Lubek J. Surgical resection and vascularized bone reconstruction in advanced stage medication-related osteonecrosis of the jaw. J Oral Maxillofac Surg. 2017;46:871–6.
39. Marx RE, Sawatari Y, Fortin M, Broumand V. Bisphosphonate-induced exposed bone (osteonecrosis/osteopetrosis) of the jaws: risk factors, recognition, prevention, and treatment. J Oral Maxillofac Surg. 2005;63:1567–75.
40. Marx RE, Cillo JE, Ulloa JJ. Oral bisphosphonate-induced osteonecrosis: risk factors, prediction of risk using serum CTX testing, prevention, and treatment. J Oral Maxillofac Surg. 2007;65:2397–410.
41. Marx RE. Reconstruction of defects caused by bisphosphonate-induced osteonecrosis of the jaws. J Oral Maxillofac Surg. 2009;67(5):107–19.
42. Rajan P, Warner A, Quick CRG. Fibular metastasis from renal cell carcinoma masquerading as deep vein thrombosis. BJU Int. 1999;84:735–6.
43. Hsu CC, Chuang YW, Lin CY, Huang YF. Solitary fibular metastasis from lung cancer mimicking stress fracture. Clin Nucl Med. 2006;31:269–71.
44. Mundy GR. Metastases to bone: causes, consequences and therapeutic opportunities. Nat Rev Cancer. 2002;2:584–93.
45. Roodman GD. Mechanism of bone metastasis. N Engl J Med. 2004;350:1655–64.
46. Carlson ER, Fleisher KE, Ruggiero SL. Metastatic cancer identified in osteonecrosis specimens of the jaws in patients receiving intravenous bisphosphonate medications. J Oral Maxillofac Surg. 2013;71:2077–86.
47. Seth R, Futran ND, Alam DS, Knott PD. Outcomes of vascularized bone graft reconstruction of the mandible in bisphosphonate-related osteonecrosis of the jaws. Laryngoscope. 2010;120:2165–71.
48. Freiberger JJ, Padilla-Burgos R. What is the role of hyperbaric oxygen in the management of bisphosphonate-related osteonecrosis of the jaw: a randomized controlled trial of hyperbaric oxygen as an adjunct to surgery and antibiotics. J Oral Maxillofac Surg. 2012;70:1573–83.
49. Ruggiero SL, Dodson TB, Fantasia J. American association of oral and maxillofacial surgeons position paper on medication-related osteonecrosis of the jaw–2014 update. J Oral Maxillofac Surg. 2014;72:1938–56.
50. Carlson ER, Basile JD. The role of surgical resection in the management of bisphosphonate-related osteonecrosis of the jaws. J Oral Maxillofac Surg. 2009;67(5):85–95.
51. Pautke C, Otto S, Reu S, Kolk A. Bisphosphonate related osteonecrosis of the jaw—manifestation in a microvascular iliac bone flap. Oral Oncol. 2011;47:425–9.
52. Vercruysse H Jr, Backer TD, Mommaerts MY. Outcomes of osseous free flap reconstruction in stage III bisphosphonate-related osteonecrosis of the jaw: systematic review and a new case series. J Craniomaxillofac Surg. 2014;42:377–86.
53. Engroff SL, Coletti D. Bisphosphonate related osteonecrosis of the palate: report of a case managed with free tissue transfer. Oral Surg Oral Med Oral Pathol Oral Radiol Endod. 2008;105:580–2.
54. Nocini PF, Saia G, Bettini G. Vascularized fibula flap reconstruction of the mandible in bisphosphonate-related osteonecrosis. Eur J Surg Oncol. 2009;35:373–9.

55. Bedogni A, Saia G, Bettini G. Long-term outcomes of surgical resection of the jaws in cancer patients with bisphosphonate-related osteonecrosis. Oral Oncol. 2011;47:420–4.
56. Bedogni A, Saia G, Ragazzo M, et al. Bisphosphonate-associated osteonecrosis can hide jaw metastases. Bone. 2007;41:942–5.
57. Pautke C, Bauer F, Otto S. Fluorescence guided bone resection in bisphosphonate-related osteonecrosis of the jaws: first clinical results of a prospective pilot study. J Oral Maxillofac Surg. 2011;69:84–91.
58. Assaf AT, Zrnc TA, Riecke B. Intraoperative efficiency of fluorescence imaging by visually enhanced lesion scope (VELscope) in patients with bisphosphonate related osteonecrosis of the jaw (BRONJ). J Craniomaxillofac Surg. 2014;42:157–64.
59. Ristow O, Pautke C. Auto-fluorescence of the bone and its use for delineation of bone necrosis. Int J Oral Maxillofac Surg. 2014;43:1391–3.

Chapter 13
Advancements in Facial Trauma

Dina Amin and Nagi Demian

Introduction

Facial trauma reconstruction is challenging due to proximity of adjacent vital structures [1–3]. Several factors have been identified for poor outcome [4, 5], such as surgical planning on two-dimensional (2D) imaging for a three-dimensional (3D) problem, difficulty in assessing intraoperative position, projection, and symmetry of repositioned skeletal anatomy and poor visualization of deep skeletal contours involving orbit and skull base [5]. This chapter will focus on the application of recent advancements in facial trauma.

Computer-Assisted Surgical Simulation

Computer-assisted surgical simulation (CASS) offers an individualized, 3D manipulation of patient's computed tomography (CT) data [5–7]. CASS technology has been combined with patient-specific implant designing and/or surgical navigation [5–7]. Atrophic and complex mandibular fractures [8, 9], orbital fractures [7], and panfacial fractures are the most common applications of CASS [9]. CASS workflow can be divided into four phases: (1) data acquisition phase, (2) planning phase, (3) surgical phase, and (4) assessment phase (Fig. 13.1) [10].

D. Amin (✉)
Oral and Maxillofacial Surgery, University of Rochester, Rochester, NY, USA

N. Demian
Oral and Maxillofacial Surgery, University of Texas Health Science Center at Huston, Houston, TX, USA
e-mail: nagi.demian@uth.tmc.edu

© The Author(s), under exclusive license to Springer Nature Switzerland AG 2023

J. C. Melville et al. (eds.), *Advancements and Innovations in OMFS, ENT, and Facial Plastic Surgery*, https://doi.org/10.1007/978-3-031-32099-6_13

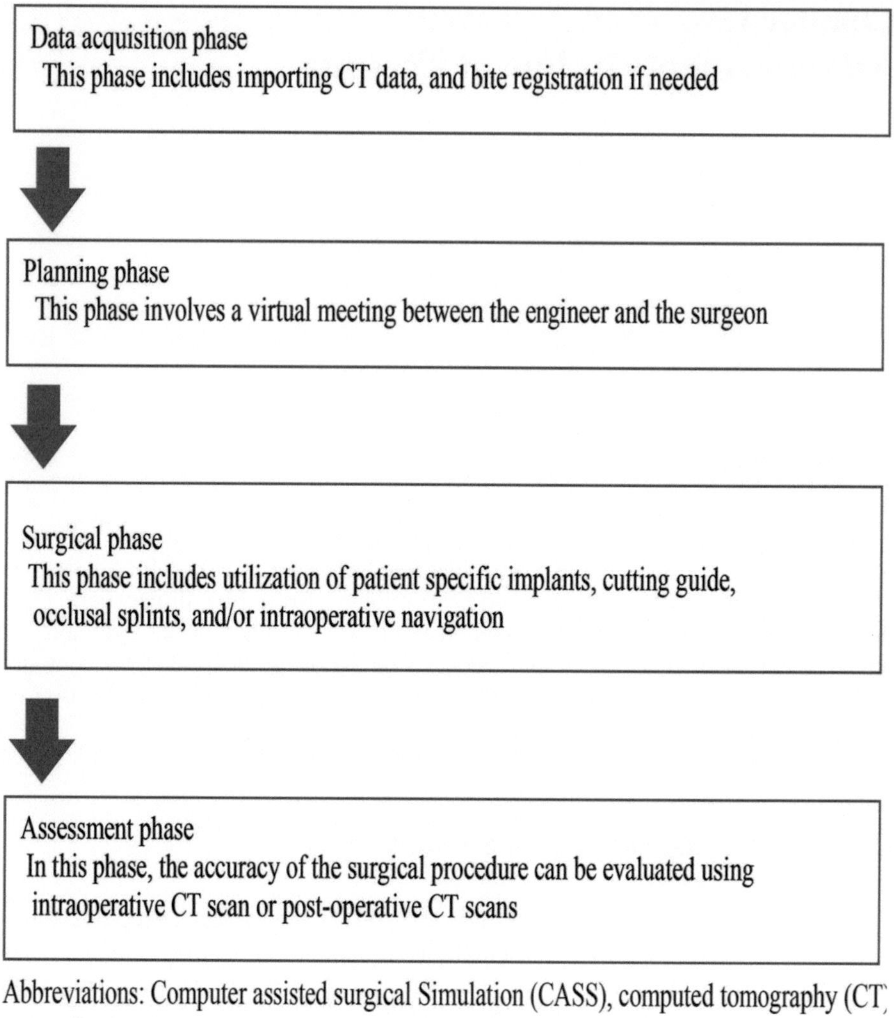

Data acquisition phase
  This phase includes importing CT data, and bite registration if needed

Planning phase
  This phase involves a virtual meeting between the engineer and the surgeon

Surgical phase
  This phase includes utilization of patient specific implants, cutting guide,
  occlusal splints, and/or intraoperative navigation

Assessment phase
  In this phase, the accuracy of the surgical procedure can be evaluated using
  intraoperative CT scan or post-operative CT scans

Abbreviations: Computer assisted surgical Simulation (CASS), computed tomography (CT)

Fig. 13.1 CASS workflow is divided into four phases

Surgical Navigation

Surgical navigation (SN) was primarily developed for neurosurgical procedures [11]. However, it has been implemented for head and neck surgery and facial fractures [12]. SN function is comparable to global positioning system (GPS) used in cars [5]. Orbital fractures, foreign body removal, and skull-base surgery are the most common applications of SN in facial trauma [13]. SN has three components: (1) localizer, an equivalent to the satellite in space; (2) surgical probe, represents the track waves emitted by GPS; and (3) CT scan dataset, an equivalent to a road map [5, 13]. NS allow precise location of an anatomic landmark with a margin of error of less than 1–2 mm. There are several types of SN systems. However, electromagnetic and optic based are the most widely used (Fig. 13.2) [5, 13].

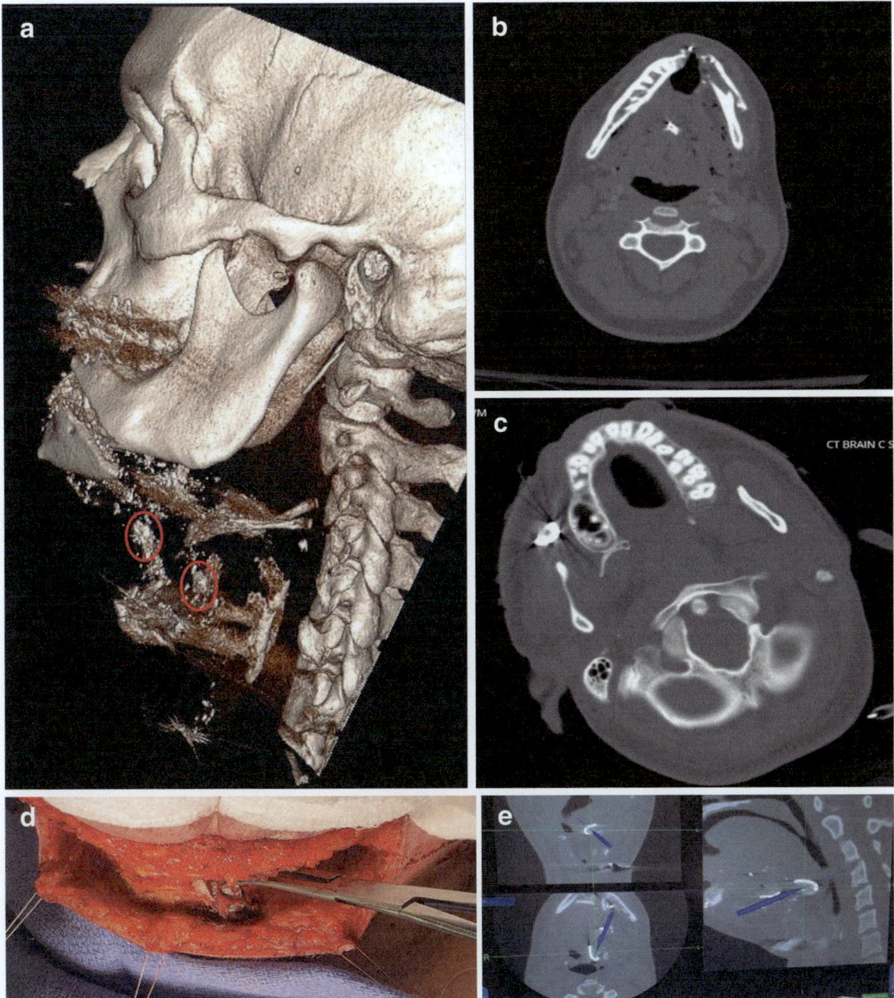

Fig. 13.2 A 25-year-old male patient sustained firearm injury (FI). FI caused comminuted symphysis and bilateral parasymphysis fractures, and four retained bullets in his neck. Lateral view (**a**) of 3D reconstruction of pre-op CT scan demonstrating mandibular fracture, track of bullet fragments extended from hyoid bone to lingual surface of mandible, and three bullets (red circles). Axial view of CT scan (**b**) showing the fourth bullet retained in the floor of the mouth. Axial view of CT scan (**c**) showing the fifth bullet retained at the level of his right maxillary sinus. Using surgical navigation, the surgeon was able to retrieve four bullets (three bullets in the neck, one in the floor of the mouth) through the transcervical approach (**d**) (yellow arrow pointing at a retrieved bullet). A screenshot of the navigation monitor showing how to locate a bullet during the procedure (**e**)

Intraoperative Computed Tomography

The use of first application of intraoperative computed tomography (ICT) was 15 years ago in management of orbitozygomatic injuries in 1999 [14]. ZMC, zygomatic arch, and orbital fractures are the most common applications. Several companies offer ICT; however the main differences between are the ability to provide an immediate 3D reconstruction of craniofacial structures and image resolution (Fig. 13.3). Several studies have shown that the use of ICT leads to accurate fracture reduction and reduces the possibility of a postoperative corrective surgery [15]. ICT can be integrated with the SN system. The main advantage is reduced take back to OR (Fig. 13.4). However, the application of ICT increases exposure to ionizing radiation, operative time, and treatment cost [16].

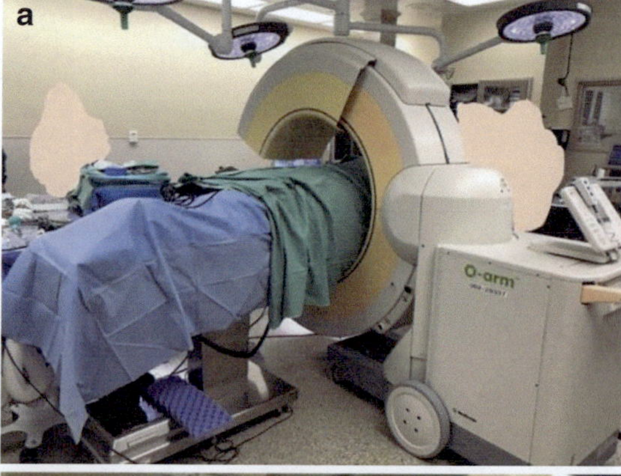
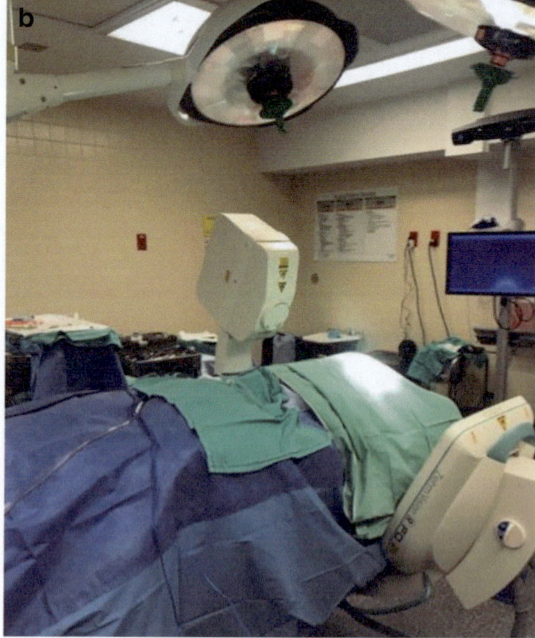

Fig. 13.3 Several companies offer intraoperative imaging systems; the main differences are radiation dose, availability of 3D reconstruction of craniofacial skeleton, and image resolution. The most used companies by authors and in the United States are the O-ARM™ (Medtronic©, Minneapolis, Minnesota) (**a**) and Ziehm Vision RFD 3D (Ziehm Imaging, Orlando, Florida) (**b**)

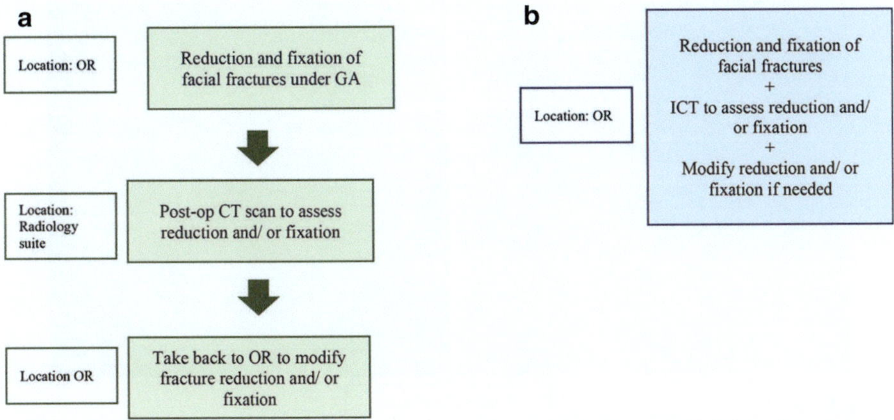

Fig. 13.4 Assessment of facial fracture reduction and/or fixation workflow, using post-op CT (**a**), using ICT (**b**). *CT* computed tomography, *GA* general anesthesia, *post-op* post-operative, *OR* operating room

Patient-Specific Implant

Advances of technology such as CASS and selective laser melting (SLM) have led to patient-specific implant (PSI) for craniomaxillofacial surgery. Several studies have shown that PSI led to decrease time to OR, intraoperative time, accurate fracture reduction, and superior outcome [17].

However, SLM technology or PSI is exceedingly expensive with long production time (7–14 days). Fracture reduction is time sensitive to prevent unfavorable long-term sequela; thus, this technology has limitation in acute setting and used in post-traumatic deformity (Fig. 13.5).

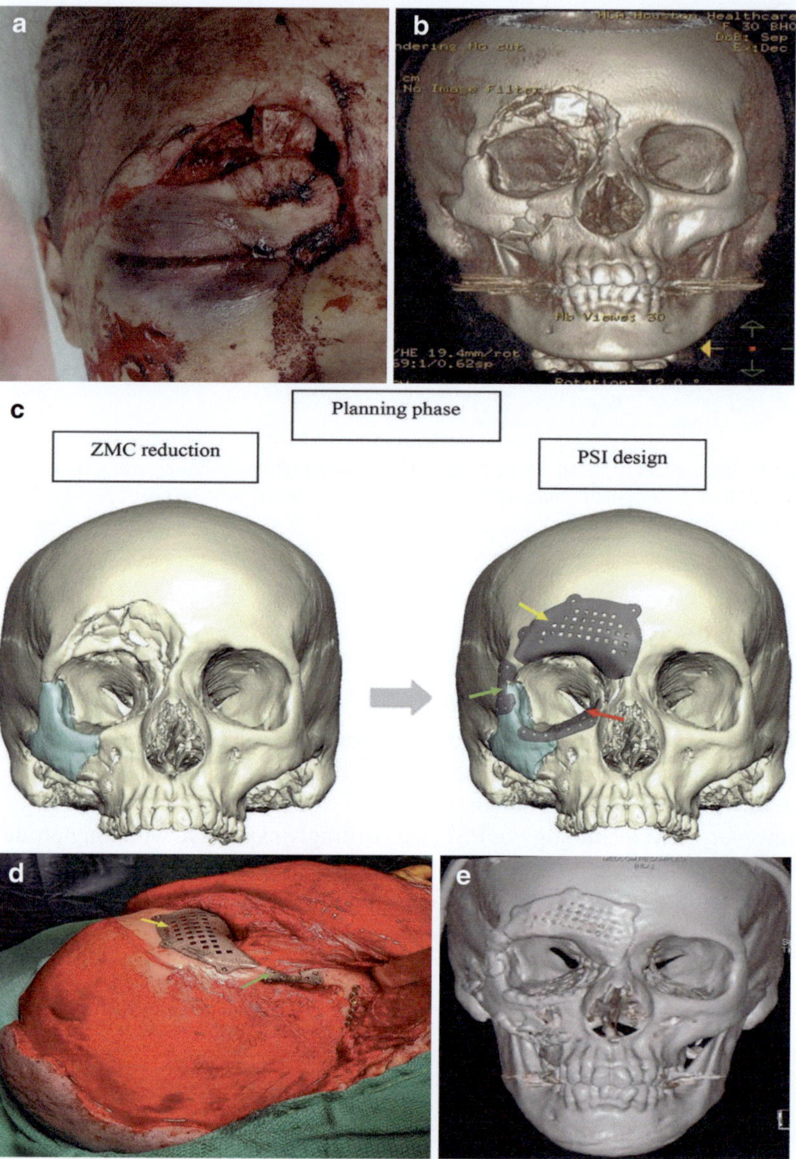

Fig. 13.5 A 35-year-old male patient sustained firearm injury (FI). FI caused right open and comminuted frontal sinus, superior orbital wall, nasoethmoidal ZMC, orbital floor, zygomatic arch fractures. Frontal view (**a**) at presentation to emergency department (ED). Frontal view of 3D reconstruction of pre-operative CT scan (**b**) showing comminuted fractures. Frontal view of a summary of CASS plan and PSI design (**c**), the right ZMC (area shaded in light blue) was reduced digitally, and three PSIs were designed to span different fractures, notice several fractures (frontal sinus, superior orbital wall, nasoethmoidal fractures) was reconstructed with one large PSI (yellow arrow), one PSI for ZMC (green arrow), and one PSI for orbital floor fracture (red arrow). Intraoperative view of two PSIs (yellow and green arrows) (**d**). Frontal view of 3D reconstruction of post-operative CT scan (**e**) showing reconstruction of the frontal sinus, superior orbital wall, nasoethmoidal, and ZMC fractures

References

1. Septa D, Newaskar VP, Agrawal D, Tibra S. Etiology, incidence and patterns of mid-face fractures and associated ocular injuries. J Maxillofac Oral Surg. 2014;13(2):115–9.
2. Lim LH, Lam LK, Moore MH, Trott JA, David DJ. Associated injuries in facial fractures: review of 839 patients. Br J Plast Surg. 1993;46(8):635–8.
3. Kieser J, Stephenson S, Liston PN, Tong DC, Langley JD. Serious facial fractures in New Zealand from 1979 to 1998. Int J Oral Maxillofac Surg. 2002;31(2):206–9.
4. Hsieh T-Y, Funamura JL, Dedhia R, Durbin-Johnson B, Dunbar C, Tollefson TT. Risk factors associated with complications after treatment of mandible fractures. JAMA Facial Plast Surg. 2019;21(3):213–20.
5. Bell RB. Computer planning and intraoperative navigation in cranio-maxillofacial surgery. Oral Maxillofac Surg Clin North Am. 2010;22(1):135–56.
6. Girod S, Keeve E, Girod B. Advances in interactive craniofacial surgery planning by 3D simulation and visualization. Int J Oral Maxillofac Surg. 1995;24(1 Pt 2):120–5.
7. Azarmehr I, Stokbro K, Bell RB, Thygesen T. Contemporary techniques in orbital reconstruction: a review of the literature and report of a case combining surgical navigation, computer-aided surgical simulation, and a patient-specific implant. J Oral Maxillofac Surg. 2020;78(4):594–609.
8. Marschall JS, Dutra V, Flint RL, et al. In-house digital workflow for the management of acute mandible fractures. J Oral Maxillofac Surg. 2019;77(10):2084.e2081–9.
9. Façanha de Carvalho E, Alkmin Paiva GL, Yonezaki F, Machado GG. Computer-aided surgical simulation in severe atrophic mandibular fractures: a new method for guided reduction and temporary stabilization before fixation. J Oral Maxillofac Surg. 2021;79(4):892.e891–7, 892.e1.
10. Markiewicz MR, Bell RB. Modern concepts in computer-assisted craniomaxillofacial reconstruction. Curr Opin Otolaryngol Head Neck Surg. 2011;19(4):295–301.
11. Mezger U, Jendrewski C, Bartels M. Navigation in surgery. Langenbecks Arch Surg. 2013;398(4):501–14.
12. Schmelzeisen R, Gellrich NC, Schramm A, Schön R, Otten JE. Navigation-guided resection of temporomandibular joint ankylosis promotes safety in skull base surgery. J Oral Maxillofac Surg. 2002;60(11):1275–83.
13. Azarmehr I, Stokbro K, Bell RB, Thygesen T. Surgical navigation: a systematic review of indications, treatments, and outcomes in oral and maxillofacial surgery. J Oral Maxillofac Surg. 2017;75(9):1987–2005.
14. Stanley RB Jr. Use of intraoperative computed tomography during repair of orbitozygomatic fractures. Arch Facial Plast Surg. 1999;1(1):19–24.
15. Alasraj A, Alasseri N, Al-Moraissi E. Does intraoperative computed tomography scanning in maxillofacial trauma surgery affect the revision rate? J Oral Maxillofac Surg. 2021;79(2):412–9.
16. Ma D, Zhang S, Pang C, Zhang W, Wang B, Liu Y. The application of intraoperative computed tomography in surgical management of temporomandibular joint ankylosis. J Oral Maxillofac Surg. 2021;79(1):90.e91–7.
17. Yang WF, Choi WS, Leung YY, et al. Three-dimensional printing of patient-specific surgical plates in head and neck reconstruction: a prospective pilot study. Oral Oncol. 2018;78:31–6.

Chapter 14
Advancements in Maxillofacial Benign Tumors and Cysts

Mari Alina Timoshchuk and Waleed Zaid

Update on World Health Organization (WHO) Odontogenic Benign Tumors and Cysts

The fifth edition of the WHO's Classification of Head and Neck Tumors was published in March 2022 [1]. Experts formulated the guidelines in the field to provide more accurate and clinically oriented classification. The main aim of these changes was to deliver a modern concise classification that properly reflects the proper entities of these lesions and reduces the need for complex molecular techniques that may not be widely available or affordable.

The 2022 fifth edition follows many of the same concepts that were introduced in the 2017 edition. In particular, the 2022 edition continues to use the odontogenic cyst classification that was introduced in the 2017 guidelines, which was previously omitted in the 2005 edition [2]. Also like the 2017 edition, the 2022 edition continued to use a simplified classification of odontogenic tumors into three main groups based on histological origin: (1) epithelial, (2) mesenchymal, and (3) mixed odontogenic tumors. Distinct from the 2017 edition update, the 2022 guidelines added

M. A. Timoshchuk
Department of Oral and Maxillofacial Surgery, School of Dentistry, Louisiana Health Sciences Center, New Orleans, LA, USA
e-mail: mtimos@lsuhsc.edu

W. Zaid (✉)
Department of Oral and Maxillofacial Surgery, School of Dentistry, Louisiana Health Sciences Center, New Orleans, LA, USA

Site Director Baton Rouge LSUHSC Oral and Maxillofacial Surgery Department, Our Lady of Lake Regional Medical Center, Baton Rouge, LA, USA
e-mail: wzaid@lsuhsc.edu

© The Author(s), under exclusive license to Springer Nature Switzerland AG 2023
J. C. Melville et al. (eds.), *Advancements and Innovations in OMFS, ENT, and Facial Plastic Surgery*, https://doi.org/10.1007/978-3-031-32099-6_14

adenoid ameloblastoma among benign epithelial odontogenic tumors and added surgical ciliated cyst to the list of jaw cysts. Additionally, the new edition text has added "essential and desirable diagnostic criteria" to simplify and emphasize key features for each pathologic entity [1].

Ameloblastoma

Odontogenic tumors (OTs) represent 2–3% of jaw lesions [3]. In the prior 2017 WHO classifications, ameloblastoma had a significant share of debate regarding its aggressive behavior. The consensus was to keep ameloblastoma as a benign epithelial odontogenic tumor despite the few reported cases of metastasizing ameloblastoma, which is defined as being ameloblastoma that is present at extraoral locations, most commonly the lungs [4, 5]. In the 2017 WHO classification, ameloblastoma was simplified to ameloblastoma, unicystic ameloblastoma, and extraosseous/peripheral ameloblastoma. The adjective "solid/multicystic" for conventional ameloblastoma was eliminated due to the lack of any biological or clinical value. Odontoameloblastoma was eliminated as it was deemed more of a descriptive term rather than having any clinical implications [1]. The 2022 WHO classifications have added adenoid ameloblastoma, which is an epithelial odontogenic neoplasm with essential diagnostic criteria that include ameloblastoma-like component, duct-like structures, whorls/morules, and a cribriform architecture. There are currently approximately 40 cases that have been reported in the literature [6]. Reports have shown locally aggressive behavior with a high recurrence rate of approximately 45.5–70% [7].

Treatment of Ameloblastoma Using Checkpoint Markers

Surgical resection with a 1 cm margin along with one added anatomical barrier is the current standard of care as more conservative approaches are linked to high recurrence rates ranging between 55% and 90% compared to 15–25% with resection [8]. Nevertheless, surgical resection is associated with a high morbidity rate without absolute elimination of the risk of recurrence. Recent in vitro studies and case reports, however, have shown that medication that targets specific genetic mutations prevalent in ameloblastomas can reduce ameloblastic cells and can potentially be used as therapeutic alternatives for patients unsuitable to undergo standard surgical resection [9]. Genetic studies show recurrent genetic mutations in the mitogen-activated protein kinase (MAPK) and sonic hedgehog (SHH) signaling pathways of ameloblastoma. Approximately 79% of ameloblastoma mutations in MAPK pathways include BRAF, RAS, and fibroblast growth factor receptor 2

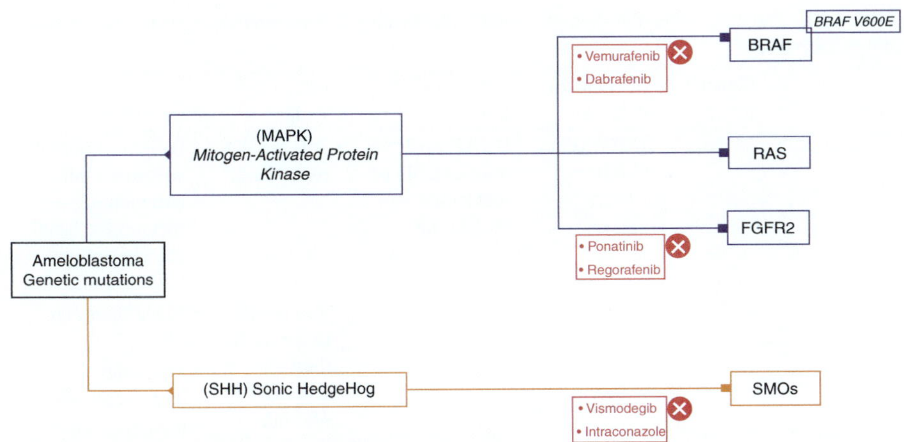

Fig. 14.1 Tumor markers and potential targeted therapies

(FGFR2) genes. Studies have found a high occurrence of BRAF V600E mutations, which involves the substitution of valine for glutamate at codon 600. Knowing the MAPK pathways activated in ameloblastomas with genetic mutations creates the potential for molecularly targeted therapies that inhibit the functions of mutated BRAF and MEK (Fig. 14.1). Potential drugs include vemurafenib and dabrafenib (inhibit mutated BRAF gene), trametinib (inhibits mutated MEK gene), and ponatinib and regorafenib (inhibit mutated FGFR2 genes). The US Food and Drug Administration (FDA) has approved the use of vemurafenib and dabrafenib for BRAF mutations and trametinib for MEK mutations [9–12]. A treatment approach has been implemented in melanoma treatment as having been proven to improve overall disease-specific survival [13].

Similar to MAPK, studies have also shown a high incidence of recurrent mutations in SMOs, a SHH pathway gene in ameloblastoma. However, SMO inhibitors, such as vismodegib and itraconazole, have not been shown to successfully treat ameloblastomas [11]. While drugs inhibiting the SHH signaling pathway are more effective in treating ameloblastomas, the most used SHH signaling pathway inhibitor, cyclopamine, can inhibit osteoblast proliferation. Thus, cyclopamine would affect bone healing and is not ideal for treating ameloblastomas [14].

The current literature on the use of medication to target specific genetic markers associated with ameloblastomas is limited to case reports and in vitro studies. Although there are more studies on the efficacy of FDA-approved medications in the treatment of melanomas, which have the same genetic mutations observed in ameloblastomas, further studies with larger sample sizes are required to determine if this approach will be widely adopted after establishing reliable long-term favorable results from using targeted molecular therapy medications in the treatment of ameloblastoma, especially with the potential side effects that might be associated with these medications (Table 14.1).

M. A. Timoshchuk and W. Zaid

Table 14.1 Targeted molecular therapy agents and currently documented dosages for the treatment of ameloblastoma

Agent	Generic name	Mechanism of action	Use	Dosage	Side effects
Vemurafenib	Zelboraf	BRAF kinase inhibitor	BRAF-positive unresectable or metastatic melanoma	• 960 mg PO twice daily	• Increased risk of squamous cell carcinoma, melanoma, basal cell carcinoma, keratoacanthomas
				• 960 mg PO twice daily, then reduced to 480 mg twice daily when side effects occurred [15, 16]	• Maculopapular rash • Follicular hyperkeratosis • Palmar-plantar erythrodysesthesia • Arthralgia • Transaminitis • QT prolongation
Dabrafenib	Tafinlar, rafinlar	BRAF kinase inhibitor	BRAF V600E mutation-positive metastatic melanoma	• 150 mg PO twice daily [17]	• New primary malignancies, increased cell proliferation in BRAF wild-type melanoma
				• 75 mg PO twice daily [18]	• Hyperkeratosis • Headache • Pyrexia • Arthralgia • Papilloma • Alopecia • Palmar-plantar erythrodysesthesia syndrome

Table 14.1   (continued)

Agent	Generic name	Mechanism of action	Use	Dosage	Side effects
Dabrafenib and trametinib (dual agent)	Tafinlar or rafinlar and mekinist	BRAF kinase inhibitor and MEK inhibitor	Unresectable or metastatic melanoma with PRAF V600E or V600K mutations	150 mg PO twice daily alongside 2 mg trametinib twice daily [19, 20]	• New primary malignancies, increased cell proliferation in BRAF wild-type melanoma
					• Major hemorrhagic events
					• Venous thromboembolism
					• Cardiomyopathy
					• Embryo-fetal toxicity, secondary skin infections hyperglycemia
					• Hemolytic anemia
					• Pyrexia
					• Chills
					• Fatigue
					• Rash
					• Nausea
					• Vomiting
					• Diarrhea
					• Abdominal pain
					• Peripheral edema
					• Cough
					• Headache
					• Arthralgia
					• Night sweats
					• Decreased appetite
					• Constipation
					• Myalgia

(continued)

Table 14.1 (continued)

Agent	Generic name	Mechanism of action	Use	Dosage	Side effects
Ponatinib	Iclusig	Multitargeted receptor tyrosine kinase inhibitor (FGFR2 gene inhibitor)	Refractory chronic myelogenous leukemia	No case studies yet	• Hypertension • Rash • Abdominal pain • Fatigue • Headache • Dry skin • Constipation • Arthralgia • Nausea • Pyrexia • Hematologic adverse reactions included thrombocytopenia, anemia, neutropenia, lymphopenia, and leukopenia
Regorafenib	Stivarga	Multi-kinase inhibitor (FGFR2 gene inhibitor)	Metastatic colorectal cancer, hepatocellular carcinoma, and gastrointestinal stromal tumors		• Severe hepatotoxicity resulting in potential liver damage • Asthenia/fatigue • HFSR • Diarrhea • Decreased appetite • Hypertension • Mucositis • Dysphonia • Infection • Pain (not otherwise specified), • Decreased weight and gastrointestinal and abdominal pain, and nausea • Rash • Fever

Odontogenic Keratocyst (OKC)

OKC arises from the cell rests of the dental lamina and represents approximately 3–20% of all odontogenic cysts of the jaw [21, 22]. It was first described by Philipsen in 1956 and was reclassified back by the WHO in 2017 as a benign cyst from a cystic neoplasm. The previously debated reason for considering it as malignancy is because of several studies that found evidence of genetic mutations. These mutations ranged between 30% in non-syndromic OKCs and 60–85% of syndromic OKCs, such as in basal cell nevus syndrome (BCNS), which have mutations in PTCH1, a marker in the SHH signaling pathway. Agaram et al. found that seven out of ten OKCs showed loss of heterozygosity in tumor suppressor genes with the most frequent allelic losses at p16, p53, PTCH, and MCC (75%, 66%, 60%, and 60%, respectively). Daughter cells were also found to contribute to a higher frequency of allelic loss [23]. Despite these mentioned factors, it was determined that this did not warrant the attachment of the tumor title to OKC [2, 24]. Regardless of nomenclature, these lesions are significant for their local aggressive growth potential, high recurrence rate, and association with syndromes such as BCNS.

PTCH1 Gene and Sonic Hedgehog Pathway

The PTCH1 gene is responsible for producing a sonic hedgehog receptor on the cell membrane called PTCH1. Normally, PTCH1 maintains smoothened, a transmembrane protein that activates GLI proteins. When SHH ligand/protein binds to PTCH1, it releases the smoothened suppression, and the activated smoothened promotes activation of transcription factors of glioma-associated oncogenes, including GLI1 [25]. GLI1 is itself a transcription factor and induces PTCH1 transcription; thus SHH signaling can create a negative feedback loop [26].

PTCH1 Mutation and BCNS

Understanding how the SHH pathway interacts with PTCH1 also sheds light on the genetic background of BCNS. BCNS is a rare autosomal-dominant condition caused by a PTCH1 mutation that releases its smoothened suppression, leading to uninhibited stimulation of the SHH. The uninhibited stimulation then leads to SHH proliferation and carcinogenesis, which explains BCNS's association with OKC and basal cell carcinomas [27]. BCNS develops through a "two-hit" mechanism. BCNS patients inherit the first "hit" when they are born with a mutation on one of the PTCH1 gene alleles, where the bulk of the mutations involve truncating the PTCH1 gene in the various germline cells. It takes, however, a second "hit" to the second and normal PTCH1 gene allele for a patient to have BCNS. This second hit may be

Table 14.2 Major and minor criteria to establish the diagnosis of BCNS based on the consensus statement from the first international colloquium on BCNS

Major criteria	Minor criteria
First degree relative with BCNS	Rib anomalies
BCC prior to 20 years old or excessive numbers of BCCs out of proportion to prior sun exposure and skin type	Skeletal malformations and radiologic changes (i.e., vertebral anomalies, kyphoscoliosis, short fourth metacarpals, and postaxial polydactyly)
Odontogenic keratocyst of the jaw prior to 20 years old	Macrocephaly
Palmar or plantar pitting	Cleft/lip palate
Lamellar calcification of the falx cerebri	Ovarian/cardiac fibroma
Medulloblastoma/neuroectodermal tumor, typically desmoplastic[a]	Lympho-mesenteric cysts
	Ocular abnormalities (i.e., strabismus, hypertelorism, congenital cataracts, glaucoma, and coloboma)

[a]This is a new major criterion that has led to the early establishment of the BCNS diagnosis as this is a finding typically diagnosed at 2 years or younger

from environmental factors such as ultraviolet light and radiation. The inherited PTCH1 mutation is transmitted as autosomal-dominant inheritance with high penetrance and inconstant expressivity leading to broad phenotypic presentation [26, 27].

Defined by Gorlin and Goltz in 1960, the classical facial features that are present in 60% of patients with BCNS include frontal bossing, macrocephaly, overall coarse facial features, and facial milia [28]. Clinical and radiographic findings are often utilized in numerous combinations as diagnostic criteria. These findings have been classified as major and minor criteria, and they are summarized in Table 14.2. The consensus from the BCNS Life Support Network suggested that a diagnosis of BCNS can be established in the following scenarios:

- The presence of one major criterion with molecular confirmation
- Two major criteria
- One major with three minor features

Despite the perception that genetic testing is the gold standard for diagnosis, it is not recommended and is rarely performed in clinical practice due to its elevated cost.

Treatment of OKC

Before diving into the treatment of OKC as surgeons, we need to understand the recurrence rate, which is reportedly between 7% and 28% after surgical treatment [29]. This recurrence rate has been attributed to various causes: the persistence of residual epithelium, the retention of daughter cysts in the walls of the original cysts or from microcysts, and the continuous intrinsic epithelial proliferation due to genetic mutation. Most recurrences occur before 5 years and decrease with time

[30, 31]. There are three primary surgical treatments employed for OKC: marsupialization and decompression, enucleation, and en bloc resection. Along with these surgical techniques, there are four main adjunct techniques to help reduce the recurrence rate and they are peripheral ostectomy, Carnoy's and modified Carnoy's solution, cryosurgery with liquid nitrogen, and 5-FU. When treatment planning a lesion that is biopsy-proven or highly suspicious for OKC, it is important to consider the timeline for dental rehabilitation. Due to the high recurrence rate of OKC, it is typically recommended to postpone reconstructive treatments until after cyst excision or a period of decompression, though there have been successful case reports of bone grafting and immediate implant placement after enucleation [32, 33]. Bone grafting has the advantage of stabilizing the blood clot, provides osteoconductive properties increasing the migration of progenitor cells, and can potentially reduce the risk of pathologic fracture. However, bone grafting can be a potential source of infection and OKCs have been shown to recur in grafted sites leading to costly and stressful re-treatment for patients [34].

In a multicenter study performed by Lim et al., 305 cysts that had undergone enucleation and simultaneous bone grafting were retrospectively investigated for factors associated with bone graft failure [35]. Bone graft failure was observed in 48 cases (15.7%) with a mean duration of surgery time to failure of 38.7 days. Graft failure was associated with younger age, smoking, preoperative infection, large cysts, impaction of the mandibular third molar in the cystic cavity, perilesional sclerosis, and the use of mixed non-autogenous and autogenous bone grafts. Similarly, Chacko et al. evaluated 44 consecutive patients with large maxillary and mandibular cysts, 20 of which were OKCs, treated with either enucleation or marsupialization with an average max lesion dimension of 58.2 mm in max dimension and follow-up of 6 months [36]. Uneventful healing and spontaneous filling of the residual cavities were obtained in all cases. Without the use of bone grafts, radiodensity of the cystic cavity recovers approximately 25% at 6 months, 58% at 9 months, 88% at 12 months, and 91–100% at 2 years [36, 37]. If bone grafting is not used, a period of 9–12 months is typically recommended depending on the original lesion size and patient factors and comorbidities before pursuing implant treatment. When considering dental rehabilitation with a lesion biopsy-proven or concerning for OKC, the patient must be informed of the risk of recurrences and weigh these with early return to function.

Marsupialization and Decompression

The concept of marsupialization and decompression was introduced by the German surgeon Partsch, who historically proposed marsupialization as a definitive treatment of cysts. Decompression involves any modality that relieves the pressure within the cyst that causes its expansion. It is alleged that cyst growth occurs from osmotic pressure and pressure resorption of the adjacent bone associated with prostaglandins and growth factors [38, 39]. The other significant advantage of marsupialization and decompression is the change in the local intracystic microenvironment by decreasing interleukin-α. Surgeons who advocate for this procedure attest to some of the benefits associated with this treatment modality, such as diminishing the cyst size and shrinking the cyst away from critical structures.

Technically, when performing a marsupialization, the surgeon needs to enter the cyst lumen and attempt to create a continuous pouch between the cyst lining and oral mucosa by suturing the cyst lining to the adjacent mucosa. The decision to marsupialize a cyst could be done during the incisional biopsy. As definitive management of OKC, marsupialization is associated with a 32.3% recurrence rate. Kolkythas et al. investigated whether decompression is associated with increased recurrence by comparing 22 patients with OKC treated either by (1) enucleation with peripheral ostectomy or resection or (2) decompression followed by enucleation and peripheral ostectomy [40]. The study found two recurrences in the decompression group compared to no recurrences in the enucleation and peripheral ostectomy group. Both recurrences, however, were themselves recurrent lesions that had previously undergone enucleation. This high recurrence rate has led clinicians to avoid marsupialization as the only surgical modality. Instead, clinicians favor combining residual cyst enucleation after the initial decompression, an approach that has reduced the recurrence rate down to 14.6% [41].

Enucleation

The definition of enucleation is to try to create a plain of separation between the cyst and the surrounding bone while preserving the surrounding osseous infrastructure. Ideally, we advocate for the cyst to be enucleated in its entirety, something that allows the pathologist to study the complete specimen. Given the lining of OKC is typically 5–6 cells thick, enucleating the cyst lining may be friable and can cause the cyst to be enucleated in pieces, especially if the cyst did not undergo previous marsupialization. Ideally, at the end of the enucleation procedure, the bone cavity should be clean from any cyst lining. The recurrence rate of enucleation alone as a surgical modality of OKC is approximately 23.1%; however, enucleation in conjunction with adjuvant therapy decreases the recurrence rate down to 11.5–17.5% [41].

En Bloc Resection

En bloc resection with or without vascularized flap reconstruction is a treatment typically reserved for cases with multiple recurrences, possibly syndromic cases, or those that have undergone malignant transformation [41, 42]. Depending on the size of the lesion, the continuity of the mandible may be preserved by performing a marginal resection. This technique results in very low recurrence rates (0–8.4%) but has a much higher patient morbidity fueling surgeons to find more conservating measures that can achieve similar recurrence outcomes [41, 43, 44]. Gosau et al. reported similar recurrence rates with enucleation with Carnoy's solution and curettage when compared to that of resection [45]. Lone et al. found a high rate of recurrence in their institution with enucleation and Carnoy's (66.6%); however, there were no recurrences in either the peripheral ostectomy with the 5-FU group or the segmental resection group [46]. Although radical resection remains the most certain option for obtaining the lowest recurrence rate compared to other modalities, it produces significant morbidity with functional and aesthetic compromises and is typically reserved for select cases.

Since the fibula free flap was introduced, the development of computer-assisted surgery has greatly increased the accuracy of mandibular reconstruction [47]. Computer-aided design and computer-aided manufacturing (CADCAM) allows surgeons to create personalized surgical devices and physical models, which greatly increases the accuracy of fibula osteotomies with respect to mandibular resections. The "Jaw in a Day" ("JIAD") technique consists of completing a virtually guided resection, a fibula reconstruction, and the insertion of an implant-retained dental prosthesis all in one operation with assistance from CADCAM technology. This technique establishes immediate restoration of form and function. The immediate fixation of the dental prosthesis also allows the patient to start dental rehabilitation in the early postoperative period. This technique will be described in greater detail in a separate chapter of this textbook.

Adjunct Therapy

This is a group of surgical steps the surgeon usually performs after the completion of the enucleation procedure, and this can be subclassified into mechanical and chemical modalities.

Peripheral Ostectomy

With this procedure, the surgeon aims to mechanically eliminate any remnants of the cyst wall or any satellite cysts by removing the bone adjacent to the cystic lining. Rotary instruments are gently applied against the cyst wall. This maneuver reduces the risk of recurrence from 23.1% to 17.5% [41, 48]. Despite the simplicity of the peripheral ostectomy maneuver, this cannot be employed in every OKC case, especially with larger cysts approaching the inferior border of the mandible or with large cysts that are prone to a pathologic fracture by just enucleation of the cyst, thin lingual cortex, or proximity to adjacent teeth.

Carnoy's Solution and Modified Carnoy's Solution

Carnoy's solution was proposed by Cutler and Zollinger back in 1933 as a fixative solution, hemostatic agent, and sclerosing agent, for the treatment of cervical cysts and fistulas in general surgery literature. Voorsmit was the first to describe the use of Carnoy's solution as an adjunct therapy in the management of OKC. The solution was a mixture of 6 mL of 100% alcohol/ethanol that allowed hardening of the tissue by the shrinking process, 3 mL of chloroform to increase the fixation speed, 1 mL of glacial acetic acid that led to tissue swelling to prevent over-hardening of the tissues, and 1 g of ferric chloride that helped with dehydration. The time-dependent penetration of Carnoy's solution was a double-edged sword: it penetrated the bone adjacent to the enucleated cyst allowing fixation of OKC remnant lining or daughter cysts, but it also possessed a risk of nerve injury, approximately 55% [46]. The recommended application time of Carnoy's solution was between 3 and 5 min. It is expected that with a 5-min application cycle of Carnoy's solution, there will be nerve penetration of 0.15 mm, 0.51 mm mucosal penetration, and approximately 1.54 mm bony penetration [49–51]. With all these properties, Carnoy's solution has proven to be a successful adjunct modality to decrease the recurrence rate of OKC between 4.5% and 11.5% [41, 52]. In 2013, the FDA Compliance Policy Guide prohibited the use of chloroform as it was proven to be carcinogenic and a reproductive toxic agent that led to the abandoning of classical Carnoy's solution that contained chloroform. This development pushed surgeons to explore the use of modified Carnoy's solution, which did not contain chloroform. When compared to classical Carnoy's solution, modified Carnoy's solution only decreased the recurrence rate of OKC to 35–45% [31]. Donnelly et al. found a similar recurrence rate reduction between classical and modified Carnoy's solution. It should be noted, however, that the group performed extractions of any necessary teeth, enucleation, peripheral ostectomy, and a 3-min application of either classical or modified Carnoy's solution when showing a comparable recurrence rate of 14% [53].

Cryosurgery Using Liquid Nitrogen

Cryosurgery affects the cellular organic component of the contacted bone while maintaining the inorganic osseous framework [54]. Cryosurgery is usually effective when the temperature is below -20°C as this leads to the formation of ice crystals, which cause damage to the intracellular and extracellular components, osmotic disturbance, and electrolyte imbalance. Cryosurgery is useful after conventional enucleation is performed and then the treatment is applied to the surrounding bony bed [55, 56]. It is expected that 1 min of cryosurgery results in approximately 1–3 mm of penetration necrosis. Cryosurgery might be associated with normal local surgical bed complications like wound dehiscence, swelling, pain, local infection, and even weakening bone, which may result in pathologic fractures [31, 56].

Bell and Derick described their cryosurgery technique as follows: after meticulous enucleation with peripheral ostectomy, the osseous bed of the OKC is isolated. Next, malleable retractors are positioned and sponges of gauze are used to insulate the soft tissues from the bony bed. Finally, with the use of the ladle and funnel, the liquid nitrogen is carefully transported to the OKC osseous bed, and a recommended three rounds of freeze-thaw are performed [55]. Cryotherapy has a higher recurrence rate than Carnoy's solution, approximately 30%, but that is followed by a steep negative gradient over time; this same trend is observed with modified Carnoy's [31, 56].

5-FU

5-FU is a chemotherapy agent classified under the antimetabolic class that was first formulated by Heidelberger, Pleven, and Duschinsky in 1957 [31, 57]. 5-FU has various mechanisms of action: first by inhibiting the enzyme thymidylate synthase and second by misincorporation of fluorinated nucleoside into both RNA and DNA instead of uracil. Inflamed OKCs are associated with low thymidylate synthase and high thymidine phosphorylase and therefore may benefit more from 5-FU application than non-inflamed OKCs [58, 59]. Additionally, 5-FU induces cell apoptosis by downregulating the SHH pathway and SMO inhibition [60]. As discussed above, the SHH signaling pathway dysregulation has been identified as the driving factor for the development of multiple basal cell carcinomas in syndromic and non-syndromic OKCs, and its treatment as a topical application for basal cell carcinoma is well established. Clinically, 5% 5-FU is used by coating a ribbon gauze and placing it in the cystic cavity after enucleation to be removed 24 h postoperatively. The advantage of using the topical form is avoiding the side effects associated with systemic use of 5-FU such as mucositis, nausea, pancytopenia, cardiac toxicity, neuropathy, and death. The main contraindication for using any form of 5-FU is dihydropyrimidine dehydrogenase (DPD) deficiency, which is the initial and rate-limiting enzyme in the catabolism of 5-FU, thus placing patients at high risk for developing severe 5-FU-associated toxicity. DPD deficiency is seen in approximately 3–5% of the general population and up to three times higher in the African-American female population, though how this translates to topical application as seen with OKC treatment is still unknown [61].

In a retrospective review conducted by Caminiti et al., 34 patients were treated with 5% topical 5-FU compared to 36 managed with modified Carnoy's solution after enucleation and peripheral ostectomy. The median follow-up time was 22 months in the 5-FU group and 27 months in modified Carnoy's group. No recurrences were identified in the 5-FU group compared to nine recurrences in modified Carnoy's solution cohort. There were no differences in the incidence of permanent nerve paresthesia between groups [62].

5-FU has been shown to be safe around vital structures. Five percent 5-FU application twice weekly for 1 month after medial maxillectomy and sphenoethmoidectomy showed no adverse effects on the infraorbital nerve or sinus mucosa [63, 64]. Lone et al. compared 9 patients treated with enucleation and modified Carnoy's solution and 11 with enucleation, peripheral ostectomy, and 5-FU with an average follow-up of 3.5 years. Five percent 5-FU application was associated with 9% temporary paresthesia and 0 recurrences compared to modified Carnoy's solution, which had 44% temporary paresthesia, 11% permanent paresthesia, and a 66.6% recurrence rate. Both 5-FU and modified Carnoy's solution were not associated with any function or cosmetic adverse events [46]. While mucosal absorption rates of 5% 5-FU are currently unclear, 20 mg/kg is the reported threshold for toxicity development providing a wide safety profile with the average 70 kg patient requiring 1400 mg of 5-FU to develop toxicity [31, 65].

In the authors' experiences, 5-FU is often more accessible than modified Carnoy's solution and technically simpler than cryotherapy allowing for reduced operating time. For biopsy-proven OKCs at our institution, patients are treated with a combination of enucleation +/− peripheral ostectomy and topical 5-FU application. During the treatment planning appointment, a script for 5% fluorouracil (Efudex) cream is provided and the patient presents to their surgery date with their prescription. Enucleation of the cyst in its entirety is performed along with concomitant through peripheral ostectomy and then non-compressed Gelfoam impregnated with 5% 5-FU is packed in the surgical bed and excess 5-FU is removed and closure is performed in the standard fashion (Fig. 14.2). This technique eliminates the need to

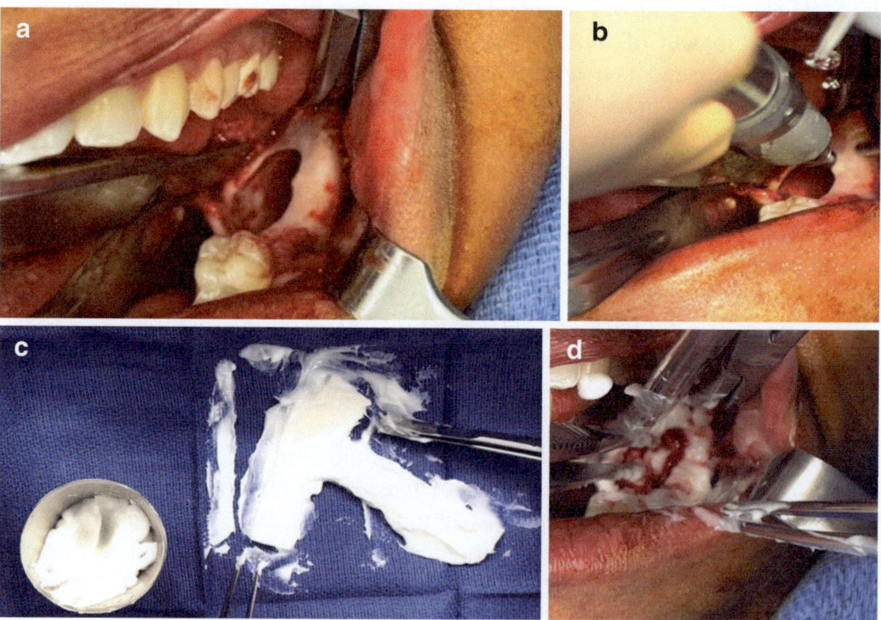

Fig. 14.2 Description of the LSU 5-FU application technique. (**a**) Mandibular OKC post-enucleation. (**b**) Peripheral ostectomy. (**c**) Non-compressed Gelfoam impregnated with 5% 5-FU. (**d**) Packing the cyst bed with Gelfoam impregnated with 5% 5-FU

remove the impregnated ¼-in. gauze with 5-FU 24 h after the original application of the technique that was described by Caminiti et al. [62].

While studies are few, they are promising showing decreased morbidity and recurrence compared to modified Carnoy's solution. Despite promising initial data, there is currently an insufficient quantity and follow-up to determine long-term recurrence rates and efficacy to make definitive conclusions regarding the effectiveness of this technique and the most appropriate protocol for its use in OKC management.

References

1. Soluk-tekkesin M, Wright JM. The world health organization classification of odontogenic lesions: a summary of the changes of the 2022 (5th) edition. Turk J Pathol. 2022;38:168–84.
2. Wright JM, Vered M. Update from the 4th edition of the World Health Organization Classification of head and neck tumours: odontogenic and maxillofacial bone tumors. Head Neck Pathol. 2017;11:68–77.
3. Philipsen HP, Reichart PA, Nikai H, Takata T, Kudo Y. Peripheral ameloblastoma: biological profile based on 160 cases from the literature. Oral Oncol. 2001;37:17–27.
4. Dissanayake RKG, Jayasooriya PR, Siriwardena DJL, Tilakaratne WM. Review of metastasizing (malignant) ameloblastoma (METAM): pattern of metastasis and treatment. Oral Surg Oral Med Oral Pathol Oral Radiol Endod. 2011;111:734–41.
5. Allen ECM, Henderson JM, Sonnet JR, Schlesinger C, Ord RA. Pulmonary metastasis of ameloblastoma: case report and review of the literature. Oral Surg Oral Med Oral Pathol Oral Radiol Endod. 2013;88:170–6.
6. Jayasooriya PR, Abeyasinghe WAMUL, Liyanage RLPR, Uthpali GN, Tilakaratne WM. Diagnostic enigma of adenoid ameloblastoma: literature review based evidence to consider it as a new sub type of ameloblastoma. Head Neck. Pathology. 2022;16:344–52.
7. Adorno-Farias D, et al. Ameloblastoma with adenoid features: a series of eight cases. Acta Histochem. 2018;120:468–76.
8. Almeida RAC, Andrade ESS, Barbalho JC, Vajgel A, Vasconcelos BCE. Recurrence rate following treatment for primary multicystic ameloblastoma: systematic review and meta-analysis. Int J Oral Maxillofac Surg. 2016;45:359–67.
9. Brown NA, et al. Activating FGFR2–RAS–BRAF mutations in ameloblastoma. Clin Cancer Res. 2014;20:5517–26.
10. Cha YH, et al. Frequent oncogenic BRAF V600E mutation in odontogenic keratocyst. Oral Oncol. 2017;74:62–7.
11. Sweeney RT, et al. Identification of recurrent SMO and BRAF mutations in ameloblastomas. Nat Genet. 2014;46:722–5.
12. Kurppa KJ, et al. High frequency of BRAF V600E mutations in ameloblastoma. J Pathol. 2014;232:492–8.
13. Flaherty KT, et al. Inhibition of mutated, activated BRAF in metastatic melanoma. New Engl J Med. 2010;363:809–19.
14. Shi HA, Ng CWB, Kwa CT, Sim QXC. Ameloblastoma: a succinct review of the classification, genetic understanding and novel molecular targeted therapies. Surgery. 2020;19:238–43.
15. Fernandes GS, Girardi DM, Bernardes JPG, Fonseca FP, Fregnani ER. Clinical benefit and radiological response with BRAF inhibitor in a patient with recurrent ameloblastoma harboring V600E mutation. BMC Cancer. 2018;18:887.
16. Broudic-Guibert M, et al. Persistent response to vemurafenib in metastatic ameloblastoma with BRAF mutation: a case report. J Med Case Rep. 2019;13:245.

17. Tan S, Pollack JR, Kaplan MJ, Colevas AD, West RB. BRAF inhibitor treatment of primary BRAF-mutant ameloblastoma with pathologic assessment of response. Oral Surg Oral Med Oral Pathol Oral Radiol. 2016;122:e5–7.
18. Faden DL, Algazi A. Durable treatment of ameloblastoma with single agent BRAFi Re: clinical and radiographic response with combined BRAF-targeted therapy in stage 4 ameloblastoma. J Natl Cancer Inst. 2017;109:djw190.
19. Kaye FJ, Ivey AM, Drane WE, Mendenhall WM, Allan RW. Clinical and radiographic response with combined BRAF-targeted therapy in stage 4 ameloblastoma. J Natl Cancer Inst. 2015;107:dju378.
20. Brunet M, Khalifa E, Italiano A. Enabling precision medicine for rare head and neck tumors: the example of BRAF/MEK targeting in patients with metastatic ameloblastoma. Front Oncol. 2019;9:1204.
21. Neville BW, Chi AC, Damm DD, Allen CM. Oral and maxillofacial pathology. Amsterdam: Elsevier Health Sciences; 2015. https://doi.org/10.1016/b978-1-4557-7052-6.00022-0.
22. Gaitán-Cepeda L, Quezada-Rivera D, Tenorio-Rocha F, Leyva-Huerta E. Reclassification of odontogenic keratocyst as tumour. Impact on the odontogenic tumours prevalence. Oral Dis. 2010;16:185–7.
23. Agaram NP, et al. Molecular analysis to demonstrate that odontogenic keratocysts are neoplastic. Arch Pathol Lab Med. 2004;128:313–7.
24. Bree AF, Shah MR, Group BC. Consensus statement from the first international colloquium on basal cell nevus syndrome (BCNS). Am J Med Genet A. 2011;155:2091–7.
25. Zwaan SED, Haass NK. Genetics of basal cell carcinoma: basal cell carcinoma genetics. Austr J Dermatol. 2009;51:81–92.
26. Lam C, Ou JC, Billingsley EM. "PTCH"-ing it together: a basal cell nevus syndrome review. Dermatol Surg. 2013;39:1557–72.
27. Bresler SC, Padwa BL, Granter SR. Nevoid basal cell carcinoma syndrome (Gorlin Syndrome). Head Neck Pathol. 2016;10:119–24.
28. Gorlin RJ, Goltz RW. Multiple nevoid basal-cell epithelioma, jaw cysts and bifid rib — a syndrome. New Engl J Med. 1960;262:908–12.
29. Antonoglou GN, Sándor GK, Koidou VP, Papageorgiou SN. Non-syndromic and syndromic keratocystic odontogenic tumors: systematic review and meta-analysis of recurrences. J Cranio-Maxillofac Surg. 2014;42:e364–71.
30. Fidele N-B, et al. Recurrence of odontogenic keratocysts and possible prognostic factors: review of 455 patients. Med Oral Patol Oral Y Cirug Bucal. 2019;24:e491–501.
31. Tay ZW, Sue WL, Leeson RMA. Chemical adjuncts and cryotherapy in the management of odontogenic keratocysts: a systematic review. Adv Oral Maxillofac Surg. 2021;3:100116.
32. Isler SC, Demircan S, Can T, Cebi Z, Baca E. Immediate implants after enucleation of an odontogenic keratocyst: an early return to function. J Oral Implantol. 2012;38:485–8.
33. Silva AGD, Alves M, Amorim M. Immediate implant following odontogenic keratocyst enucleation – clinical case. Clin Oral Implants Res. 2019;30:395.
34. Ogunsalu C, et al. Odontogenic keratocyst in Jamaica: a review of five new cases and five instances of recurrence together with comparative analyses of four treatment modalities. West Indian Med J. 2007;56:90–5.
35. Lim H-K, Kim J-W, Lee U-L, Kim J-W, Lee H. Risk factor analysis of graft failure with concomitant cyst enucleation of the jaw bone: a retrospective multicenter study. J Oral Maxillofac Surg. 2017;75:1668–78.
36. Chacko R, Kumar S, Paul A, Arvind. Spontaneous bone regeneration after enucleation of large jaw cysts: a digital radiographic analysis of 44 consecutive cases. J Clin Diagn Res. 2015;9:ZC84-9.
37. Chiapasco M, Rossi A, Motta JJ, Crescentini M. Spontaneous bone regeneration after enucleation of large mandibular cysts: a radiographic computed analysis of 27 consecutive cases. J Oral Maxillofac Surg. 2000;58:942–8.

38. Pogrel MA. Decompression and marsupialization as a treatment for the odontogenic keratocyst. Oral Maxillofac Surg Clin. 2003;15:415–27.
39. Harris M. Odontogenic cyst growth and prostaglandin-induced bone resorption. Ann R Coll Surg. 1978;60:85–91.
40. Kolokythas A, Fernandes RP, Pazoki A, Ord RA. Odontogenic keratocyst: to decompress or not to decompress? A comparative study of decompression and enucleation versus resection/peripheral ostectomy. J Oral Maxillofac Surg. 2007;65:640–4.
41. Al-Moraissi EA, et al. What surgical treatment has the lowest recurrence rate following the management of keratocystic odontogenic tumor?: a large systematic review and meta-analysis. J Cranio-Maxillofac Surg. 2017;45:131–44.
42. Zaid WY, Alshehry S, Zakhary G, Yampolsky A, Kim B. Use of vascularized myo-osseous fibula free flap to reconstruct a hemimandibular defect with a concomitant skull defect arising from stock condylar prosthesis displacement into the middle cranial fossa. J Oral Maxillofac Surg. 2019;77(1316):e1–1316.e12.
43. Kaczmarzyk T, Mojsa I, Stypulkowska J. A systematic review of the recurrence rate for keratocystic odontogenic tumour in relation to treatment modalities. Int J Oral Maxillofac Surg. 2012;41:756–67.
44. Chrcanovic BR, Gomez RS. Recurrence probability for keratocystic odontogenic tumors: an analysis of 6427 cases. J Cranio-Maxillofac Surg. 2017;45:244–51.
45. Gosau M, et al. Two modifications in the treatment of keratocystic odontogenic tumors (KCOT) and the use of Carnoy's solution (CS)—a retrospective study lasting between 2 and 10 years. Clin Oral Investig. 2010;14:27–34.
46. Lone PA, Wani NA, Janbaz ZA, Bibi M, Kour A. Topical 5-fluorouracil application in management of odontogenic keratocysts. J Oral Biol Craniofac Res. 2020;10:404–6.
47. Levine JP, et al. Jaw in a day: total maxillofacial reconstruction using digital technology. Plast Reconstr Surg. 2013;131:1386–91.
48. Cassoni A, et al. Keratocystic odontogenic tumor surgical management: retrospective analysis on 77 patients. Eur J Inflamm. 2013;12:209–15.
49. Voorsmit RACA, Stoelinga PJW, van Haelst UJGM. The management of keratocysts. J Maxillofac Surg. 1981;9:228–36.
50. Lal B, et al. Role of Carnoy's solution as treatment adjunct in jaw lesions other than odontogenic keratocyst: a systematic review. Br J Oral Maxillofac Surg. 2021;59:729–41.
51. Cutler EC, Zollinger R. The use of sclerosing solutions in the treatment of cysts and fistulae. Am J Surg. 1933;19:411–8.
52. Dashow JE, et al. Significantly decreased recurrence rates in keratocystic odontogenic tumor with simple enucleation and curettage using Carnoy's versus modified Carnoy's solution. J Oral Maxillofac Surg. 2015;73:2132–5.
53. Donnelly LA, et al. Modified Carnoy's compared to Carnoy's solution is equally effective in preventing recurrence of odontogenic keratocysts. J Oral Maxillofac Surg. 2021;79:1874–81.
54. Bradley PF, Fisher AD. The cryosurgery of bone. An experimental and clinical assessment. Br J Oral Surg. 1975;13:111–27.
55. Bell RB, Dierks EJ. Treatment options for the recurrent odontogenic keratocyst. Oral Maxillofac Surg Clin N Am. 2003;15:429–46.
56. Schmidt BL, Pogrel MA. The use of enucleation and liquid nitrogen cryotherapy in the management of odontogenic keratocysts. J Oral Maxillofac Surg. 2001;59:720–5.
57. Duschinsky R, Pleven E, Heidelberger C. The synthesis of 5-fluoropyrimidines. J Am Chem Soc. 1957;79:4559–60.
58. Ledderhof NJ, Caminiti MF, Bradley G, Lam DK. Topical 5-fluorouracil is a novel targeted therapy for the keratocystic odontogenic tumor. J Oral Maxillofac Surg. 2017;75:514–24.
59. Leichman CG, et al. Quantitation of intratumoral thymidylate synthase expression predicts for disseminated colorectal cancer response and resistance to protracted-infusion fluorouracil and weekly leucovorin. J Clin Oncol. 1997;15:3223–9.

60. Wang Q, et al. Down-regulation of Sonic hedgehog signaling pathway activity is involved in 5-fluorouracil-induced apoptosis and motility inhibition in Hep3B cells. Acta Biochim Biophys Sin. 2008;40:819–29.
61. Mattison LK, et al. Increased prevalence of dihydropyrimidine dehydrogenase deficiency in African-Americans compared with Caucasians. Clin Cancer Res. 2006;12:5491–5.
62. Caminiti MF, El-Rabbany M, Jeon J, Bradley G. 5-Fluorouracil is associated with a decreased recurrence risk in odontogenic keratocyst management: a retrospective cohort study. J Oral Maxillofac Surg. 2021;79:814–21.
63. Knegt PP, Ah-See KW, Velden L-AVD, Kerrebijn J. Adenocarcinoma of the ethmoidal sinus complex: surgical debulking and topical fluorouracil may be the optimal treatment. Arch Otolaryngol Head Neck Surg. 2001;127:141–6.
64. Mackie S, Malik T, Khalil H. Endoscopic resection and topical 5-fluorouracil as an alternative treatment to craniofacial resection for the management of primary intestinal-type sinonasal adenocarcinoma. Minim Invasive Surg. 2010;2010:750253.
65. Prado CMM, et al. Body composition as an independent determinant of 5-fluorouracil–based chemotherapy toxicity. Clin Cancer Res. 2007;13:3264–8.

Chapter 15
Update and Advancements in Facial Plastics

Parul Sinha, Brian H. Cameron, and Tang Ho

Introduction

The field of facial plastic and reconstructive surgery is witnessing a myriad of technological advances in both surgical and nonsurgical techniques. This chapter aims to provide an overview of the recent innovations and practice trends for different procedures within the facial plastic and reconstructive surgery specialty that aim to improve care, quality of life, and patient satisfaction.

P. Sinha
Division of Facial Plastic and Reconstructive Surgery, Department of Otorhinolaryngology Head and Neck Surgery, University of Texas Health Science Center in Houston, Houston, TX, USA
e-mail: Parul.Sinha@uth.tmc.edu

B. H. Cameron
Department of Otorhinolaryngology-Head and Neck Surgery, University of Texas Health Science Center in Houston, McGovern Medical School, Houston, TX, USA
e-mail: Brian.H.Cameron@uth.tmc.edu

T. Ho (✉)
Department of Otorhinolaryngology-Head and Neck Surgery, University of Texas Health Science Center in Houston, McGovern Medical School, Houston, TX, USA

Division of Facial Plastic and Reconstructive Surgery, Department of Otorhinolaryngology Head and Neck Surgery, University of Texas Health Science Center in Houston, Houston, TX, USA
e-mail: Tang.Ho@uth.tmc.edu

© The Author(s), under exclusive license to Springer Nature Switzerland AG 2023
J. C. Melville et al. (eds.), *Advancements and Innovations in OMFS, ENT, and Facial Plastic Surgery*, https://doi.org/10.1007/978-3-031-32099-6_15

Rhinoplasty and Nasoseptal Reconstruction

Surgical rhinoplasty has remained as the preferred technique for improving nasal form and function. However, nonsurgical rhinoplasty is gaining popularity for certain indications. Nonsurgical rhinoplasty allows facial plastic surgeons to address selected nasal deformities in a relatively safe, less invasive manner in an office setting and allows for a faster recovery time [1]. The indications include camouflaging of the dorsal and nasal side wall imperfections, alteration of the nasal tip projection or rotation, elongation of nasal length, augmentation of a deep radix (Fig. 15.1), lowering of alar rims for retraction, or correction of minor contour imperfections following a previous rhinoplasty [2, 3]. The procedure is most commonly performed with synthetic dermal fillers such as hyaluronic acid. Autologous materials such as fat, cartilage, and platelet-rich fibrin have also been used for augmentation of the nasal soft tissue envelope [4]. Other nonsurgical rhinoplasty techniques use botulinum toxin either alone or in combination with filler injection to correct certain nasal aesthetic deformities. It is used to target muscles at the base and sides of the nose,

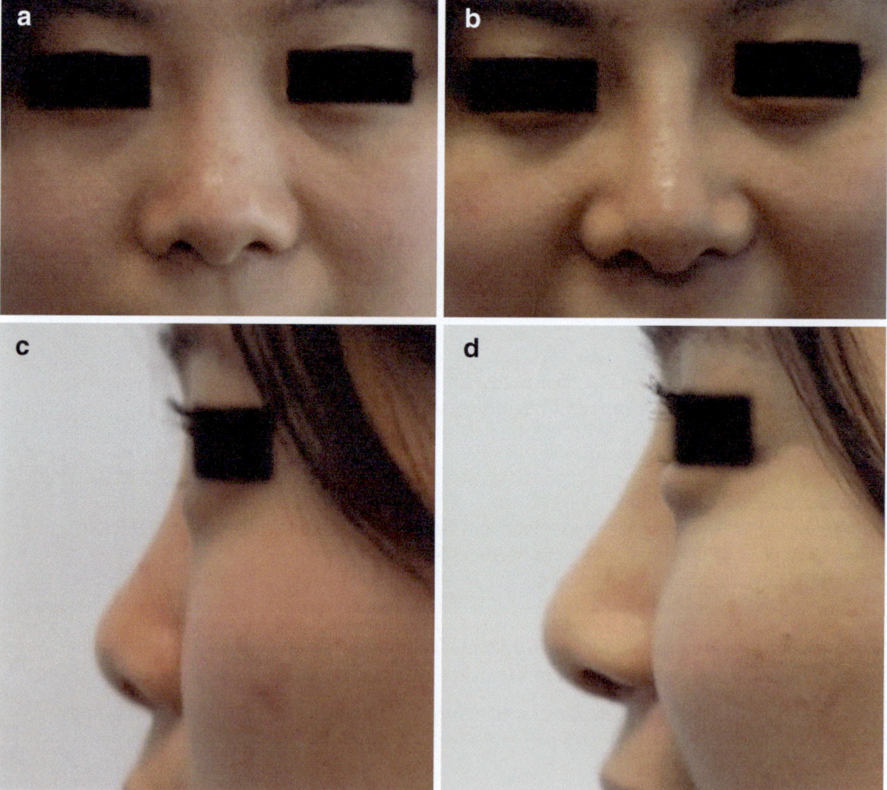

Fig. 15.1 Nonsurgical rhinoplasty for dorsal augmentation of a deep radix using hyaluronic acid fillers in a 20-year-old female. Frontal view, (**a**) pre-injection, (**b**) post-injection. Left profile view, (**c**) pre-injection, (**d**) post-injection

mainly depressor nasi septi and levator labii superioris alaeque nasi, to improve undesirable ala or upper lip appearances, that sometimes are more noticeable with smile or articulation. Overactivity of the paired depressor nasi septi muscles at the nasal base can cause rotation and the drooping of the nasal tip, while that of levator labii superioris alaeque nasi can cause tip rotation and upper lip elevation. By reducing overactivity of these muscles, botox injections can improve the nasal tip projection in patients with tip ptosis [5] and improve the upper lip appearance in patients with excess dental show. Caution is recommended with injection of the levator labii superioris alaeque nasi in older patients as it can cause droopiness of the upper lip ptosis further increasing the upper lip length.

In addition to nasal aesthetics, nonsurgical rhinoplasty technique also finds application in improving nasal function [3]. Intranasal placement of fillers at the internal nasal valve or scroll area has been described as a nonsurgical technique to correct nasal valve collapse and improve nasal airflow. External placement at the nasal sidewalls is also reported to improve nasal breathing by reducing dynamic collapse of the nose. Similar to surgical rhinoplasty however, it is critical to discuss and set realistic patient expectations and increased infection risk. Vascular necrosis is one of the notable complications about which patients should always be counseled in addition to the need of revision and repeated procedures. Overall, good patient satisfaction scores have been demonstrated with the nonsurgical rhinoplasty techniques, but long-term results are lacking [5].

The field of rhinoplasty is currently also seeing a re-emergence of the structural preservation concept, originally described in the beginning of the twentieth century, mainly for managing deformities of the nasal dorsum and the tip. The basic principles of preservation rhinoplasty advocate to elevate the nasal soft tissue envelope in a subperichondrial–subperiosteal dissection with preservation of the nasal ligaments, minimize cartilage resection through reorientation, and maintain the patient's natural dorsum contours. When applied to dorsal hump deformities, the term "dorsal preservation rhinoplasty (DPR)" is used. The DPR technique includes preservation of the bony-cartilaginous dorsum without interrupting the osseocartilaginous interface. In contrast to the conventional dorsal hump takedown with an osteotome or a rasp, DPR emphasizes preservation of the dorsal configuration of the upper lateral cartilage with its attachments. Application of the DPR technique is considered to preserve the nasal bridge, avoid creation of an open roof deformity, and minimize time and effort to reconstruct the middle vault following hump reduction [6]. Two methods, the "let down" and the "push down," are described to address the bony vault in dorsal preservation. The "let down" technique involves removal of a bony strip at the nasofacial groove, and the "push down" involves sagittal osteotomies to overlap the bones. Transverse and radix osteotomies are used to mobilize the nasal pyramid. Due to the need for precise alteration of the osseocartilaginous vault without disruption of the keystone area, adoption of newer instrumentation using ultrasonic piezo technology in combination with the DPR is another of the recent trends. The piezoelectric instrument is used both to make precise osteotomies and septal cartilage resection and to drill controlled holes for suture stabilization between the bony dorsum and septum [7]. The potential complications of DPR include residual/recurrent hump, saddling of the nasal dorsum, bony pyramid asymmetries, cerebrospinal fluid leak, and radix step-off. Patient selection is key to the use of this technique and conventional methods are still recommended for patients with wide dorsum, low radix, and severely deviated dorsum along with underlying septal deformity [6]. Knowledge of the preservation rhinoplasty techniques is a desirable element in the armamentarium of a rhinoplasty surgeon who can combine it with the concepts of structural grafting to obtain the most favorable and long-lasting aesthetic and functional outcomes while optimally maintaining integrity of patient's native tissue structure.

Upper Lip Lift

The shape, projection, and volume of upper lip are important features of the facial aesthetics and symmetry and, thus, central to perception of youth and beauty. Aging results in relative elongation of the philtrum and inversion of vermilion with atrophy of the red lip. Wider and fuller lips in relation to the facial width with a slightly convex profile and greater vermilion height are desirable upper lip attributes in females [8]. Due to its age- and gender-specific features, the upper lip lift has gained popularity as a component of both facial rejuvenation and facial feminization processes. Nonsurgical upper lip augmentation to improve structure and volume is achieved with injectable hyaluronic acid fillers of smooth consistency. It allows for immediate outcomes, no scarring, no need of postoperative recovery, and reversibility. However, the effects usually last for 6–8 months and repetitive sessions are required. The risks of nonsurgical augmentation include the adverse effects from fillers such as asymmetry, bruising, swelling, herpes simplex virus infections, and the rare event of vascular compromise that should be promptly recognized and managed. Surgical upper lip augmentation involves two methods, lip implantation and subnasal lip lift. Surgical lip implantation is an option to increase volume in younger patients with a normal cutaneous upper lip length and is most commonly performed with a soft, malleable, silicone implant that is available in 3-, 4-, and 5-mm diameters. The procedure is usually performed under local anesthesia in which small incisions are placed at each of the commissures and a submucosal pocket is developed at the wet and dry lip border to position the implant. Surgical subnasal lip lift is usually employed in individuals with an elongated cutaneous lip associated with lip thinning. The goals of the lip lift are to reduce the height of the cutaneous upper lip, increase the visible red vermilion, and enhance projection with appropriate dental show and minimal scarring [9]. The subnasal lip lift, also known as the "bull-horn/gull wing" lip lift (Fig. 15.2), uses a curved skin excision along the nasal sill and bilateral alar skin creases to remove the upper lip skin, followed by skin and subcutaneous tissue advancement to reduce the distance from the nasal base to the vermilion border [9]. The amount of skin

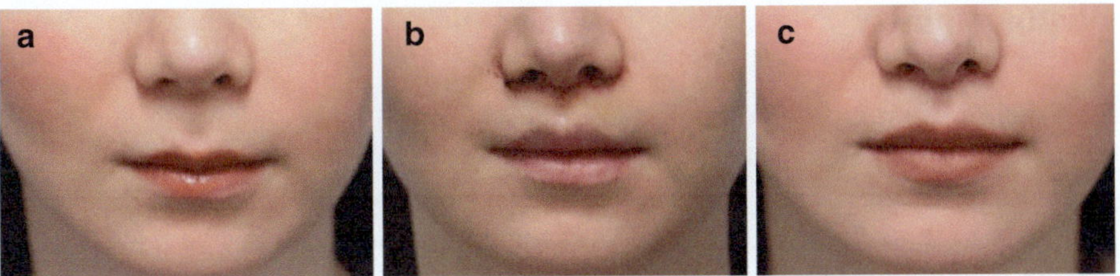

Fig. 15.2 (**a**) Preoperative image of a 29-year-old female with long philtral length and reduced vermilion show. (**b**) Postoperative image after subnasal upper lip lift at 1 week showing the "bull-horn" scar along the nasal base, reduced philtral length, and improved vermilion show. (**c**) Postoperative image at 3 months showed stable lip lift with well-concealed scar

excised varies but usually averages between 4 and 6 mm of the skin. The scar usually is well concealed with meticulous incision planning and good dermal apposition. For individuals with an unsatisfactory visible scar persisting up to 6 months, adjunctive interventions of dermabrasion and laser therapy can be offered in addition to scar creams and silicone sheets. Over-resection with excessive dental show or a "gummy smile" and under-corrections can result as complications of the surgical subnasal lip lift along with form asymmetry such as side-to-side height disparities of the cupid's bow peak [9]. While under-correction and asymmetry can be addressed with revision surgical lip lift, it is difficult to treat the deformities resulting from over-resection. Hence, accurate measurements and incision markings before local anesthetic infiltration are recommended to minimize these complications.

Some recent modifications in techniques to the traditional surgical subnasal lip lift include a deeper and more extensive release of the upper lip that may include separation of the deeper attachments of the orbicularis oris and a more definitive suspension with anchoring of the muscle edge at the premaxillary periosteum [10–12]. These modifications are considered to create longer-lasting results with a more favorable concealment of the subnasal scar [12]. Other surgical options used for upper lip augmentation include the use of autologous fat, sternocleidomastoid muscle, and dermal and fascia grafts mostly in individuals with baseline side-to-side asymmetry in lip size who may benefit from but are not interested in surgical lip implantation. These surgical techniques can be associated with gradual resorption with subsequent form asymmetry owing to differential resorption from side to side [13].

In summary, the upper lip lift can be a significant component of facial rejuvenation and feminization procedures. With a variety of surgical and nonsurgical options available, satisfactory outcomes with minimal complications require appropriate selection of patient and the technique. A meticulous preoperative planning and precise surgical technique are critical in patients undergoing surgical lip lift as some of the changes can be irreversible.

Blepharoplasty

Restoration of youthful eyelid aesthetics is one of the most commonly performed procedures in patients seeking facial rejuvenation [14]. "Nonsurgical" blepharoplasty involving lasers and fillers has been described to address aging of the periorbital tissues in selected patients [15]. Recently, another noninvasive device using plasma technology has been reported to improve dermatochalasis and periorbital rhytids by induction of new collagen formation through controlled thermal damage [15]. Although acceptable outcomes can be achieved with nonsurgical measures, surgical blepharoplasty remains the gold standard for addressing aesthetics of the eyelids and the periorbita region.

Upper eyelid blepharoplasty addresses excessive skin and upper lid sulcus deflation. Lower eyelid blepharoplasty focuses on the lower eyelid–malar complex involving laxity of the eyelid skin, orbital septum, canthal tendons, and orbicularis muscles that commonly manifest as pseudoherniation of fat, tear trough deformity, malar festoons, etc. For both upper and lower eyelids, there has been a practice shift toward tissue preservation and/or augmentation compared to the traditional techniques of aggressive skin, orbicularis, and fat excision [14]. For upper eyelid blepharoplasty, the surgical considerations are relatively consistent with some recent trends that further refine the approach by favoring graded removal of the nasal fat pad with preservation or repositioning of the central fat. These trends are supported by studies that show the nasal fat compartment to become more prominent with age, while the central compartment tends to involute [16]. These techniques are considered to optimally preserve the orbital volume and minimize iatrogenic hollowing of the superior sulcus [16]. For lower eyelid blepharoplasty, the surgical considerations can be more nuanced and complex in comparison to upper blepharoplasty as it involves not only the rejuvenation of lower eyelid but also recreation of a youthful lower eyelid–malar interface. The favored approach for lower eyelid blepharoplasty remains largely surgeon-dependent. However, in addition to conservative skin and fat excision with orbicularis preservation, the current trends favor enhancement of eyelid volume with orbital and suborbicularis oculi fat (SOOF) repositioning and fat transposition [16]. The preservation and transposition of fat are purported to restore the volume loss associated with aging changes in the lower eyelid–malar area and minimize the risk of lid retraction and iatrogenic enhancement of the tear trough deformity. Mobilization of herniated fat pads (Fig. 15.3) to areas of depression improves the periorbital volume [17]. Autogenous microfat grafting or use of autogenous dermis fat grafts are other options both to minimize post-blepharoplasty hollowing and to augment the lower eyelid–malar interface in patients who are not candidates for traditional blepharoplasty. A recent survey among oculoplastic surgeons showed that a majority (80%) perform fat repositioning, and of those, about 70% perform it in the supraperiosteal plane [16]. In addition to fat repositioning, there is a growing trend to routinely perform adjunctive procedures including lateral canthoplasty or canthopexy at the time of blepharoplasty to minimize lower eyelid malposition. In short, there may not be a single "one-size-fits-all" surgical approach

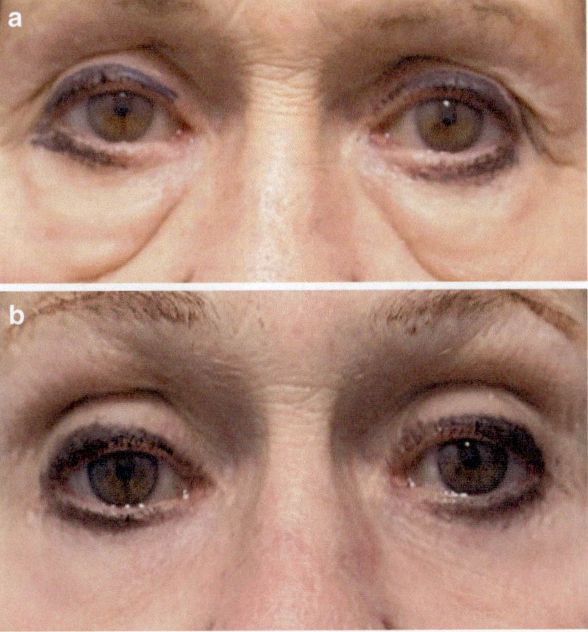

Fig. 15.3 Images of a 75-year-old female with bilateral lower eyelid fat pseudoherniation and tear trough deformity who underwent lower eyelid blepharoplasty with fat transposition. (**a**) Preoperative, (**b**) postoperative

to blepharoplasty, but awareness of the surgical trends and customizing their application based on careful assessment of an individual's features of excessive skin, fat herniation, orbital vector, tear troughs, and malar festoons are essential to achieve optimal outcomes for eyelids rejuvenation.

Facial Rejuvenation

As skin ages, a variety of physiologic changes take place. The dermis and epidermis thin and fibroblasts decrease resulting in decreased collagen and hyaluronic acid production. As a result, the skin loses elasticity and volume. Facial rejuvenation techniques aim to remedy these changes, restoring skin elasticity and restoring lost volume using a combination of noninvasive and invasive methods.

Laser and Light-Based Rejuvenation

Laser technology has been utilized for facial rejuvenation since the 1980s, evolving from ablative full-field CO_2 lasers to a wide range of fractional/non-ablative lasers. Laser and other light-based technology rejuvenate the skin by utilizing a specific wavelength of energy, which targets specific chromophores (typically water), causing local tissue injury and coagulation of tissue. Full-field lasers produce dramatic visible results but are often associated with long recovery times and high rates of post-inflammatory hyperpigmentation and often have limited use in darker skin tones (Fitzpatrick 4 and up). Fractional laser technology was introduced in the mid-2000s for facial resurfacing with the purpose of improved tissue precision and less thermal damage, which allowed for faster healing and reduced complications [18, 19]. Fractional laser delivers smaller pulses of energy in a grid pattern with islands of healthy tissue in between treated skin. Fractionated CO_2 (10,000 nm) and Erbium:YAG (2940 nm) are mainstays of current facial resurfacing treatment. Erbium is thought to result in pure ablation of tissue with minimal collateral heat transfer and damage to melanocytes and thus can be used in darker skin tones. Though Erbium:YAG does not result in as much coagulation as CO_2 lasers, both technologies produce similar results for facial rejuvenation with a similar rate of complication [19]. Traditionally, laser facial resurfacing has been either ablative or non-ablative, in which ablative laser targets the damaged external layers for epidermal renewal, while the non-ablative lasers penetrate deeper to direct the energy at a precise depth below the intact skin surface for deep dermal rejuvenation. The use of laser in facial rejuvenation has been revolutionized with integration of newer technology of hybrid fractional lasers that delivers both ablative and non-ablative wavelengths at the same treatment zone for optimal results. The hybrid Erbium:YAG fractional laser delivers an ablative (2940 nm) wavelength to address outer skin texture and pore size issues with a sequential non-ablative (1470 nm) wavelength that addresses the deeper photoaging and other dermal pigment issues and also stimulates collagen formation. This technology allows each wavelength to be tuned independently for precise coverage and depth to vaporize tissue in a controlled manner to achieve effective outcomes. The use of hybrid fractional laser has gained wide popularity and significant improvement in facial rejuvenation has been observed, especially in cases of photoaging and dyschromia, with decreased recovery time and pain [18, 20]. Though there are limited studies examining long-term outcome of the hybrid laser technology, it does appear to offer a viable option with promising early results and enhanced wound healing.

Radiofrequency Micro-Needling

Laser rejuvenation relies on externally applied photothermal energy, resulting in temperatures highest at the skin surface. This is of particular importance to patients with darker skin tones, as they are at increased risk of the post-inflammatory hyperpigmentation complications, even with the use of fractional technology. Additionally, lasers rely on the pilosebaceous unit to replenish damaged skin cells. These functional units are limited in certain regions of the face and, particularly, the neck. Radiofrequency micro-needling is an alternative technique for facial rejuvenation and skin tightening that utilizes electrothermal energy directed through the epidermis and dermis with small needles. The first radiofrequency micro-needling device was introduced in the early 2000s for aesthetic use, and since then multiple devices have been developed to further refine the technology for application in facial rejuvenation. The radiofrequency micro-needling technique allows for deposition of energy deeper in tissues with minimal epidermal heating and thus is not limited by skin tone and presence of pilosebaceous units. The radiofrequency micro-needling method creates high local dermal temperatures ranging from 65 to 100°C, which causes denaturing of type I collagen resulting in thickened and contracted collagen fibers and increased skin tension [21]. Micro-needling can be done with both insulated and non-insulated tips, manual versus mechanical insertion, and variable versus fixed needles, all of which affect the precision with which a provider can deliver electrothermal energy to the dermis and overlying epidermis. Radiofrequency micro-needling overall appears to have minimal patient downtime with few complications. While studies have shown radiofrequency micro-needling to achieve good clinical results in facial rejuvenation and acne scar treatment, there is no evidence yet of its therapeutic superiority compared with other available techniques. However, its use could be considered in patients with darker skin phototypes and areas of the face and neck with low pilosebaceous units [21].

Platelet-Rich Fibrin/Autologous Nanofat Graft

While laser and micro-needling technologies aim to contract existing collagen, autologous products like platelet-rich fibrin (PRF) and fat grafting rejuvenate the face by augmenting existing soft tissue and regenerating lost ones. Platelet-rich fibrin acts in a similar fashion to the more established platelet-rich plasma (PRP). Platelet-rich plasma induces the migration of stem cells and the secretion of local growth factors through the release of platelet alpha granules. The growth factors are localized at the intended site through interaction with newly formed clot. Together these processes result in increased fibroblast production and collagen formation, augmenting volume loss and improved skin laxity. Platelet-rich fibrin attempts to improve upon PRP by utilizing a naturally formed fibrin scaffold to guide clot formation and confine localized growth factors to local tissues. While PRP utilizes bovine-derived additives to facilitate clot formation, PRF creates the fibrin scaffold spontaneously and without additives. This results in a more durable scaffold that protects degradation of growth factors and helps sustain growth factor release attracting more mesenchymal stem cells [22]. By prolonging the growth factor release, the duration of their effects is increased (up to 7 days for some factors), and the lack of additives reduces the risk of adverse reactions [22]. Due to these benefits, PRF can be used in a variety of settings. The gel-like consistency of the fibrin matrix not only attracts mesenchymal stem cells but also stimulates the growth of fibroblasts and increases collagen production. This allows providers to use it as a filler material where repeated treatments have shown improvement in rhytids and hollowing tear troughs [22]. Some providers have also used it in combination with hyaluronic acid with improved results compared to either product alone [22]. Furthermore, there is also evidence to suggest that PRF can improve outcomes when used in cases of scarring and fat grafting [23].

A variety of materials have been used to augment lost facial tissue that accompanies aging or acquired facial deformities. Fat grafting has been utilized in facial rejuvenation since the early 2000s as a means of restoring lost facial volume. While other filler options offer temporary results, fat grafting can potentially be a permanent option for volume restoration. Fat grafting classically utilizes both the adipocyte and non-adipocyte components of fat known as the stromal vascular fraction. This contains adipose-derived stem cells, endothelial cells, monocytes, macrophages, granulocytes, and lymphocytes. After harvest, the fat is emulsified into fluids with various fat particle sizes and function, such as millifat, microfat, and nanofat. Within the last decade, nanofat grafting has gained traction in facial rejuvenation. Nanofat grafts are first harvested and then emulsified and filtered, creating a solution consisting of only mesenchymal stem cells and devoid of adipocytes. The mechanism is unclear, but this liquid has multiple regenerative properties including increased collagen production, neovascularization, and thickening of the dermis [24]. This technique is of particular benefit in the subcutaneous tissues of the eyelid, as there is no fat present in this region and there is no need for large adipocytes to provide structural augmentation but can also provide benefit in other regions of the face. Nanofat has been used in conjunction with other techniques (e.g., laser, PRF) and may achieve improved outcomes with improved healing in facial rejuvenation cases.

Face Lift: Deep Plane Rhytidectomy and Thread Lift

Surgical facelift or "rhytidectomy" to restore a youthful shape, contour, and volume in the aging face remains one of the most common aesthetic surgeries in the United States. In 2019, it was noted to be the sixth most common aesthetic procedure. While rhytidectomy continues to be a mainstay in facial rejuvenation with the techniques that have long been described, the concept of deep plane rhytidectomy has grown in popularity in recent years. In this technique, skin flap elevation first begins in the subcutaneous plane in the auricular region and then the plane between the superficial musculoaponeurotic system (SMAS) and the parotidomasseteric fascia is entered for elevation of a composite skin/SMAS flap by making an incision in the SMAS from above the angle of mandible up to the lateral orbital rim. The sub-SMAS plane of dissection allows for direct release of the key facial retaining ligaments (zygomatic, maxillary, masseteric, mandibular, and cervical) attached to the SMAS, resulting in maximal mobilization of the superficial soft tissue that is carried anteriorly toward the oral commissure, medially into the premaxillary space and nasofacial crease, and inferiorly along the zygomatic muscles to the nasolabial fold. Furthermore, the deep plane technique is also considered to improve jowling by addressing the pseudoherniated buccal fat in which a small fascial incision is made to excise a conservative amount of buccal fat. Extreme caution during deep plane dissection is warranted in order to avoid injury to the facial nerve branches particularly the buccal and zygomatic. With resuspension of the SMAS, the deep plane technique exerts tension in a vertically oblique manner at the level of fascia and not skin and therefore is believed to reduce the risk of skin flap necrosis by allowing a tension free skin closure. The debate regarding the optimal facelift technique is ongoing, but the deep plane rhytidectomy is posited to produce improved aesthetic results. Objective comparisons are limited, but studies suggest when compared to SMAS plication, a deep plane approach can produce better and sustained aesthetic outcomes (especially in the midface) while reducing the need for corrective procedures [25, 26]. As the deep plane is relatively avascular, it is thought that dissection in this plane reduces the risk of postoperative hematoma; however this plane is closer to the facial nerve branches putting them more at risk of injury (3.6%) compared to more superficial dissections, particularly for the buccal branch in the malar region [27].

Though the outcomes of facial rejuvenation are more definitive and sustained with the procedure of rhytidectomy, the trend of minimally invasive, nonsurgical, facelift using dissolvable thread is becoming increasingly popular as an alternative in patients who do not wish to undergo surgery. The thread lift procedures for the face and neck are performed in the office settings within a limited amount of time and have a quick recovery period (Fig. 15.4). The use of thread lift technique started in the 1990s, but innovations have been made in the suture material (resorbable vs. permanent) and design through the years including addition of barbs and cones. The main types of thread lift sutures are polydioxanone (PDO), polypropylene, poly-L-lactic acid (PLLA), polyglycolic acid (PLGA), and polycaprolactone, of which absorbable PDO and polypropylene are most common in use. The utilized thread materials in current use are fully resorbable and slow-degrading that come in different forms—smooth, intertwined, or with uni- or bidirectional barbs and cones. Thread lifts using these suture materials, particularly cone-based or ones with molded barbs, are thought to induce an immune reaction that stimulates fibroblast activation and collagen formation for skin lift and tightness [28]. By utilizing barbed sutures, the number of points of fixation is increased, thus reducing skin relaxation. The barbs also form a fibrous capsule, adhering to the dermis and subcutaneous tissue, aiding in the long-term lifting effect. This technique has been shown to achieve considerable skin lift with good patient satisfaction particularly in the midface region; however results have limited longevity (1–2 years) [28], as the anchor points loosen with facial movements and gravity exerts its effects over time. Appropriate selection of patients with mild to moderate skin laxity and adequate skin thickness and who do not desire drastic changes to their appearance and have realistic expectations will maximize results and patient satisfaction with nonsurgical thread lifts. Bruising edema, asymmetry, skin dimpling and infection are relatively rare but can occur as potential side effects. Knowledge of facial anatomy is essential for safety and efficacy of the procedure.

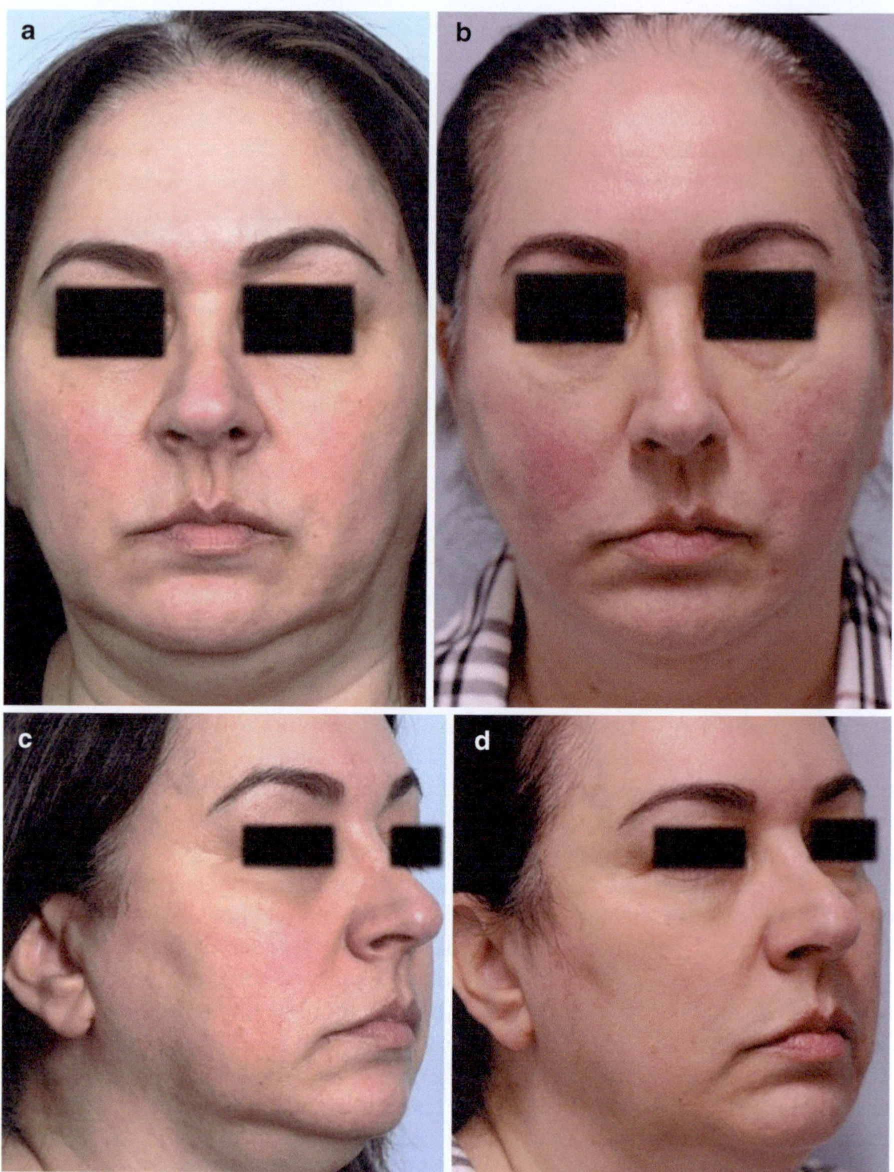

Fig. 15.4 Images of a 55-year-old female patient undergoing the thread facelift procedure. Frontal view of pre- and immediate post-thread lift (**a**, **b**), left profile view of pre- and immediate post-thread lift (**c**, **d**)

Hair Restoration

Hair loss affects a significant portion of population with a prevalence cited as high as 85% among males and 40% among females [29]. It results in reduced self-esteem and is often a source of psychological distress in affected men and women. Medical treatment including finasteride and minoxidil are shown to only delay progression of hair loss and promote some partial growth. The recent advancements in surgical hair transplantation have made this procedure a safe and effective method to restore a more natural and youthful hair pattern in patients that meet candidacy. There are two hair transplantation techniques, the follicular unit transplantation (FUT) and follicular unit extraction (FUE) techniques. These techniques have largely supplanted the historical surgical options in hair loss treatment of plug grafts, scalp reductions, and transposition flaps. The FUE technique is the more commonly applied approach due to its cited advantages that include increased number of harvestable grafts, ability to target follicles of a specific size, diameter or pigmentation, increased freedom to adopt any hairstyle due to minimal scarring, reduced postoperative pain, and faster postoperative healing. The use of additional modalities such as platelet-rich plasma injections, lasers, and stem cells are considered to further enhance the survival and appearance of hair transplants. Another recent innovation in the field of hair restoration is introduction of robotic technology to maximize patient outcomes. There is a FDA-approved robotic device developed specifically for the FUE procedure in male patients. The robot scans and digitizes the visual characteristics of the donor area and analyzes each follicular unit including the follicular unit density and hair angulation. The robotic arm has a dual-chamber needle for harvest of the selected follicular units that includes a sharp tip to enter the skin and a surrounding coring blunt punch that then goes deeper into the tissue to limit the chance of transection [30]. Studies comparing the robotic versus manual techniques are lacking; however, the proposed advantages of the robotic system include a more accurate and faster graft harvest, decreased follicular transection rate, and increased implantation accuracy at the recipient site [29]. More recently, advancements in the FUE techniques have allowed expansion of hair transplantation to the non-scalp hair-bearing regions of the face including beard, eyebrows, and sideburns.

Candidates for facial hair restoration in the beard, moustache, and sideburns are usually males with hair paucity that is either of primary origin or secondary to scarring, burn, and iatrogenic procedures such as laser hair removal or cleft lip repair [31]. It is also sought by patients undergoing gender transformation surgery. The FUE technique is often preferred as it avoids a linear scar. Scalp is the donor area with the occiput being used in cases requiring smaller grafts and extension into the parietal area for larger cases. Depending on the exact design and density, graft counts can range from 250 to 300 grafts to each sideburn, 400–800 grafts to the mustache and goatee, and 300–500 grafts per cheek. Patients seeking eyebrow transplantation are females with thinning of the eyebrows from over-plucking, aging, or genetic causes [31]. A high degree of experience and dexterity is recommended to perform microscopic dissection of the harvested donor hairs that usually includes one- and two-hair follicular units from the occipital scalp. Scalp hair transplantation for facial hair restoration is shown to achieve natural outcomes and a high regrowth percentage using the optimal techniques in appropriate patients [31]. Adoption of advanced hair transplantation techniques allows facial plastic surgeons to offer patients a comprehensive scalp and facial hair restoration with a goal to attain the best possible natural and preferred outcomes.

Facial Reinnervation

The functional and psychosocial distress from facial paralysis is known to cause a significant negative impact on an individual's quality of life. Advances have been made over the last few decades in surgical techniques to achieve dynamic facial reanimation in patients with long-standing paralysis. The dynamic reanimation is mainly achieved through nerve grafting or transfer of nerve and functional muscle. These procedures encompass cross-facial nerve grafting, motor nerve transposition using the masseteric and/or hypoglossal nerves, temporalis muscle/tendon transfer, and microvascular transposition of gracilis free flap. Of all the abovementioned procedures, gracilis transfer and innervation by the ipsilateral masseteric nerve have emerged as the preferred approach that results in significantly improved facial symmetry and smile and oral commissure excursion. Novel bioelectrical interfaces using the tissue engineering technology are currently being developed for application in patients with chronic facial paralysis [32]. Use of such technology can complement the innovative surgical techniques and has potential to improve not only the facial and smile asymmetry but also the dynamic movement of the brow and eyelid. We refer readers to the chapter in this volume on motor nerve reconstruction of the facial nerve for further details on facial reinnervation.

References

1. Harb A, Brewster CT. The nonsurgical rhinoplasty: a retrospective review of 5000 treatments. Plast Reconstr Surg. 2020;145:661–7.
2. Keyhan SO, Ramezanzade S, Bohluli B, Fallahi HR, Mirzahoseini S, Nahai F. Autologous fat injection for augmentation rhinoplasty: a systematic review. Aesthetic Surg J Open Forum. 2021;3(2):ojab010. https://pubmed.ncbi.nlm.nih.gov/33987531/. Accessed 26 Nov 2021.
3. Mehta U, Fridirici Z. Advanced techniques in nonsurgical rhinoplasty. Facial Plast Surg Clin North Am. 2019;27(3):355–65. https://pubmed.ncbi.nlm.nih.gov/31280849/. Accessed 26 Nov 2021.
4. Rohrich R, Alleyne B, Novak M, Bellamy J, Chamata E. Nonsurgical rhinoplasty. Clin Plast Surg. 2022;49(1):191–5. https://pubmed.ncbi.nlm.nih.gov/34782136/. Accessed 26 Nov 2021.
5. Williams LC, Kidwai SM, Mehta K, Kamel G, Tepper OM, Rosenberg JD. Nonsurgical rhinoplasty: a systematic review of technique, outcomes, and complications. Plast Reconstr Surg. 2020;146:41–51.

6. Toriumi DM, Kovacevic M. Dorsal preservation rhinoplasty: measures to prevent suboptimal outcomes. Facial Plast Surg Clin North Am. 2021;29(1):141–53. https://pubmed.ncbi.nlm.nih.gov/33220839/. Accessed 4 Dec 2021.
7. Göksel A, Patel PN, Most SP. Piezoelectric osteotomies in dorsal preservation rhinoplasty. Facial Plast Surg Clin North Am. 2021;29(1):77–84.
8. Kar M, Muluk NB, Bafaqeeh SA, Cingi C. Is it possible to define the ideal lips? Acta Otorhinolaryngol Ital. 2018;38(1):67. https://pubmed.ncbi.nlm.nih.gov/29756617/. Accessed 7 Nov 2021.
9. Salibian AA, Bluebond-Langner R. Lip lift. Facial Plast Surg Clin North Am. 2019;27(2):261–6. https://pubmed.ncbi.nlm.nih.gov/30940392/. Accessed 6 Nov 2021.
10. Spiegel JH. The modified bullhorn approach for the lip-lift. JAMA Fac Plast Surg. 2019;21(1):69–70. https://pubmed.ncbi.nlm.nih.gov/30326516/. Accessed 6 Nov 2021.
11. Talei B. The modified upper lip lift: advanced approach with deep-plane release and secure suspension: 823-patient series. Facial Plast Surg Clin North Am. 2019;27(3):385–98. https://pubmed.ncbi.nlm.nih.gov/31280853/. Accessed 6 Nov 2021.
12. Li YK, Ritz M. The modified bull's horn upper lip lift. J Plast Reconstr Aesthet Surg. 2018;71(8):1216–30.
13. De Joseph LM, Agarwal A, Greco TM. Lip augmentation. Facial Plast Surg Clin North Am. 2018;26(2):193–203. https://pubmed.ncbi.nlm.nih.gov/29636150/. Accessed 7 Nov 2021.
14. Drolet BC, Sullivan PK. Evidence-based medicine: blepharoplasty. Plast Reconstr Surg. 2014;133(5):1195–205.
15. Cantisani C, Amori P, Vitiello G, Tirant M, Thuong VN, Lotti T, et al. Nonsurgical blepharoplasty. Dermatol Ther. 2019;32(6):e13119.
16. Kossler AL, Peng GL, Yoo DB, Azizzadeh B, Massry GG. Current trends in upper and lower eyelid blepharoplasty among American Society of Ophthalmic Plastic and Reconstructive Surgery Members. Ophthal Plast Reconstr Surg. 2018;34(1):37–42.
17. Bhattacharjee K, Ghosh S, Ugradar S, Azhdam AM. Lower eyelid blepharoplasty: an overview. Indian J Ophthalmol. 2020;68(10):2075–83. https://pubmed.ncbi.nlm.nih.gov/32971612/. Accessed 11 Dec 2021.
18. Marcus BC. Nonablative and hybrid fractional laser skin rejuvenation. Facial Plast Surg Clin North Am. 2020;28(1):37–44. https://www.ncbi.nlm.nih.gov/pubmed/31779940.
19. Ansari F, Sadeghi-Ghyassi F, Yaaghoobian B. The clinical effectiveness and cost-effectiveness of fractional CO2 laser in acne scars and skin rejuvenation: a meta-analysis and economic evaluation. J Cosmet Laser Ther. 2018;20(4):248–51. https://www.ncbi.nlm.nih.gov/pubmed/29384405.
20. Waibel S, Pozner J, Robb C, Tanzi E. Hybrid fractional laser: a multi-center trial on the safety and efficacy for photorejuvenation. J Drugs Dermatol. 2018;17(11):1164–8. https://www.ncbi.nlm.nih.gov/pubmed/30481954.
21. Weiner SF. Radiofrequency microneedling: overview of technology, advantages, differences in devices, studies, and indications. Facial Plast Surg Clin North Am. 2019;27(3):291–303.
22. Karimi K, Rockwell H. The benefits of platelet-rich fibrin. Facial Plast Surg Clin North Am. 2019;27(3):331–40. https://www.ncbi.nlm.nih.gov/pubmed/31280847.
23. Mahapatra S, Kumar D, Subramanian V, Chakrabarti SK, Deb KD. Study on the efficacy of platelet-rich fibrin matrix in hair follicular unit transplantation in androgenetic alopecia patients. J Clin Aesthet Dermatol. 2016;9(9):29–35. https://www.ncbi.nlm.nih.gov/pubmed/27853485.
24. Xu P, Yu Q, Huang H, Zhang WJ, Li W. Nanofat increases dermis thickness and neovascularization in photoaged nude mouse skin. Aesthet Plast Surg. 2018;42(2):343–51. https://www.ncbi.nlm.nih.gov/pubmed/29380024.
25. Kamer FM, Frankel AS. SMAS rhytidectomy versus deep plane rhytidectomy: an objective comparison. Plast Reconstr Surg. 1998;102(3):878–81. https://www.ncbi.nlm.nih.gov/pubmed/9727459.
26. Adamson PA, Dahiya R, Litner J. Midface effects of the deep-plane vs the superficial musculoaponeurotic system plication face-lift. Arch Facial Plast Surg. 2007;9(1):9–11. https://www.ncbi.nlm.nih.gov/pubmed/17224481.

27. Wulu JA, Spiegel JH. Is deep plane rhytidectomy superior to superficial musculoaponeurotic system plication facelift? Laryngoscope. 2017;128(8):1741–2. https://www.ncbi.nlm.nih.gov/pubmed/29280491.
28. Ali YH. Two years' outcome of thread lifting with absorbable barbed PDO threads: innovative score for objective and subjective assessment. J Cosmet Laser Ther. 2018;20(1):41–9. https://www.ncbi.nlm.nih.gov/pubmed/28863268.
29. Zito PM, Raggio BS. Hair transplantation. Treasure Island, FL: StatPearls; 2021. https://www.ncbi.nlm.nih.gov/books/NBK547740/. Accessed 3 Nov 2021.
30. Rose PT. Advances in hair restoration. Dermatol Clin. 2018;36(1):57–62. https://pubmed.ncbi.nlm.nih.gov/29108547/. Accessed 3 Nov 2021.
31. Bared A. What's new in facial hair transplantation?: effective techniques for beard and eyebrow transplantation. Facial Plast Surg Clin North Am. 2019;27(3):379–84. https://pubmed.ncbi.nlm.nih.gov/31280852/. Accessed 3 Nov 2021.
32. Langhals NB, Urbanchek MG, Ray A, Brenner MJ. Update in facial nerve paralysis: tissue engineering and new technologies. Curr Opin Otolaryngol Head Neck Surg. 2014;22(4):291–9. https://pubmed.ncbi.nlm.nih.gov/24979369/. Accessed 7 Jan 2021.

Chapter 16
Innovative Treatment Modalities for Craniofacial Reconstruction

Vasudev Vivekanand Nayak iD**, Daniel Boczar** iD**, Paulo G. Coelho** iD**, Andrea Torroni** iD**, Christopher M. Runyan** iD**, James C. Melville** iD**, Simon Young** iD**, Bruce Cronstein** iD**, Roberto L. Flores** iD**, and Lukasz Witek** iD

V. V. Nayak
Department of Biochemistry and Molecular Biology, University of Miami Miller School of
Medicine, New York, NY, USA
e-mail: vxn188@miami.edu

D. Boczar
Department of Surgery, University of Washington, Seattle, WA, USA
e-mail: Boczad01@uw.edu

P. G. Coelho
Department of Biochemistry and Molecular Biology, University of Miami Miller School of
Medicine, Miami, FL, USA

Division of Plastic Surgery, Department of Surgery, University of Miami Miller School of
Medicine, Miami, FL, USA
e-mail: pgc51@med.miami.edu

A. Torroni · R. L. Flores
Hansjörg Wyss Department of Plastic Surgery, NYU Grossman School of Medicine,
New York, NY, USA
e-mail: andrea.torroni@nyumc.org; roberto.Flores@nyulangone.org

C. M. Runyan
Department of Plastic Surgery, Wake Forest University School of Medicine,
Winston-Salem, NC, USA
e-mail: crunyan@wakehealth.edu

J. C. Melville · S. Young
Bernard and Gloria Pepper Katz Department of Oral and Maxillofacial Surgery, School of
Dentistry, The University of Texas Health Science Center at Houston, Houston, TX, USA
e-mail: James.C.Melville@uth.tmc.edu; Simon.Young@uth.tmc.edu

B. Cronstein
Department of Medicine, NYU Grossman School of Medicine, New York, NY, USA
e-mail: bruce.cronstein@nyumc.org

L. Witek (✉)
Biomaterials Division, NYU College of Dentistry, New York, NY, USA

Hansjörg Wyss Department of Plastic Surgery, NYU Grossman School of Medicine,
New York, NY, USA

Department of Biomedical Engineering, NYU Tandon School of Engineering,
Brooklyn, NY, USA
e-mail: lukasz.witek@nyu.edu

Introduction

The craniomaxillofacial (CMF) region is comprised of a complex system of soft and hard tissues. The primary function of the intracranial space is to accommodate the brain, while the oral cavity, which is anatomically encompassed by the cranial base and the mandible, enables respiration, speech, and mastication [1, 2]. Defects affecting this musculoskeletal structure of the midface comprise a large number of cases requiring CMF surgery. In the year 2020, 256,085 maxillofacial surgeries, 35,387 head and neck reconstructions, and 68,915 reconstructive surgeries were performed to address congenital deformities [3].

Cleft palate (e.g., anterior alveolar defect of the maxilla) has been reported to affect 1 in 600 newborns [4] and requires alveolar bone grafting traditionally harvested from the iliac crest. Hemifacial microsomia (HFM) and Pierre Robin sequence are both associated with micrognathia, which may cause tongue-based airway obstruction, and are often treated with mandibular distraction osteogenesis, requiring two separate operations with morbidities including facial scarring and potential nerve damage. Treacher Collins syndrome is another disorder associated with congenital absence of the zygoma necessitating autologous bone grafting. Craniosynostosis is a condition involving premature fusion of the cranial sutures that may lead to increased intracranial pressure. If left untreated, patients can potentially suffer from developmental delays or intellectual disabilities, malocclusion, dysphagia, and speech abnormalities [5]. Treatment modalities for this condition include cranial expansion surgery requiring autologous split cranial bone graft or autograft (native tissue) to adequately expand the skull without leaving critical size defects [6].

For many CMF bony defects, autografts, to date, are considered the "gold standard" reconstructive modality. Although an effective treatment modality, autografts are associated with multiple disadvantages including a limited quantity of available donor tissue, donor site morbidity, and the potential for infection at the site of surgery, along with cost [7]. Specifically, cleft repair with harvested autogenous iliac crest has been known to cause short- and long-term donor site pain and sensory disturbances [8]. HFM treatment using autogenous grafting procedures typically entails longer surgical procedures, greater surgical mobility, and asymmetry between the reconstructed side and the normal, unoperated, contralateral side [9]. Reconstructive surgery in the case of Treacher Collins syndrome involves using calvarial bone grafts, especially for zygomatic reconstruction. One primary limitation of this treatment modality is the resorption of the bone graft, seen in a majority of patients [10, 11]. Furthermore in the case of craniosynostosis treatment, the likely presence of critically sized defects necessitates the use of devices, grafts, and implants, to aid in the healing process [12].

A requirement for grafts or implants used in the reconstruction of CMF defects is the capacity to restore the bony defect while maintaining the three-dimensional (3D) skeletal architecture. Thus, the field of CMF surgery has evolved toward utilization of customized treatment plans for patients to improve outcomes in terms of physiology, function, and aesthetics, post-recovery. Such challenges have warranted the search for alternative materials and modalities that are not limited in quantity, are biocompatible, have the capacity to be tailored specific to the patient and anatomic location, and are augmented with biologic factors to facilitate bone regeneration. This chapter focuses on the re-purposing of bulk materials that have been previously utilized for bony defect regeneration through the application of additive manufacturing techniques to advance CMF reconstruction in both pediatric and adult patients.

New Materials and Methods

Ceramics are synthesized solid inorganic materials that are crystalline in nature. Bioceramics are a subset of this class, which are biocompatible, bioinert, bioactive, or bioresorbable. Calcium phosphate (CaP)-based materials have garnered increased attention dating back to the early 1960s as they can be utilized as resorbable and implantable devices/materials in their bulk form [13–18]. CaP-based ceramics have a reliable safety profile and excellent biocompatibility [5]. Among the different CaP ceramics available, β-tricalcium phosphate (β-TCP) ($Ca_3(PO_4)_2$) and hydroxyapatite (HA) ($Ca_{10}(PO_4)_6(OH)_2$) have been widely utilized for bony defect regeneration [19]. Devices manufactured using HA or β-TCP have traditionally been fabricated through molding or casting. The process involves using a die to produce parts for a specific application. While the accuracy of parts generated remains satisfactory, the process is laborious to carry out for each patient or anatomic location requiring a customized, fit-and-fill graft. Furthermore, casting a part with controlled pore spacing and distribution is difficult, especially in small scaffolds. Such limitations have prompted the search for alternative manufacturing techniques that can more readily facilitate the production of patient-specific devices.

In the most recent form of additive manufacturing, 3D printing (3DP)—the sequential layer-by-layer addition of material, custom medical devices/scaffolds have been designed and fabricated using computer-aided design (CAD). While this form of rapid prototyping has evolved considerably in recent years in various surgical fields, its presence in CMF surgery has demonstrated substantially greater advances. One reason for such growth has been attributed to the paucity of clinically available patient-specific tissue engineering-based therapies [4]. Further advances in 3DP technology have been due to increased accuracy and stability of printed materials by simultaneously reducing post-processing steps required prior to implantation. Additive manufacturing (AM) of metals and polymers are relatively older techniques, whereas 3DP of ceramics through solid free-form fabrication (SFFF) or robocasting, is a newer and emerging method to fabricate resorbable, porous scaffolds through the use of ceramic-based slurries [20]. HA and β-TCP are two such CaP-based ceramics that can be extruded in a controlled fashion [21]. In their bulk form, both materials exhibit valuable biocompatibility and osseoconduction in vivo. HA, which is the primary inorganic component of bone, has been reported to show ~2% resorption annually [22]. Such low resorption kinetics have rendered HA unfavorable in terms of a resorbable grafting material. β-TCP on the other hand has been shown to fully resorb within a period between 6 and 18 months depending on various factors (i.e., volume, shape, porosity, and surface characteristics) of the construct [23]. This has driven researchers to develop new workflows using β-TCP slurries to produce 3DP customized fit-and-fill scaffolds.

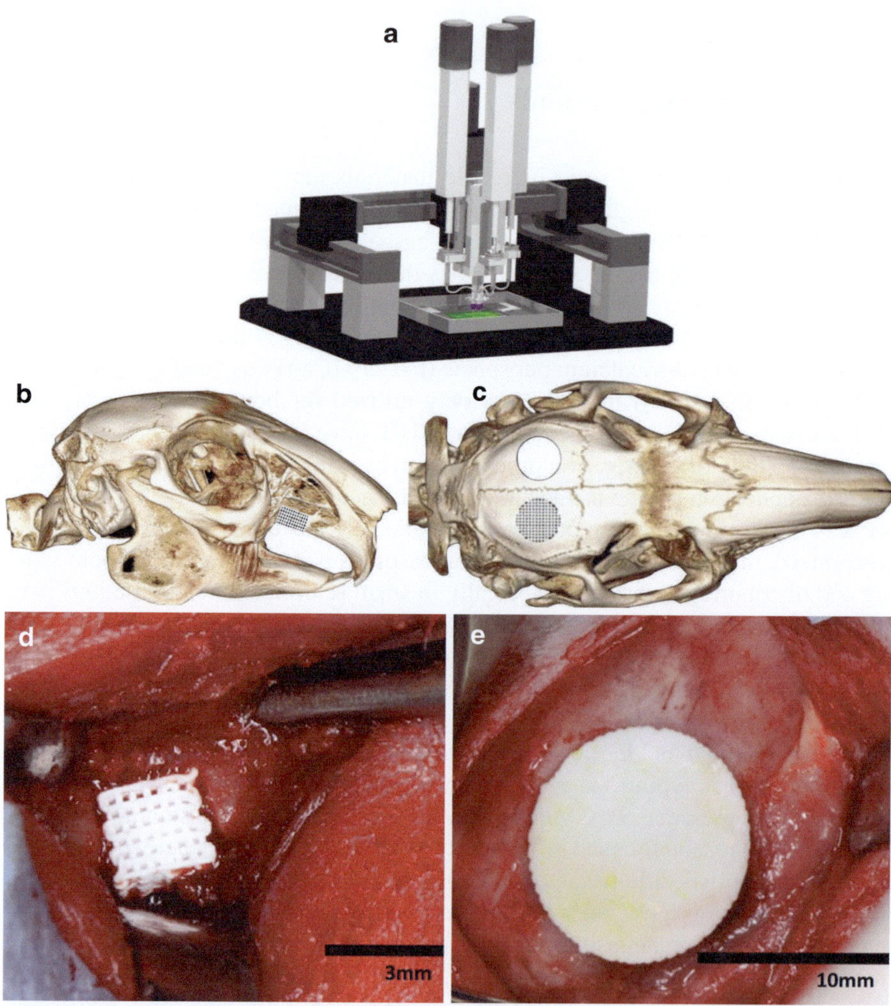

Fig. 16.1 (**a**) CAD rendering of custom-built solid free-form fabrication 3D printer. (**b**) Schematic depicting alveolar cleft model. (**c**) Schematic depicting calvarial defect model, intraoperative image of fit-and-fill reconstruction of (**d**) cleft and (**e**) calvarial defect with scaffold. (Reproduced with permission from Shen C, Wang MM, Witek L, Tovar N, Cronstein BN, Torroni A, et al. Transforming the Degradation Rate of β-tricalcium Phosphate Bone Replacement Using 3-Dimensional Printing. Annals of Plastic Surgery. 2021;87(6))

The 3D printing workflow for ceramics is multifaceted consisting of the following steps (Fig. 16.1):

1. *Pre-processing:* This step includes computer-aided design (CAD) and successive computer-aided manufacturing (CAM) to generate digital part files. With the introduction of 3D printing, CAD has seen significant development with its synergistic integration to hardware like micro-computed tomography (microCT) and volumetric rendering software tools such as AMIRA or mimics for isolation and refinement of the region of interest. The digitally reconstructed 3D computer-generated solid is then exported to stereolithography (.STL) format through discretization after which is it digitally sliced and meshed into a multilayered three-dimensional (3D) object. This slicing process converts the surface data of the .STL file into machine level ".gcode" comprising of coordinate-related instructions along with auxiliary commands such as feed rate, print speed, etc. This is especially useful to tailor the scaffold lattice parameters, namely, pore spacing, layer height, and rod size. Once the details have been set, the ".gcode" is exported to the SFFF printer.

2. *Printing:* SFFF printers consist of a stationary platform equipped with a moveable gantry. Commonly these printers consist of multiple extrusion nozzles to deposit both primary and secondary, fugitive support materials simultaneously. While there are various protocols published in the literature to synthesize a colloidal mixture or slurry of β-TCP, a previously established protocol combines powdered β-TCP powder with controlled amounts of antiflocculants, dispersive agents, and viscosifiers to generate a shear thinning gel [5, 21, 24]. The extruders of the SFFF printer follow a tool path in the x-, y-, and z-axes from the file while depositing the colloidal gel onto a substrate.

3. *Post-processing:* This type of fabrication method requires a single post-processing step. Ceramics are generally brittle without heat treatment, causing problems with handling and usage. To overcome this, ceramic scaffolds are heat treated (sintered) to solidify the constructs. The heating leads to shrinkage and subsequent densification of the construct for it to achieve the required mechanical properties for surgical handling. Subsequently, prior to implantation scaffolds are also sterilized in an autoclave at approximately 121°C before surgical implantation.

Bioactive Molecules (rhBMP-2, Adenosine, and Dipyridamole)

With the introduction of tissue engineering-based approaches, the embryonic process of tissue generation has been further recapitulated using mesenchymal stem cells (MSCs), growth factors (GFs), and cytokines [25–27]. Similarly, the unique combination of 3D-printed grafting materials and bioactive molecules can further enhance the rate of bone formation and regeneration, potentially reducing the time needed to return to form and function. Such results are possible due to increased osteoblast activity and subsequent reduction in osteoclast activity while also leading to scaffold resorption [4]. One such innovation that has resulted from the amalgamation of various surgical techniques is the use of recombinant human bone morphogenetic protein-2 (rhBMP-2) for the reconstruction of segmental CMF defects [28].

Bone regeneration is a complex process with a primary goal being osseoinduction [4]. Recombinant human bone morphogenetic protein-2 (rhBMP-2) is one commercially available FDA-approved osteogenic agent. Its use in preclinical in vivo models has shown considerably faster bone regeneration when compared to scaffolds implanted without such bioactive molecules. Unfortunately, its share of drawbacks such as ectopic bone formation and premature suture fusion [29–34] has limited its use. In contrast, adenosine, commonly termed "the retaliatory metabolite," has gained popularity as an osteogenic agent capable of promoting higher levels of bone regeneration. The mechanism of action of adenosine is by attenuating activity of a wide array of cell types as a protective mechanism [35, 36]. Regulatory effects of adenosine such as induced protective vasodilatory and negative inotropic effects on stressed cardiac vessels and tissue have been reported for over a century [7]. While tissues are stressed, adenosine is present in higher quantities (e.g., in septic patients [35]). Adenosine receptors A_1 (ligation of which plays a role in osteoclast formation), A_{2A} (activation of which inhibits osteoclastogenesis), A_{2B} (agonism of which influences osteogenic differentiation), and A_{3A} (agonism of which has been reported to cause downregulation in bone resorption) cause systemic effects since they are present throughout almost every tissue [7]. However, in unstressed tissues, its activity is limited by its lower extracellular presence (~1 µM/L) and short half-life due to the aforementioned receptors being left inactivated even with continuous blockage of adenosine deaminase enzyme [19, 35].

Due to these shortcomings, the search for alternatives mainly through pharmacological manipulation has led research groups to the selection of dipyridamole (DIPY) as a suitable bioactive molecule. DIPY has been FDA approved for clinical

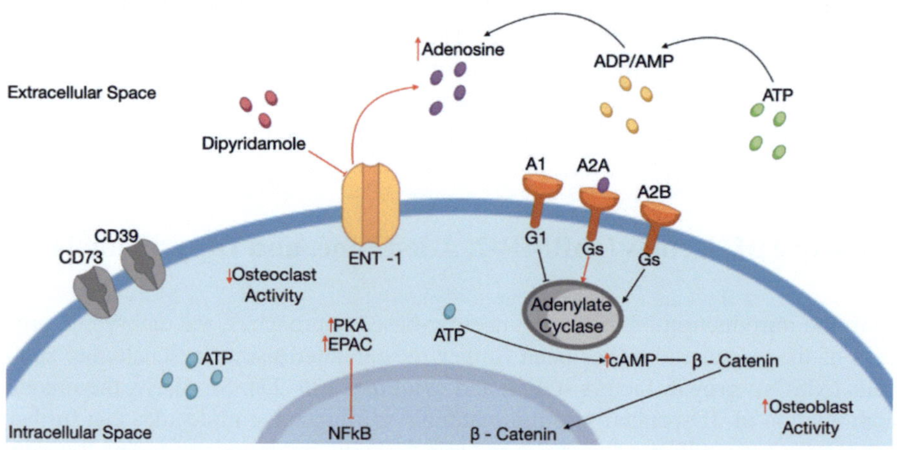

Fig. 16.2 Schematic depicting how adenosine receptor activation alters osteoclast and osteoblast activity. (Adapted from Lopez CD, Witek L, Torroni A, Flores RL, Demissie DB, Young S, et al. The role of 3D printing in treating craniomaxillofacial congenital anomalies. Birth Defects Res. 2018;110(13):1055–64)

use and has already been established as a drug in cardiac stress testing and antiplatelet therapy [37–39]. DIPY, an adenosine A_{2A} receptor indirect agonist, functions through type 1 equilibrative nucleoside transporter (ENT1) to block the reuptake of adenosine into cells causing extracellular accumulation (Fig. 16.2). With the hypothesis that DIPY can enhance bone formation while avoiding the common side effects of rhBMP-2, several tissue engineering strategies have been developed to treat critical-sized defects in immature and mature skeletal models.

Tissue Engineering Strategies: Evidence in a Small Translational Model

Research shows that bioactive ceramic scaffolds can be used to fill critically sized segmental defects and bridge defects with newly regenerated bone as early as 8 weeks in vivo. Furthermore, simultaneous scaffold degradation with bone formation and remodeling has been observed over 6 months [20]. In vivo studies have also enabled important insights into the role of adenosine indirect agonists on bone regeneration. To test the hypothesis that DIPY enhances bone regenerative capabilities of already osseoconductive ceramic 3DP constructs, β-TCP scaffolds were utilized in critical-sized calvarial defects in a A_{2A} knockout (KO) murine model [33] (Fig. 16.3). The bone regenerative capacity of DIPY was leveraged via local delivery to the defect site, thereby avoiding systemic effects while simplifying release kinetics [4]. Significantly increased bone formation was recorded for the scaffold group loaded with DIPY prior to implantation, when compared to the experimental group without the bioactive molecule.

A_{2A} receptor activation was determined to be a critical mechanism of action for bone as A_{2A} receptor knockouts failed to regenerate the cranial bone defects. Conversely, the control groups showed favorable healing, thereby highlighting the role the A_{2A} receptor plays in bone regeneration [40]. While 3DP scaffolds composed of β-TCP alone can restore bone defects, the addition of DIPY significantly increases osteogenic potential. Loading a 3D-printed (3DP) bioactive ceramic scaffold that serves as a carrier of an osseoinductive molecule like DIPY has paved the way for new tissue engineering strategies [41–43]. Research has since been conducted making extensive use of DIPY as an osseoinductive coating on fit-and-fill 3DP β-TCP scaffolds to treat critically sized defects induced in the calvaria, cleft, and mandible of translational models at multiple length scales.

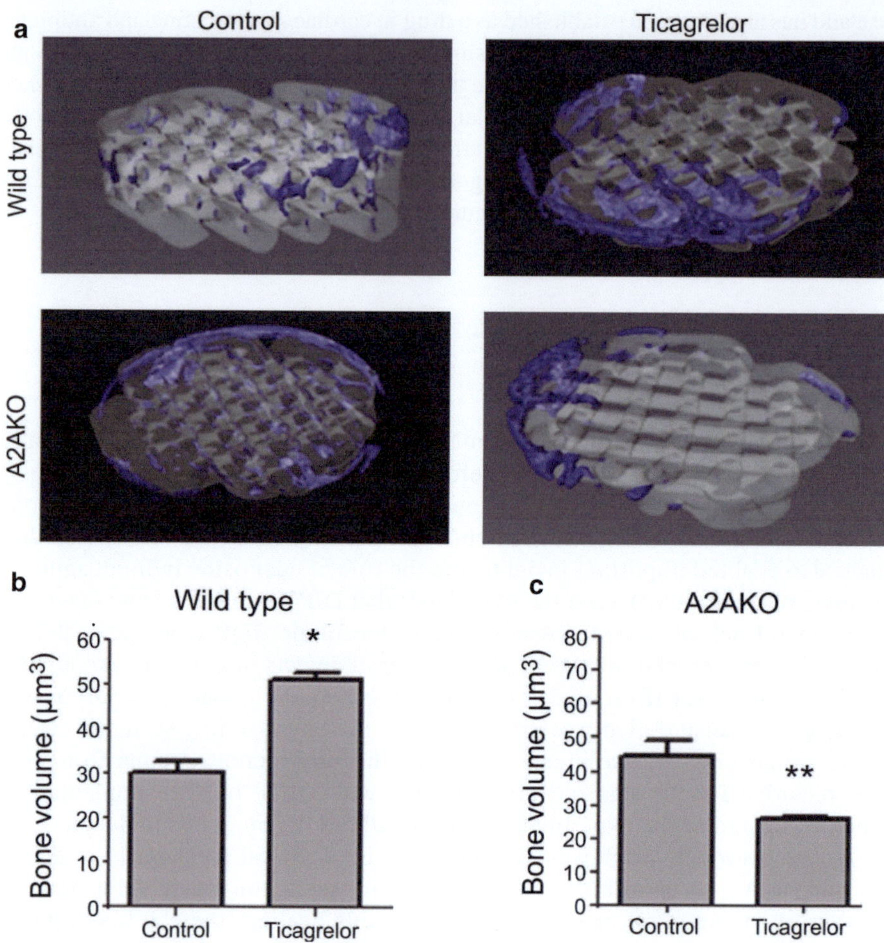

Fig. 16.3 (**a**) Volumetric reconstruction of bone and scaffold of the collagen-coated scaffold for both wild-type and A2A KO groups. Volume of new bone formation within the scaffolds at the site of trephination for (**b**) wild-type and (**c**) A2A KO groups. (Data presented as mean ± SEM). (Reproduced with permission from Mediero A, Wilder T, Reddy VS, Cheng Q, Tovar N, Coelho PG, et al. Ticagrelor regulates osteoblast and osteoclast function and promotes bone formation in vivo via an adenosine-dependent mechanism. FASEB J. 2016;30(11):3887–900)

Preclinical Translational Models

Skeletally Mature Translational Models

Murine models used in previous studies posed a concern during the quantitative and qualitative analysis of the effect of DIPY. Specifically, no attempt was made to isolate the effect of DIPY on different bone healing tissue contributors, specifically the bone defect margin, dura, and pericranium, due to the model's constraints in size [33, 34]. Alternatively, a larger preclinical sheep model was selected for implantation of scaffolds designed with a cap (a solid barrier on the ectocortical side) to minimize the infiltration of pericranium while allowing for contact between the dura and an open, porous, lattice-based interior scaffold structure [34]. 3DP ceramic scaffolds comprised of 100% β-TCP were printed for inlay reconstruction of a surgically induced calvarial defect (Fig. 16.4). Specifically, custom 3DP scaffolds with lattice-based porosity were designed and printed such that the lattice structure faced toward the dural surface. Scaffolds were either augmented only with collagen,

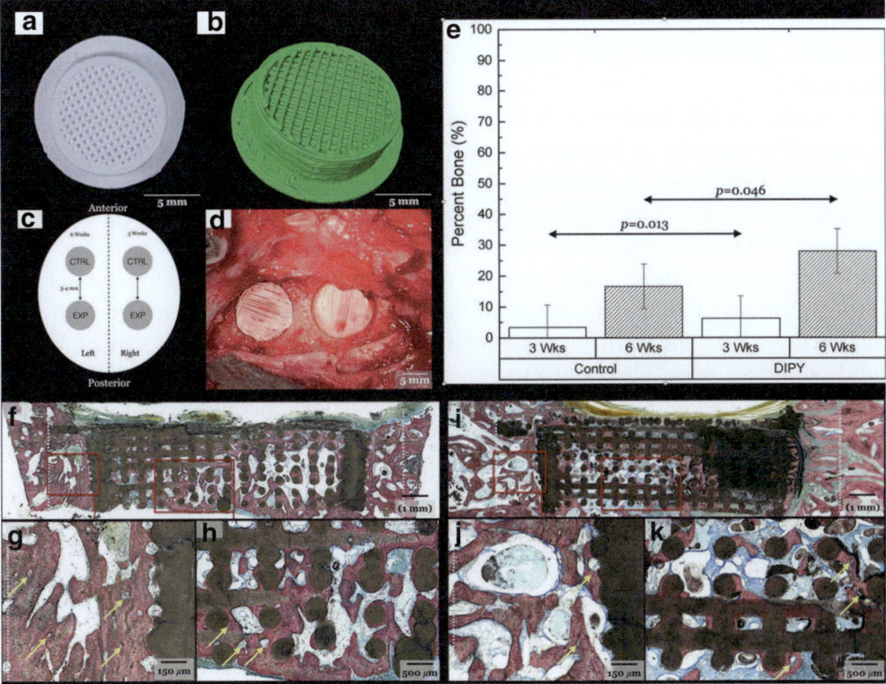

Fig. 16.4 (**a**) Inferior surface of the scaffold, (**b**) 3D reconstruction of the scaffold created using Amira 6.3 software (Visage Imaging GmbH, Berlin, Germany), (**c**) schematic representation of experimental design, (**d**) intraoperative photograph showing scaffold placement, (**e**) graph depicting the percentage of bone formation (error bars indicate 95% confidence intervals), (**f**) representative histologic image from animals in the control group at the 6-week time point, (**g**) magnification of abundant bone growth between the defect margin and wall of the scaffold with a primary osteon highlighted (yellow arrow), (**h**) angiogenesis (green arrows), (**i**) representative histologic image from animals in the DIPY group at the 6-week time point, (**j**) close-up depicting significant bony infill within the space between the defect margin and wall of the scaffold, with several osteons highlighted (yellow arrows) that provide evidence of lamellar reorganization, (**k**) angiogenesis and osteon development is evident (green arrows) and more prevalent in the DIPY group. (Reproduced with permission from Bekisz JM, Flores RL, Witek L, Lopez CD, Runyan CM, Torroni A, et al. Dipyridamole enhances osteogenesis of three-dimensionally printed bioactive ceramic scaffolds in calvarial defects. J Craniomaxillofac Surg. 2018;46(2):237–44)

which served as the control group or coated with collagen and then subsequently immersed in a 100 µM concentration DIPY solution. Two ipsilateral 11-mm calvarial defects were induced in sheep ($n = 5$) with trephines. Defects were filled with either a control or a DIPY-augmented scaffold, and the surgery was repeated on the contralateral side after 3 weeks. Following euthanasia, defects were evaluated through microCT and histomorphometric analysis for bone, scaffold, and soft tissue quantification within the defect. No histologic evidence of ectopic bone formation or inflammation was observed within the defects. Significantly higher osteogenesis was seen in DIPY-coated scaffolds compared to controls both at the 3-week ($p = 0.013$) and 6-week time points ($p = 0.046$) [34]. Furthermore, the most significant difference in results pertaining to bone regeneration was observed centrally within the interface between the 3DPBC scaffold and the dura mater, with a bone formation increase of ~85% when compared to control scaffolds at the 6-week time point.

In studies employing 3DP β-TCP scaffolds in load-bearing applications, the regenerative capacity of bioceramic scaffolds has yielded favorable results. In one such study, full-thickness, unilateral defects were induced in skeletally mature New Zealand White rabbits (NZWR) at the segmental mandibular body. β-TCP scaffolds demonstrated bone regeneration at 8 weeks in vivo [44] (Fig. 16.5). Scaffolds were seen to bridge the entire defect span despite the presence of physiological loading during masticatory function. Intramembranous-like healing was observed with vascularized woven bone formation around the scaffold indicating close contact. While good outcomes were observed in studies utilizing skeletally mature models, the challenges for regenerating skeletally immature bone are much different. For example, an alveolar cleft defect of the primary palate creates structural instability of the maxillary arch that could lead to an inability to support tooth eruption and cause facial asymmetry [19]. Current tissue engineering approaches must also be modified by considering the constraints of a growing maxillofacial skeleton. Thus, alternative therapies must be explored and employed such that premature suture fusion is not induced.

Skeletally Immature Translational Model

In scenarios involving cleft palate reconstruction in pediatric patients, autologous bone graft from the calvaria, iliac crest, and costal cartilage is limited by the volume and shape of harvestable bone, donor site morbidity, and in some instances a risk of infection. The ideal pediatric bone replacement would effectively fit and fill the defect site and restore structure and function while preserving harmonious growth. To test this hypothesis, a study was conducted in NZWR where unilateral 3.5 mm × 3.5 mm, full-thickness defects were created in the maxilla to simulate an alveolar cleft [45]. Defects were treated with custom 3D-printed scaffolds coated with bovine type 1 collagen and augmented with either 100, 1000, or 10,000 µM DIPY. Euthanasia at the 8-week time point revealed dose-dependent bone

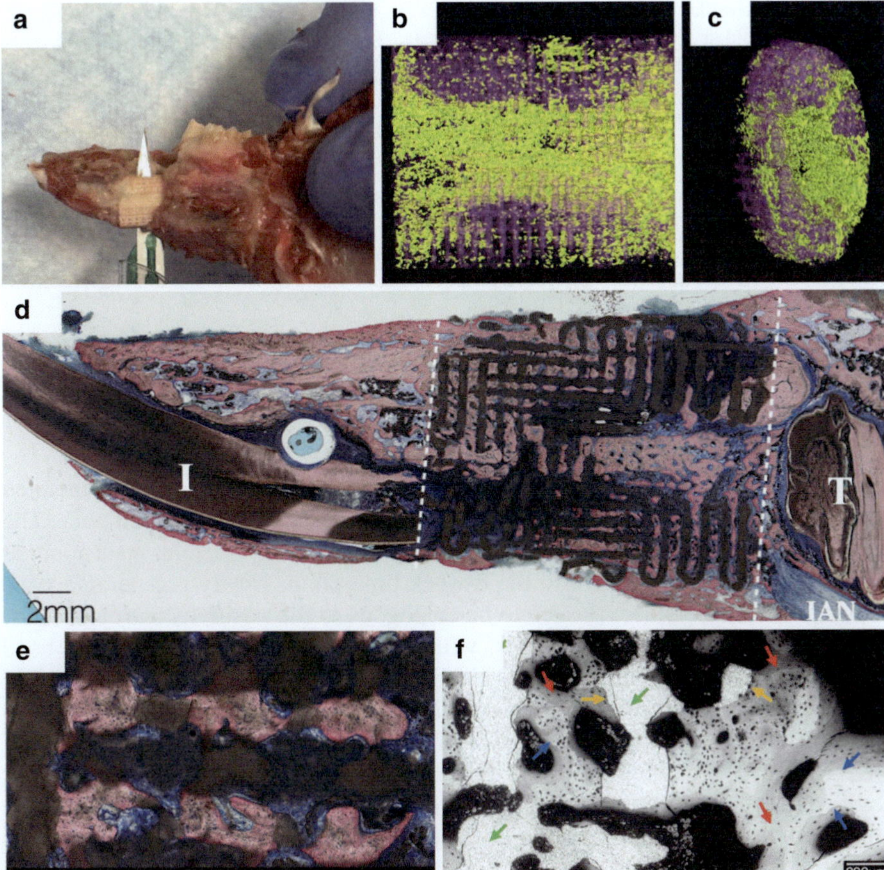

Fig. 16.5 (**a**) Scaffold integration with rabbit mandible, (**b**) lengthwise 3D reconstruction of scaffold, (**c**) end of scaffold with bony infiltration of lumen (scaffold in purple, bone in yellow), (**d**) sagittal histologic slice of scaffold in continuity with rabbit mandible, (**e**) high magnification from (**d**) demonstrating porous ingrowth, and highly cellular and vascularized woven bone structure, as well as newer, organized lamellar bone formation depicted by arrows. I, incisor; T, tooth; IAN, inferior alveolar nerve (color version of figure is available online). (**f**) Electron microscopy depicting scaffold struts (green arrows) and new bone formation throughout scaffold interstices (red arrows). New woven bone is seen filling sites of scaffold degradation (yellow arrows) and regions of lamellar reorganization juxtaposed with immature woven bone are evident (blue arrows, lamellar as brighter bone, woven is darker). (Reproduced with permission from Lopez CD, Diaz-Siso JR, Witek L, Bekisz JM, Cronstein BN, Torroni A, et al. Three-dimensionally printed bioactive ceramic scaffold osseoconduction across critical-sized mandibular defects. Journal of Surgical Research. 2018;223:115–22)

Fig. 16.6 (**a**) Alveolar cleft with scaffold at 8 weeks. Scaffold (black) lattice with bone growth (pink). Suture patency is noted as well in lower magnification (blue arrow) and (**b**) cranial sutures patent (yellow arrows) at 8 weeks evident with new bone growth in and around scaffold lattice structure (green arrows) [45, 46]

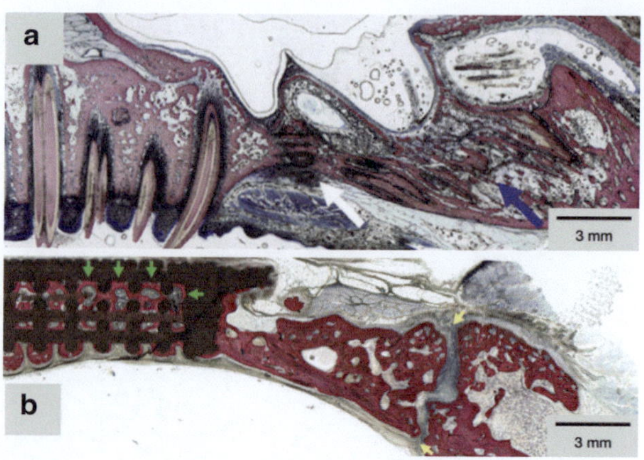

regeneration with no evidence of maxillary suture fusion (Fig. 16.6a). Regenerated bone density was increased compared to native contralateral unoperated bone. The long-term analysis revealed that there was substantial scaffold resorption at 24 weeks (6 months) relative to the 8-week time point. Newly regenerated bone using the 3DP scaffolds was seen to be analogous to the positive control animals, treated with autologous bone grafts, with no signs of asymmetry, ectopic bone growth, or morbidity. Furthermore, alveolar bone tissue was seen to ultimately remodel similar to native bone density without detriment to function when given enough time. Similarly, in an 8-week bilateral calvarial defect study involving NZWR, scaffold-induced bone growth was statistically greater than bone growth in empty defects ($p = 0.02$). Histologic analysis revealed patent calvarial sutures with no ectopic bone formation, among all (100, 1000, and 10,000 µM) DIPY concentrations [46] (Fig. 16.6b).

While the previously conducted studies have provided foundational evidence of effectiveness of 3DP β-TCP scaffolds in regenerating pediatric craniofacial defects, pediatric clinical applications would require successful implementation in a large, preclinical, translational animal model (e.g., swine). A recent study conducted on 6-week-old Göttingen minipigs served as an excellent pediatric preclinical animal model due to similarities to human bone morphology, regeneration, and wound healing [47, 48]. Unilateral calvarial defects (~1.4 cm) were created. Two groups of animals were implanted with scaffolds with or without a cap (both groups coated

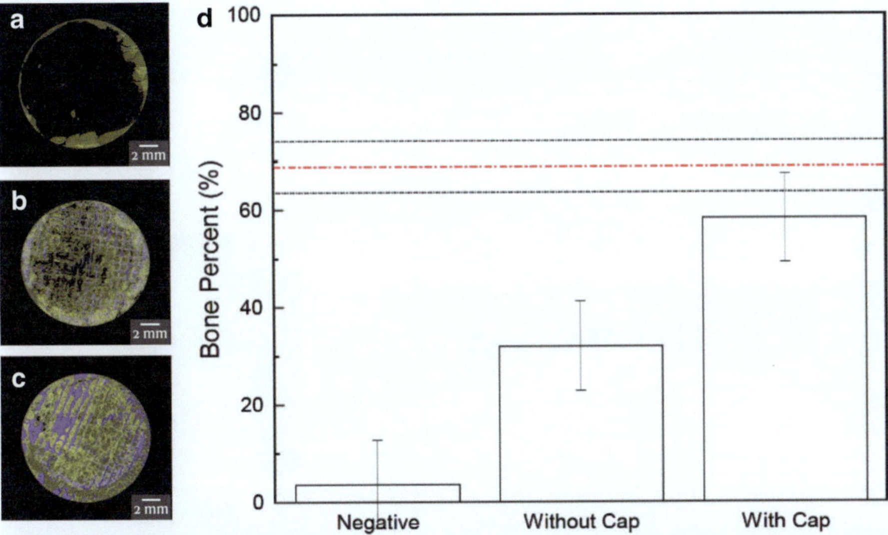

Fig. 16.7 3D reconstruction of the bone (yellow) and remaining scaffold (purple) in the defect site after 12 weeks of healing in a (**a**) negative control, (**b**) a defect that had been filled with a scaffold without a cap, (**c**) a defect that had been filled with a scaffold with a cap. (**d**) Bar graph presenting the mean (±95% CI) of bone that filled the defect sites in each group after 12 weeks of healing compared to the average bone density of native bone (red line). The horizontal dashed red line denotes the mean with corresponding 95% CI shown by the black horizontal lines

with 1000 μM DIPY), while a third group served as the negative control (no scaffold) (Figs. 16.7a and 16.8a). Animals were euthanized 12 weeks postoperatively. Defects repaired with scaffolds with caps yielded a significantly higher bone volume fraction (Fig. 16.7d) compared to defects repaired without caps ($p \leq 0.001$) (Figs. 16.7b, c, 16.8b, b.1, c, c.1).

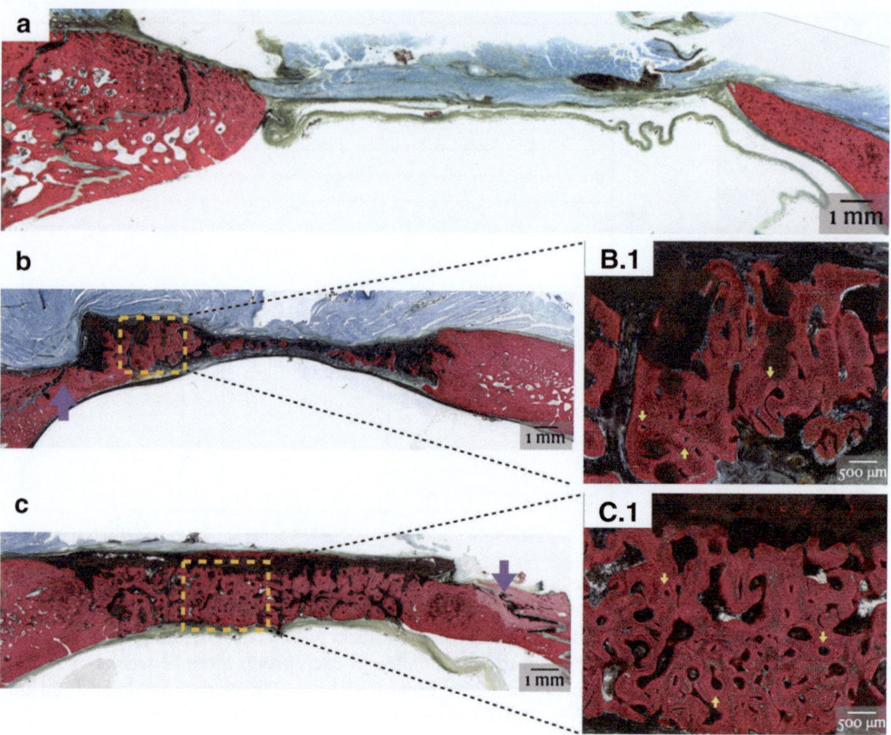

Fig. 16.8 Nondecalcified histologic sections of a (**a**) negative control after 12 weeks of healing. No bridging bone was seen across any of the unfilled defect sites, (**b**) defect filled with a scaffold that that did not contain a cap after 12 weeks of healing. Vascularized woven and lamellar bone formed throughout the defect site and cranial sutures remained patent (purple arrow). (**b.1**) Areas of mature, organized bone (yellow arrows) can be seen in the higher magnified portion of the slide. (**c**) Defect filled with a scaffold that included a cap after 12 weeks of healing. Vascularized woven and lamellar bone formed throughout the defect site and cranial sutures remained patent (purple arrow). (**c.1**) Areas of mature, organized bone (yellow arrows) can be seen in the higher magnified portion of the slide

Future Outlook

The field of CMF surgery has evolved from its sole purpose of treating a disease. With technological advancements in the field where new techniques and materials are continuously being developed, there has been an evolving need for innovative and comprehensive surgical care. To enable such advancements to proceed from bench to bedside deployment, a robust understanding of regenerative medicine and materials along with excellent surgical judgment is required. In the field of reconstructive surgery and more specifically the field of CMF, limited volume or poor bone quality has been a factor, which has warranted further research for alternatives. 3DP of porous, bioactive, and biocompatible CaP ceramic scaffolds thus far has shown excellent results in repairing critically sized bony defects. 3DP implants have not only shown an ability to perform the desired function of bone healing but have also induced favorable responses in the presence of physiological loads. Significant bone healing has hence been recorded in anatomic locations such as the mandible. Furthermore, the combination of 3DP scaffolds and $A_{2A}R$ activation has proven fruitful in augmenting bone growth in calvarial defects in large translational models without any changes to suture biology. Similar responses have been observed in alveolar cleft and calvarial defects in the growing craniofacial skeleton. With these advancements, however, come several challenges which surgeons should be aware of, in addition to fully understanding the principle components of tissue engineering: scaffolds, bioactive agents, and stem cell therapies. While scaffolds and pharmaceutical bioactive molecules have been explored and have shown favorable results, clinical deployment of stem cell therapies has not yet demonstrated desired outcomes [49, 50]. As such, regulatory concerns pose a major challenge in the deployment of some of these techniques for clinical trials. Nevertheless, the relative ease of 3DP, abundant material availability, and most importantly, proven, complete re-establishment of form and function at skeletal defect sites warrant further investigation, especially through direct translation in patients.

Acknowledgments The work presented in this chapter was supported by NIH/NIAMS (MPI-Cronstein, Coelho) R01AR068593, R01AR068593-S1, NIH/NICHD (MPI-Coelho, Flores, Crosntein, and Witek) R21R33HD090664, DoD (MPI-Rodriguez, Coelho) W81XWH-16-1-0772, and an Osteo Science Foundation Peter Geistlich Research Award (MPI-Coelho, Kasper, Young, and Witek). Dr. Coelho is a co-inventor of the 3D-printing technology presented in this chapter (Patent #: US20150150681A1).

References

1. Lanza RP. Principles of tissue engineering. 5th ed. London: Academic Press; 2020.
2. Seper L, Piffkó J, Joos U, Meyer U. Treatment of fractures of the atrophic mandible in the elderly. J Am Geriatr Soc. 2004;52(9):1583–4.
3. American Society of Plastic Surgeons. 2020 Plastic surgery statistics. Arlington Heights, IL: American Society of Plastic Surgeons; 2020. https://www.plasticsurgery.org/documents/News/Statistics/2020/plastic-surgery-statistics-full-report-2020.pdf.
4. Witek L, Colon RR, Wang MM, Torroni A, Young S, Melville J, et al. 24 - Tissue-engineered alloplastic scaffolds for reconstruction of alveolar defects. In: Mozafari M, Sefat F, Atala A, editors. Handbook of tissue engineering scaffolds, vol. 1. New Delhi: Woodhead Publishing; 2019. p. 505–20.
5. Lopez CD, Witek L, Torroni A, Flores RL, Demissie DB, Young S, et al. The role of 3D printing in treating craniomaxillofacial congenital anomalies. Birth Defects Res. 2018;110(13):1055–64.
6. Wang MM, Flores RL, Witek L, Torroni A, Ibrahim A, Wang Z, et al. Dipyridamole-loaded 3D-printed bioceramic scaffolds stimulate pediatric bone regeneration in vivo without disruption of craniofacial growth through facial maturity. Sci Rep. 2019;9(1):18439.
7. Lopez CD, Diaz-Siso JR, Witek L, Bekisz JM, Gil LF, Cronstein BN, et al. Dipyridamole augments three-dimensionally printed bioactive ceramic scaffolds to regenerate craniofacial bone. Plast Reconstr Surg. 2019;143(5):1408–19.

8. Gimbel M, Ashley RK, Sisodia M, Gabbay JS, Wasson KL, Heller J, et al. Repair of alveolar cleft defects: reduced morbidity with bone marrow stem cells in a resorbable matrix. J Craniofac Surg. 2007;18(4):895.

9. Wang RR, Andres CJ, Wang RR, Andres CJ. Hemifacial microsomia and treatment options for auricular replacement: a review of the literature. J Prosthet Dent. 1999;82(2):197–204.

10. Plomp RG, van Lieshout MJS, Joosten KFM, Wolvius EB, van der Schroeff MP, Versnel SL, et al. Treacher Collins Syndrome: a systematic review of evidence-based treatment and recommendations. Plast Reconstr Surg. 2016;137(1):191.

11. Fan KL, Federico C, Kawamoto HK, Bradley JP. Optimizing the timing and technique of Treacher Collins orbital malar reconstruction. J Craniofac Surg. 2012;23(7 Suppl 1):2033–7.

12. Shen C, et al. Three-dimensional printing for craniofacial bone tissue engineering. Tissue Eng A. 2020;26(23–24):1303–11.

13. Dawood A, Marti Marti B, Sauret-Jackson V, Darwood A. 3D printing in dentistry. Br Dent J. 2015;219(11):521–9.

14. Baker MI, Eberhardt AW, Martin DM, McGwin G, Lemons JE. Bone properties surrounding hydroxyapatite-coated custom osseous integrated dental implants. J Biomed Mater Res B Appl Biomater. 2010;95(1):218–24.

15. Ducheyne P, De Groot K. In vivo surface activity of a hydroxyapatite alveolar bone substitute. J Biomed Mater Res. 1981;15(3):441–5.

16. Ducheyne P, Hench LL, Kagan A II, Martens M, Bursens A, Mulier JC. Effect of hydroxyapatite impregnation on skeletal bonding of porous coated implants. J Biomed Mater Res. 1980;14(3):225–37.

17. Ducheyne P, Van Raemdonck W, Heughebaert JC, Heughebaert M. Structural analysis of hydroxyapatite coatings on titanium. Biomaterials. 1986;7(2):97–103.

18. Duheyne P, Beight J, Cuckler J, Evans B, Radin S. Effect of calcium phosphate coating characteristics on early post-operative bone tissue ingrowth. Biomaterials. 1990;11(8):531–40.

19. Lopez CD, Witek L, Flores RL, Torroni A, Rodriguez ED, Cronstein BN, et al. 3D printing and adenosine receptor activation for craniomaxillofacial regeneration. In: Melville JC, Shum JW, Young S, Wong ME, editors. Regenerative strategies for maxillary and mandibular reconstruction: a practical guide. Cham: Springer International Publishing; 2019. p. 255–67.

20. Tovar N, Witek L, Atria P, Sobieraj M, Bowers M, Lopez CD, et al. Form and functional repair of long bone using 3D-printed bioactive scaffolds. J Tissue Eng Regen Med. 2018;12(9):1986–99.

21. Witek L, Smay J, Silva NRFA, Guda T, Ong JL, Coelho PG. Sintering effects on chemical and physical properties of bioactive ceramics. J Adv Ceram. 2013;2(3):274–84.

22. Moore WR, Graves SE, Bain GI. Synthetic bone graft substitutes. ANZ J Surg. 2001;71(6):354–61.

23. Shen C, Wang MM, Witek L, Tovar N, Cronstein BN, Torroni A, et al. Transforming the degradation rate of β-tricalcium phosphate bone replacement using 3-dimensional printing. Ann Plast Surg. 2021;87(6):e153.

24. Smay JE, Lewis JA. Solid free-form fabrication of 3-D ceramic structures. Ceramics and composites processing methods. 1st ed. Hoboken, NJ: Wiley; 2012. p. 459–84.

25. Melville JC, Nassari NN, Hanna IA, Shum JW, Wong ME, Young S. Immediate transoral allogeneic bone grafting for large mandibular defects. Less morbidity, more bone. A paradigm in benign tumor mandibular reconstruction? J Oral Maxillofac Surg. 2017;75(4):828–38.

26. Melville JC, Shum JW, Young S, Wong ME. Regenerative strategies for maxillary and mandibular reconstruction: a practical guide. New York, NY: Springer; 2019.

27. Jäger M, Herten M, Fochtmann U, Fischer J, Hernigou P, Zilkens C, et al. Bridging the gap: bone marrow aspiration concentrate reduces autologous bone grafting in osseous defects. J Orthop Res. 2011;29(2):173–80.

28. Melville JC, Tursun R, Green JM III, Marx RE. Reconstruction of a post-traumatic maxillary ridge using a radial forearm free flap and immediate tissue engineering (bone morphogenetic

protein, bone marrow aspirate concentrate, and cortical-cancellous bone): case report. J Oral Maxillofac Surg. 2017;75(2):438.e1–6.

29. Costa MA, Barbosa A, Neto E, Sá-e-Sousa A, Freitas R, Neves JM, et al. On the role of sub-type selective adenosine receptor agonists during proliferation and osteogenic differentiation of human primary bone marrow stromal cells. J Cell Physiol. 2011;226(5):1353–66.

30. Mediero A, Cronstein BN. Adenosine and bone metabolism. Trends Endocrinol Metab. 2013;24(6):290–300.

31. Mediero A, Frenkel SR, Wilder T, He W, Mazumder A, Cronstein BN. Adenosine A2A receptor activation prevents wear particle-induced osteolysis. Sci Transl Med. 2012;4(135):135ra65.

32. Mediero A, Wilder T, Perez-Aso M, Cronstein BN. Direct or indirect stimulation of adenosine A2A receptors enhances bone regeneration as well as bone morphogenetic protein-2. FASEB J. 2015;29(4):1577–90.

33. Mediero A, Wilder T, Reddy VS, Cheng Q, Tovar N, Coelho PG, et al. Ticagrelor regulates osteoblast and osteoclast function and promotes bone formation in vivo via an adenosine-dependent mechanism. FASEB J. 2016;30(11):3887–900.

34. Bekisz JM, Flores RL, Witek L, Lopez CD, Runyan CM, Torroni A, et al. Dipyridamole enhances osteogenesis of three-dimensionally printed bioactive ceramic scaffolds in calvarial defects. J Craniomaxillofac Surg. 2018;46(2):237–44.

35. Martin C, Leone M, Viviand X, Ayem ML, Guieu R. High adenosine plasma concentration as a prognostic index for outcome in patients with septic shock. Crit Care Med. 2000;28(9):3198–202.

36. Cronstein BN, Kramer SB, Weissmann G, Hirschhorn R. A new physiological function for adenosine: regulation of superoxide anion production. Trans Assoc Am Phys. 1983;96:384–91.

37. Fitz Gerald GA. Dipyridamole. N Engl J Med. 1987;316(20):1247–57.

38. Patrono C, Coller B, Dalen JE, Fuster V, Gent M, Harker LA, et al. Platelet-active drugs: the relationships among dose, effectiveness, and side effects. Chest. 1998;114(5 Suppl):470s–88s.

39. Monagle P, Chan AK, Goldenberg NA, Ichord RN, Journeycake JM, Nowak-Göttl U, et al. Antithrombotic therapy in neonates and children: antithrombotic therapy and prevention of thrombosis: American College of Chest Physicians Evidence-Based Clinical Practice Guidelines. Chest. 2012;141(2):e737S–801S.

40. Ishack S, Mediero A, Wilder T, Ricci JL, Cronstein BN. Bone regeneration in critical bone defects using three-dimensionally printed β-tricalcium phosphate/hydroxyapatite scaffolds is enhanced by coating scaffolds with either dipyridamole or BMP-2. J Biomed Mater Res B Appl Biomater. 2017;105(2):366–75.

41. Carragee EJ, Hurwitz EL, Weiner BK. A critical review of recombinant human bone morpho-genetic protein-2 trials in spinal surgery: emerging safety concerns and lessons learned. Spine J. 2011;11(6):471–91.

42. Spiro AS, Beil FT, Baranowsky A, Barvencik F, Schilling AF, Nguyen K, et al. BMP-7-induced ectopic bone formation and fracture healing is impaired by systemic NSAID application in C57BL/6-mice. J Orthop Res. 2010;28(6):785–91.

43. Kinsella CR, Cray JJ, Durham EL, Burrows AM, Vecchione L, Smith DM, et al. Recombinant human bone morphogenetic protein-2-induced craniosynostosis and growth restriction in the immature skeleton. Plast Reconstr Surg. 2011;127(3):1173–81.

44. Lopez CD, Diaz-Siso JR, Witek L, Bekisz JM, Cronstein BN, Torroni A, et al. Three dimensionally printed bioactive ceramic scaffold osseo conduction across critical-sized mandibular defects. J Surg Res. 2018;223:115–22.

45. Lopez CD, Coelho PG, Witek L, Torroni A, Greenberg MI, Cuadrado DL, et al. Regeneration of a pediatric alveolar cleft model using three-dimensionally printed bioceramic scaffolds and osteogenic agents: comparison of dipyridamole and rhBMP-2. Plast Reconstr Surg. 2019;144(2):358.

46. Maliha SG, Lopez CD, Coelho PG, Witek L, Cox M, Meskin A, et al. Bone Tissue engineering in the growing calvaria using dipyridamole-coated, three-dimensionally-printed bioceramic

scaffolds: construct optimization and effects on cranial suture patency. Plast Reconstr Surg. 2020;145(2):337e–47e.
47. McGovern JA, Griffin M, Hutmacher DW. Animal models for bone tissue engineering and modelling disease. Dis Model Mech. 2018;11(4):dmm033084.
48. Li Y, Chen SK, Li L, Qin L, Wang XL, Lai YX. Bone defect animal models for testing efficacy of bone substitute biomaterials. J Orthop Transl. 2015;3(3):95–104.
49. Weinand C, Neville CM, Weinberg E, Tabata Y, Vacanti JP. Optimizing biomaterials for tissue engineering human bone using mesenchymal stem cells. Plast Reconstr Surg. 2016;137(3):854–63.
50. Cooper GM, Miller ED, Decesare GE, Usas A, Lensie EL, Bykowski MR, et al. Inkjet-based biopatterning of bone morphogenetic protein-2 to spatially control calvarial bone formation. Tissue Eng Part A. 2010;16(5):1749–59.

Chapter 17
Tissue Engineering in Maxillofacial Reconstruction: Past, Present, and Future

Jeffrey S. Marschall, Mark E. Wong, Simon Young , Robert E. Marx,
Chi T. Viet, Anthony B. Morlandt, and James C. Melville

Introduction: Basic Principles of Maxillomandibular Tissue Engineering and Reconstruction

Reconstruction of maxillomandibular defects resulting from trauma or tumor ablation is a ubiquitous, formidable, and controversial challenge for maxillofacial surgeons. The maxillofacial region is a complex and highly visible region with

J. S. Marschall (✉)
Department of Oral and Maxillofacial Surgery, University of Iowa Hospital and Clinics,
Iowa City, IA, USA
e-mail: jsmarschall@uiowa.edu

M. E. Wong
Bernard & Gloria Pepper Katz Department of Oral and Maxillofacial Surgery, University of
Texas School of Dentistry Houston, Houston, TX, USA
e-mail: Mark.E.Wong@uth.tmc.edu

S. Young · J. C. Melville
Department of Oral and Maxillofacial Surgery, The University of Texas Health Science
Center at Houston, Houston, TX, USA
e-mail: Simon.Young@uth.tmc.edu; James.C.Melville@uth.tmc.edu

R. E. Marx
Department of Oral and Maxillofacial Surgery, University of Miami School of Medicine,
Florida, USA

C. T. Viet
Oral and Maxillofacial Surgery, Loma Linda University, Loma Linda, CA, USA
e-mail: chi.viet@LLU.edu

A. B. Morlandt
Oral and Maxillofacial Surgery, University of Alabama at Birmingham,
Birmingham, Alabama, USA
e-mail: morlandt@uab.edu

J. C. Melville et al. (eds.), *Advancements and Innovations in OMFS, ENT, and
Facial Plastic Surgery*, https://doi.org/10.1007/978-3-031-32099-6_17

specialized functions. The obvious functions of speech, deglutination, mastication, facial expression, and airway maintenance play a critical role in a patient's quality of life. Furthermore, the cosmesis of this region plays, perhaps, an equal or greater role in the patient's quality of life. Taken together, reconstruction of this anatomic area must consider and recapitulate these functions and restore the patient to his/her presurgical state.

The fundamental considerations of maxillomandibular reconstruction are often the size and location of the defect. Taking this further, one must also consider the tissues missing from the defect. Although focus is generally centered toward bony reconstruction, the astute surgeon must consider reconstruction of all tissues missing. For example, if a post-ablative defect results in missing teeth, nerve, and bone, the surgeon should be inclined to replace the teeth, nerve, and bone. Collectively, these concepts guide the reconstructive approach. Recently, the principles of tissue engineering (Fig. 17.1); that is, using scaffolds, cells, and bioactive molecules (cytokines and growth factors) to promote regeneration of missing tissues is starting to change the way surgeons approach reconstructing these defects. This chapter will describe the past, present, and future applications of maxillomandibular reconstruction and tissue engineering.

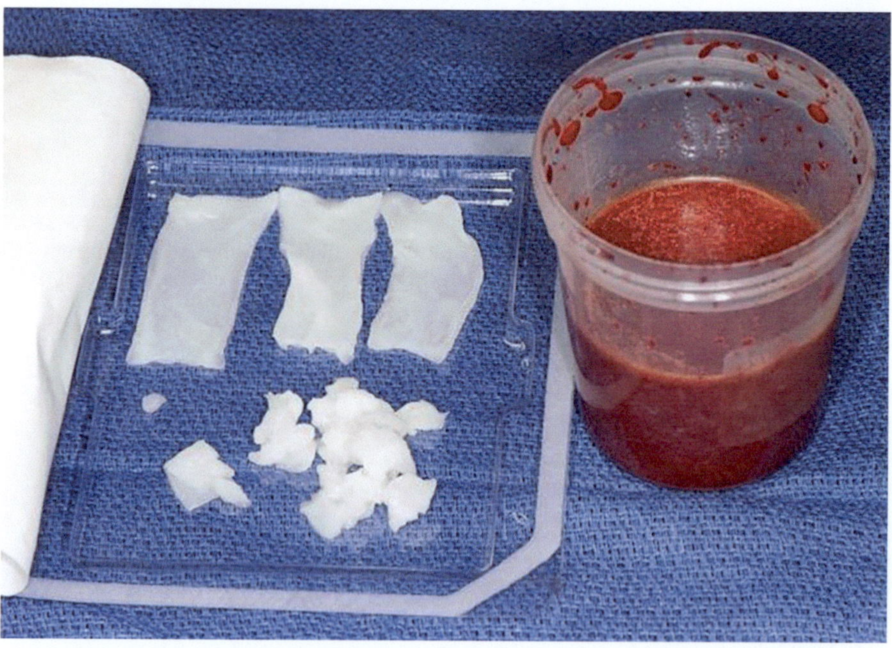

Fig. 17.1 The tissue-engineered triangle in clinical application osteoconductive (allogeneic bone), osteoinductive (rh-BMP2), and osteogenic (mesenchymal and stem cells from bone marrow)

Traditional Non-vascular Bone Grafts

Non-vascularized free bone grafts have stood the test of time and are an excellent solution for reconstructing bony defects of the maxillofacial skeleton, although they have limitations. Non-autogenous grafts are available to surgeons as allografts (donor is same species) or as xenografts (bone from different species, i.e., bovine/porcine) [1].

Allografts and xenografts are available as mineralized, demineralized, fresh, frozen, or freeze-dried [1]. These grafts go through extensive processing to remove antigenic components and to ensure sterility. Due to this processing, these grafts function biologically as osteoconductive scaffolds. Particulate and block allo/xenografts are used for small dentoalveolar bony defects (i.e., socket preservation technique; guided bone regeneration). Recently, tissue engineering technology using particulate allografts in conjunction with autogenous marrow and recombinant bone morphogenetic protein (rh-BMP) has been used to reconstruct large mandibular defects [2]. Furthermore, new specially processed cellularized bone matrices (e.g., Vivigen, LifeNet Health) have been used to reconstruct large mandibular defects [3]. This will be discussed in greater detail later in this chapter.

Autogenous free bone grafts remain the gold standard for many situations in maxillomandibular reconstruction. Non-vascular free bone grafts have traditionally been used for reconstruction of mandibular defects less than 6 cm in length in healthy soft tissue beds that have not been subjected to radiation [4, 5]. Recently, the long-standing "6-cm rule" is being challenged [2, 3, 6, 7]. Autogenous non-vascular bone grafts can be harvested as cancellous bone and marrow and cortical and corticocancellous bone. Common locations include the anterior and posterior iliac crest and proximal tibia.

The anterior and posterior iliac crests are common sites to harvest autogenous free bone grafts. Indeed, Obwegeser demonstrated transoral iliac crest bone grafting to be successful in a series of cases as far back as 1966 [8]. One of the advantages of harvesting grafts from this region is the versatility. Surgeons have the option of particulate cancellous grafts, cortical block grafts, or corticocancellous block grafts. Immobilization is key for any graft to prevent resorption and failure; block grafts allow for screw fixation and complete immobilization. The anterior iliac crest is generally a more common site for harvest. The anterior iliac crest can yield approximately 50 cm^3 of uncompressed cancellous bone or a cortical block of 5 × 3 cm [9–11]. The bone harvested from the anterior iliac crest is excellent for fracture nonunions, alveolar clefts, sinus lifting, and filling in mandibular defects with or without titanium mesh. The complications associated with anterior iliac crest graft harvest range from 1% to 25% and are most commonly hematoma, seroma, infection, and nerve injuries [12]. If larger amounts (greater than 60 cm^3 of uncompressed cancellous bone) of the bone are required, the posterior iliac crest is preferred. One hundred cubic centimeter of uncompressed bone may be harvested [11]. The primary downside to harvesting bone from the posterior iliac crest is that the patient needs to be placed in the prone position, which can add substantial time to a procedure.

The proximal tibia bone graft is an excellent source for cancellous bone. This procedure is relatively easy to perform with a low complication rate [13]. Twenty five cubic centimeter of cancellous bone can be harvested from a single site [13]. However, this rate is variable. Interestingly an investigation by Engelstad and Morse demonstrated that the proximal tibia yielded a significantly greater mean volume of compressed cancellous bone when compared to the anterior iliac crest [14]. Cancellous bone from the proximal tibia has been demonstrated to be a predictable graft for a variety of mandibular defects both large and small [3, 6, 15].

Growth Factors for Maxillomandibular Reconstruction

Bone repair can be divided into three distinct phases: (1) the inflammatory phase, (2) the repair phase, and (3) the remodeling phase [16, 17]. These phases are carefully orchestrated by a plethora of growth factors and the cells these factors recruit. Growth factors can be used to enhance each of these biological processes. Furthermore, growth factors are essential for generalized cell fate processes (replication, migration, differentiation, etc.); development of materials that deliver specific growth factor(s) can help modify and enhance these processes. These growth factors, when considered in the context of oral and maxillofacial surgery, are broadly classified as blood-borne bioactive modifiers (e.g., PRP and PRF) and recombinant growth factors. Perhaps the first clinically relevant source of growth factors that was used on a wide scale was platelet-rich plasma (PRP) [18]. PRP is easily assessable and contains several biologically relevant growth factors, including platelet-derived growth factor, transforming growth factor beta, fibroblast growth factor, insulin-like growth factors 1 and 2, and vascular endothelial growth factor [19, 20]. One of the drawbacks of PRP is the widely varying concentration of growth factors and delivery kinetics. Growth factor release from PRP occurs rapidly. Growth factors are sequestered within the extracellular matrix, and cells need sustained delivery of these factors over many days to weeks [21]. Platelet-rich fibrin (PRF) was developed to mimic a more physiologic growth factor release profile [22]. As mentioned above, tissue engineering requires the presence of a three-dimensional scaffold for cells that can differentiate into the tissues that are missing; ideally growth factors would be present within the matrix to help recruitment and differentiation of these cells. The fibrin within PRF serves as a scaffold; platelets and leukocytes are present within the matrix that has plethora of bioactive growth factors. Furthermore, because the growth factors are within the fibrin matrix in PRF, the release kinetics mimic what is seen physiologically [20]. These characteristics have led to a wide use of PRF clinically; PRF has been used as an adjunct for reconstructing large mandibular resections [3, 6], guided bone regeneration [23], sinus augmentation [24], and other dentoalveolar procedures.

Bone morphogenetic proteins (BMPs) were initially identified in the 1960s. Part of the transforming growth factor-β superfamily, BMPs are a class of some 20 proteins that have been demonstrated to induce angiogenesis, cell death, inflammation, and bone and cartilage formation [25]. Specifically, BMP-2 has been demonstrated to be one of the most osteogenic growth factors [26]. BMP-2 binds to its cell surface receptor on undifferentiated mesenchymal cells and activates the SMAD family of transcription factors [25]. Ultimately, this leads to osteoblast differentiation, osteoblast chemotaxis, osteogenesis, and extracellular matrix production [25]. BMP-2's osteoinductivity is particularly useful when combined with allografts or xenografts that do not have intrinsic osteoinduction; this potentially accelerates the ingrowth of native bone cells making these alloplastic materials more similar to autografts [27–30]. BMP-2 is available clinically as rh-BMP-2 (Infuse, Medtronic). Recent studies demonstrate that rhBMP-2 while using an absorbable collagen sponge along with allo- and/or xenografts has comparable and, in some cases, superior results compared to the gold standard autografts in alveolar cleft grafting [31], alveolar bone regeneration [29, 32, 33], and critically sized maxillary and mandibular bone defects [33, 34]. Complications associated with rhBMP-2 use are generally seen in spinal fusion cases versus cases of maxillofacial reconstruction [35]. Complications associated with maxillofacial use are severe edema/swelling, erythema, and dysphagia [36, 37]. These complications are self-limiting and generally do not affect the success rate of the graft.

Current Methods of Maxillofacial Tissue Engineering

In the history of mandibular reconstruction, in situ tissue engineering was only introduced within the past 20 years. It has mostly replaced autogenous non-vascularized block grafts and non-vascularized cancellous marrow grafts.

Non-vascularized block grafts are noted for their dual morbidity and poor long-term bone regeneration, that is, pain, bleeding, and complications at both the donor and recipient sites and resorption of the graft due to incomplete and/or delayed revascularization. Autogenous cancellous marrow grafts regenerate a full graft volume of bone and are durable. Along with free microvascular osteocutaneous grafts, it has been in common utilization from the 1990s to the present. However, cancellous marrow graft's donor site morbidity, increased operating time, and increased hospital stay, although less than a free vascular osteocutaneous graft, were significantly more than an in situ tissue-engineered graft that had no donor site and less than half of the operating time and hospital stay of a cancellous marrow graft (Table 17.1). In situ tissue-engineered grafts also have only one third of the operating time and one fifth of the hospital stay of a microvascular osteocutaneous graft (Table 17.1). These advantages of in situ tissue-engineered grafts in addition to the patient's earlier return to work and family have catapulted in situ tissue-engineered grafts to a common and growing utilization in mandibular reconstructions.

Table 17.1 Comparison of cortical cancellous graft (autogenous), tissue engineering (rhBMP-2 + allogeneic bone), and free fibula microvascular reconstruction

Continuity Defects 6 cm or Greater			
	CCM	**In-Situ Tissue Engineering**	**Fibula**
Continuity	145/151 (96%)	266/277 (96%)	128/138 (93%)
Vertical Height	140/151 (93%)	260/277 (94%)	66/138 (48%)
Donor Site	151/151 (100%)	0 (0%)	138/138 (100%)
Average OR Time	5.7 h	3.7 h	10.4 h
Hospital Stay	4.2 days	1.7 days	11.3 days
Cost	$41,300	$21,400	$89,000

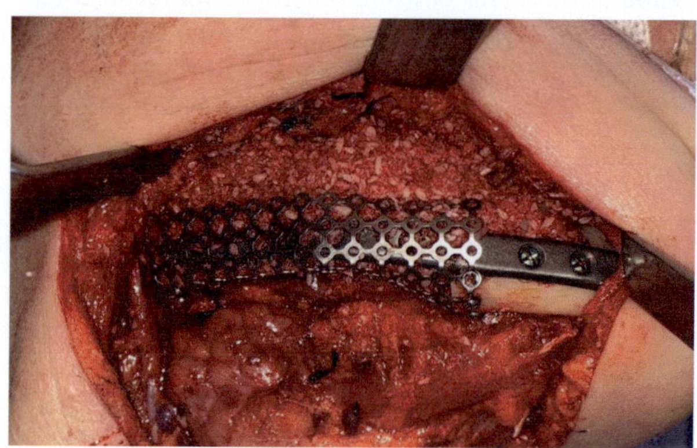

Fig. 17.2 Large tissue-engineered graft in particulate form condensed into post-ablative defect

Tissue engineering can eliminate donor site morbidity, reduce operating times and overall costs, and return patients back to their work and families sooner. As stated above, the cornerstone of tissue engineering is delivering cells, growth factors, and a scaffold to regenerate a target tissue. Current methods of maxillofacial tissue engineering have been referred to as "in situ tissue engineering" (Figs. 17.2, 17.3, 17.4, 17.5, and 17.6) [7]. Currently, clinicians can access autogenous stem and progenitor cells via bone marrow aspirate concentrate (BMAC). BMAC is obtained at the point of care and can yield a clinically significant amount of mesenchymal stem cells (MSCs) and osteoprogenitor cells (OPCs) [38]. Combined with an immediate centrifugation method, the percentage of MSCs can be exponentially increased [39]. Another important component to the tissue engineering triangle is the scaffold. Particulate allogeneic bone can be utilized as a biological scaffold. Lastly, rhBMP-2 is used to provide the required cellular signals to promote tissue (i.e., bone)

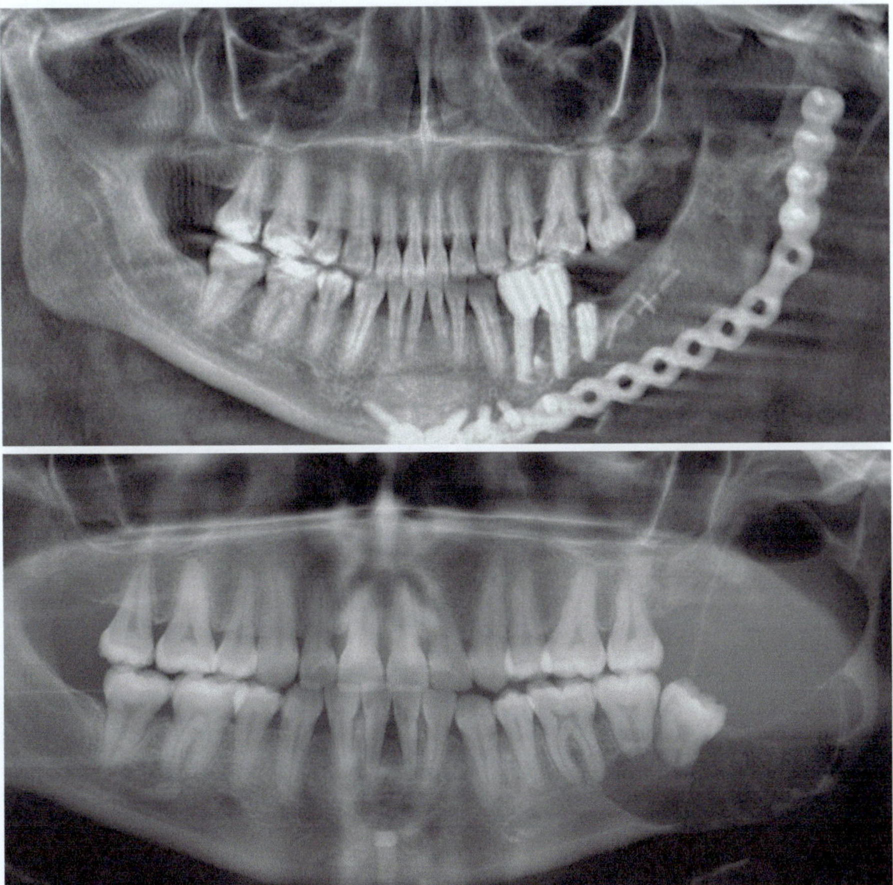

Fig. 17.3 Immediate reconstruction with tissue-engineered grafts are reliable and predicable with proper surgical technique and most importantly adequate soft tissue coverage

regeneration [40]. Using this composite tissue-engineered grafting method, Melville et al. demonstrated success in 30 of 34 patients with large mandibular continuity defects [7]. The synergistic relationship between BMAC and rhBMP-2 has been studied at the histologic level [41]. Using animal models, Egashria et al. showed that the use of BMAC will accelerate the bone formation rate in the early transplantation phase when rhBMP-2 has been used concurrently and will allow for a reduction of the rhBMP-2 dosage [41].

Although the free fibula flap is an excellent option for composite, hemi/complete mandibular defects or patients who have been radiated, donor site morbidity and the cost of the procedure should be considered. A retrospective, multicenter study reported mean hospital charges and duration for 42 patients who received a fibula free flap of $140,747 and 10.5 days, respectively [42]. The advantages of in situ

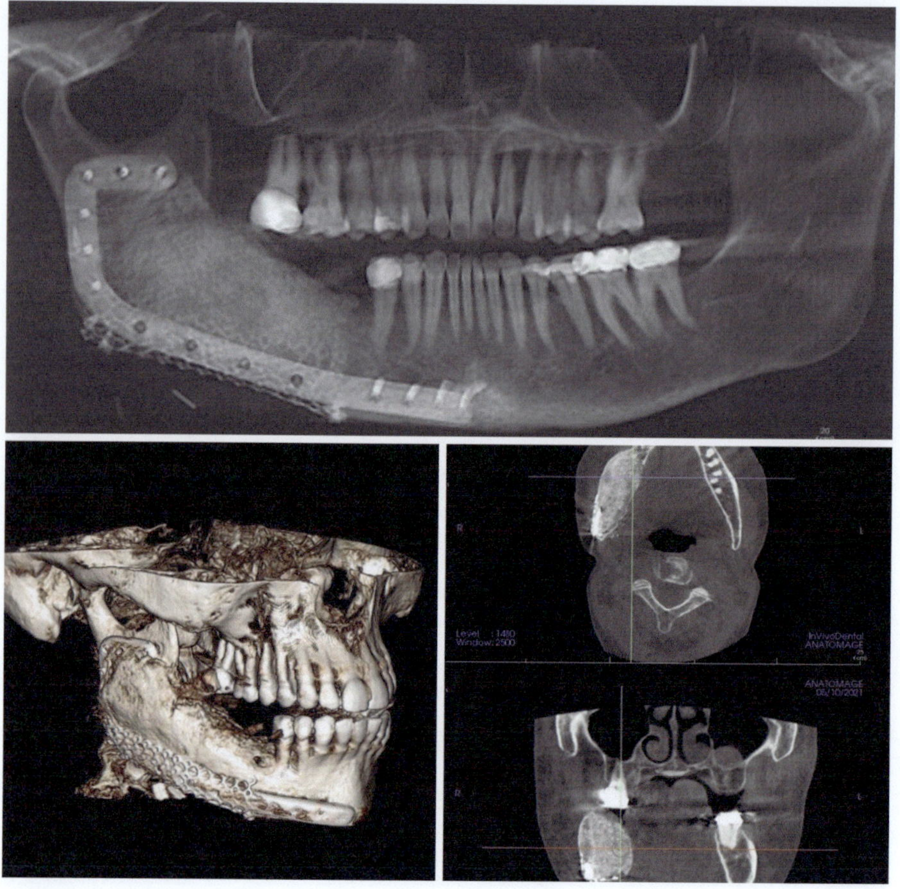

Fig. 17.4 Tissue-engineered grafts are excellent for reconstruction of nature shape and contours of the mandible. Ideal shape and dimensions are propagated by masticatory muscle attachment and function

tissue engineering composite graft are severalfold; first, there is much lower morbidity especially when compared to free flap harvest. Furthermore, there are lower healthcare costs and proven surgical efficiency [7].

The Cells

The specifics of in situ tissue engineering for mandibular reconstruction have been worked out to predictably regenerate genetically normal human bone that matures and remodels as do other parts of the skeleton. The cells are derived from a bone

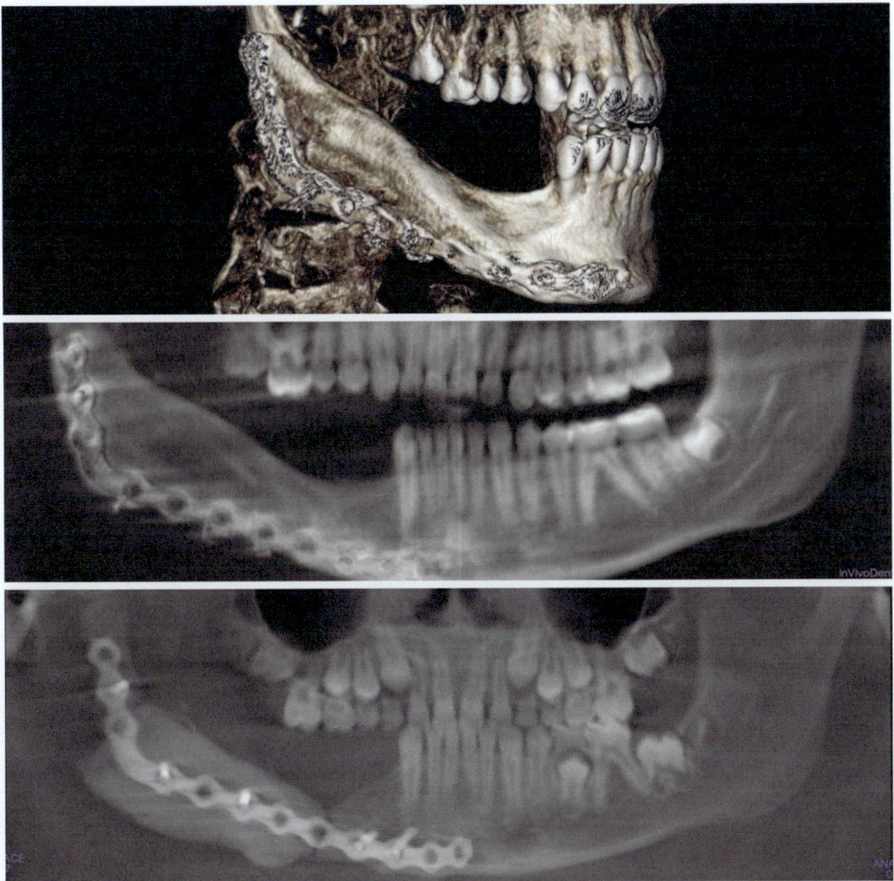

Fig. 17.5 Excellent regeneration of mandible with secondary grafting. Size and shape of mandibular regeneration is 100% on soft tissue bed

marrow aspirate (BMA) that has in the past been centrifuged to concentrate the osteoprogenitor cells (OPCs) and mesenchymal stem cells (MSC). However, recent studies have identified a 20% or greater death rate of OPC and MSC due to the g-forces of centrifugation. Today, the preferred bone marrow harvesting devices do not use centrifugation and those with flexible cannulas produce the higher yields of OPC/MSC as shown by cultured explants referred to as colony-forming units-fibroblast-like (CFU-f). Such higher yields of stem cells have been shown to regenerate bone faster and produce more bone and bone with a greater mineral content. Therefore, yields of CD34+ cells should be on the order of 330×10^3 cells/mL and grow 3000 or more viable bone-producing cells documented by CFU-f (Table 17.2).

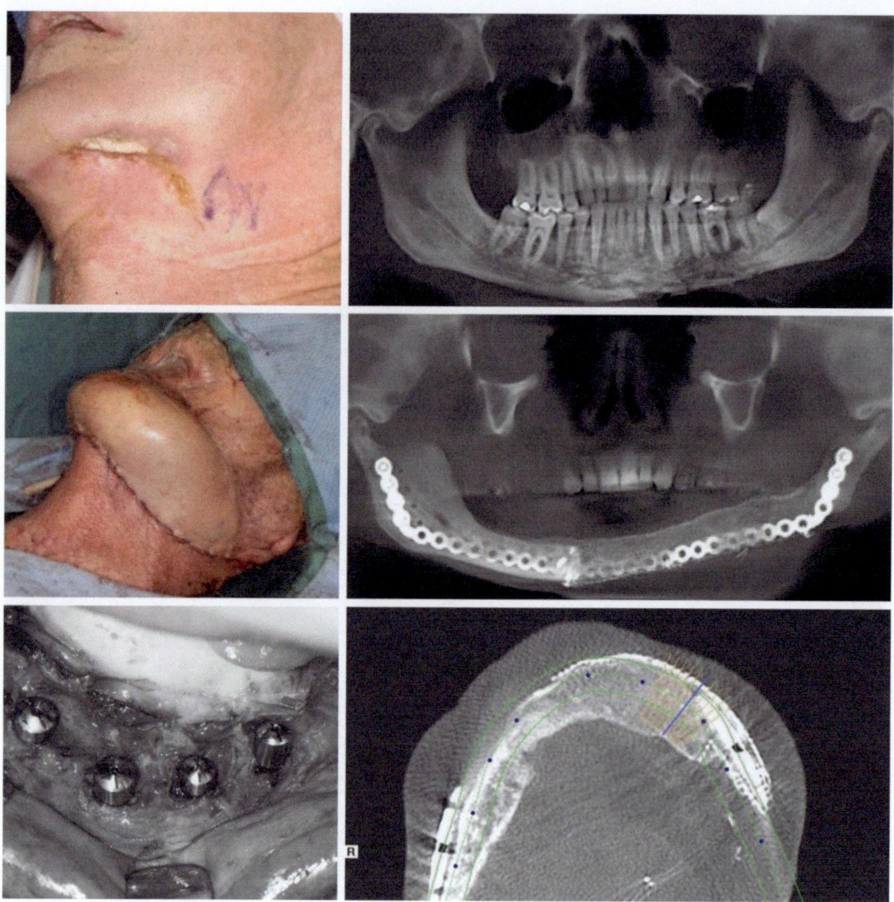

Fig. 17.6 Osteoradionecrosis patient with multiple failed salvage surgeries. Successfully reconstructed with anterior lateral thigh free flap and tissue-engineered graft. By optimizing biology, we expect once difficult cases to become routine and predictable

Table 17.2 Stem cell counts

	Volume	CD34+ 10^3/ml	CD105+ 10^3/ml	CFUF /ml
BMAC	**10 mL**	172	114	1,234
Straight Needle	**10 mL**	252	173	2,060
Flex Metrics	**10 mL**	334	396	3,095
Δ FM vs. SN		82	228	1,035

The Signal

The signal is a recombinant human bone morphogenetic protein-2/acellular collagen sponge (rhBMP-2/ACS Infuse Bone Graft® Medtronic). The dose of rhBMP-2/ACS has been determined to be 1 mg/1 cm length of mandibular bony continuity defect. The rhBMP-2/ACS acts over the first 21 days of the graft with its greatest activity being within the first 14 days. As a specific bone morphogen, it will induce the required proliferation of the OPC/MSCs in the BMA and their differentiation and actual bone production. By day 21, the rhBMP-2/ACS has been used and is no longer present. However, osteoid and a complete revascularization of the graft have occurred. The graft now goes into a self-remodeling cycle toward maturity, which can be seen radiographically as a consolidation.

The Matrix

The matrix is a cancellous freeze-dried mineralized allogeneic bone, with a particle size of 100–300 μm. The matrix also includes the proteins in the bone marrow plasma, fibrin, fibronectin, and vitronectin, as well as the exosomes in the bone marrow plasma released by the OPC/MSCs prior to harvesting. One such exosomal protein, stromal-derived activation factor 1-alpha (SDAF1-alpha), is a critical support protein for stem cells.

The proteins in the bone marrow plasma connect and bind the allogeneic bone particles together. It is on this surface that the new bone will regenerate and fuse together with adjacent niduses of bone formation that are recognized radiographically as the graft consolidates and becomes more mineral dense. By the time of maturity at 6 months, the graft can receive dental implants with good primary stability. At that time, all the allogeneic bone particles have been resorbed and replaced by the patient's own bone. The bone is all the patient's own bone. It will osseointegrate implants, it will heal, it will respond to orthodontic tooth movement, and it will grow normally in growing children without overgrowth or undergrowth.

During composite resection of the mandible (and other areas of the facial skeleton), the bone, soft tissue, nerve, and teeth are removed. Recently, nerve allografts have become available, which have demonstrated excellent results [43]. However, if a patient wishes to have complete reconstruction and dental rehabilitation completed in a single surgery, currently, the only option is the "Jaw-in-a-Day" procedure.

Future Methods of Maxillofacial Tissue Engineering

The future of maxillofacial tissue engineering and bone regeneration has been centered around several areas: first, 3D printing of bioactive scaffolds to provide tailored osteoconduction [44] and second the delivery of specific bioactive molecules from materials [16].

Over the last decade, the geometric design of implants on several orders of magnitude has been demonstrated to play a profound role on osteoconduction and ultimately bone healing [45]. The original studies were completed with metallic implants. More recently, these principles have been translated to biomolecules that are much more osteogenic such as calcium phosphate-based bioactive ceramics [46]. Usually calcium phosphate-based bio-ceramics are powder based. The advent of 3D printing has led to the development of personalized scaffolds by using CAD/CAM methods. Promising data is being developed utilizing 3D-printed bioactive β-tricalcium phosphate scaffolds that selectively stimulate A2AR receptors. Another area of future development is the use of layer-by-layer deposition of robotic printed hydrogels and cells with precise position of growth factor presenting matrices and microtissues [16]. For example, a custom-tailored material could selectively release the factors required for ideal bone healing, that is, migration-inducing growth factors, proliferation-inducing growth factors, and lastly, differentiation-inducing growth factors (Fig. 17.6) [16].

Conclusion

Maxillomandibular reconstruction is a controversial and essential component to craniomaxillofacial surgery. The basic and clinical science behind reconstruction of ablative and traumatic defects has progressed considerably. Progenitor and stem cell use in in situ tissue engineering today is in its infancy. For now, bone regeneration has led the way. The next horizon is cartilage, which is already underway with intra-joint injections of stem cells. The skin and oral mucosa are very doable but are only at the beginning stages. Teeth and major organs (i.e., kidney, liver, and heart) are a very long way off in the future due to the complexity of these organs. Treatment of stroke through intraarterial stem cell injections and even intravenous injections for lung congestion in COVID cases has shown significant benefit in a few cases. However, FDA and their governmental restrictions limit its expansion.

References

1. Khan SN, Cammisa FP Jr, Sandhu HS, et al. The biology of bone grafting. J Am Acad Orthop Surg. 2005;13(1):77–86.
2. Melville JC, Nassari NN, Hanna IA, et al. Immediate transoral allogeneic bone grafting for large mandibular defects. Less morbidity, more bone. A paradigm in benign tumor mandibular reconstruction? J Oral Maxillofac Surg. 2017;75(4):828–38.
3. Marschall JS, Kushner GM, Flint RL, Jones LC, Alpert B. Immediate reconstruction of segmental mandibular defects with nonvascular bone grafts: a 30-year perspective. J Oral Maxillofac Surg. 2020;78(11):2099.e1–9.
4. Pogrel MA, Podlesh S, Anthony JP, Alexander J. A comparison of vascularized and nonvascularized bone grafts for reconstruction of mandibular continuity defects. J Oral Maxillofac Surg. 1997;55(11):1200–6.

5. Foster RD, Anthony JP, Sharma A, Pogrel MA. Vascularized bone flaps versus nonvascularized bone grafts for mandibular reconstruction: an outcome analysis of primary bony union and endosseous implant success. Head Neck. 1999;21(1):66–71.

6. Marschall JS, Flint RL, Kushner GM, Alpert B. Management of mandibular osteomyelitis with segmental resection, nerve preservation, and immediate reconstruction. J Oral Maxillofac Surg. 2019;77(7):1490–504.

7. Melville JC, Tran HQ, Bhatti AK, et al. Is reconstruction of large mandibular defects using bioengineering materials effective? J Oral Maxillofac Surg. 2020;78(4):661.e1–1.e29.

8. Obwegeser HL. Simultaneous resection and reconstruction of parts of the mandible via the intraoral route in patients with and without gross infections. Oral Surg Oral Med Oral Pathol. 1966;21(6):693–705.

9. Zouhary KJ. Bone graft harvesting from distant sites: concepts and techniques. Oral Maxillofac Surg Clin North Am. 2010;22(3):301–16, v.

10. Peleg M, Sawatari Y, Marx RN, et al. Use of corticocancellous allogeneic bone blocks for augmentation of alveolar bone defects. Int J Oral Maxillofac Implants. 2010;25(1):153–62.

11. Gangwani P, Aziz SR, Marchena JM. Traditional use of autogenous and non-autogenous grafts in head and neck reconstruction: principles of conventional bone grafting. In: Melville JC, Shum JW, Young S, Wong ME, editors. Regenerative strategies for maxillary and mandibular reconstruction: a practical guide. Cham: Springer International Publishing; 2019. p. 13–24.

12. Almaiman M, Al-Bargi HH, Manson P. Complication of anterior iliac bone graft harvesting in 372 adult patients from May 2006 to May 2011 and a literature review. Craniomaxillofac Trauma Reconstr. 2013;6(4):257–66.

13. Kushner GM. Tibia bone graft harvest technique. Atlas Oral Maxillofac Surg Clin North Am. 2005;13(2):119–26.

14. Engelstad ME, Morse T. Anterior iliac crest, posterior iliac crest, and proximal tibia donor sites: a comparison of cancellous bone volumes in fresh cadavers. J Oral Maxillofac Surg. 2010;68(12):3015–21.

15. Benson PD, Marshall MK, Engelstad ME, Kushner GM, Alpert B. The use of immediate bone grafting in reconstruction of clinically infected mandibular fractures: bone grafts in the presence of pus. J Oral Maxillofac Surg. 2006;64(1):122–6.

16. Lienemann PS, Lutolf MP, Ehrbar M. Biomimetic hydrogels for controlled biomolecule delivery to augment bone regeneration. Adv Drug Deliv Rev. 2012;64(12):1078–89.

17. Rahn BA. Direct and indirect bone healing after operative fracture treatment. Otolaryngol Clin N Am. 1987;20(3):425–40.

18. Marx RE, Carlson ER, Eichstaedt RM, et al. Platelet-rich plasma: growth factor enhancement for bone grafts. Oral Surg Oral Med Oral Pathol Oral Radiol Endod. 1998;85(6):638–46.

19. Freymiller EG, Aghaloo TL. Platelet-rich plasma: ready or not? J Oral Maxillofac Surg. 2004;62(4):484–8.

20. Kobayashi E, Fluckiger L, Fujioka-Kobayashi M, et al. Comparative release of growth factors from PRP, PRF, and advanced-PRF. Clin Oral Investig. 2016;20(9):2353–60.

21. Zisch AH, Lutolf MP, Ehrbar M, et al. Cell-demanded release of VEGF from synthetic, biointeractive cell ingrowth matrices for vascularized tissue growth. FASEB J. 2003;17(15):2260–2.

22. Dohan Ehrenfest DM, Del Corso M, Diss A, Mouhyi J, Charrier JB. Three-dimensional architecture and cell composition of a Choukroun's platelet-rich fibrin clot and membrane. J Periodontol. 2010;81(4):546–55.

23. Dohan DM, Choukroun J, Diss A, et al. Platelet-rich fibrin (PRF): a second-generation platelet concentrate. Part III: leucocyte activation: a new feature for platelet concentrates? Oral Surg Oral Med Oral Pathol Oral Radiol Endod. 2006;101(3):e51–5.

24. Inchingolo F, Tatullo M, Marrelli M, et al. Trial with platelet-rich fibrin and bio-Oss used as grafting materials in the treatment of the severe maxillar bone atrophy: clinical and radiological evaluations. Eur Rev Med Pharmacol Sci. 2010;14(12):1075–84.

25. Reddi AH. Bone morphogenetic proteins and skeletal development: the kidney-bone connection. Pediatr Nephrol. 2000;14(7):598–601.

26. Cicciu M, Herford AS, Cicciu D, Tandon R, Maiorana C. Recombinant human bone morphogenetic protein-2 promote and stabilize hard and soft tissue healing for large mandibular new bone reconstruction defects. J Craniofac Surg. 2014;25(3):860–2.
27. Herford AS. The use of recombinant human bone morphogenetic protein-2 (rhBMP-2) in maxillofacial trauma. Chin J Traumatol. 2017;20(1):1–3.
28. Herford AS, Cicciu M. Recombinant human bone morphogenetic protein type 2 jaw reconstruction in patients affected by giant cell tumor. J Craniofac Surg. 2010;21(6):1970–5.
29. Herford AS, Lowe I, Jung P. Titanium mesh grafting combined with recombinant human bone morphogenetic protein 2 for alveolar reconstruction. Oral Maxillofac Surg Clin North Am. 2019;31(2):309–15.
30. Herford AS, Lu M, Buxton AN, et al. Recombinant human bone morphogenetic protein 2 combined with an osteoconductive bulking agent for mandibular continuity defects in nonhuman primates. J Oral Maxillofac Surg. 2012;70(3):703–16.
31. Hammoudeh JA, Fahradyan A, Gould DJ, et al. A comparative analysis of recombinant human bone morphogenetic protein-2 with a demineralized bone matrix versus iliac crest bone graft for secondary alveolar bone grafts in patients with cleft lip and palate: review of 501 cases. Plast Reconstr Surg. 2017;140(2):318e–25e.
32. McKay WF, Peckham SM, Badura JM. A comprehensive clinical review of recombinant human bone morphogenetic protein-2 (INFUSE Bone Graft). Int Orthop. 2007;31(6):729–34.
33. Cicciu M, Herford AS, Stoffella E, Cervino G, Cicciu D. Protein-signaled guided bone regeneration using titanium mesh and Rh-BMP2 in oral surgery: a case report involving left mandibular reconstruction after tumor resection. Open Dent J. 2012;6:51–5.
34. Herford AS, Boyne PJ. Reconstruction of mandibular continuity defects with bone morphogenetic protein-2 (rhBMP-2). J Oral Maxillofac Surg. 2008;66(4):616–24.
35. Hustedt JW, Blizzard DJ. The controversy surrounding bone morphogenetic proteins in the spine: a review of current research. Yale J Biol Med. 2014;87(4):549–61.
36. Boyne PJ. Animal studies of application of rhBMP-2 in maxillofacial reconstruction. Bone. 1996;19(1 Suppl):83S–92S.
37. Shah MM, Smyth MD, Woo AS. Adverse facial edema associated with off-label use of recombinant human bone morphogenetic protein-2 in cranial reconstruction for craniosynostosis. Case report. J Neurosurg Pediatr. 2008;1(3):255–7.
38. Hernigou P, Dubory A, Roubineau F, et al. Allografts supercharged with bone-marrow-derived mesenchymal stem cells possess equivalent osteogenic capacity to that of autograft: a study with long-term follow-ups of human biopsies. Int Orthop. 2017;41(1):127–32.
39. Pittenger MF, Mackay AM, Beck SC, et al. Multilineage potential of adult human mesenchymal stem cells. Science. 1999;284(5411):143–7.
40. Ramly EP, Alfonso AR, Kantar RS, et al. Safety and efficacy of recombinant human bone morphogenetic protein-2 (rhBMP-2) in craniofacial surgery. Plast Reconstr Surg Glob Open. 2019;7(8):e2347.
41. Egashira K, Sumita Y, Zhong W, et al. Bone marrow concentrate promotes bone regeneration with a suboptimal-dose of rhBMP-2. PLoS One. 2018;13(1):e0191099.
42. Sweeny L, Rosenthal EL, Light T, et al. Outcomes and cost implications of microvascular reconstructions of the head and neck. Head Neck. 2019;41(4):930–9.
43. Zuniga JR, Williams F, Petrisor D. A Case-and-control, multisite, positive controlled, prospective study of the safety and effectiveness of immediate inferior alveolar nerve processed nerve allograft reconstruction with ablation of the mandible for benign pathology. J Oral Maxillofac Surg. 2017;75(12):2669–81.
44. Coelho PG, Jimbo R, Tovar N, Bonfante EA. Osseointegration: hierarchical designing encompassing the macrometer, micrometer, and nanometer length scales. Dent Mater. 2015;31(1):37–52.
45. Steigenga JT, Al-Shammari KF, Nociti FH, Misch CE, Wang HL. Dental implant design and its relationship to long-term implant success. Implant Dent. 2003;12(4):306–17.
46. Bekisz JM, Flores RL, Witek L, et al. Dipyridamole enhances osteogenesis of three-dimensionally printed bioactive ceramic scaffolds in calvarial defects. J Craniomaxillofac Surg. 2018;46(2):237–44.

Chapter 18
The New Norm: Examining Quality of Life with Trigeminal Nerve Deficits and New Standards of Nerve Repair—A Systematic Review and Meta-analysis

Victoria A. Manon, Huy Q. Tran, Ramzey Tursun, Paulo G. Coelho iD,
Lukasz Witek, Mark E. Wong, Simon Young iD, **and James C. Melville** iD

V. A. Manon · H. Q. Tran
Bernard and Gloria P. Katz Department of Oral and Maxillofacial Surgery, University of
Texas Health Science Center at Houston, Houston, TX, USA
e-mail: victoria.a.manon@uth.tmc.edu; huy.q.tran@uth.tmc.edu

R. Tursun
Clinical Surgery, University of Miami, Miami, FL, USA

Oral, Head & Neck Oncologic, University of Miami, Miami, FL, USA

Microvascular Reconstructive Surgery, University of Miami, Miami, FL, USA

Division of Oral Maxillofacial Surgery, DeWitt Daughtry Family Department of Surgery,
Leonard M. Miller School of Medicine, University of Miami, Miami, FL, USA

Security Forces Hospital, Riyad, Saudi Arabia

P. G. Coelho
School of Medicine, New York University, New York, NY, USA
e-mail: pc92@nyu.edu

L. Witek
Department of Biomaterials and Biomimetics, New York University College of Dentistry,
New York, NY, USA

Department of Biomedical Engineering, New York University Tandon School of Engineering,
New York, NY, USA

Craniomaxillofacial Orthopaedic Biomaterials Regenerative Applications Lab, New York, NY, USA
e-mail: lw901@nyu.edu

M. E. Wong
Department of Oral and Maxillofacial Surgery, School of Dentistry, University of Texas
Health Science Center at Houston, Houston, TX, USA
e-mail: Mark.E.Wong@uth.tmc.edu

S. Young · J. C. Melville (✉)
Department of Oral and Maxillofacial Surgery, The University of Texas Health Science
Center at Houston, Houston, TX, USA
e-mail: Simon.Young@uth.tmc.edu; James.C.Melville@uth.tmc.edu

© The Author(s), under exclusive license to Springer Nature
Switzerland AG 2023
J. C. Melville et al. (eds.), *Advancements and Innovations in OMFS, ENT, and
Facial Plastic Surgery*, https://doi.org/10.1007/978-3-031-32099-6_18

Introduction

Continuous advances in surgical techniques and immunotherapies are anticipated to improve survival rates of patients with head and neck cancer, placing even greater emphasis on maxillofacial reconstruction by surgeons. While much of this attention has been directed toward the restoration of muscular and bony structures, increased patient longevity has directed focus toward the reconstruction of resected nerves following resection of pathology. The purpose of this review was to discuss the impact of inferior alveolar nerve (IAN) and/or lingual nerve (LN) resection on quality of life and examine the numerous reconstructive options now available to practitioners.

Methods

A literature review was conducted to determine the qualitative and quantitative effects of IAN and/or LN resection on quality of life (QoL), using scales such as the Medical Research Council Scale (MRCS) and/or the Oral Health Impact Questionnaire (OHIP). We also searched for data regarding the relationship of time to nerve reconstruction and improvement in functional sensory recovery and overall QoL. In accord with the policy of the institutional review board of the University of Texas Health Sciences Center at Houston (UTHealth), institutional review board approved of this study.

Results

Persistent paresthesia and/or anesthesia of the IAN or LN results in significantly reduced quality of life with psychosocial and physical implications. Patients report interferences in their ability to socialize (i.e., retaining food particles on the face or drooling) and difficulties with employment. Other psychological implications include increased social anxiety and symptoms of clinical depression. When addressed within 9 months of injury or resection, reconstruction of the inferior alveolar and/or lingual nerves via direct neurorrhaphy, autografts, or processed allogeneic grafts has successfully demonstrated marked improvements in patients' functional sensory recovery and overall quality of life.

Conclusion

The results of this review indicate that timely reconstruction of the inferior alveolar and/or lingual nerves can lead to significant improvements in functional sensory recovery and patient quality of life. When reviewing options for reconstruction of maxillomandibular and oral structures, consideration of nerve reconstruction should also be prioritized.

Background

The inferior alveolar (IAN) and lingual (LN) nerves are branches of the mandibular nerve, the third branch of the trigeminal nerve (cranial nerve V). When functioning normally, the IAN provides sensation to the lower teeth and lip, while the LN provides general sensory innervation to the anterior two-thirds of the tongue. Upon exiting the mandible at the mental foramen, the IAN continues as the mental nerve providing sensation to the front of the chin and lower lip. These functions facilitate daily activities such as chewing, smiling, and tasting, which play an important role in social interactions. Damage to the IAN or LN during surgery can result in anesthesia or paresthesia of the affected structures, therefore interfering with daily activities and the patient's quality of life. Injury of these structures occurs most commonly during lower third molar extractions, but certain procedures, such as mandibular resections for benign or malignant pathology, may also require the resection of these nerves. While reconstruction of bone and soft tissue defects has been extensively studied and is a common procedure for most oral surgeons, reconstruction of the nerves is less common and not always considered by surgeons, which can leave patients with persistent functional sensory deficits.

Various techniques are available to the surgeon for reconstruct of the IAN and/or LN; if possible, nerve reconstruction should be implemented during the primary reconstruction, particularly after mandibular resections for benign and malignant head and neck pathology. As advances are made in surgery, chemoradiation, and now immunotherapy, patient survival rates for head and neck cancer have increased from 53% in the 1970s to 66% in 2010 [1]. Surgical management of benign and malignant pathology of the maxillomandibular region includes resection of the affected structures, often including the IAN and LNs. Improvements in survival rates have motivated surgeons and their patients to pursue additional surgeries to reconstruct the residual defects. This should include reconstruction of the resected neural structures to improve the surviving patients' quality of life. While direct neurorrhaphy can be used for nerve transections where nerve stumps are in close proximity, this requires approximation of the free nerve stumps without tension and is not feasible for larger spanning defects. Autogenous grafts, commonly requiring harvest of the sural nerve, may be successfully used in younger patients but can result in donor site morbidity, including the additional surgical site and sensory deficits in the distribution of the harvested nerve. Decellularized allogenic nerve grafts, such as the AxoGen AVANCE graft, can be used to successfully reconstruct neural defects over distances of 5–70 mm without tension, donor site morbidity, or immunosuppression. Nerve reconstruction techniques have demonstrated greater functional sensory recovery (FSR) with early intervention as compared to delayed or no intervention. Patients that do not receive early intervention often report persistent neurosensory disturbances, affecting their overall quality of life [2–6]. While early intervention is advocated over delayed intervention, Robinson et al. found that there was no correlation in outcome measures and timing of repair for lingual nerve injuries [7]. Instead they found that early or delayed intervention did not reduce the

Table 18.1 Medical Research Council Scale (MRCS) for neurosensory recovery

Score	Parameter	FSR
S0	No recovery	No
S1	Recovery of deep cutaneous pain	No
S1+	Recovery of some superficial pain	No
S2	Recovery of some superficial pain and tactile sensation	No
S2+	S2 with over-response	No
S3	S2+ without over-response and 2-PD >15 mm	Yes, clinical recovery
S3+	S3, plus 2-PD = 7–15 mm	Yes
S4	S3+, plus 2-PD = 2–6 mm	Yes, complete recovery

number of patients with dysesthesia, but reduced the quality of their symptoms. Patients that do not receive surgical intervention often report persistent neurosensory disturbances, affecting their overall quality of life.

Patients with residual deficits of the IAN and/or LN consistently report higher levels of dissatisfaction and poorer quality of life. Objective measures of functional sensory recovery include neurosensory testing instruments and survey. The Medical Research Council Scale (MRCS) is commonly used, although this measure does not assess the patient's self-perceptions of quality of life or impact on daily activities. The MRCS uses neurosensory tests, such as two-point discrimination, brushstroke directional sensation, contact detection, and pain and temperature nociception, and scores the recovery on a scale from S0 to S4 (Table 18.1) [8, 9]. While these measures are crucial for the evaluation, documented measurements of the patients' subjective experiences are less likely to be collected and discussed. Other methods can be used to assess subjective sensory recovery, such as surveys or the visual analogue scale (scale, 0–10, with 0 = completely anesthetic and 10 = normal sensation). Various surveys have been designed and can be used to collect this information; the Oral Health Impact Questionnaire (OHIP) and Short Form Health Survey (SF-36) are widely used today [10, 11]. The OHIP, originally developed by Slade in 1977, is a 49-question survey used to evaluate the patient's perceptions of their functional disability, physical pain, physical disability, psychological disability, social disability, psychological discomfort, and handicap. The OHIP-14 is an abbreviated, 14-question version of the OHIP. The SF-36 can be used to measure health-related quality of life using eight subcategories of physical and mental components. The physical component score (PCS) includes physical functioning, role-physical, bodily pain, and general health. The mental component score (MCS) includes patient perceptions of vitality, social functioning, role-emotional, and mental health. These scores quantify the patients' self-perceptions of physical and mental health-related quality of life [12]. Patients with persistent neurosensory disturbances evaluated using the OHIP and/or SF-36 after IAN and/or LN damage are found to report consistently higher levels of dissatisfaction in each category. These studies demonstrate that these patients have poorer quality of life as compared to those that do not have these neurosensory disturbances [10–12].

The purpose of this paper is to discuss the decreased quality of life observed in patients with IAN and LN neurosensory disturbances and encourage practitioners to consider neural reconstruction in the effort to improve the lives of their patients. Advances in the management of head and neck cancer have increased the survival rates of patients requiring major resections of the mandible and associated neural structures, and this improvement has led to the need for reconstruction of the patient's maxillomandibular defects. Failure to reconstruct the patient's IAN and/or LN leads to persistent neurosensory disturbances, reducing the patient's quality of life. When possible, immediate reconstruction of the nerves should be seriously considered during surgical planning. The surgeon should be aware of the psychosocial impact nerve deficits can have and should discuss this, as well as treatment options, with the patient.

Review of Literature

How Does This Problem Impact and Affect the Afflicted Population and How Can It Be Measured?

Patients with persistent neurosensory disturbances after IAN and/or LN damage consistently report reduced quality of life related to their injuries. When evaluated using the OHIP-14 and/or SF-36, patients consistently report more functional/physical limitations and psychological discomfort and disabilities as compared to those that did not suffer the same injury [10–12]. Reported functional/physical limitations include difficulty eating, speech deterioration, inability to detect food on the lip when eating, and unawareness of drooling [12, 13]. Negative impacts of these physical limitations have social implications including the patients' ability to socialize with others, their ability to enjoy their food, and their difficulties with employment [12, 14]. The psychosocial implications of these difficulties can impact the patients' self-perceptions, leading to increased social anxiety, difficulty managing emotions of anger and irritability, and even clinical depression [10, 14]. While neurosensory recovery is an important parameter to record when these injuries occur, understanding the patients' physical and psychological disabilities that resulted from this injury is equally as important to understand and document.

The surgeon's ability to elicit and discuss the aforementioned problems can help them properly inform the patient of complications associated with IAN and/or LN injury prior to surgery and to manage the afflicted patient postoperatively. Patel et al. conducted interviews with five afflicted patients, finding many were dissatisfied with the initial consent process, their injury, and postoperative management [12]. Many questioned the informed consent process and stated they felt they were not properly informed of the quality of life implications associated with neural damage. They expressed a desire for more information preoperatively and on the recovery prognosis. This indicates a need for a more comprehensive, preoperative discussion regarding the impact on quality of life that neurosensory deficits can cause. Many also expressed significant frustration and anger associated with the injury, indicating that they felt they were not appropriately managed initially after the injury. Patel et al. found that the average time of referral to a specialist was 7 months postoperatively (range 3 weeks to 18 months). Patients indicated that they would like disclosure of their neurosensory prognosis and prompt management. Given the physical and psychosocial implications of these injuries, there is a need to improve postoperative management, including early referral to a specialist, surgical intervention, and management of patient expectations [12, 15, 16]. In accord with the policy of the institutional review board of the University of Texas Health Sciences Center at Houston (UTHealth), institutional review board approved this study.

Available Surgical Interventions

Surgical intervention of neural injuries is critical for improvement of functional sensory recovery and improvement of quality of life. Once the surgeon identifies a nerve injury or knows that treatment will require transection of neural structures, prompt initial management is necessary for clinical success and patient satisfaction [2–7]. Indications for trigeminal nerve repair include observed nerve transection, lack of clinical improvement of paresthesia for >3 months, development of neuropathy due to nerve entrapment or neuroma formation, presence of a foreign body, worsening paresthesia or dysesthesia, and hypoesthesia affecting patient's quality of life [3]. Techniques for neural repair or reconstruction include direct neurorrhaphy, autogenous nerve grafts, vascularized free flaps, and decellularized allogenic nerve grafts.

Direct neurorrhaphy is the direct repair of the proximal and distal nerve stumps. The most commonly used method for direct nerve repair of the IAN or LN is the epineural suture technique. Successful surgical outcomes, defined as return of useful sensory function, are best achieved with timely repair (within 9 months from the time of injury) and tension-free approximation of the nerve ends. In a retrospective study of 222 lingual nerve repairs, Bagheri et al. found that 90.5% of patients achieved useful sensory recovery or complete return of sensation with use of this technique [2]. Patients that sought surgical intervention after 9 months were significantly less likely to achieve any meaningful sensory recovery. The study also found that age and preoperative symptoms were important determinants of surgical success. For every year above the age of 45, the chances of obtaining functional sensory recovery decreased 5.5%; preoperative numbness, as compared to preoperative pain, was a negative indicator for return of sensation.

Autogenous nerve grafting, considered the gold standard for peripheral nerve grafting, allows tension-free approximation when larger defects are present [17, 18]. The surgeon must consider the following factors when determining the choice of a donor nerve graft: accessibility, length required, diameter of donor nerve compared to host nerve, patient reference, and fascicular number and pattern. The two most commonly used autogenous nerve grafts are the sural and great auricular nerves (GAN). There is some debate as to the appropriate length for the use of certain nerve grafts. The great auricular nerve in the upper lateral neck has been the most frequently harvested for nerve defects of less than 3 cm, while the sural nerve in the lower extremity is more suitable for longer nerve defects [19]. Wolford recommends that the GAN should only be used to reconstruct defects up to 1.5 cm in length and that the sural nerve should be used for defects up to 2.5 cm [17, 19]. Although the graft can successfully be used to create a tension-free nerve repair, it can be difficult to achieve ideal donor to recipient match and is associated with donor site morbidity [17]. Despite harvesting the nerve from a donor site, Miloro and Stoner found that most patients under the age of 38 tolerated harvest of the sural nerve without significant neurosensory disturbances or morbidity of the donor site if functional sensory recovery was achieved at the trigeminal nerve [20].

Microvascular free tissue transfer offers great versatility in the selection of tissue for reconstruction of head and neck defects. The utilization of vascularized free flaps is indicated when extensive soft tissue and bone are included in tumor ablation or an avulsive injury that requires reconstruction. The nerves contained in the following vascularized free flaps may be used for nerve repair:

- The medial antebrachial [21] or the lateral cutaneous nerve of forearm [22]. In a study of 22 patients who had glossectomy for oral carcinoma, Kuriakose found that 77% of patients had sensory recovery within 8 months after reconstruction with a radial forearm free flap via the lateral antebrachial cutaneous nerve [23].
- The long thoracic nerve can be harvested when performing a scapula latissimus dorsi free flap. Schultes et al. found that all five patients had progressive return of sensation when the long thoracic nerve was used to reconstruct the mental nerve [24]. Pressure sensation returned for the five patients at 3–4 months postoperatively. Pain sensation returned thereafter 2 months, with conversion to hyperesthesia, lessening to normal after months 5 and 6. Four of the five patients were able to discriminate between sharp and blunt sensations after the fifth month, the last patient after 7 months. At 6–7 months, all patients were able to discriminate between two points and recovered senses of vibration and light touch in the original region of the mental nerve distribution. After 9 months, four patients had bilateral equal sensitivity.
- A case report by Tanaka et al. found that the lateral sural cutaneous nerve can be anastomosed to the distal end of the remnant lAN using an epineural repair [25]. The mandible was reconstructed with a fibula free flap that included the sural nerve. The proximal ends of the right and left IAN were re-approximated to the proximal and distal ends of the sural nerve. Sensations were measured using Semmes-Weinstein monofilaments. Tanaka et al. found that sensory recovery was first noted after 5 months and the quantitative results of the Semmes-Weinstein test 45 months after surgery ranged from 2.83 to 4.08.

Nerve allografts are decellularized conduits that serve as a temporary scaffold for neural regeneration [26]. The decellularized allogenic nerve graft provides an unlimited source of graft with no associated donor site morbidity and reduces the risk of immune rejection [17, 27]. Processed nerve allografts may be safely and effectively used to reconstruct trigeminal sensory nerve defects between 5 and 70 mm. Miloro et al. found that patients that had reconstruction of the IAN or LN with allogeneic grafts reported a satisfaction score of 8.9 on the visual analogue scale, as compared to the reported score of 8.1 for patients that had undergone direct repair. He also reported an accelerated rate of functional sensory recovery as compared to direct neurorrhaphy or no intervention [28]. The study noted that indirect graft nerve repair, using an allograft (AVANCE nerve graft), is associated with improved objective and subjective nerve outcomes compared with direct nerve repair [28]. Zuniga also reported that of his 16 patients reconstructed with an allogeneic nerve graft, 14 (87%) of them saw improvements in sensory function (87%) [29]. Salomon reported a similar finding, stating that 85.7% of his patients reconstructed with the allogeneic nerve graft achieved some return of tactile sensation and superficial pain without over-response [9]. Numerous publications have confirmed the safety and efficacy of using a cadaveric peripheral nerve allograft (AVANCE, Axogen Corporation, Alachua, FL) to reconstruct the inferior alveolar nerve (IAN) following non-ablative and ablative mandibular resection, mostly for benign disease [1, 28–30]. Risks associated with the reconstruction include failure to gain FSR; this approach is not associated with the donor site morbidity of autologous nerve grafts. It is important to note that even if only some sensation is regained, this would be an improvement as opposed to no attempt at nerve reconstruction and, consequently, no change in neurosensory function [17, 31]. It has been proposed that acellular processed nerve allografts may replace autogenous nerve grafts [30].

Conclusions

Iatrogenic injury or resection of the IAN and/or LNs as a result of oral and maxillofacial procedures can result in devastating physical and psychosocial complications for the patient, reducing their overall quality of life. These injuries can negatively impact the patients' ability to eat and enjoy their food and impair social interactions via deterioration of speech, sensory limitations causing retention of food on the face and drooling, and increased self-conscious awareness associated with their disabilities. Psychological consequences of these impairments may lead to clinical depression. It is imperative that these potential complications and their associated functional/sensory implications are discussed preoperatively and that they are managed promptly and appropriately when they occur. Attention to the patient's psychosocial and functional disabilities deserves attention in order to achieve holistic patient care.

Surgeons are encouraged to document functional sensory loss after these injuries and perceived quality of life using patient surveys such as the OHIP-14 or SF-36. Once physical and/or psychological disabilities are observed and documented, prompt intervention or referral is crucial for successful clinical outcomes and patient satisfaction. Various treatment options are available to the head and neck surgeon: direct neurorrhaphy, autogenous nerve grafts, vascularized free flaps, and decellularized allogenic nerve grafts. Use of these techniques can result in significant functional sensory recovery, improving the patients' overall quality of life. When possible, the surgeon is encouraged to consider maxillomandibular reconstruction not only of the bone and soft tissues but also of the sensory nerves necessary for human function.

References

1. Tursun R, Green JM III. Immediate microsurgical bone and nerve reconstruction in the irradiated patient: a case report. J Oral Maxillofac Surg. 2017;75(6):1302.e1301–7.
2. Bagheri SC, et al. Retrospective review of microsurgical repair of 222 lingual nerve injuries. J Oral Maxillofac Surg. 2010;68(4):715–23.
3. Ziccardi VB. Microsurgical techniques for repair of the inferior alveolar and lingual nerves. Atlas Oral Maxillofac Surg Clin North Am. 2011;19(1):79–90.
4. Bagheri SC, et al. Microsurgical repair of the inferior alveolar nerve: success rate and factors that adversely affect outcome. J Oral Maxillofac Surg. 2012;70(8):1978–90.
5. Erakat MS, et al. Interval between injury and lingual nerve repair as a prognostic factor for success using type I collagen conduit. J Oral Maxillofac Surg. 2013;71(5):833–8.
6. White H, Rosenthal E. Static and dynamic repairs of facial nerve injuries. Oral Maxillofac Surg Clin North Am. 2013;25(2):303–12.
7. Robinson PP, et al. Current management of damage to the inferior alveolar and lingual nerves as a result of removal of third molars. Br J Oral Maxillofac Surg. 2004;42(4):285–92.
8. Doucet JC, et al. Concomitant removal of mandibular third molars during sagittal split osteotomy minimizes neurosensory dysfunction. J Oral Maxillofac Surg. 2012;70(9):2153–63.
9. Salomon D, et al. Outcomes of immediate allograft reconstruction of long-span defects of the inferior alveolar nerve. J Oral Maxillofac Surg. 2016;74(12):2507–14.
10. Leung YY, et al. Trigeminal neurosensory deficit and patient reported outcome measures: the effect on quality of life. PLoS One. 2013;8(10):e77391.
11. Cakir M, et al. Effects of inferior alveolar nerve neurosensory deficits on quality of life. Niger J Clin Pract. 2018;21(2):206–11.
12. Patel N, et al. Quality of life following injury to the inferior dental or lingual nerve – a cross-sectional mixed-methods study. Oral Surg. 2018;11(1):9–16.
13. Sandstedt P, Sorensen S. Neurosensory disturbances of the trigeminal nerve: a long-term follow-up of traumatic injuries. J Oral Maxillofac Surg. 1995;53(5):498–505.
14. Pogrel MA, et al. Long-term outcome of trigeminal nerve injuries related to dental treatment. J Oral Maxillofac Surg. 2011;69(9):2284–8.
15. Tolle T, et al. Patient burden of trigeminal neuralgia: results from a cross-sectional survey of health state impairment and treatment patterns in six European countries. Pain Pract. 2006;6(3):153–60.
16. Smith JG, et al. The psychosocial and affective burden of posttraumatic neuropathy following injuries to the trigeminal nerve. J Orofac Pain. 2013;27(4):293–303.
17. Wolford LM, Rodrigues DB. Autogenous grafts/allografts/conduits for bridging peripheral trigeminal nerve gaps. Atlas Oral Maxillofac Surg Clin North Am. 2011;19(1):91–107.
18. Dodson TB, Kaban LB. Recommendations for management of trigeminal nerve defects based on a critical appraisal of the literature. J Oral Maxillofac Surg. 1997;55(12):1380–6; discussion 1387.
19. Meyer RA. Improving quality of life for oral cancer patients. J Oral Maxillofac Surg. 2018;76(3):468.

20. Miloro M, Stoner JA. Subjective outcomes following sural nerve harvest. J Oral Maxillofac Surg. 2005;63(8):1150–4.
21. McCormick SU, Buchbinder, McCormick SA, Stark M. Microanatomic analysis of the medial antebrachial nerve as a potential donor nerve in maxillofacial grafting. J Oral Maxillofac Surg. 1994;52(10):1022–5.
22. Shibahara T, et al. Morphologic changes in forearm flaps of the oral cavity. J Oral Maxillofac Surg. 2000;58(5):495–9.
23. Kuriakose MA, et al. Sensate radial forearm free flaps in tongue reconstruction. Arch Otolaryngol Head Neck Surg. 2001;127(12):1463–6.
24. Schultes G, Gaggl A, Kärcher H. Vascularized transplantation of the long thoracic nerve for sensory reinnervation of the lower lip. Br J Oral Maxillofac Surg. 2000;38(2):138–41.
25. Tanaka K, et al. Bilateral inferior alveolar nerve reconstruction with a vascularized sural nerve graft included in a free fibular osteocutaneous flap after segmental mandibulectomy. Head Neck. 2016;38(5):E111–4.
26. Sedaghati T, Jell G, Seifalian AM. Nerve regeneration and bioengineering. Regenerative medicine applications in organ transplantation. London: Academic Press; 2014. p. 799–810.
27. Chaimanakarn S, Sakdejayont W. Inferior alveolar and lingual nerve microneurosurgery. Mahidol Dental J. 2019;39(1):41–52.
28. Miloro M, Ruckman P III, Kolokythas A. Lingual nerve repair: to graft or not to graft? J Oral Maxillofac Surg. 2015;73(9):1844–50.
29. Zuniga JR. Sensory outcomes after reconstruction of lingual and inferior alveolar nerve discontinuities using processed nerve allograft—a case series. J Oral Maxillofac Surg. 2015;73(4):734–44.
30. Yampolsky A, et al. Efficacy of acellular nerve allografts in trigeminal nerve reconstruction. J Oral Maxillofac Surg. 2017;75(10):2230–4.
31. Akbari M, Miloro M. The inferior alveolar nerve: to graft or not to graft in ablative mandibular resection? J Oral Maxillofac Surg. 2019;77(6):1280–128.

Chapter 19
Trigeminal Nerve Reconstruction in Maxillofacial Surgery

Raymond P. Shupak, Jeffrey Hartgerink, Cheuk Sun Edwin Lai,
Simon Young [iD], Alexis M. Linnebur, Zachary S. Peacock,
Srinivasa R. Chandra, Ashish Patel, and James C. Melville [iD]

R. P. Shupak (✉)
Department of Oral Medicine and Maxillofacial Surgery, Geisinger Commonwealth School
of Medicine, Geisinger Health System, Danville, PA, USA
e-mail: rshupak@geisinger.edu

J. Hartgerink
Chemistry and Bioengineering, Rice University, Houston, TX, USA

Undergraduate Studies, Rice University, Houston, TX, USA
e-mail: jdh@rice.edu

C. S. E. Lai
Rice University, Houston, TX, USA
e-mail: cl95@rice.edu

S. Young · J. C. Melville
Department of Oral and Maxillofacial Surgery, The University of Texas Health Science
Center at Houston, Houston, TX, USA
e-mail: Simon.Young@uth.tmc.edu; James.C.Melville@uth.tmc.edu

A. M. Linnebur
Carle Foundation Hospital, Urbana, IL, USA
e-mail: alexis.linnebur@carle.com

Z. S. Peacock
Oral and Maxillofacial Surgery, Massachusetts General Hospital (MGH), Boston, MA, USA
e-mail: zpeacock@partners.org

S. R. Chandra
Oral and Maxillofacial Surgery, Oregon Health Sciences School of Dentistry,
Portland, OR, USA
e-mail: chandrsr@ohsu.edu

A. Patel
Oral, Head and Neck Surgery, Head and Neck Surgical Associates, Portland, OR, USA
e-mail: Patela@head-neck.com

© The Author(s), under exclusive license to Springer Nature
Switzerland AG 2023
J. C. Melville et al. (eds.), *Advancements and Innovations in OMFS, ENT, and
Facial Plastic Surgery*, https://doi.org/10.1007/978-3-031-32099-6_19

Introduction

Surgeons often encounter peripheral nerve injuries in practice. This is especially true when operating in the head and neck region where there is a rich supply of cranial and spinal nerves. As the largest cranial and peripheral sensory nerve, the trigeminal nerve is one of the most commonly injured [1, 2]. Main branches of the trigeminal nerve, namely, the mental, inferior alveolar, lingual, and infraorbital nerves, are highly susceptible to damage. Injury often results from trauma, iatrogenic injury following routine surgery, or planned ablative procedures. Regardless of the etiology, trigeminal nerve injury results in neurosensory disturbances that have detrimental effects on patients' quality-of-life.

Damage to the trigeminal nerve can result in worrisome dysesthesias (pain, hypersensitivity, burning, numbness, tingling, and itching) that significantly affect patients' well-being [3]. Dysesthesias can alter normal functions such as speech, taste, swallowing, mastication, and maintenance of saliva within the oral cavity [4]. Additionally, pain catastrophizing, depression, psychological disability, and discomfort have been associated with inferior alveolar and lingual nerve injury [5].

In order to appropriately treat and rehabilitate patients, accurate classification of trigeminal nerve injury is required. Currently, there is inconsistency in the clinical grading of trigeminal nerve injury with several classification systems used for clinical care and research including Seddon, Sunderland, and the Medical Research Council Scale. In a recent study, Miloro et al. surveyed oral and maxillofacial surgeons and found inconsistency, lack of surgeon confidence, and need for a uniform grading system to communicate and guide trigeminal nerve injury and treatment [6]. Expert consensus suggests that clinicians utilize neurosensory testing to calculate Medical Research Council Scale (MRCS) grading scores, allowing for valid comparison and outcome measurement [6]. The objective of trigeminal reconstructive surgery is to meaningfully restore patient sensation with consistent and reliable protocols to achieve functional sensory recovery (FSR). This correlates to an MRCS grade 3.0 or greater [3].

Historical Perspective on Trigeminal Nerve Reconstruction and Repair

Historical mention of nerve anatomy and injury dates back to Greco-Roman times with descriptions from Hippocrates (460–370 BCE). At that time, it was universally believed that nerve tissue could not unite, and therefore, early attempts of nerve repair were not undertaken [7, 8]. It was not until the seventh century with Paul of Aegina (626–696 CE) that text descriptions of nerve handling and postulations of nerve repair exist. The first suitable description of direct nerve suturing techniques was in the thirteenth century by Lanfranchi at Bologna Medical School. Centuries then passed without significant evolution from these early descriptions.

Modern nerve surgery evolved quickly during the nineteenth and twentieth century in part due to increased traumatic nerve injury occurring during wartime. In their descriptions and texts, individuals such as Langenbeck, Vulpian, and Létiévant advanced the field of peripheral nerve repair, thus setting the foundation for those to follow [7]. Further work by individuals such as Mitchell, Woolsey, Tinel, Elsberg, Babcock, Dandy, Seddon, and Sunderland laid the foundation of how we currently understand, classify, and surgically treat peripheral nerve injury [7].

Within the scope of oral and maxillofacial surgery, cranial nerve repair literature began to appear during the mid-twentieth century. Surgeons began to push the forefront of peripheral nerve repair with the advent and refinement of microsurgical techniques in the 1950s and 1960s. Case series of direct nerve repair and autogenous nerve grafting techniques for trigeminal and facial nerve repair detailed promising results [9–11]. During the latter part of the twentieth and early twenty-first century, surgical approaches, materials, and techniques continued to advance. Many utilized autogenous sources as interpositional grafts when direct nerve repair was impossible. Most recently, nerve allografts became available, which reduced donor site morbidity. Commercially available allografts and scaffold connectors/protectors now play a major role in trigeminal nerve microneurosurgery.

Current Practices and Outcomes of Peripheral Trigeminal Nerve Repair

Pathophysiology of Nerve Damage

Peripheral nerve damage can result from trauma, tumor, thermal, ischemic, chemical, infectious, inflammatory, or iatrogenic injury. Seddon describes three degrees of nerve injury [12]. The least severe form of nerve injury, neuropraxia, results in localized reversible conduction blockade. Complete nerve recovery can be expected within weeks to months. More severe damage results in axonotmesis. This is characterized by axonal and myelin disruption with its connective tissue framework preservation. These forms of injury are more severe and result in varying degrees of recovery. Neurotmesis is the most severe and results from contusion, stretch, or laceration. With this form of injury, there is little to no potential for full recovery when left untreated.

In axonotmesis and neurotmesis, Wallerian degeneration occurs shortly after injury. Wallerian degeneration describes the process of retrograde degeneration of the distal end of the injured nerve. This results in disruption of the distal axonal skeleton and membrane. This is followed by myelin sheath degradation clearance by macrophages and Schwann cells. If terminally injured, the nerve cell undergoes apoptosis; otherwise, it enters the regeneration phase. This phase is a complex multifactorial process resulting in a growth cone at the distal aspect of injury to support axonal branching and outgrowth. If the distal endoneurium remains in close approximation after injury, it can direct axonal growth back to its target. If not, there is potential for incomplete functional regeneration and neuroma formation. Unlike the central nervous system (CNS), peripheral nerve injury lends itself to a better environment for axonal regeneration [13].

Current Options for Trigeminal Nerve Repair and Reconstruction

Surgeons have multiple options when repairing trigeminal nerve injuries. The type of repair is dictated by the type, severity, and size of defect. When direct repair is feasible, end-to end coaptation (i.e., neurorrhaphy) is performed under magnification utilizing non-tissue reactive microsuture (e.g., 8-0 to 10-0 Nylon) in a tension-free manner [2, 3, 14]. More recently, the literature supports the utilization of connectors to protect the direct repair as it shields the regeneration process from the deleterious effects of the wound bed [15]. When direct repair is not possible (extended continuity defects or repairs under tension), interpositional grafts are required.

Saphenous, medial antebrachial cutaneous, sural, or greater auricular nerves were historically utilized as interpositional grafts. Donor site morbidity, incomplete functional return, and the increasing availability of alternative options have decreased the use of autografts [13]. First-generation nerve conduits (silicone/polytetrafluoroethylene) were introduced to guide axonal regrowth and protect from the infiltration of connective tissue in the wound bed. These conduits often require secondary removal and can result in nerve compression syndromes.

Second-generation nerve conduits were subsequently developed to mitigate the pitfalls of non-resorbable materials. These conduits are both resorbable and biocompatible avoiding a second-stage procedure. Materials such as polyglycolic acid, type I collagen, polycaprolactone, and N-fibroin have been studied as conduits for peripheral nerve repair with mixed efficacy [13]. Third-generation nerve conduits containing neurotrophic factors, stem cells, extracellular matrix (ECM) proteins, and other neuroactive substances are being studied and may guide and stimulate peripheral nerve repair.

There has been a significant trend in current practice to repair and reconstruct trigeminal nerve injury with nerve allograft (AxoGen, Alachua, FL) [2–4, 14, 16]. Avance™ is a processed human nerve that is treated via a combination of detergent decellularization, chondroitin sulfate proteoglycan degradation, chondroitinase treatment, and gamma-irradiation sterilization [17]. The nerve allograft is brought into the operative field and neurorrhaphy is performed at the proximal and distal nerve stump via AxoGuard™ nerve connectors. The connector is comprised of porcine small intestinal submucosa, which allows for a tension-free coaptation. It can prevent aberrant axonal growth and protects the nerve regeneration process from inflammation at the repair site [2, 17].

Surgeons must also consider the timing of trigeminal nerve reconstruction. Timing to repair/reconstruction remains controversial in the literature [18–20]. Consensus dictates that the surgeon immediately repairs a witnessed trigeminal nerve injury. There is also a trend toward immediate reconstruction of planned ablative defects when feasible. Early repair (i.e., within 3–6 months from injury) of trigeminal nerve injuries and its effect on neurosensory recovery was studied in a recent systematic review and meta-analysis [19]. The review showed mixed results in obtaining functional sensory recovery with early intervention. However, the meta-analysis showed higher combined success rates (93% versus 78.5%) and higher odds of improvement in the early versus late (>6 months) group. The optimal time for repair is still being elucidated [19].

Current Practices: Inferior Alveolar, Long Buccal, and Mental Nerve Repair and Reconstruction

The inferior alveolar nerve (IAN) and mental nerve (MN) are among the most commonly reconstructed divisions of the trigeminal nerve. The authors' preference is direct tension-free repair utilizing AxoGuard connectors when possible (Fig. 19.1). Approaches to the IAN are performed both intraorally or transcutaneous based on extent and position of injury. Virtual surgical planning can be employed to aid in nerve locating, repair, and reconstruction. The authors utilize a combination of interposition allograft (Avance™, AxoGen) with proximal and distal nerve connectors in situations where a segmental nerve defect exists (AxoGuard™, AxoGen) (Figs. 19.2 and 19.3).

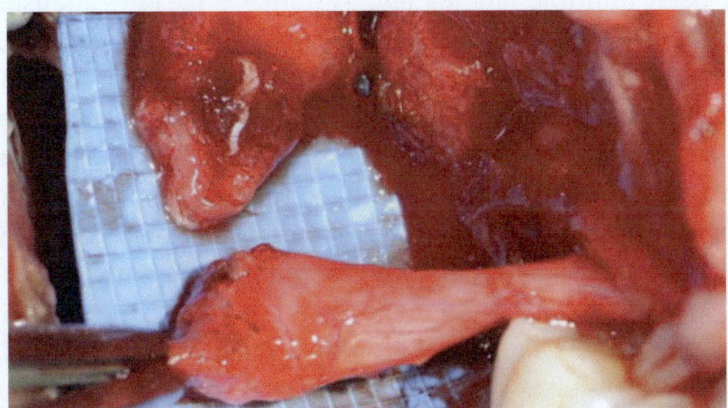

Fig. 19.1 A transected trigeminal nerve branch showing proximal and distal nerve stumps within proximity for direct repair. The site of injury is identified, dissected, and prepared for primary neurorrhaphy. If the proximal and distal ends of the nerve can be coapted in a tension free manner, a direct repair or preferentially a nerve connector can be utilized. Care is taken to not cause additional axonal damage during manipulation. The epineurium is handled with microsurgical instrumentation

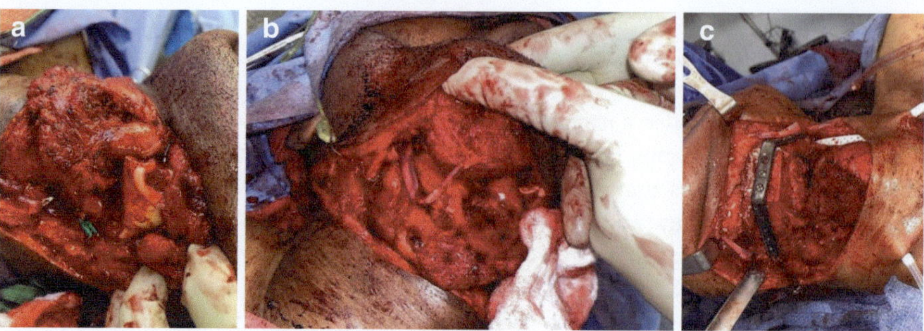

Fig. 19.2 A planned ablative procedure with immediate nerve reconstruction of the inferior alveolar nerve. (**a**) The proximal inferior alveolar nerve is identified after mandibulectomy. Avance™ nerve graft is used with proximal and distal Axoguard™ nerve connectors. The proximal nerve coaptation is performed first. (**b**) The mental nerve stump is identified and neurorrhaphy is performed. (**c**) A fibula free flap is inset around the segmental inferior alveolar nerve reconstruction

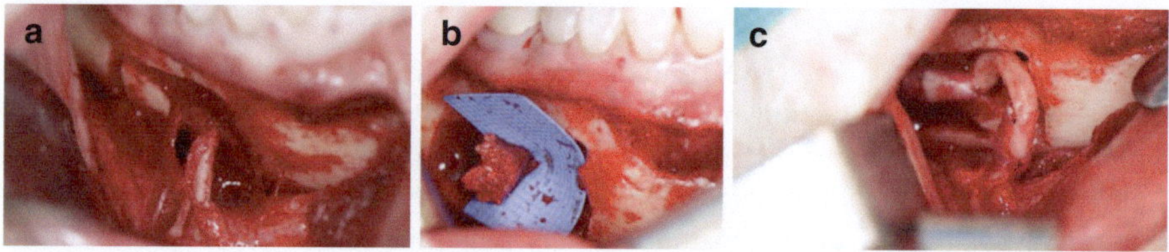

Fig. 19.3 A mental nerve injury is identified. (**a**) The proximal and distal nerve stumps are dissected and identified. (**b**) A buccal decortication is performed to gain access to additional length of inferior alveolar nerve. (**b**) The inferior alveolar nerve is removed from the canal and trimmed to healthy nerve tissue. (**c**) An interpositional allogenic nerve graft is used via a connector-assisted repair to reconstruct the mental nerve injury

There have been multiple studies and systematic reviews focusing on inferior alveolar nerve repair and reconstruction outcomes [1, 4, 16, 19–21]. Rates in the literature support 80% or more excellent FSR when direct repair is undertaken [4, 20]. When interpositional grafts are utilized, nerve autografts appear to have slightly lower rates of FSR in comparison to direct repair [4, 20]. Allogenic nerve sources for inferior alveolar nerve reconstruction have received much attention. FSR rates for IAN reconstructions utilizing allogenic sources are reported from 88% to 100%. The success rates appear to be higher when immediate reconstruction is performed [4, 16, 21].

The long buccal nerve is a terminal sensory branch of the mandibular division of the trigeminal nerve. It is close to local and regional infiltrative techniques routinely used in oral maxillofacial surgery. It runs on the surface of the buccinator muscle with sensory innervation from the commissure of the mouth and the buccal mucosa and around the posterior dental segment of the mandible. Anatomically the buccal nerve passes between the superior and inferior heads of the lateral pterygoid muscles and descends on the mandibular ramus onto the buccinator. Its final sensory plexus is with the facial nerve and the infraorbital nerve and the mental nerve.

Current Practices: Lingual Nerve Repair and Reconstruction

Damage to the lingual nerve affects tongue sensation, taste, and speech. The lingual nerve is typically approached intraorally when the repair is secondary to damage from dentoalveolar surgery (Fig. 19.4). The lingual nerve can also be approached in trans-cervical fashion when damaged or sacrificed during an ablative procedure (Fig. 19.5). Like the IAN, lingual nerve repair has shown to be successful in providing patients with functional sensory recovery [1, 4, 20]. Direct repair has shown success rates as high as 95% in the literature. Both autografts and allografts have also demonstrated success above 80–90%. Non-biological conduits have lower success rates than direct repair or grafting (need reference(s)—such as pogrel using vein grafts).

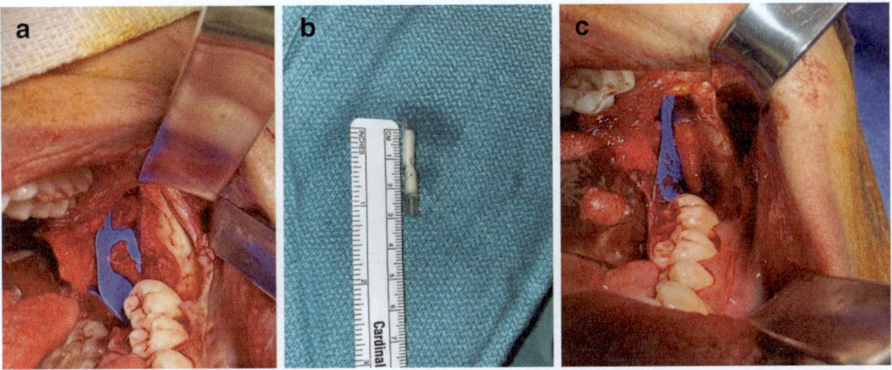

Fig. 19.4 Lingual nerve injury following third molar surgery. (**a**) The lingual nerve is approached intraorally. A lingual flap is elevated and the proximal and distal ends of the injured lingual nerve are identified. (**b**) An allogenic interpositional nerve graft is prepared with two nerve connectors prior to being brought into the surgical field. (**c**) The interpositional graft is secured to the proximal and distal nerve stumps

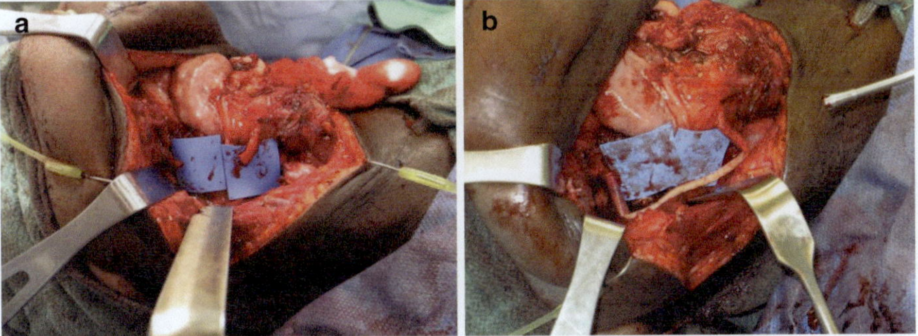

Fig. 19.5 Transcervical approach to a planned lingual nerve resection associated with an ablative procedure. (**a**) The proximal and distal lingual nerve stumps are identified and preserved. (**b**) The sacrificed lingual nerve is reconstructed with a combination of Avance™ and Axoguard™ products

Current Practices: Infraorbital Nerve (IO) Repair and Reconstruction

Recent reports detail immediate reconstruction of the second division of the trigeminal nerve. Infraorbital nerve repair planning and technique are similar to the inferior alveolar and lingual nerve. Aside from direct repair, studies have emerged detailing successful neurosensory recovery utilizing nerve allografts at the time of ablative maxillary procedures [18, 22]. In a small retrospective cohort, one group reported 100% FSR of three patients undergoing immediate allograft reconstruction of the infraorbital nerve at 6 months [18].

Measuring Outcomes and Controversies in Trigeminal Nerve Reconstruction

Peripheral trigeminal nerve repair and reconstruction have come a long way since Hippocrates. However, controversies still exist, and further research is needed to optimize patient outcomes. There is continued need for adequately powered prospective, multicenter studies. The Registry of Avance® Nerve Graft's Utilization and Recovery Outcomes Post Peripheral Nerve Reconstruction (RANGER®) has been established in one such attempt. This registered clinical trial (NCT01526681) aims to provide data for outcome analysis Avance™ assisted repairs. Trigeminal nerve reconstruction is included in the registry, which will hopefully aid in answering some of the clinical questions that still exist.

In a recent article by Pogrel, the author reports on long-term outcome data following the sacrifice of the inferior alveolar nerve during mandibular resection [23]. In his retrospective review, the author reports on sensation recovery without nerve reconstruction in 30 patients. The author found 29 of the 30 patients regained some sensation in the IAN distribution. Additionally, 70% of the subjects had a return of function at the MRCS S3 level. The author noted that subjects adapted well to the loss of sensation and had little effect on quality of life. Even though the author asks readers to interpret the results with caution, the study highlights the need for well-designed studies evaluating both the short-term and long-term benefits of trigeminal reconstruction after ablation utilizing the latest tools and techniques.

Future Developments

The use of autografts and allografts to repair human trigeminal nerve injuries has resulted in 70–90% successful recovery that surpasses the performance of any second-generation nerve conduit [4, 24]. However, autografts have multiple limitations including the sensory loss of secondary surgical sites and the risk of neuroma formation [25, 26]. Allografts, on the other hand, have high costs and potential limited availability, particularly on demand. Hence, third-generation nerve conduits are being actively studied with potential to replace autografts and allografts to achieve optimal surgical outcomes.

As successful peripheral nerve regeneration requires biochemical and structural cues, the main objectives of third-generation nerve conduits involve initiating/extending the regenerative phase after nerve injuries and recapitulating the native environment of nerve tissues [26, 27]. Many tissue engineering strategies such as growth factors, stem cell therapy, and intraluminal architecture are currently employed to enhance the rate of nerve regeneration. Each methodology plays a vital role in developing future treatments, with its advantages/limitations summarized in Table 19.1.

Growth factors facilitate nerve regeneration via their interactions with cell surface receptors, which trigger intracellular signal transduction, including the mitogen-activated protein kinase pathway [26, 28, 29]. As a result, neurons undergo axonal outgrowth and less apoptosis. After nerve injuries, the production of neurotrophic factors is only upregulated for a few hours to days, insufficient for regenerating larger nerve defects [27, 30]. In rabbit IAN injury models, injections of human

Table 19.1 Overview of common tissue engineering strategies found in third-generation nerve conduits

Strategy	Working principle	Advantages	Limitations
Growth factors (NGF/hbFGF)	Interact with cell surface receptors to stimulate axonal outgrowths	1. Easy to use	1. Short shelf-lives
		2. Readily available	2. Tumorigenesis
			3. Hyperalgesia
Stem cells (ADSCs/NSCs)	Dynamic and long-term release of a combination of neurotrophic factors	1. Self-renewal	1. Unclear long-term metabolic activities
		2. Able to differentiate into specialized cells	2. High costs
			3. Time-consuming
			4. Tumorigenesis
Intraluminal architecture (matrices/hydrogels)	Provide directional guidance/structural support for axon elongation/adhesion	1. Mimic native microenvironment	1. Low bioactivity
		2. Low cost	
		3. Low immunogenicity	
		4. Few side effects	

nerve growth factor and basic fibroblast growth factor (FGF) near surgical sites show limited improvement in myelination and jaw-opening reflex thresholds, respectively [31–33]. It is hypothesized that the supplemental growth factors quickly decrease in concentration below the triggering threshold of surface receptors. To improve the efficacy of growth factor treatments, researchers have investigated different entrapment strategies to control the release of growth factors [26, 34]. Growth factors can be chemically attached to the nerve conduits to prolong their release [35, 36]. Multiple vehicles including microspheres [37, 38] and nanoparticles [39–41] have been loaded with growth factors and localized within nerve conduits for sustained delivery. Furthermore, matrix-like materials can mix with neurotrophic factors before in situ injection within the nerve conduits to achieve physical entrapment [42, 43]. In rat sciatic nerve resection models, these spatiotemporal delivery approaches lead to better axon counts, gastrocnemius muscle retention, and electrical conduction [35–43]. The use of growth factors is quick and simple but unsuitable for long-term regeneration due to short shelf-lives. The common side effects found in preclinical studies consist of tumorigenesis and hyperalgesia at surgical sites [28, 44, 45].

Peripheral nerve regeneration is complex and difficult to mimic by the controlled release of growth factors alone [26, 27]. In vivo, regeneration involves interaction between multiple neurotropic factors, cytokines, Schwann cells, and macrophages. Introducing stem cells to surgical sites replenishes damaged cells during nerve injures and supports continuous release of multiple growth factors that facilitate nerve regeneration and angiogenesis [46]. Adipose stem cells (ADSCs), harvested from patients' fat tissues, have been reported to accelerate sciatic nerve regeneration in rodent models [47–49]. When encapsulated in gelatin methacrylate (GelMA) gels, ADSCs resulted in better electrophysiological performance and myelination than acellular conduits after 16-week implantation [48]. Similar improvements were also observed in another study that embedded ADSCs within dual-layer conduits made of poly(caprolactone) and GelMA [49]. Further immunofluorescence staining showed that some ADSCs stayed well encapsulated for 6 weeks [49]. In addition to these direct encapsulation methodologies, ADSCs can be differentiated to express Schwann cell-like behaviors and biomarkers before use [47, 50, 51]. These differentiated ADSCs and autografts shared comparable measurements in nerve density and the amplitude of compound muscle action potential (CMAP) in a 16-week study [50]. Alternatively, neural stem cells (NSCs), derived from induced pluripotent stem cells, can differentiate into Schwann-like cells and enhance functional recovery and axon count of resected rat sciatic nerves after 12 weeks [52]. When encapsulated into GelMA and implanted into injured spinal cords, NSCs promote axonal regeneration and inhibit glial scar formation [53]. The self-renewal and multipotent characteristics of ADSCs and NSCs allow them to be cultured into large quantities of specialized cells [26, 47]. Harvesting patients' own stem cells also reduces the risk of immune rejection. However, stem cells' long-term metabolic activity and viability after in vivo implantations remain unclear. High costs, time-consuming procedures, and the inherent tumorigenicity associated with stem cell therapy are challenging roadblocks that need to be overcome before clinical use [26, 47, 54].

Intraluminal architecture, present in autografts and allografts, is not present in second-generation conduits. Some research in third-generation conduits focuses on adding solid structures [55–57], microporous matrices [58, 59], and nanofibrous hydrogels [60–67] within the conduits to promote cellular adhesions and direct axonal outgrowth. Regenerated axons can orient themselves and grow within spaces between solid structures such as multichannels [55, 56] and bundled rods [57]. Yet, solid structures reduce cross-sectional area that could be occupied by axons. Microporous matrices maximize the available area by creating a greater number of micro-size canals. For example, a honeycomb architecture fabricated from unidirectional freezing demonstrated accelerated sciatic nerve regeneration [58, 59]. Moreover, nanofibrous hydrogels better mimic the characteristics of uninjured nerve tissues due to their resemblance to extracellular matrix, large water content, and physiologically relevant material stiffness [68–70]. In rodent sciatic nerve transection models, the use of fibrin and silk hydrogels in conduits results in faster neurite elongation and greater amplitude of CMAP respectively after 4-week implantation when compared to hollow conduits [60–63]. Alternatively, some studies investigate the neuroregenerative potential of self-assembling peptides, customized with biomimetic motifs from growth factors that introduce bioactivity in synthetic hydrogels [70]. Peptide amphiphiles with RGDS (integrin binding) and Ile-Lys-Val-ala-Val (IKVAV) (laminin-mimetic) peptide sequences have more cell density than the negative control after 12 weeks in sciatic nerve regeneration [64]. Álvarez et al. fine-tuned the linkage sequence of peptide amphiphiles and added a FGF mimetic sequence, which yielded better neuronal extension and motor functional recovery in a murine spinal cord injury model [65]. In a study from our lab using a nerve crush injury model in rats, multidomain peptide hydrogels showed improved motor recovery and significant remyelination after 15 days [66]. The internal modification of third-generation conduits has potentially fewer side effects than growth factors and cell therapies, but faces challenges with reduced bioactivity.

The future of trigeminal nerve reconstruction will involve third-generation nerve conduits with the implementations of growth factors, stem cells, and/or internal architecture, along with 3D bioprinting to regenerate convoluted and large-scale nerve defects. Further advancement and combinations of these approaches would supersede the clinical outcomes of autografts and allografts with fewer side effects. Most of the nerve conduit research is tested in rodent models, with a few exceptions in canine, feline, and leporine models [33, 71–73]. As the pathophysiology and recovery process of large animal and primate resemble those of humans, third-generation nerve conduits must be validated by large animal studies before human clinical trials to ensure the safety and efficacy of these conduits [74].

References

1. Weyh A, Pucci R, Valentini V, Fernandes R, Salman S. Injuries of the peripheral mandibular nerve, evaluation of interventions and outcomes: a systematic review. Craniomaxillofac Trauma Reconstr. 2021;14(4):337–48.
2. Kaleem A, Amailuk P, Hatoum H, Tursun R. The trigeminal nerve injury. Oral Maxillofac Surg Clin North Am. 2020;32(4):675–87. https://doi.org/10.1016/j.coms.2020.07.005.
3. Meyer RA, Bagheri SC. Microsurgical reconstruction of the trigeminal nerve. Oral Maxillofac Surg Clin North Am. 2013;25(2):287–302. https://doi.org/10.1016/j.coms.2013.01.002.
4. Ducic I, Yoon J. Reconstructive options for inferior alveolar and lingual nerve injuries after dental and oral surgery: an evidence-based review. Ann Plast Surg. 2019;82(6):653–60.
5. Smith JG, Elias L-A, Yilmaz Z, Barker S, Shah K, Shah S, et al. The psychosocial and affective burden of posttraumatic stress neuropathy following injuries to the trigeminal nerve. J Orofac Pain. 2013;27(4):293–303.
6. Miloro M, Zuniga JR, Meyer RA. How many oral surgeons does it take to classify a nerve injury? J Oral Maxillofac Surg. 2021;79(7):1550–6. https://doi.org/10.1016/j.joms.2021.01.006.
7. Walters BC. History of peripheral nerve repair. Vol. 1, Nerves and nerve injuries. London: Elsevier; 2015. p. 23–36. https://doi.org/10.1016/B978-0-12-410390-0.00002-0.
8. Belen D, Aciduman A, Er U. History of peripheral nerve repair: may the procedure have been practiced in Hippocratic School? Surg Neurol. 2009;72(2):190–3. https://doi.org/10.1016/j.surneu.2008.03.030.
9. Wessberg GA, Wolford LM. Bilateral microneurosurgical reconstruction of inferior alveolar nerves via autogenous sural nerve transplantation. Oral Surg Oral Med Oral Pathol. 1981;52(5):465–70.
10. Mozsary PG, Middleton RA. Microsurgical reconstruction of the lingual nerve. J Oral Maxillofac Surg. 1984;42(7):415–20.
11. Hausamen JE, Samii M, Schmidseder R. Indication and technique for the reconstruction of nerve defects in head and neck. J Maxillofac Surg. 1974;2(C):159–67.
12. Seddon HJ. A classification of nerve injuries. Br Med J. 1942;2(4260):237–9.
13. Gaudin R, Knipfer C, Henningsen A, Smeets R, Heiland M, Hadlock T. Approaches to peripheral nerve repair: generations of biomaterial conduits yielding to replacing autologous nerve grafts in craniomaxillofacial surgery. Biomed Res Int. 2016;2016:3856262.
14. Shanti RM, Ziccardi VB. Use of decellularized nerve allograft for inferior alveolar nerve reconstruction: a case report. J Oral Maxillofac Surg. 2011;69(2):550–3. https://doi.org/10.1016/j.joms.2010.10.004.
15. Ducic I, Safa B, De Vinney E. Refinements of nerve repair with connector-assisted coaptation. Microsurgery. 2017;37(3):256–63.
16. Zuniga JR, Williams F, Petrisor D. A case-and-control, multisite, positive controlled, prospective study of the safety and effectiveness of immediate inferior alveolar nerve processed nerve allograft reconstruction with ablation of the mandible for benign pathology. J Oral Maxillofac Surg. 2017;75(12):2669–81. https://doi.org/10.1016/j.joms.2017.04.002.
17. AxoGen. 2022. https://www.axogeninc.com.
18. Callahan N, Miloro M, Markiewicz MR. Immediate reconstruction of the infraorbital nerve after maxillectomy: is it feasible? J Oral Maxillofac Surg. 2020;78(12):2300–5. https://doi.org/10.1016/j.joms.2020.07.211.
19. Suhaym O, Miloro M. Does early repair of trigeminal nerve injuries influence neurosensory recovery? A systematic review and meta-analysis. Int J Oral Maxillofac Surg. 2021;50(6):820–9. https://doi.org/10.1016/j.ijom.2020.10.002.
20. Kushnerev E, Yates JM. Evidence-based outcomes following inferior alveolar and lingual nerve injury and repair: a systematic review. J Oral Rehabil. 2015;42(10):786–802.
21. Miloro M, Zuniga JR. Does immediate inferior alveolar nerve allograft reconstruction result in functional sensory recovery in pediatric patients? J Oral Maxillofac Surg. 2020;78(11):2073–9. https://doi.org/10.1016/j.joms.2020.06.033.

22. Rath EM. Surgical treatment of maxillary nerve injuries. The infraorbital nerve. Atlas Oral Maxillofac Surg Clin North Am. 2001;9(2):31–41.
23. Pogrel MA. Recovery of sensation over the distribution of the inferior alveolar nerve following mandibular resection without nerve reconstruction. J Oral Maxillofac Surg. 2021;79(10):2143–6. https://doi.org/10.1016/j.joms.2021.04.029.
24. Le Donne M, Jouan R, Bourlet J, Louvrier A, Ducret M, Sigaux N. Inferior alveolar nerve allogenic repair following mandibulectomy: a systematic review. J Stomatol Oral Maxillofac Surg. 2021;123:233–8. https://doi.org/10.1016/j.jormas.2021.04.007.
25. Kehoe S, Zhang XF, Boyd D. FDA approved guidance conduits and wraps for peripheral nerve injury: a review of materials and efficacy. Injury. 2012;43(5):553–72. https://doi.org/10.1016/j.injury.2010.12.030.
26. López-Cebral R, Silva-Correia J, Reis RL, Silva TH, Oliveira JM. Peripheral nerve injury: current challenges, conventional treatment approaches, and new trends in biomaterials-based regenerative strategies. ACS Biomater Sci Eng. 2017;3(12):3098–122. https://doi.org/10.1021/acsbiomaterials.7b00655.
27. Scheib J, Höke A. Advances in peripheral nerve regeneration. Nat Rev Neurol. 2013;9(12):668–76. https://doi.org/10.1038/nrneurol.2013.227.
28. Aloe L, Rocco ML, Bianchi P, Manni L. Nerve growth factor: from the early discoveries to the potential clinical use. J Transl Med. 2012;10(1):1–15. https://doi.org/10.1186/1479-5876-10-239.
29. Li R, Li DH, Zhang HY, Wang J, Li XK, Xiao J. Growth factors-based therapeutic strategies and their underlying signaling mechanisms for peripheral nerve regeneration. Acta Pharmacol Sin. 2020;41(10):1289–300. https://doi.org/10.1038/s41401-019-0338-1.
30. Rotshenker S. Wallerian degeneration: the innate-immune response to traumatic nerve injury. J Neuroinflammation. 2011;8:109. https://doi.org/10.1186/1742-2094-8-109.
31. Wang L, Zhao Y, Cheng X, et al. Effects of locally applied nerve growth factor to the inferior alveolar nerve histology in a rabbit model of mandibular distraction osteogenesis. Int J Oral Maxillofac Surg. 2009;38(1):64–9. https://doi.org/10.1016/j.ijom.2008.11.010.
32. Hergt AC, Beck-Broichsitter BE, Raethjen J, et al. Nerve regeneration techniques respecting the special characteristics of the inferior alveolar nerve. J Cranio-Maxillofac Surg. 2016;44(9):1381–6. https://doi.org/10.1016/j.jcms.2016.06.020.
33. Nemoto A, Akashi Y, Nakajima K, et al. The effects of recombinant human basic fibroblast growth factor on nerve regeneration in a partial defect inferior alveolar nerve model in rabbits. J Oral Maxillofac Surg Med Pathol. 2021;33(3):348–53. https://doi.org/10.1016/j.ajoms.2020.12.003.
34. Sarker MD, Naghieh S, McInnes AD, Schreyer DJ, Chen X. Regeneration of peripheral nerves by nerve guidance conduits: influence of design, biopolymers, cells, growth factors, and physical stimuli. Prog Neurobiol. 2018;171(July):125–50. https://doi.org/10.1016/j.pneurobio.2018.07.002.
35. Madduri S, Feldman K, Tervoort T, Papaloïzos M, Gander B. Collagen nerve conduits releasing the neurotrophic factors GDNF and NGF. J Control Release. 2010;143(2):168–74. https://doi.org/10.1016/j.jconrel.2009.12.017.
36. Ma F, Xu F, Li R, et al. Sustained delivery of glial cell-derived neurotrophic factors in collagen conduits for facial nerve regeneration. Acta Biomater. 2018;69:146–55.
37. Roam JL, Yan Y, Nguyen PK, et al. A modular, plasmin-sensitive, clickable poly(ethylene glycol)-heparin-laminin microsphere system for establishing growth factor gradients in nerve guidance conduits. Biomaterials. 2015;72:112–24. https://doi.org/10.1016/j.biomaterials.2015.08.054.
38. Wood MD, Gordon T, Kim H, et al. Fibrin gels containing GDNF microspheres increase axonal regeneration after delayed peripheral nerve repair. Regen Med. 2013;8(1):27–37.
39. Giannaccini M, Calatayud MP, Poggetti A, et al. Magnetic nanoparticles for efficient delivery of growth factors: stimulation of peripheral nerve regeneration. Adv Healthc Mater. 2017;6(7):1601429. https://doi.org/10.1002/adhm.201601429.

40. Chen X, Ge X, Qian Y, et al. Electrospinning multilayered scaffolds loaded with melatonin and Fe3O4 magnetic nanoparticles for peripheral nerve regeneration. Adv Funct Mater. 2020;30(38):1–12. https://doi.org/10.1002/adfm.202004537.
41. Wei Z, Hong FF, Cao Z, Zhao SY, Chen L. In situ fabrication of nerve growth factor encapsulated chitosan nanoparticles in oxidized bacterial nanocellulose for rat sciatic nerve regeneration. Biomacromolecules. 2021;22(12):4988–99. https://doi.org/10.1021/acs.biomac.1c00947.
42. Mokarram N, Merchant A, Mukhatyar V, Patel G, Bellamkonda RV. Effect of modulating macrophage phenotype on peripheral nerve repair. Biomaterials. 2012;33(34):8793–801. https://doi.org/10.1016/j.biomaterials.2012.08.050.
43. Mokarram N, Dymanusb K, Srinivasan A, et al. Immunoengineering nerve repair. Proc Natl Acad Sci U S A. 2017;114(26):E5077–84. https://doi.org/10.1073/pnas.1705757114.
44. Khodorova A, Nicol GD, Strichartz G. The TrkA receptor mediates experimental thermal hyperalgesia produced by nerve growth factor: modulation by the p75 neurotrophin receptor. Neuroscience. 2017;340:384–97. https://doi.org/10.1016/j.neuroscience.2016.10.064.
45. Hayakawa Y, Sakitani K, Konishi M, et al. Nerve growth factor promotes gastric tumorigenesis through aberrant cholinergic signaling. Cancer Cell. 2017;31(1):21–34. https://doi.org/10.1016/j.ccell.2016.11.005.
46. Li Y, Fraser D, Mereness J, et al. Tissue engineered neurovascularization strategies for craniofacial tissue regeneration. ACS Appl Bio Mater. 2022;5(1):20–39. https://doi.org/10.1021/acsabm.1c00979.
47. Khalifian S, Sarhane KA, Tammia M, et al. Stem cell-based approaches to improve nerve regeneration: potential implications for reconstructive transplantation? Arch Immunol Ther Exp. 2015;63(1):15–30. https://doi.org/10.1007/s00005-014-0323-9.
48. Hu Y, Wu Y, Gou Z, et al. 3D-engineering of cellularized conduits for peripheral nerve regeneration. Sci Rep. 2016;6(August):1–12. https://doi.org/10.1038/srep32184.
49. Sun AX, Prest TA, Fowler JR, et al. Conduits harnessing spatially controlled cell-secreted neurotrophic factors improve peripheral nerve regeneration. Biomaterials. 2019;203:86–95. https://doi.org/10.1016/j.biomaterials.2019.01.038.
50. di Summa PG, Kalbermatten DF, Pralong E, Raffoul W, Kingham PJ, Terenghi G. Long-term in vivo regeneration of peripheral nerves through bioengineered nerve grafts. Neuroscience. 2011;181:278.
51. Wang Y, Zhao Z, Ren Z, et al. Recellularized nerve allografts with differentiated mesenchymal stem cells promote peripheral nerve regeneration. Neurosci Lett. 2012;514(1):96–101. https://doi.org/10.1016/j.neulet.2012.02.066.
52. Onode E, Uemura T, Takamatsu K, et al. Bioabsorbable nerve conduits three-dimensionally coated with human induced pluripotent stem cell-derived neural stem/progenitor cells promote peripheral nerve regeneration in rats. Sci Rep. 2021;11(1):1–13. https://doi.org/10.1038/s41598-021-83385-9.
53. Fan L, Liu C, Chen X, et al. Directing induced pluripotent stem cell derived neural stem cell fate with a three-dimensional biomimetic hydrogel for spinal cord injury repair. ACS Appl Mater Interfaces. 2018;10(21):17742–55. https://doi.org/10.1021/acsami.8b05293.
54. Lee AS, Tang C, Rao MS, Weissman IL, Wu JC. Tumorigenicity as a clinical hurdle for pluripotent stem cell therapies. Nat Med. 2013;19(8):998–1004. https://doi.org/10.1038/nm.3267.
55. Arcaute K, Mann BK, Wicker RB. Fabrication of off-the-shelf multilumen poly(Ethylene glycol) nerve guidance conduits using stereolithography. Tissue Eng Part C Methods. 2010;17(1):27–38. https://doi.org/10.1089/ten.tec.2010.0011.
56. Yao L, de Ruiter GCW, Wang H, et al. Controlling dispersion of axonal regeneration using a multichannel collagen nerve conduit. Biomaterials. 2010;31(22):5789–97. https://doi.org/10.1016/j.biomaterials.2010.03.081.
57. Koh HS, Yong T, Teo WE, et al. In vivo study of novel nanofibrous intra-luminal guidance channels to promote nerve regeneration. J Neural Eng. 2010;7(4):046003. https://doi.org/10.1088/1741-2560/7/4/046003.

58. Singh A, Asikainen S, Teotia AK, et al. Biomimetic photocurable three-dimensional printed nerve guidance channels with aligned cryomatrix lumen for peripheral nerve regeneration. ACS Appl Mater Interfaces. 2018;10(50):43327–42. https://doi.org/10.1021/acsami.8b11677.

59. Huang L, Zhu L, Shi X, et al. A compound scaffold with uniform longitudinally oriented guidance cues and a porous sheath promotes peripheral nerve regeneration in vivo. Acta Biomater. 2018;68:223–36. https://doi.org/10.1016/j.actbio.2017.12.010.

60. Du J, Liu J, Yao S, et al. Prompt peripheral nerve regeneration induced by a hierarchically aligned fibrin nanofiber hydrogel. Acta Biomater. 2017;55:296–309. https://doi.org/10.1016/j.actbio.2017.04.010.

61. Yang S, Zhu J, Lu C, et al. Aligned fibrin/functionalized self-assembling peptide interpenetrating nanofiber hydrogel presenting multi-cues promotes peripheral nerve functional recovery. Bioact Mater. 2022;8:529–44. https://doi.org/10.1016/j.bioactmat.2021.05.056.

62. Magaz A, Faroni A, Gough JE, Reid AJ, Li X, Blaker JJ. Bioactive silk-based nerve guidance conduits for augmenting peripheral nerve repair. Adv Healthc Mater. 2018;7(23):e1800308. https://doi.org/10.1002/adhm.201800308.

63. Wei GJ, Yao M, Wang YS, et al. Promotion of peripheral nerve regeneration of a peptide compound hydrogel scaffold. Int J Nanomedicine. 2013;8:3217–25. https://doi.org/10.2147/IJN.S43681.

64. Li A, Hokugo A, Yalom A, et al. A bioengineered peripheral nerve construct using aligned peptide amphiphile nanofibers. Biomaterials. 2014;35(31):8780–90. https://doi.org/10.1016/j.biomaterials.2014.06.049.

65. Álvarez Z, Kolberg-Edelbrock AN, Sasselli IR, et al. Bioactive scaffolds with enhanced supramolecular motion promote recovery from spinal cord injury. Science. 2021;374(6569):848–56. https://doi.org/10.1126/science.abh3602.

66. Lopez-Silva TL, Cristobal CD, Lai CSE, Leyva-Aranda V, Lee HK, Hartgerink JD. Self-assembling multidomain peptide hydrogels accelerate peripheral nerve regeneration after crush injury. Biomaterials. 2021;265:120401. https://doi.org/10.1016/j.biomaterials.2020.120401.

67. Wu X, He L, Li W, et al. Functional self-assembling peptide nanofiber hydrogel for peripheral nerve regeneration. Regen Biomater. 2017;4(1):21–30. https://doi.org/10.1093/rb/rbw034.

68. Leach JB, Brown XQ, Jacot JG, Dimilla PA, Wong JY. Neurite outgrowth and branching of PC12 cells on very soft substrates sharply decreases below a threshold of substrate rigidity. J Neural Eng. 2007;4(2):26–34. https://doi.org/10.1088/1741-2560/4/2/003.

69. Wheeldon I, Farhadi A, Bick AG, Jabbari E, Khademhosseini A. Nanoscale tissue engineering: spatial control over cell-materials interactions. Nanotechnology. 2011;22(21):212001. https://doi.org/10.1088/0957-4484/22/21/212001.Nanoscale.

70. Levin A, Hakala TA, Schnaider L, Bernardes GJL, Gazit E, Knowles TPJ. Biomimetic peptide self-assembly for functional materials. Nat Rev Chem. 2020;4(11):615–34. https://doi.org/10.1038/s41570-020-0215-y.

71. Wang X, Hu W, Cao Y, Yao J, Wu J, Gu X. Dog sciatic nerve regeneration across a 30-mm defect bridged by a chitosan/PGA artificial nerve graft. Brain. 2005;128(8):1897–910.

72. Sufan W, Suzuki Y, Tanihara M, et al. Sciatic nerve regeneration through alginate with tubulation or nontubulation repair in cat. J Neurotrauma. 2001;18(3):329–38. https://doi.org/10.1089/08977150151070991.

73. Takata M, Murayama M, Sasaki K, Shibahara T. Histomorphometric observations of surgical methods for partial amputation injury of the inferior alveolar nerve using polyglycolic acid. J Oral Maxillofac Surg Med Pathol. 2018;30(2):95–110. https://doi.org/10.1016/j.ajoms.2017.10.001.

74. Ribitsch I, Baptista PM, Lange-Consiglio A, et al. Large animal models in regenerative medicine and tissue engineering: to do or not to do. Front Bioeng Biotechnol. 2020;8(August):1–28. https://doi.org/10.3389/fbioe.2020.00972.

Chapter 20
Gender-Affirming Facial Surgery: Office-Based Procedures

Abigail Frazier, Poolak Bhatt, and Elda Fisher

Transgender care has become a critical point of discussion within healthcare spheres. With the number of patients seeking gender-affirming care on the rise, it is crucial to provide insight into transgender populations, along with a thorough understanding of medical and surgical techniques to meet the needs of transgender patients. This chapter aims to briefly investigate the definition of gender dysphoria, the basic World Professional Association for Transgender Health (WPATH) criteria for gender-affirming care and the application of gender-affirming surgery as it applies to office-based procedures for facial gender affirmation.

Transgender Populations

Terminology

Over the last few decades, transgender terminology has rapidly evolved to reflect the growing needs of the community. It is critical for surgeons to understand fundamental differences in terminology to successfully treat this population. Perhaps most crucial to the discussion of gender-affirming surgery is distinguishing between gender nonconformity and gender dysphoria. It is well established that biological

A. Frazier · P. Bhatt · E. Fisher (✉)
Division of Craniofacial and Surgical Care, ASoD, University of North Carolina at Chapel Hill, Chapel Hill, NC, USA

Residency Program in Oral and Maxillofacial Surgery, University of North Carolina Hospitals, Chapel Hill, NC, USA
e-mail: Abigail.Frazier@unchealth.unc.edu; Poolak.Bhatt@unchealth.unc.edu; elda.fisher@unc.edu

J. C. Melville et al. (eds.), *Advancements and Innovations in OMFS, ENT, and Facial Plastic Surgery*, https://doi.org/10.1007/978-3-031-32099-6_20

sex and gender are exclusive entities, with sex referring to specific chromosomes and genitalia that identify people as either "male" or "female" at birth and gender referring to the internal feelings of masculinity or femininity experienced by each person. From these definitions, each culture has adopted both spoken and unspoken protocols dictating how a person's gender should align with their birth sex [1]. While the majority of the population has a gender identity that conforms with their biological sex, a subset of people do not share this experience. Interestingly, there is a growing body of evidence suggesting one's brain has anatomic findings that reflect their preferred biological sex rather than their assigned biological sex [2]. As a person's gender identity, role, or expression begins to contrast with gender norms for a given sex, they are considered transgender/gender nonconforming. While gender nonconformity is a blanket statement for the extent one's gender expression deviates from cultural norms, gender dysphoria is the marked stress and discomfort resulting from the inconsistency between birth sex and gender identity [3]. It is within the gender dysphoria population that gender-affirming surgeons find themselves tasked to address surgical needs to alleviate distress on the road to acceptance for their desired gender expression and identity.

Validation and support for the transgender community begin long before the surgery date. In addition to understanding transgender terminology, the proper use of pronouns is vital to generating trust and respect with patients. Misgendering patients continues to serve as a barrier to healthcare access for the transgender community [3–5]. To counteract this issue, it is recommended that gender-affirming surgeons make inclusive questions and language part of their daily routine, including asking each patient their preferred pronouns. Proactive measures are the foundation for building relationships and achieving long-term treatment goals.

Epidemiology

The question that arises during gender-affirming surgery discussions is that of need. *What is the prevalence of people who identify as transgender, and how many have gender dysphoria that requires medical and surgical intervention?* In the United States, most recent studies have identified anywhere between 0.4% and 3% of the population identify themselves as transgender [6, 7]. This equates to, at the very least, over one million people in the United States who are transgender. International studies over the years have discovered the prevalence of those living with gender dysphoria to range from 1:11,900 to 1:45,000 for male-to-female individuals (MtF) and 1:30,400 to 1:200,000 for female-to-male (FtM) individuals [3]. Though studies range in their methodology, there is a common theme among scholars: the population of transgender and those living with gender dysphoria is grossly underestimated. Reasons for this discrepancy include but are not limited to access to healthcare, discrimination and fear surrounding gender nonconforming individuals, and lack of education to both healthcare providers and the public [3, 6, 7]. Since it is assumed the true population of transgender individuals is underrepresented, the question becomes not whether the need exists, but how can surgeons advocate for transgender patients through medical and surgical intervention.

Inaccurate representation of the transgender population is in part due to discrimination in healthcare environments. Roughly one-third of transgender patients have reported some form of harassment or outright denial of service in a medical setting, causing many transgender people to postpone medical care altogether [2]. There are, therefore, health disparities unique to the transgender population such as higher than average rates of HIV, drug, and alcohol dependence found in transgender populations. Notably, with the absence of regular care to monitor hormone therapy, one in four transgender people have turned to self-prescribing illegally obtained cross-sex hormones to manage their dysphoria [2]. Further, without adequate attention to the subject, transgender patients who should be screened for cancer/disease associated with sex are overlooked. Not only is this dangerous if pathological processes go undiagnosed, but without transgender-competent providers, transgender patients who are screened for organ-associated disease processes can experience further physical and emotional distress when the screening does not affirm their gender [3]. Finally, suicide and suicidal ideation are alarmingly high in this population and should be addressed in the context of psychosocial considerations as a whole.

In the United States, the annual rate for suicidal ideation is 4%. This is a staggering contrast to the transgender community, where reports of suicidal ideation reach as high as 50% of the population [8]. The reason behind such a stark contrast is multifactorial but is centered around the psychosocial pain and stress faced by the transgender community due to discrimination within society. Transgender people are twice likely to be refused a job compared to cis-LGB (lesbian, gay, and bisexual individuals who identify with their assigned birth gender) employees, have 2.2× greater risk of homelessness than non-LGBT (lesbian, gay, bisexual, transgender) individuals, experience 71.1 violent victimizations per 1000 people compared to 19.2 per 1000 non-LGBT people, and are overall more likely to experience prejudice and bullying from peers and family [3, 9, 10, 11]. The levels of anxiety, depression, eating disorders, self-harm, and suicidal ideation are influenced heavily by the experiences transgender people have in their daily lives. It is important to be cognizant of health disparities and psychosocial considerations in the transgender community to educate, refer to specialists, and support them in continuity of care.

Gender-Affirming Care

With a broad understanding of transgender terminology and epidemiology, the discussion can appropriately shift to medical interventions and their associated criteria for transgender patients. The current authority on transgender treatment guidelines is The Standards of Care Version 7, researched and constructed by the World Professional Association for Transgender Health (WPATH). In short, this document functions "to provide clinical guidance for health professionals to assist transsexual, transgender, and gender-nonconforming people with safe and effective pathways to achieving lasting personal comfort with their gendered selves, in order to maximize their overall health, psychological well-being, and self-fulfillment." [3] An important aspect of these guidelines are criteria for hormonal and surgical intervention. For both hormonal and surgical intervention, it is required to have (1) persistent, well-documented gender dysphoria (12 months for surgical intervention), (2) the capacity to make fully informed decision and to consent for treatment, (3) age of majority in a given country, and (4) reasonably well-controlled medical or mental health concerns if present. Additional requirements for surgery include (1) referrals from a qualified mental health professional, (2) hormone therapy, and (3) 12 continuous months of living in a gender role that is congruent with their gender identity. The 12-month criteria serve as an evidence-based timeline to give patients ample time to socially adjust to the desired gender role before undergoing irreversible interventions [3].

Given the above criteria, most gender dysphoria patients who present for gender-affirming facial surgery consultations have had hormone and other surgical therapy. For hormone therapy, dosage and regimen vary greatly depending on the person and predisposing risks for complications. For feminizing medications, a combination of estrogen and anti-androgens are most commonly used. Given the risk of venous thromboembolism (VTE) associated with high-dose exogenous estrogen, transdermal estrogen is recommended, and anti-androgen medications minimize the amount of estrogen needed to suppress testosterone [3]. Common anti-androgenic hormones include spironolactone (Aldactone), cyproterone (Androcur), GnRH agonists (Eligard, Lupron Depot), and 5-alpha reductase inhibitors (Avodart, Propecia). For masculinizing hormones, testosterone is sufficient, although progestins can be used in the early stages for a short time to aid in menstrual cessation [3]. The degree/rate of physical effects and development of risks depends on the medication(s) of choice, dose, and route of administration. Risks as defined by the standard of care are categorized by "likely increased risk," "possible increased risk," and "no increased risk or inconclusive." Feminizing hormones are associated with a likely increased risk of complications like VTE and hypertriglyceridemia, but there is currently no increased risk of breast cancer. Masculinizing hormones are associated with a likely increased risk of complications like polycythemia, male pattern balding, and sleep apnea, but there is currently no evidence to support risk of breast, cervical, ovarian, or uterine cancer [3]. These risks and other potential risks are summarized in Table 20.1. In general and although highly variable, physical changes are expected to occur over the course of 2 years [3] (Table 20.1).

Table 20.1   Risk of various diseases associated with feminizing and masculinizing hormones

Feminizing hormones	Masculinizing hormones	
• Breast cancer	• Breast cancer • Cervical cancer • Decreased bone density • Ovarian cancer • Uterine cancer	No known increased risk of these outcomes
• Hyperprolactinemia • Hypertension • Prolactinoma • Type 2 diabetes	• Cardiovascular disease • Elevated liver enzymes • Exacerbation of psychiatric disorder • Hyperlipidemia • Hypertension • Type 2 diabetes	Possible increased risk
• Cholelithiasis • Elevated liver enzymes • Hyperlipidemia • Venous thromboembolism • Weight gain	• Acne • Andogenic alopecia • Polycythemia • Weight gain • Obstructive sleep apnea	Increased risk

The Facial Skeletal and Soft Tissue Differences

The foundation for facial feminization surgical planning must be a sound knowledge of anatomy and its variations between men and women. Over the years, anthropometric and cephalometric studies have determined facial sex differences are most noticeable in the forehead/supraorbital ridges, orbital borders, malar eminences, nose, mandible, and neck form [12, 13]. It is important to note there are other variables that affect facial shape and proportions besides gender, such as race and age; however, for the purpose of this discussion, craniofacial and soft tissue standards are compared only between males and females.

The craniofacial skeleton has distinct bony that are the target of facial feminization procedures. Overall, the male face is wider and longer in regard to both the skeletal and soft tissue due to the length of exposure to and amount of testosterone during development. There are standard measurements that delineate the general differences in facial width and height between men and women: Fig. 20.1.

Not only is the male face larger overall, but variations exist within each facial third. With the upper facial third, the forehead and orbital rims differ between males and females. In females, their forehead slope tends to be more vertical, they have more obtuse nasofrontal angle, and less projection of lateral orbital rims. The angulation in the forehead slope is measured relative to the vertical plane through the glabella [13].

The supraorbital and lateral orbital rims normally project 5–10 mm beyond the anterior corneal plane and are far more pronounced in men than women [13]. In addition, the nasion in males is deeper than in females [6]. As a result, the nasofrontal angle in men is more acute than in females [13] (Fig. 20.2).

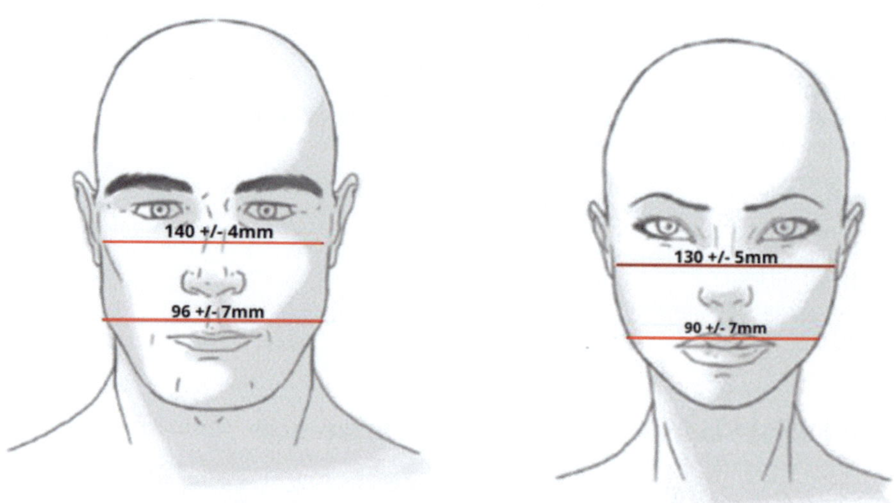

Fig. 20.1 Masculine and feminine craniofacial skeletal measurement norms. (**a**) Bizygomatic width, the widest portion of the face [13]: male: 140 mm+/−4 mm; female: 130 mm+/−5 mm (**b**) Bigonial width, generally 70–75% of the bizygomatic width [13]: skeletal: male: 96+/−7 mm; female: 90+/−7 mm

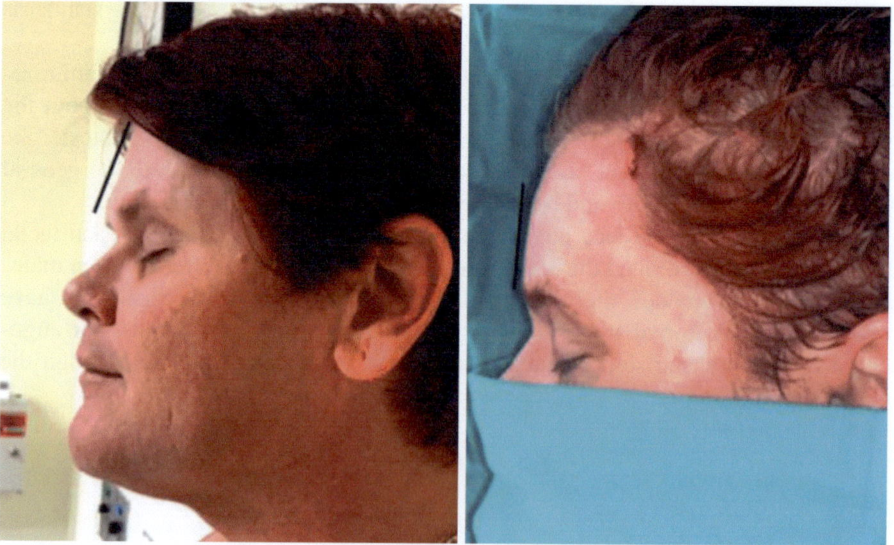

Fig. 20.2 Preoperative (left) and postoperative (right) lateral view demonstrating increase in nasofrontal angle postoperatively in facial feminization surgery

The segments analyzed in the lower facial third include the mandible and the chin. The measurements of mandibular height and length in terms of generalized facial size differences have previously been discussed. In addition to overall size of the mandible, the mandibular plane and gonial angles are compared. While these are different landmarks for standardized measurements, they often correlate. These angles tend to be sharper and more defined in males [14] (Fig. 20.3).

Paralleling the greater mandibular size found in males, the male chin is wider than in females. In the female skeleton, the transition from gonial angles to the chin follows a smoother contour than in men, ending in a single chin point (single light reflection). Males, on the other hand, have a more rectangular chin morphology and are considered to have a double chin point (double light reflection) [13]. The chin is also projected further anterior in males, as demonstrated by Riolo et al. [14] (Fig. 20.4).

The final element of the craniofacial skeleton often used as an objective for facial feminization surgery is the thyroid cartilage. Adam's apple changes in response to levels of testosterone during puberty with the development of secondary sex characteristics [14]. It increases along the sagittal dimension, lengthening the vocal cords and deepening the voice [15]. This change in the sagittal dimension is due to the interlaminar angle between the thyroid cartilage and is classically more acute in males, causing the laryngeal prominence to protrude to a greater degree than in females [15].

In addition to differences in the craniofacial skeleton, soft tissue differences between men and women are also evaluated for facial feminization surgery. Beginning with facial hair, there are several distinctions between the male and female face. First, only males typically have facial hair due to higher levels of testosterone. Men also tend to have an "M-shaped" hairline that is at baseline higher than the female hairline [12].

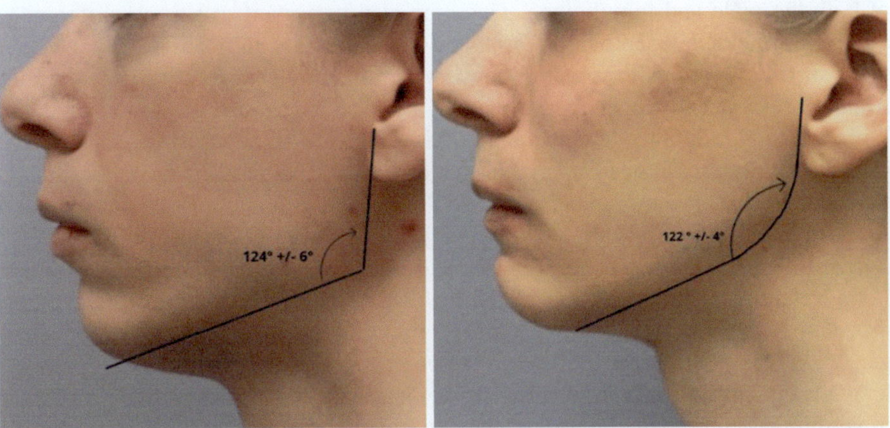

Fig. 20.3 Gonial angle, posterior border of the ramus to the mandibular plane [13]. Preoperative (left) and postoperative (right) facial feminization surgery lateral views of mandibular gonial angle. Superimposed normative angle measurements for males and females. Male: 124°+/−6°, female: 122°+/−4°

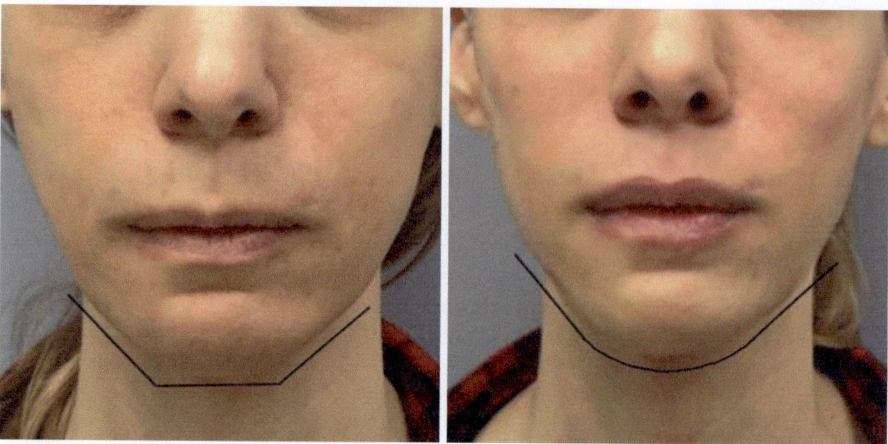

Fig. 20.4 Frontal view chin. Preoperative (left) and postoperative (right) facial feminization surgery demonstrating wider chin in the preoperative masculine face and narrowed, more-rounded chin contour in the postoperative feminine face

Forehead height, nasion to trichion:

Male: 70 mm

Female: 64 mm

As men age, their hairline shape becomes more pronounced as their hairline recedes at an earlier age on the lateral aspect than in the midline [12]. The male and female eyebrows also differ in both position and shape. The male eyebrow is positioned horizontally on the supraorbital rim, while the female eyebrow is naturally arched with an apex is 8–10 mm superior to the supraorbital rim [12, 13].

It has already been addressed that the zygomatic arch width is the widest portion of both the male and female face. There are also important soft tissue differences within the midface; specifically, the Ogee curve varies significantly between men and women. The transition of the bony zygoma laterally to the maxilla centrally results in a convexity over the cheek and a concavity toward the lower midface. From looking at the face at a 45° angle, this double curve is called the Ogee curve [16]. It is more pronounced in females as females tend to have more malar fat volume, while men have more buccal fat pad volume and is a marker of a youthful and aesthetically pleasing feminine face [6] (Fig. 20.5).

The lips also demonstrate soft tissue differences between men and women. Length, volume, and projection of the lips are considered for facial feminization procedures. Overall, women have a greater lip volume under the influence of estrogen [6]. While there is no significant difference in lower lip length, the upper lip length is typically shorter in females: [8] Females also have an increased proportion of vermilion height to overall lip height, resulting in greater vermillion exposure [8] (Fig. 20.5).

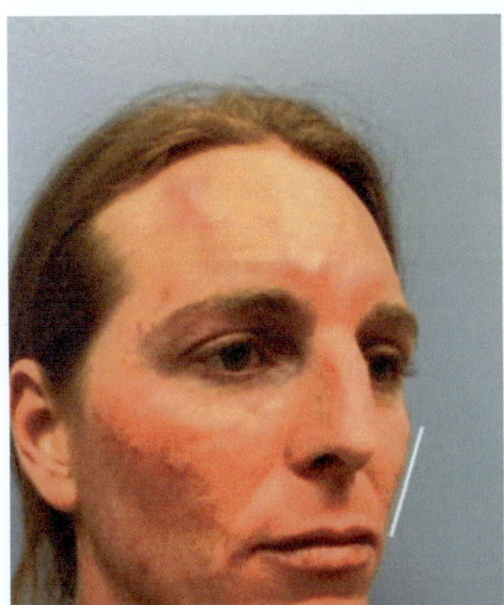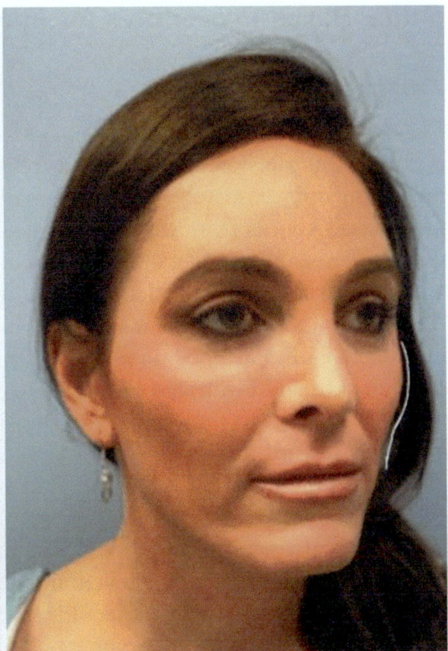

Fig. 20.5 Three/four view Preoperative (left) and postoperative (right) facial feminization surgery demonstrating Ogee curve in the feminine postoperative face and decreased upper lip length with increased vermillion show

Upper lip height, subnasale to stomion superius:
Male: 22+/−2 mm
Female: 20+/−2 mm
All of facial feminization surgery must be guided by a sound understanding of differences between the male and female face. With these standards in mind, surgical technique can be explored. The primary surgical procedures for facial feminization address skeletal differences and include front-orbital recontouring and anterior frontal sinus wall setback, lateral orbital recontouring, rhinoplasty, malar implants, genioplasty, gonial angle reduction, and tracheal shave "Adam's apple reduction." Facial masculinization procedures are typically less common because testosterone supplementation in the FtM patient results in growth of facial hair, coarser features, and recession of the hairline. As a result, "passing" as their preferred gender identity is generally easier in this population. However, masculinization procedures typically include advancement genioplasty, mandibular angle implants, and neurotoxins to the forehead to masculinize the brows.

Common procedures performed in-office under local anesthesia or sedation are detailed in the remaining portion of this chapter. One exception is hairline advancement, which is often performed in office but typically also requires hair transplantation techniques to optimize outcomes.

Office-Based Procedures for Facial Gender Affirmation

Tracheal Shave

A curvilinear incision is marked in a crease of the neck cephalad to the cartilage and measuring approximately 2.5 cm. A smaller incision is most ideal to hide the scar in the crease. Access from this point instead of at a site in the submental region (as used in access for platysmaplasty) provides easier access and exposure to the cartilage while keeping the healed incision hidden in a natural neck crease (Fig. 20.6). The incision site and subcutaneous tissues adjacent to the laryngeal cartilage are infiltrated with 1% lidocaine 1:00 K epinephrine. A #15 blade is used to incise through skin and infiltrated tissue. Dissection in the subcutaneous plane continues with iris scissors to undermine the skin incision for closure. Dissection continues inferiorly toward the laryngeal cartilage and careful dissection deeply through the platysma will reveal paired infrahyoid muscles. Care should be taken in to also avoid vascular structures including the anterior jugular vein and its tributaries. Bipolar electrocautery is preferred. The infrahyoid muscles are released at the midline in the longitudinal plane revealing the perichondrium of the laryngeal cartilage. In some cases, particularly in the older subset of patients, the cartilage has calcified. The superior aspect of the laryngeal cartilage is incised bilaterally along the superior aspect and at the midline to just below the most prominent portion of the

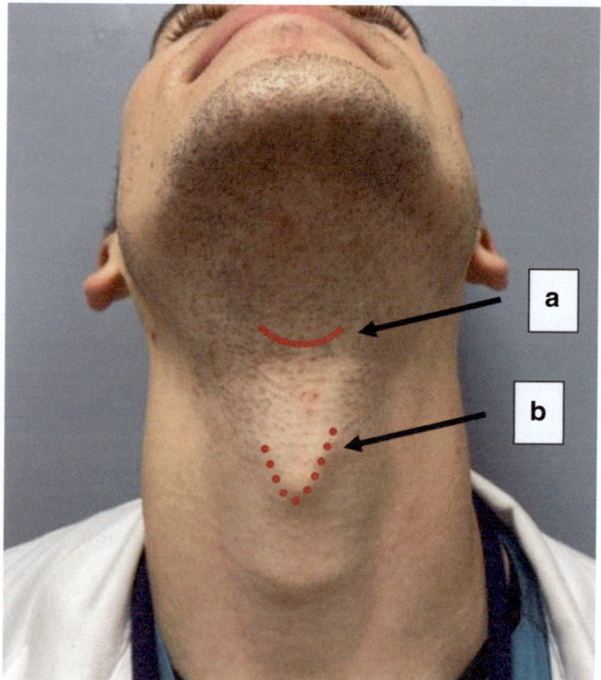

Fig. 20.6 Anterior view of masculine neck with Adam's apple prominence. (**a**) Incision site in neck crease. (**b**) Area of anticipated cartilage excision

cartilage. A woodson or caudal elevator is used to dissect into the subperichondrial plane onto the cartilage. If the cartilage is still immature, the incision may incise completely into the cartilage, making dissection under the perichondrium more difficult, so it is important to minimize pressure on the #15 blade with an effort to incise only through the perichondrium. Once a perichondrial plane has been elevated, the upper half of the laryngeal cartilage should be exposed. This should reveal the area for cartilage removal that comprises the laryngeal prominence and the bilateral superior wings of the cartilage.

The excision should be in the shape of a "V" and include the laryngeal prominence as long as the laryngeal prominence is superior to the insertion of the vocal cords. In most cases, however, this can be predetermined in two ways. First preoperative CT scan can demonstrate the site of insertion of the vocal folds into the anterior aspect of the cartilage. Second, the site of insertion can be marked at the time of intubation of the video laryngoscopy that is used for endotracheal tube placement. A syringe loaded with methylene blue and with a 19G needle can be visualized by entering through the skin at the anticipated level of the vocal cords. The video laryngoscope will demonstrate the needle at the site of the vocal cords, and a small amount of methylene blue is injected here to mark the site of the chords on the external surface of the laryngeal cartilage. This technique gives the surgeon a marked hard stop for cartilage removal on the anterior aspect of the prominence. In general, chord insertion is at the approximately 2/5 to ½ way point from the superior prominence to the inferior border of the cartilage. Measuring with a ruler and marking this site is also an acceptable method to avoid disinsertion of the chords (Fig. 20.7).

The area intended for excision and/or reduction is marked with a surgical pen. Removal can be completed in variety of ways. A #15 or #11 blade is used to remove noncalcified cartilage. Rongeurs can remove the cartilage and prominence quickly,

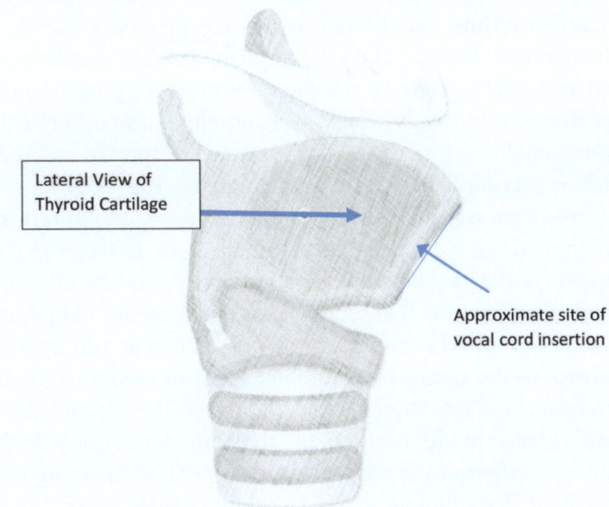

Fig. 20.7 Schematic lateral view of thyroid cartilage indicating site of vocal cord insertion inferior to the most prominent aspect of the thyroid cartilage and approximately 2/5 to ½ distance from notch to inferior border

as can a round diamond bur. This author prefers the use of an ultrasonic cutting device to ensure that there is minimal damage to the perichondrium. Cartilage burring or shaving can continue below the marked level of the chords, but the surgeon should be cautious to avoid thinning this area too much. A good marker for thinning is that cartilage becomes a little purplish or mauve, and this indicates a necessary stopping point of reduction to avoid voice changes. Once the area planned for excision has been removed, the tissues are replaced and the patient is viewed from the lateral angle to ensure that adequate removal has been completed. The margins of the excised areas are then smoothed with a bone file and wound is thoroughly irrigated.

Closure begins by closing the perichondrium back over the laryngeal cartilage. This step is tedious and difficult because the perichondrium is thin and often difficult to reapproximate; however, this is an imperative step to ensure that raw cartilage is not exposed to the subcutanenous tissues and results in scarring of the cartilage directly to the skin. This leaves a tell-tale motion defect upon swallowing where the skin is obviously tethered over the cartilage and does not move freely upon swallowing (tracheostomy defect). The perichondrium is closed with 5-0 monocryl. The infrahyoid strap muscles are then reapproximated at the midline with a running interlocking 4-0 vicryl suture. Closure of the skin is then completed with 5-0 monofilament.

Gonial Angle Reduction

Several methods exist to narrow the width of the lower face at the level of the gonial angles. The goal is to achieve a tapered feminine face with proportionate bigonial width to bizygomatic width and increased mandibular plane angle. This ratio for bizygomatic to bigonial width should be approximately 70% for a feminine face. The masculine mandibular angles are generally flared, and lateral shaving of the mandibular angles can be accomplished with bur reduction (either rasp or pineapple-shaped bur) to remove the laterally projecting portion of the angles. This author's preferred method, however, is a complete ostectomy of the mandibular angles from the gonial notch to the posterior aspect of the ramus. Access for either of the methods is accomplished in the same manner (Fig. 20.8).

An intraoral incision is completed along the anterior ramus along the external oblique ridge measuring approximate 3 cm. Dissection is competed along the lateral aspect of the ramus with the patient in a closed mouth position to optimize exposure and visualization. Dissection continues in the subperiosteal plane to expose the entire mandibular angle. A toe-out or bower retractor is placed on the posterior aspect of the ramus to define the superior extent of the ostectomy on the posterior ramus. If the intention is only for lateral shaving, this can be completed at this time, with care to avoid traumatizing the periosteum lying deep to the masseter muscle as injury to the muscle will result in significant bleeding and difficult visualization of the field. To completely excise the mandibular angles, the area of excision is marked.

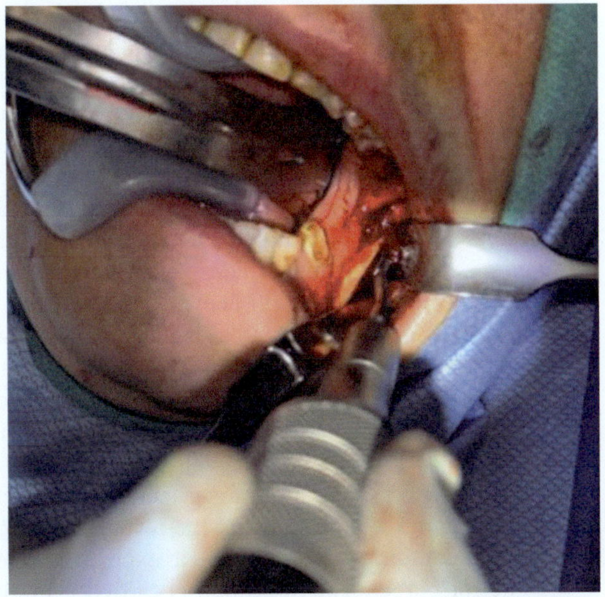

Fig. 20.8 Intraoperative view of access for lateral gonial angle reduction

This can be completed with preformed 3D guides or simply by direct visualization and marking of the area. A reciprocating saw, IVRO saw, or piezoelectric saw is used to remove the demarcated angle to the gonial notch. Preoperative planning of some form is imperative since the ostectomy should be completed at least 5 mm from the inferior alveolar canal. Osteotomes are often necessary to complete the fracture. Once the gonial angle has been removed, or the lateral reduction completed, the site is smoothed with a rasp or bone file. The body of the mandible may also need lateral reduction for a more feminine facial taper, but this should be minimal since the lower face tissues are supported by the mandible, and removal of the bony support will result in increased sagging and jowling of facial tissues and overall contribute to facial aging. In some cases, the mandibular width reduction should be accompanied by rhytidectomy to re-suspend the facial tissues in a superolateral vector.

The site is fully irrigated and closed with running interlocking chromic gut sutures.

Genioplasty

The primary rational for genioplasty for gender affirmation in the male to female patient is to decrease the chin width. While there are no masculine or feminine standards for chin width, the overall goal of the surgical procedure is to create a tapered face. The masculine chin is wider and boxy, while the feminine chin is narrow, tapered to point, and projected.

Width reduction genioplasty can be accomplished without 3D planning and standard genioplasty techniques; however, 3D planning is optimal since the central portion planned for excision may be coincident with the insertion of the tongue musculature at the genial tubercle. Accidental excision of the genial tubercle can be catastrophic and result in glossoptosis, postoperative airway compromise, and obstructive apnea. Therefore, it is imperative that either the genial tubercle is not included in the resection area or the muscle insertions at that site are re-positioned and suspended by the remaining mandibular bone or titanium plate.

Titanium or hybrid cutting guides are useful and time-saving for width narrowing genioplasty. The guides will demarcate the area of excision of the central portion for excision and the sites for the standard mandibular ostectomy. This ostectomy should be at least 5 mm below the bilateral mental foramina.

The procedure begins with standard genioplasty incision from the level of the lower premolar teeth posteriorly progressing anteriorly into the lip mucosa and submucosa and down through the mentalis muscle. The incision should be anterior enough to allow for enough proximal mentalis muscles and a cuff of 2–3 mm of non-attached gingival al tissues on the alveolar aspect of the wound for closure. Dissection is completed down to bone to expose the anterior aspect of the mandible to the inferior border. The dissection is carried laterally and the mental nerved is identified and retracted superiorly. The central wedge for excision is marked and a reciprocating saw, oscillating saw, or piezoelectric or ultrasonic bone cutting device is used to create vertical osteotomies for the planned excision. A screw is placed at this site and a suture or hemostat is placed on the screw to avoid retraction of this central wedge into the floor of the mouth once the wedge osteotomy is completed. The planned horizontal osteotomy through the entire anterior portion of the mandible is completed with a reciprocating saw. If necessary, osteotomes are used to complete the posterior aspect of the cuts. The central wedge is then removed and lateral pieces are reapproximated and held in place with the inferior lateral holes of a square or rectangular titanium plate (Fig. 20.9).

If projection of the chin is also indicated, the plate is also bent to accomplish the desired chin projection. Projection of the chin is typically aesthetically favorable if the gonial angles have been resected – this helps to enhance the jaw contour and

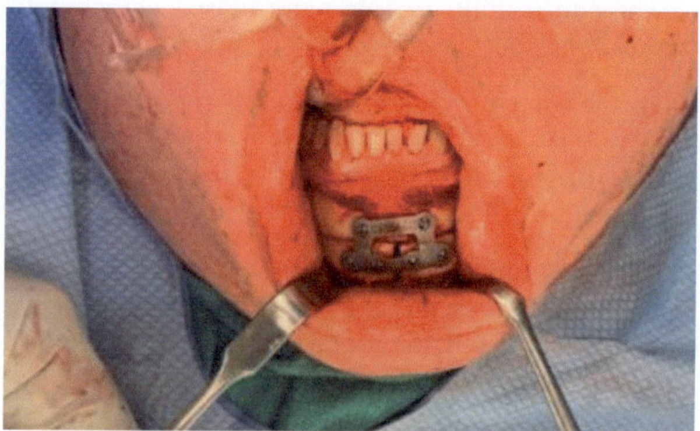

Fig. 20.9 Intraoperative view of width reduction genioplasty after placement of titanium fixation plate

suspend the soft tissues that can contribute to jowling. If there is significant vertical space between the new chin position and the native bone, interpositional grafts from the mandibular angles can be inserted here. The plate is secured with titanium screws and the suprahyoid musculature is suspended to the inferior aspect of the titanium plate with long-lasting resorbable sutures.

Attention is then turned to the bilateral inferior borders of the mandible. Excision of the wedge of bone produces a step deformity of the inferior cortex. An egg-shaped bur should be used to smooth the defect and produce a more discreet contour from native bone to the newly medially advanced portion of the anterior mandible. The wound is then thoroughly irrigated. The mentalis muscle is carefully reapproximated with 3-0 vicryl, followed by closure of the mucosa with chromic gut.

Lip Lift

The lip lift procedure is an ideal procedure for in-office gender affirmation in the male to female transgender patient. The procedure can be completed under local anesthesia or sedation. It is generally well tolerated and typically takes less than 1 h to complete.

The masculine upper lip is longer than that of the feminine lip, and aging will contribute to the overall upper lip length. This combination makes the lip lift procedure both important and highly effective in gender affirmation surgery for the male to female patient.

Lip length is measured preoperatively, and lengths in excess of 20 mm are generally masculine and unaesthetic. Additionally, if less than 8 mm of vermillion is shown at rest, then the patient would likely benefit from a lip lift procedure. The lip lift has two main effects, (1) decreasing the overall upper lip length and (2) increasing the amount of pink vermillion demonstrated at rest.

The bullhorn incision is preferred because the scar is easily hidden in the natural limits of the aesthetic subunit. The lip is marked preoperatively and a defined area of excision is measured to create a final lip length of approximately one-third of the total height of the lower face height. This is typically around 14 mm. Excision of too much skin from this area is problematic, since there will be too much tooth show and may result a gummy smile.

Once the area of excision is marked, local anesthesia is injected at bilateral inferior orbital blocks with 2% lidocaine 1:100 k epi and local infiltration at the incision site only. This ensures that the tissues are not distorted with local infiltration.

A #15 blade is used to create the bullhorn subnasal incision (Fig. 20.10). The inferior tissue is undermined in the subcutaneous plane. The paired columellar arteries are encountered and cauterized. Once dissection is completed to the vermillion border, a single 4-0 vicryl suture can be used horizontally at the level of the cupids bow to re-establish philtral columns. Alternatively, in highly aged or atrophic lips lacking architecture, philtral columns can be created with running 5-0 vicryl

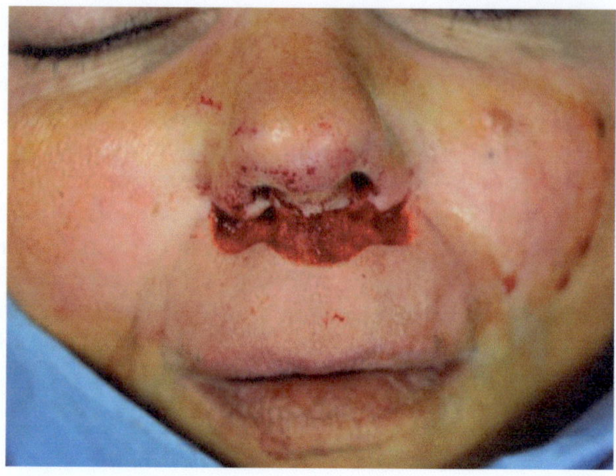

Fig. 20.10 Intraoperative photo of bullhorn-shaped incision for feminizing upper lip lift

suture in the subdermal plane from each cupids bow peak to the corresponding lateral columella. Deep 4-0 vicryl sutures are used to close the incision followed by 6-0 monofilament suture in the skin.

Use of Injectable Medicines in Gender Affirmation

The use of injectable medicines such as neurotoxins and hyaluronic acid fillers can be important adjuncts in facial gender affirmation. In the male to female patient, neurotoxins are beneficial reducing horizontal and vertical forehead rhytids and raising the brows for a more arched and feminine position so that the apex of the brow is positioned 1 cm above the orbital rim and the tail at approximately 12 mm above the rim. This can be accomplished with neurotoxin injections to the forehead, glabella, and lateral orbicularis oculi muscles. Conversely in the female to male transgender patient, neurotoxin can be delivered throughout the forehead only without treatment of the forehead depressors. This lowers the brows uniformly into a horizontal position onto the orbital rim and creates the appearance of a prominent frontal bone projection at the level of the brow. Neurotoxin is also beneficial for the male to female for lip projection and eversion. 4–8 units of neurotoxin into the upper portion of the orbicularis oris creates a temporary lip lift and exposes more vermillion. Similarly, injection of neurotoxin into the depressor septi muscle at can rotate the nasal tip upward and create a slightly more feminine nose projection for those patients with downturned nasal tip.

Hyaluronic acid and other fillers are also a useful adjunct for gender affirmation. Creating an Ogee curve and feminine cheek with heavy body filler in the malar region can be highly feminizing. Lip augmentation with filler is also typically indicated in transfeminine patients and can be completed either before or after surgical lip lifting. In many cases, malar implants or dermal-fat lip grafts can be a more permanent solutions in these areas, and these procedures are often coupled with

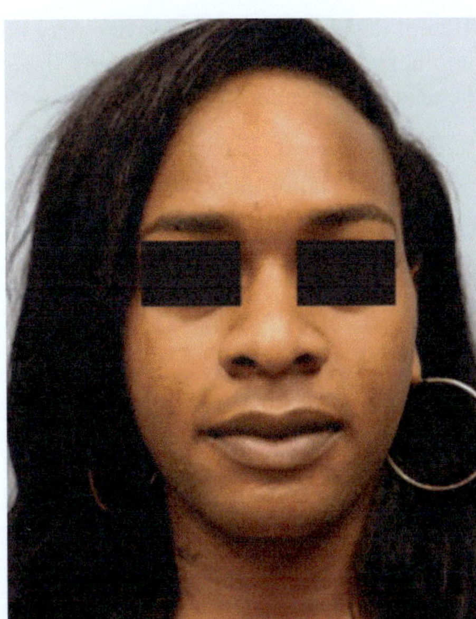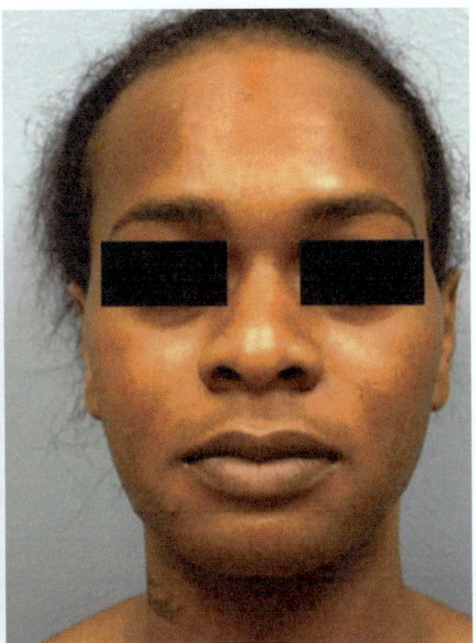

Fig. 20.11 Before (left) and after (right) feminizing cheek injections with hyaluronic acid filler. Note more rounded malar projection post-filler placement and improvement in facial taper from midface to lower face

other feminization procedures. The use of resorbable fillers offers the patients the unique opportunity for instant results and time to see if they are interested in a more permanent solution. For female to male patients, fillers are used for augmenting the mandibular angle projection laterally and for temporary chin augmentation (Fig. 20.11).

Summary

The facial gender transition process is a long one. Certainly there are some centers performing all surgical procedures at one time, but a long-standing relationship with the patient can be beneficial for several reasons. (1) A gradual transition is sometimes more accepted by the patient and their close contacts. (2) The wait for funding or insurance coverage can delay major surgery, so office adjunctive procedure such as these mentioned here can allow the patient to have a an easier social transition while awaiting major skeletal recontouring procedures. (3) Fine-tuning skeletal recontouring can be completed with in-office procedures that both improve the appearance of aging and also target minor soft tissue differences between the masculine and feminine face. (4) Completing these procedures in office allows time to develop a rapport and understanding with your patients who, similar to many cosmetic/aesthetic patients, often have different desires for outcomes; one may be interested in ultra-feminized face, while another may want to focus on only those features that are highly masculinizing and causing misgendering in public areas.

References

1. Joseph A, Cliffe C, Hillyard M, Majeed A. Gender identity and the management of the transgender patient: a guide for non-specialists. J R Soc Med. 2017;110(4):144–52.
2. Houssayni S, Nilsen K. Transgender competent provider: identifying transgender health needs, health disparities, and health coverage. Kansas J Med. 2019;11(1):15–9.
3. The World Professional Association for Transgender Health. Standards of care for the health of transsexual, transgender, and gender-nonconforming people, version 7. Int J Transgend. 2012;13(4):165–232.
4. Baldwin A, Dodge B, Schick VR, Light B, Schnarrs PW, Herbenick D, Fortenberry JD. Transgender and genderqueer individuals' experiences with health care providers: what's working, what's not, and where to we go from here? J Health Care Poor Underserved. 2018;29(4):1300–18.
5. Eisenberg ME, McMorris BJ, Rider GN, Gower AL, Coleman E. "It's king of hard to go to the doctor's office if you're hated there." A call for gender-affirming care from transgender and gender diverse adolescents in the United States. Health Soc Care Community. 2020;28:1082–9.
6. Hohman MH, Teixeira J. Transgender surgery of the head and neck. In: StatPearls [Internet]. Treasure Island, FL: StatPearls Publishing; 2021. p. 1–26.
7. Flores AR, Herman JL, Gates GJ, Brown TNT. How many adults identify as transgender in the United States? Los Angeles, CA: Williams Institute; 2016. p. 1–13.
8. Yarns BC, Abrams JM, Meeks TW, Sewell DD. The mental health of older LGBT adults. Curr Psychiatry Rep. 2016;18(60):5.
9. Sears B, Mallory C, Flores AR, Conron KJ. LGBT people's experiences of workplace discrimination and harassment. Los Angeles, CA: Williams Institute; 2021. p. 4.
10. Flores AR, Langton L, Meyer IH, Romero AP. Victimization rates and traits of sexual and gender minorities in the United States: results from the National crime victimization survey, 2017. Sci Adv. 2020;6(6):10.
11. Romero AP, Goldberg SK, Vasquez LA. LGBT people and housing affordability, discrimination, and homelessness. Los Angeles, CA: Williams Institute; 2020. p. 1–31.
12. Hage JJ, Becking AG, Graaf FH, Tuinzing DB. Gender-confirming facial surgery: considerations on the masculinity and femininity of faces. Plast Reconstr Surg. 1997;99(7):1800. 1803
13. Naini FB. Facial aesthetics: concepts & clinical diagnosis. Hoboken, NJ: Wiley; 2011.
14. Fitzpatrick TH, Siccardi MA. Anatomy, head and neck, Adam's apple, vol. 2. Treasure Island, FL: StatPearls Publishing; 2021.
15. Flynn W, Vickerton P. Anatomy, head and neck, larynx cartilage, vol. 2. Treasure Island, FL: StatPearls Publishing; 2021.
16. Ko AC, Korn BS, Kikkawa DO. The aging face. Surv Ophthalmol. 2017;62(2):193.

Chapter 21
Advancements in Dermal Substitutes for Head and Neck Reconstruction

Sarah Anne Wong, Dina Amin, Jonathon Jundt, Michael R. Markiewicz, Simon Young (iD), Allen Cheng, and James C. Melville (iD)

Introduction

Head and neck soft tissue reconstruction is critical to restoring patient health and quality of life following conditions such as trauma, vascular disease, or cancer [1]. Care must be taken to not only restore original function but also esthetics. Thus, the

S. A. Wong
Oral and Craniofacial Sciences Graduate Program, School of Dentistry, University of California, San Francisco, CA, USA
e-mail: Sarah.Wong@ucsf.edu

D. Amin
Division of Oral and Maxillofacial Surgery, Emory University School of Medicine, Dallas, TX, USA
e-mail: damin@exchange.tamu.edu

J. Jundt
Bernard and Gloria Pepper Katz Department of Oral and Maxillofacial Surgery, School of Dentistry, The University of Texas Health Science Center at Houston, Houston, TX, USA
e-mail: Jonathon.Jundt@uth.tmc.edu

M. R. Markiewicz
Department of Oral and Maxillofacial Surgery, School of Dental Medicine, University at Buffalo, Buffalo, NY, USA
e-mail: mrm25@buffalo.edu

S. Young · J. C. Melville (✉)
Department of Oral and Maxillofacial Surgery, The University of Texas Health Science Center at Houston, Houston, TX, USA
e-mail: Simon.Young@uth.tmc.edu; James.C.Melville@uth.tmc.edu

A. Cheng
Head and Neck Surgical Associates, Oral, Head and Neck Cancer Center Program, Legacy Cancer Institute, Portland, OR, USA
e-mail: chenga@hnsa1.com

J. C. Melville et al. (eds.), *Advancements and Innovations in OMFS, ENT, and Facial Plastic Surgery*, https://doi.org/10.1007/978-3-031-32099-6_21

ideal reconstructive therapy must not only restore proper tissue mobility, strength, and elasticity to carry out everyday functions and withstand common stresses (0.33–1.28 MPa), but it must also prevent moisture loss, infection, and cicatrix formation and provide a cosmetic, symmetrical, and well color-matched outcome [2]. Although soft tissue reconstruction procedures, such as skin grafting, have been performed for several centuries, over recent decades, surgeons and scientists have collaborated to develop a variety of new tools and techniques that can be used for soft tissue reconstruction [1].

Current soft tissue reconstructive therapies include local advancement flaps, microvascular free tissue transfer, split- and full-thickness skin grafting, negative pressure therapy, and dermal substitutes. It is important to note that these techniques vary in the tissue layers they replace. Local flaps and free tissue transfers not only replace all three layers of the skin (epidermis, dermis, and hypodermis), but they can also include any combination of skin, fascia, muscle, and bone. Their significant clinical success has been attributed in large part to the maintenance of a vascular supply to transplanted tissues, either by retaining local vascular connections (local flaps) or through anastomosis of transplanted arteries/veins with local blood vessels (free tissue transfers). In contrast, skin grafts do not provide immediate vascular perfusion to the transplanted tissues. Rather, they rely on the gradual formation of local vascular connections at the graft-wound bed interface. Unlike flaps, skin grafts only replace the layers of the skin and do not include additional tissues such as fascia, muscle, or bone. Skin grafts can be either split-thickness, including epidermis with a variable amount of dermis, or full-thickness, including all layers of the skin. As will be explored in greater depth later in this chapter, dermal substitutes include a wide variety of decellularized allografts, xenografts, and fully synthetic matrices that primarily serve to replace or augment the dermal layer of the skin. Although they are typically used in conjunction with skin grafting, some have been successfully used alone, as the primary reconstruction modality, and can effect reconstruction of full-thickness epithelial defects. In comparison, negative pressure therapy does not replace any layers of the skin. Rather, it is a technique that uses a vacuum device to exert light, evenly distributed pressure on the wound surface and a conduit for fluid removal from the wound site. The negative pressure created by the vacuum helps draw the edges of the wound together and secure any skin grafts or flaps that may be present. It also helps to maintain a moist and warm environment conducive to wound healing and to reduce wound edema and infection. The above-listed techniques are often used in combination and are selected based on the complexity of each case, which is determined by factors such as anatomical location, depth, and size of the soft tissue defect, vascular supply, the presence or absence of infection, and systemic comorbidities.

Dermal substitutes have been a prolific area of study in recent decades and have been increasingly used for soft tissue reconstruction in the head and neck. Although flap and skin grafting techniques are often preferred, dermal substitutes have demonstrated clinical success both when used as the primary reconstruction modality and when used in combination with standard surgical techniques [3]. In contrast to flap and skin grafting, which require a second surgical site, have limited donor tissue availability, and cause donor site morbidity, dermal substitutes provide a promising therapeutic alternative, particularly for large soft tissue defects. Dermal substitutes have also demonstrated greater clinical success than some autologous tissue engineering strategies such as cultured epidermal autografts (CEA) and micrografts. Although these techniques have the theoretical advantage of reduced rejection, they also pose significant disadvantages that hinder their clinical use such as high cost, procedural complexity that often requires a lab facility, and multiple stages of treatment resulting in prolonged treatment duration [4, 5]. These autologous constructs are often fragile and require additional scaffolding in order to provide sufficient mechanical strength. Additionally, CEAS have demonstrated increased risk of infection [6]. In contrast, dermal substitutes, which are not derived from autologous tissues, have been shown to achieve reconstruction of full-thickness epithelial defects while improving pliability and decreasing scar formation [7].

There is a wide spectrum of available dermal substitutes that range from allografts and xenografts to completely synthetic devices (Table 21.1). Dermal substitutes are traditionally divided into two categories: biologic and bioartificial. Biologic substitutes consist of allografts and xenografts that are entirely derived from living organisms and must undergo strict processing, including lyophilization, gamma irradiation, and de-cellularization, in order to render them safe for implantation. In contrast, bioartificial substitutes are either completely or partially synthetic [9]. Dermal substitutes promote wound repair through the process of constructive remodeling [3]. During this process, the body gradually replaces the dermal substitute with new tissue, creating a neodermis that resembles the native tissue present prior to injury. Dermal substitutes achieve this through mechanical and molecular means. They serve as scaffolds that provide directional guidance for tissue regeneration, increase tissue inosculation, and promote plasma imbibition. They also act as reservoirs for molecular signals that stimulate regenerative processes. The extracellular matrix (ECM) of dermal substitutes contains a rich supply and variety of growth factors that are released upon matrix degradation, including vascular endothelial growth factor (VEGF), platelet-derived growth factor (PDGF-AA, PDGF-BB), transforming growth factor (TGFα, TGFβ1), basic fibroblast growth factor (bFGF), epidermal growth factor (EGF), placental growth factor (PlGF), granulocyte colony-stimulating factor (G-CSF), anti-inflammatory interleukins (IL-4, 6, 8, 10), and tissue inhibitors of metalloproteinases (TIMP 1, 2, 4) [10]. Additionally, peptide fragments often referred to as matricryptins, matrikinins, or matricryptic peptides are generated upon enzymatic breakdown of the device ECM [11, 12]. These peptides often demonstrate bioactivities unique to and more potent than their native, full-length forms [13]. This combination of molecular signals stimulates a wide array of repair processes including angiogenesis, cell migration, differentiation, adhesion, and in some cases immunomodulation. This series of events mimics the natural repair process, and, indeed, many of the growth factors commonly found in dermal substitute ECM are also found in the ECM of natural tissues at different stages of repair.

In this chapter, we review the use of dermal substitutes for soft tissue maxillofacial reconstruction, including the most commonly used products, their clinical

Table 21.1 Currently available dermal substitutes. Modified from [8]

Substitute type	Commercial forms	Description	Uses
Autografts	Cultured skin substitutes (CSS)	Autologous fibroblasts and keratinocytes on a biopolymer sponge	Full-thickness burns
	Epicel®	Cultured epidermal autograft	Adult and pediatric patients with deep dermal or full-thickness burns. Can be used alone or in conjunction with split-thickness skin grafts
	Recell®	RECELL's autologous cell harvesting device can be used by a licensed healthcare professional to prepare an autologous RES® regenerative epidermal suspension for direct application to burns	Acute, partial-thickness thermal burn wounds in adult patients. Can be applied in combination with meshed autograft for acute full-thickness burn wounds in pediatric and adult patients
Allografts	AlloDerm®	Cadaveric skin with acellular dermal matrix and intact basement membrane	Full-thickness burns, nasal reconstruction, facial soft-tissue defect augmentation, free-flap donor site coverage, wound bed graft, implant to repair and replace damaged or inadequate integumental tissue, abdominal wall reconstruction, breast reconstruction, vaginal repair
	Amniofix®	Dehydrated human amnion/chorion membrane Available in sheet, fenestrated, and wrap configurations	Debridements, dehiscence, flap donor sites, ulcers (including decubitus, diabetic foot, and venous leg ulcers), trauma, burns, management of chronic neuropathic pain, nerve repair, cardiac tissue repair following myocardial infarction, plantar fasciitis, osteoarthritis, amputations, pilonidal cysts, port sites, urothelial tissue repair Particularly effective for comorbid patients with complex defects or delayed healing
	BioTissue®	Cryopreserved human amniotic membrane Comes in a variety of forms: Prokera®, AmnioGraft®, AmnioGuard®, Neox®100, Clarix®100, Neox®1 K, Clarix®1 K	Prokera®, AmnioGraft®, and AmnioGuard® formulations are for use in treating ocular surfaces Neox®100, Clarix®100, Neox®1 K, and Clarix®1 K are for treating acute, chronic, partial, and full-thickness wounds
	Stratagraft®	Allogeneic cultured keratinocytes and dermal fibroblasts in murine collagen	Deep partial-thickness burns

Xenografts and biosynthetic grafts	ACell®	Porcine urinary bladder mucosal matrix. Consists of two layers, a lamina propria and a basement membrane Comes in a variety of forms: Cytal®, Gentrix® (sheets), MicroMatrix® (particulate)	Partial- and full-thickness wounds, ulcers (pressure, venous, diabetic, chronic vascular), surgical wounds (donor sites/grafts, post-Mohs surgery, post-laser surgery, wound dehiscence), traumatic wounds (abrasions, lacerations, second-degree burns, skin tears), tunneled and undermined wounds, and noninfected draining wounds Particularly effective when treating wounds challenged with bacterial infection
	Biobrane®	Bioartificial dressing consisting of a silicone membrane bonded to a nylon mesh to which porcine dermal collagen peptides have been bonded	Temporary dressing to cover clean partial-thickness burn wounds and split-thickness donor sites
	EZ Derm™	Aldehyde cross-linked porcine dermis	Partial-thickness wounds, burns, donor sites, chronic vascular ulcers, temporary coverage for wounds prior to grafting, test graft prior to autografting, protective coverage over meshed autografts
	Integra®	Bioartificial device consisting of two layers, an inner bovine collagen matrix and an outer silicone layer	Full-thickness burns, neck scar contractures, scar reduction in buccal defects created when harvesting mucosal grafts for urethral reconstruction, tongue coverage following partial glossectomies, nonhealing osteoradionecrosis, medication-related osteonecrosis of the jaw, coverage of exposed bone, tendon, cartilage, and joints
	Kerecis® MariGen™	Decellularized fish skin	Partial- and full-thickness wounds, pressure ulcers, chronic vascular ulcers, diabetic ulcers, traumatic wounds (including abrasions, lacerations, and skin tears), surgical wounds (including donor site/grafts, post-Mohs surgery, podiatric, and wound dehiscence), draining wounds
	MatriDerm®	Acellular bovine dermal matrix consisting of collagen and elastin	Burns, wounds (including traumatic, acute, and chronic), post-Mohs surgery, donor sites/grafts, mucosal defects
	OASIS®	Porcine small intestinal submucosa extracellular matrix	Partial- and full-thickness wounds, ulcers (including pressure, venous, chronic vascular, and diabetic), tunneled, undermined wounds, trauma wounds (including abrasions, lacerations, second-degree burns, skin tears), draining wounds, surgical wounds (including donor sites/grafts, post-Mohs surgery, post-laser surgery, podiatric, wound dehiscence)
	Permacol™	Porcine dermal collagen	Temporary coverage of partial-thickness burns, hernia, and abdominal wall repair

indications, recommended methods of application, and future developments. Although a comprehensive list of currently available dermal substitutes is available in Table 21.1, an exhaustive review of all available products is not our goal. Rather, we aim to compare and contrast the most commonly used dermal substitutes, highlighting their similarities and differences in design and application, in order to aid our readers in selecting the ideal product for each clinical situation. For the purposes of this chapter, we have limited our discussion to soft tissue reconstruction of the scalp, face, neck, and oral cavity.

Common Indications for Dermal Substitutes and Global Principles of Use

The most commonly used substitutes include Integra Wound Matrix System, AlloDerm, ACell, and AmnioFix. Primary indications for their use include treatment of flap donor sites, scar reduction in acute wounds, granulation bed development in avulsive wounds, moisture loss prevention, basement membrane replacement in burn wounds, closure of complex chronic wounds associated with diabetes, radiation, or high velocity, and treatment of recalcitrant chronic wounds that have been repeatedly operated [1, 4, 7, 14–19]. Additional uses for dermal substitutes include rhinoplasty, temporal hollowing, and other volume replacement indications [20]. Dermal substitutes can also be used as biological barriers such as in the prevention of Frey syndrome. In this case, following surgical dissection of the parotid gland, dermal substitutes are applied to separate the parotid bed from the overlying skin, thus preventing the development of aberrant neural connections between the regenerating parasympathetic axons in the parotid gland and sweat glands in the overlying skin [21].

There are several principles that should be applied when using any dermal substitute. Wound bed preparation is paramount to ensuring graft survival. It must be free of necrotic tissue and devitalized bone prior to matrix placement. Vascular supply is critical to new tissue formation. Thus, a wound bed with adequate blood supply must be exposed. This is particularly challenging when the wound bed primarily consists of bone since a bony layer with punctate bleeding must be exposed without damaging underlying structures such as the brain. While debriding to establish this bony layer, it is important to minimize excessive trauma to the bone. This can be accomplished by reserving the use of electric burrs for initial stages of decortication followed by the use of rongeurs or curettes to gradually remove residual cortical and underlying trabecular bone until punctate bleeding is achieved [3]. The outer margin of bony debridement should extend beyond the soft tissue margin of the wound by several millimeters in order to provide adequate peripheral tissue interaction with the dermal substitute [3].

The vast majority of dermal substitutes also require that the wound be free of infection. However, some substitutes such as ACell's porcine urinary bladder matrix have been successfully used under bacterial challenge [3, 11, 12, 22, 23]. Depending on the case, additional materials may need to be removed from the wound bed prior to matrix placement. For example, in some patients with neurosurgical scalp wounds, especially those who have undergone older meningioma procedures, the materials historically used to treat cranial defects can sometimes interfere with scalp wound healing. Thus, these materials may need to be removed from the exposed wound in order for stable healing to occur [3].

Once inserted, dermal substitutes must achieve intimate contact with the host tissue since the constructive remodeling repair process occurs at the interface between the dermal substitute and the wound bed. The device must remain immobilized, and secondary dressings should be applied to secure the device and reduce fluid loss in order for healing to successfully progress. Most dermal substitutes require a secondary dressing that typically consists of silicone sheets, or sutured dressings. Optimal secondary dressings should be determined by wound location, size, depth, and user preference. If adequate hydration is not maintained, healing will be delayed. Indeed, if healing is slow and the device appears dry, one should first attempt to increase the moisture of the dermal substitute device before seeking further treatment [3]. Increased hydration of the wound site can be attained by using hydrogels or Telfa-type dressings [3]. Inner dressings with petrolatum-impregnated gauze or a damp saline layer may also be applied to increase moisture retention at the wound site.

For scalp wounds, it is often customized to shave a 3–4 cm rim of hair around the defect. It was believed that this practice improves wound hygiene as well as placement of secondary dressings [3]. However, more recently, studies have shown that hair shaving neither benefits the surgery itself nor confers any benefit against postoperative infection. In fact, data now suggests that hair removal may lead to higher rates of infection [24]. Due to its cosmetic value to patients, it is recommended that hair removal be avoided or minimized as much as possible [24].

Below we explore each of the most commonly used dermal substitutes, listing their specific indications, optimized instructions for application, as well as clinical examples of their use. Recommended protocols are based on instructions from manufacturers. However, they have been modified to include suggested techniques that, from our experience, have resulted in the best outcomes.

Integra Wound Matrix System

Developed in the 1980s, the Integra Wound Matrix System became the first commercially available dermal substitute. Initially developed as an alternative to skin grafting in burn patients, it has since expanded its application to include routine use in several head and neck reconstructive procedures including treatment of neck scar contractures, reduction of scarring in buccal defects created when harvesting mucosal grafts for urethral reconstruction, tongue coverage following partial glossectomies, and in cases of nonhealing osteoradionecrosis and medication-related osteonecrosis of the jaw [9]. Integra has also been used to cover exposed bone, tendon, cartilage, and joints [25].

Integra is a bioartificial device consisting of two layers, an inner layer of bovine collagen matrix and an outer layer of silicone. The bovine collagen serves to promote tissue inosculation and the development of neodermis, whereas the silicone provides an environmental barrier to reduce moisture loss for up to 2–3 weeks postplacement. Following removal of the silicone layer, a thin split thickness skin graft is often recommended. Integra has been shown to significantly reduce scar formation and to produce a smooth neodermis that readily incorporates with secondary skin grafting.

Below is our recommended protocol for using the Integra matrix system as well as a clinical example demonstrating its use in treating a scalp injury due to dog bite (Fig. 21.1).

Integra Recommended Protocol

1. Using sterile technique, peel open the outer pouch and gently drop the inner foil pouch onto a sterile surface. Lay the foil pouch flat and peel open.
2. Remove the product, including the protective polyethylene sheets.
3. While holding the product by the tab, remove one polyethylene cover sheet then turn the product and remove the second.
4. Using the tab, place the product in a basin of sterile saline. Carefully remove the tab from the product while rinsing for 1–2 min. Keep the product in the basin until ready for insertion into the wound.
5. Prepare the wound bed using standard procedures, ensuring that the wound is free of necrotic tissue or debris. Note: It is important that the wound edges contain viable tissue. Surgically debride in order to obtain this if needed.
6. Cut the device to size and immediately apply following wound bed preparation. Note: It is critical that the collagen layer be in direct contact with the prepared wound. Take care to not apply the product upside down. The silicone layer, identified by black threads, must face the outer surface, away from the wound bed. If placed properly, the black threads identifying the silicone layer will be clearly visible after matrix placement.
7. Firmly secure the Integra matrix using surgical staples, sutures, or other mechanical means. All air bubbles should be carefully removed in order to promote direct contact with the wound.
8. (Optional) Negative pressure wound therapy can be applied at this time. Apply according to manufacturer's instructions, paying close attention to contraindications, warnings, and precautions.
9. Use appropriate secondary dressings to ensure device adherence and to protect the wound area.

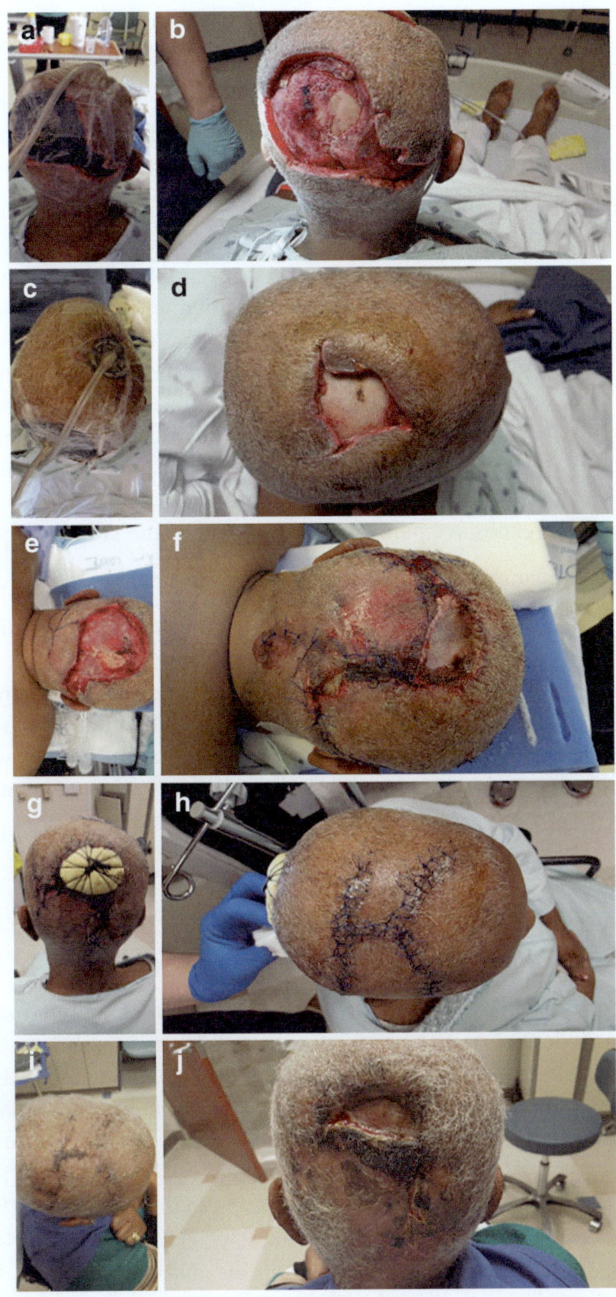

Fig. 21.1 Integra Wound Matrix System used to treat a scalp wound due to dog bite in a 59-year-old female. (**a**, **c**) Negative pressure wound therapy of scalp defects. (**b**, **d**) Scalp wounds following negative pressure therapy. Scalp wounds (**e**) pre- and (**f**) post-local advancement flap surgery. (**g**–**h**) Application of Integra Wound Matrix System in residual defect. Note the outer black threads that identify the silicone layer of the matrix. (**i**, **j**) Two weeks post-surgery (Images courtesy of Dr. Jonathon Jundt)

Integra Postoperative Management

1. Change the secondary dressings as needed. The frequency at which secondary dressing are changed will depend upon the volume of exudate produced, the type of dressing used, and the clinician's need to inspect the wound for signs of infection or healing.
2. Removing the Integra silicone layer:

   (a) If the edges of the matrix are loose before full healing has occurred, carefully trim away the loose silicone leaving the attached silicone in place. Repeat until the entire wound has healed.
   (b) Remove the silicone layer once the underlying tissue has healed, typically 14–28 days. Note: It is normal for the matrix to be loose in some spots.
   (c) When removing the silicone layer, start at one corner and pull gently. Note: Healed tissue can easily peel away along with the silicone layer.
   (d) Stop and wait 1–2 additional days if bleeding occurs or patient reports excessive pain. Forced removal of the silicone layer may result in reinjury.

3. If using negative pressure wound therapy:

   (a) The device will need to be removed during dressing changes. Take care not to disrupt the Integra matrix during this process.
   (b) Discontinue use of negative pressure wound therapy when the Integra collagen matrix has integrated with surrounding tissues and the silicone layer has separated. Using negative pressure therapy will likely reduce the time required for wound healing. Healing without negative pressure therapy typically occurs in 14–28 days.

AlloDerm

Introduced in 1994 as a treatment for full-thickness burns, AlloDerm was one of the first dermal matrix products reported in the literature [26]. It currently has a wide variety of applications including rhinoplasty, facial soft-tissue defect augmentation, abdominal wall reconstruction, alloplastic breast reconstruction, radial forearm free-flap donor site coverage, and vaginal repair [27]. In the field of maxillofacial surgery, AlloDerm is primarily used as a wound bed graft or as an implant to repair and replace damaged or inadequate integumental tissue [9].

AlloDerm is a human acellular dermal graft that is biochemically intact [27]. The use of this device often requires the application of an overlying skin graft. The device has two distinct surfaces, a "dermal" side and a "basement membrane" side. The dermal side exhibits greater plasma imbibition and is placed in contact with the most vascularized surface. The basement membrane surface serves as an attachment site for migrating stem cells from the overlying skin autograft.

AlloDerm Recommended Protocol

1. Open the outer foil bag, and remove the inner Tyvek pouch. Both the foil bag and Tyvek pouch should be kept out of the sterile field. Using sterile technique, open the inner Tyvek pouch and remove the enclosed matrix. Do not remove the paper backing at this time.
2. Completely immerse the matrix in sterile saline for at least 5 min or until the backing separates from the AlloDerm matrix.

   (a) Warming the saline solution as high as 37 °C and gently rocking the rehydration bath to provide slight mechanical motion will speed the rehydration process. It is important NOT to heat the saline solution above 37 °C.
   (b) If simultaneously rehydrating multiple matrix pieces, ensure that the pieces do not overlap or stick together as this may slow the rehydration process. Instead, rehydrate matrices in separate containers.
   (c) Ensure that the AlloDerm matrix remains fully submerged by weighing it down with a sterile object, such as sterile forceps.
   (d) If the AlloDerm matrix does not achieve complete rehydration, gently wipe/rub both sides of the matrix with a sterile gloved hand to remove excess cryoprotectant material that may be preventing the rehydration fluid from contacting the AlloDerm matrix.

3. Aseptically remove and discard the paper backing once it separates from the matrix.
4. Transfer the matrix to a second bath sufficiently filled with rehydration fluid. As before, ensure that the matrix is completely submerged, and soak the matrix until it is fully rehydrated (this may take up to 40 min for thicker grafts).

   (a) The graft should be soft and pliable throughout once it is fully rehydrated. Once this has been achieved, the graft is ready for implantation and should be inserted within 4 h of rehydration.

5. Trim AlloDerm matrix to required dimensions prior to insertion.
6. Determine the proper orientation of the AlloDerm matrix, and insert as appropriate.

   (a) Identify the distinct surfaces of the AlloDerm matrix once it has been rehydrated by adding a drop of blood to both sides and rinsing with rehydration solution. The dermal side will appear bloody, whereas the basement membrane side will appear pink. When applying AlloDerm to a wound bed during grafting procedures, the dermal side should be placed in direct contact with the wound bed, and the basement membrane side should face in the opposite direction, toward the surface of the wound. When AlloDerm is used as an implant, the dermal side of the matrix should be placed against the most vascularized tissue.

7. Following AlloDerm insertion, place an overlying skin autograft, and secure using preferred techniques.

8. Place an inner dressing of petrolatum-impregnated gauze to reduce moisture loss, and secure using appropriate outer secondary dressings. A damp saline layer may also be applied to increase moisture retention at the wound site.

AlloDerm Postoperative Management

1. During the first few postoperative days, the outer dressing layers may require frequent changing in order to prevent accumulation of fluid and bacteria. It is critical that the AlloDerm matrix and overlying autograft remain undisturbed in order to achieve sufficient revascularization and re-epithelization. To prevent reinjury, do not disturb the inner dressing of petrolatum-impregnated gauze for at least 7 days, after which use extreme care when removing the inner dressing. Prior to removing the inner dressing, generously apply petrolatum-based ointment to prevent adherence and to reduce stress applied to the grafted areas. Soaking the wound area with saline may also be effective when removing the dressing.
2. Around day 7 post-surgery, it is normal for the AlloDerm graft to appear white/yellow in some areas. It is also common for the skin autograft to appear whiter than the surrounding epidermis and to only weakly adhere at this time.
3. Continue to redress the surgical site with antibiotic-impregnated fine mesh gauze or other nonadherent dressings until the graft has fully re-vascularized and re-epithelized. A damp saline layer is no longer necessary at this time.
4. If all or part of the autograft is removed with the dressing, this does not always require regrafting. If sufficient epidermal cells have migrated from the autograft to the basement membrane, regrafting will not be needed.
5. If using a meshed graft, epithelial cell growth under the thin dermal layer of the autograft may cause it to detach. Regrafting may not be needed if sufficient epidermal cells have seeded the surface of the AlloDerm matrix to provide sufficient wound coverage prior to autograft detachment. The surface of the AlloDerm matrix should be carefully examined to determine if regrafting is required.
6. Protective dressings may be eliminated as the cornified layer of the newly formed skin is established (10–14 days). At this point, bathing with mild soaps and limited activity may commence.

ACell (Cytal, Gentrix, MicroMatrix)

ACell is derived from porcine urinary bladder mucosa (UBM). It is the only commercially available form of UBM and consists of two layers, a lamina propria that promotes cellular infiltration and neovascularization and a basement membrane layer that supports cell proliferation and neodermis formation. ACell comes in several formulations, including sheet (Cytal, Gentrix) and particulate forms (MicroMatrix).

ACell's sheet formulations come in 3-, 6- (Cytal® Surgical Sheets), and 8-layered varieties (Gentrix® Surgical Thick Sheets). These formulations take longer to degrade than the MicroMatrix powder and provide a sustained response that lasts over the course of 1 week or longer, depending on the degree to which the device is packed into the wound. The suture-holding capacity of ACell's sheet formulations make them useful in securing the skin margins of an open wound, reducing skin closure tension, and retaining other ACell formulations placed deeper in the wound.

ACell's MicroMatrix is created by grinding Cytal Surgical Sheets into powder. Due to its small particle size, this formulation has a rapid breakdown, resulting in a faster and more robust healing response. MicroMatrix can be applied directly as a powder or mixed with saline to create a thick injectable slurry. MicroMatrix has been useful in treating chronic wounds where stimulation of a robust healing response is needed as well as wounds in patients who are poor surgical candidates [3].

Some wounds, such as those of the scalp and forehead, heal slower and often require several applications of ACell devices in order to achieve complete closure or to reach sufficient healing to permit skin grafting. Treatment with MicroMatrix can be applied serially with alternate day treatments or with single placement of a large volume. It has been noted that applying larger amounts of ACell as well as simultaneous placement of multiple formulations of the device at the time of initial wound bed preparation leads to better outcomes with fewer revision surgeries and improved patient comfort [3].

In addition to the above, ACell devices have numerous clinical indications including partial and full-thickness wounds, a variety of ulcers (pressure, venous, diabetic, chronic vascular), surgical wounds (donor sites/grafts, post-Mohs surgery, post-laser surgery, wound dehiscence), traumatic wounds (abrasions, lacerations, second-degree burns, skin tears), tunneled and undermined wounds, and noninfected draining wounds [9].

Unlike most dermal substitutes, ACell has demonstrated clinical success when treating wounds challenged with bacterial infection [28]. Studies have shown that treatment with UBM promotes an anti-inflammatory (M2) macrophage phenotype, reducing the ratio of pro-inflammatory (M1) to anti-inflammatory (M2) macrophages [29]. This is significant since M1 macrophages are associated with scar formation, whereas M2 macrophages have been associated with tissue remodeling and improved wound repair [29]. Clinically, it has been noted that patients treated with ACell experience decreased swelling, scarring, and pain both at early and late stages of healing [3]. Furthermore, while treatment with ACell does not restore skin appendages, wounds healed using this device are amenable to hair follicle grafting procedures [3].

Below is our recommended ACell protocol along with clinical examples of using this dermal substitute to treat radial forearm (Figs. 21.2 and 21.3) and fibula flap donor sites (Fig. 21.4).

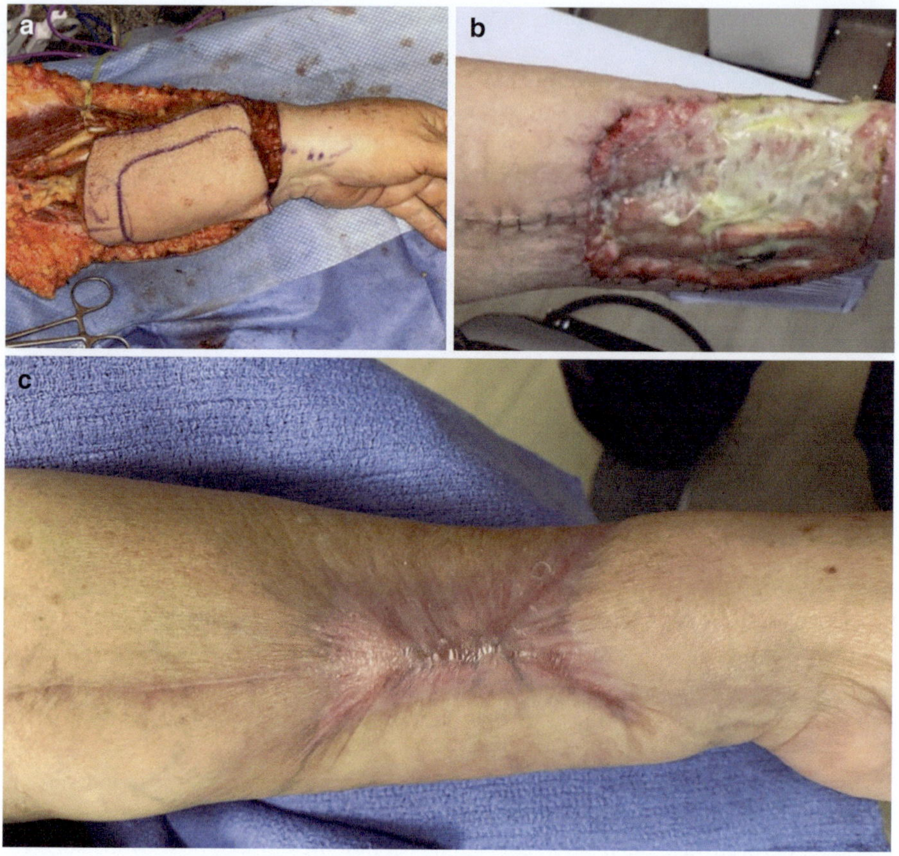

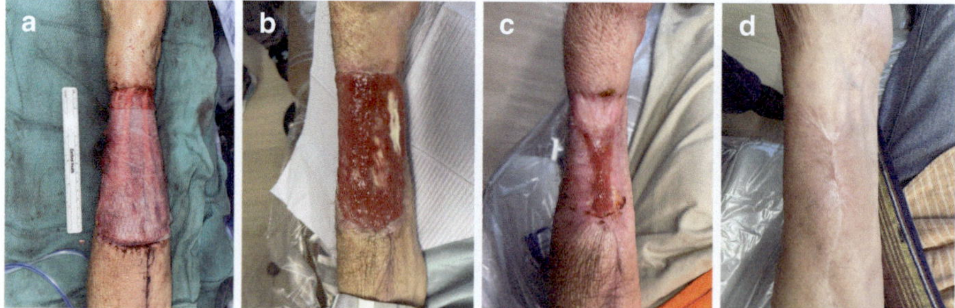

Fig. 21.2 ACell used to treat a radial forearm flap donor site. (**a**) Radial forearm flap harvested from donor site. (**b**) Flap donor site after placement of ACell Cytal Wound Matrix. (**c**) Complete neo-epithelization 3 months post-surgery (Images courtesy of Dr. James Melville)

Fig. 21.3 ACell used to treat a radial forearm flap donor site. (**a**) Placement of Cytal Wound Matrix dermal substitute. Progression of wound healing at (**b**) 2 weeks and (**c**) 3 months following application of dermal substitute. (**d**) Complete neo-epithelization achieved 4 months post-surgery (Images courtesy of Dr. James Melville)

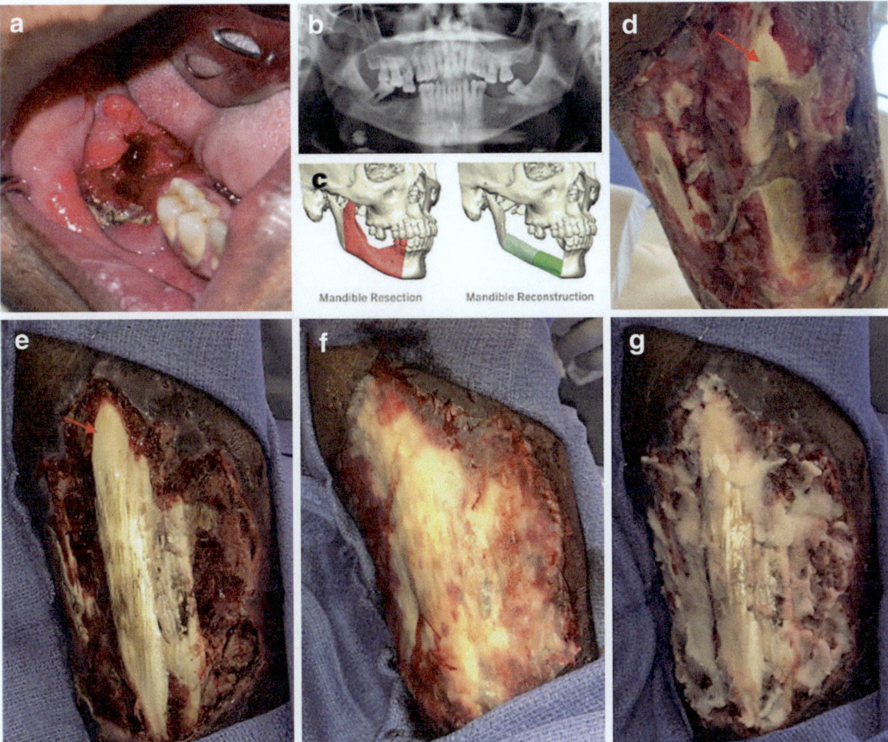

Fig. 21.4 ACell used to treat a nonhealing fibula flap donor site in a 70-year-old male with past medical history of hypertension, congested heart failure (ejection fraction (EF) 31.55%), and myocardial infarction (MI). Patient was diagnosed with stage IV oral squamous cell carcinoma of the right mandibular gingiva (T4aN3bM0). (**a**) Intraoral clinical picture showing 4.5 × 6 cm erosive ulcer in the right mandibular gingiva. (**b**) Orthopantomogram showing cortical bone erosion around tooth number 32. (**c**) The patient was treated with composite resection of the mandible, bilateral neck dissection (right neck levels I-IV, left neck levels I-III), osteo-cutaneous free fibula flap (FFF), and split-thickness skin graft (STSG) for reconstruction. (**d**) On the second postoperative week, the patient presented with failed STSG on his lower limb with tendon exposure (red arrow). (**e**) Under general anesthesia, STSG area was debrided (tendon exposure noted with red arrow). (**f**) 10 × 15 cm 6-layer Cytal wound matrix was used to reconstruct the ESD, which was secured with 3/0 chromic sutures. (**g**) MicroMatrix (1000 mg) was mixed with 5CC of saline to form a paste and applied on top of the Cytal wound matrix. (**h**) Two weeks later, granulation tissue was observed covering the exposed tendon (yellow arrows). Clinical pictures show healing progression at postoperative weeks 4 (**i**) and 5 (**j**). Complete tendon coverage with granulation tissue was achieved (Images courtesy of Dr. Dina Amin)

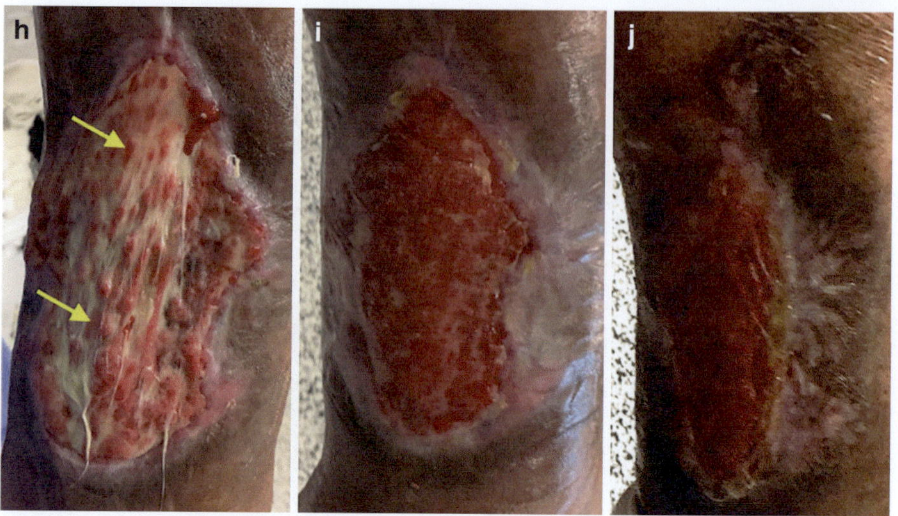

Fig. 21.4 (continued)

ACell Recommended Protocol: Intended for Sheet Formulations

1. Prepare the wound bed using standard procedures. Debride as needed to ensure that the wound is free of exudate and debris.
2. Using sterile technique, open device packaging and remove device from inner pouch.
3. Prior to insertion, hydrate device with either room temperature sterile saline (0.9%) or sterile lactated Ringer's solution. The ACell device must be hydrated for a minimum of 2 min and no longer than 45 min.
4. Cut the device to size, ensuring complete wound coverage.
5. Insert device directly into the wound bed.
6. Apply an overlying nonadherent dressing, and secure using preferred methods. For a wet wound, apply an absorptive dressing, and secure dressings using preferred methods. For a dry wound, apply a hydrogel dressing to retain moisture, and secure dressing using preferred methods.

ACell Postoperative Management

1. At a minimum, inspect the primary dressing every 7 days. During inspection, remove any exudate, and apply new ACell device to any non-covered areas of the wound. If a new device is applied, cover it with a new secondary dressing.
2. Change secondary dressings as needed without removing any of the remaining ACell device that is present on the wound surface.

3. A caramel-colored gel and a pungent odor will be produced as the ACell device is resorbed. When washing the wound surface, gently rinse so that the caramel-colored gel remains on the wound surface.
4. Continue the above postoperative management on a weekly basis until the wound has epithelized or until the desired wound state has been achieved.

AmnioFix

AmnioFix is an allograft derived from dehydrated human amniotic and chorionic membranes (dHACM). The high concentration of cytokines and growth factors found within these extraembryonic tissues significantly contributes to the wound healing response elicited by the AmnioFix device [10]. This dermal substitute comes as a lightweight, opaque, thin collagenous membrane that consists of two layers: a basement membrane layer and a stromal matrix.

dHACM-based dermal substitutes, such as AmnioFix, are particularly known for their success in healing chronic, nonhealing wounds, i.e., wounds that either fail to respond to standard treatment or show <40–50% healing within 3–4 weeks post-treatment [10]. This includes classic chronic wounds such as diabetic foot ulcers and venous leg ulcers. Although the mechanism is not fully understood, it is believed that the collagen-rich ECM of these dermal substitutes serves as a "sacrificial substrate" that reduces the activity of matrix metalloproteinases (MMPs), which are classically present in high numbers in many chronic wounds. dHACM-based devices, such as AmnioFix, have a > 90% success rate in achieving chronic wound closure within 12 weeks [10]. Of the dHACM-based products, Amniofix has the lowest reported complication rate, the most common complication being infection [10].

Due to their anti-inflammatory and pain mitigation properties, dHACM-based products have been used to treat inflammatory conditions such as plantar fasciitis and osteoarthritis [10, 30]. Other indications include urothelial tissue repair, management of chronic neuropathic pain, nerve repair, and cardiac tissue repair following myocardial infarction [10]. Regarding head and neck applications of dHACM-based devices, they have been successfully used to treat superficial and deep partial-thickness facial burns in both adult and pediatric patients, ocular surface pathologies (ocular burns, symblepharon, pterygium, corneal and conjunctival tumors, persistent epithelial defects with ulceration), and facial dermabrasions [31–37].

AmnioFix Recommended Protocol

1. Using sterile technique, open the outer pouch and place the inner pouch onto a sterile field.
2. Have an assistant slowly peel open the corner of the inner pouch, and present the allograft to the surgeon. The surgeon should grasp the allograft with sterile gloves or non-toothed, sterile forceps.

3. Prior to hydration, cut the allograft to the desired size using sharp scissors.
4. Place the allograft into the surgical site. Be sure to properly orient the allograft so that the embossed lettering reads correctly from left to right. The orientation of the allograft may vary depending on the surgical indication.
5. Hydrate the allograft with sterile saline, while it is in the surgical site. This should be done by applying several drops of sterile saline to the allograft at 1–2 min intervals for a period of 5–10 min. As the allograft becomes hydrated, the embossed lettering will begin to fade. It may take several minutes for the lettering to completely fade.
6. Following the recommended 5–10 min of hydration, visually inspect and manipulate the allograft to determine whether complete hydration has been achieved. Some allografts may require additional time.
7. Use absorbable and nonabsorbable suture material and/or tissue adhesives to secure the allograft to the surgical site.
8. Apply secondary dressings as needed.

AmnioFix Postoperative Management

1. Regularly inspect surgical site to determine progression of healing and to monitor for signs of infection.
2. If exudate is present, gently remove and irrigate the wound with sterile saline. Take care not to disturb the allograft and surrounding tissues.
3. Replace secondary dressings as needed, taking care not to disturb the underlying allograft and surrounding tissues.
4. Application of a new allograft may be required if the wound does not achieve complete re-epithelialization.

Conclusion

Dermal substitutes provide an excellent treatment option for head and neck soft tissue reconstruction both when used as the primary reconstructive modality and when combined with adjunctive procedures. The use of these substitutes has been particularly beneficial to medically complex patients, such as those on anticoagulants, as well as younger patients who would rather avoid two- or three-stage flap reconstructive procedures. In recent decades, numerous dermal substitutes have been developed that vary in their design and composition. However, they all serve to promote wound healing through the process of constructive remodeling by providing a scaffold that supports re-epithelization, neovascularization, and fibroblast infiltration while supplying an array of growth factors, cytokines, and chemokines that are released into the wound site as the dermal substitutes are gradually resorbed and replaced with natural tissue. Integra Wound Matrix System, AlloDerm, ACell, and AmnioFix are among the most commonly used dermal substitutes in the field of head and neck soft tissue reconstruction. These devices are simple to use, have a long shelf life (~5 years), do not interfere with commonly used dressing materials, and have demonstrated consistent clinical success. Some reports even suggest that the use of dermal substitutes reduces the overall cost of treatment, especially in the context of chronic, recalcitrant wounds [10]. Although dermal substitutes have a high per unit cost, the overall expense is similar if not reduced when considering the increased rate of healing and lower rate of complications/clinical sequelae [10]. One study went so far as to recommend the use of dermal substitutes, specifically the use of amniotic membrane, in developing countries as its use in treating superficial and deep partial-thickness burns significantly reduced hospital stay and overall costs [34].

Future developments in tissue engineering hold great promise in advancing the field of dermal substitutes. In recent years, hydrogel-based skin substitutes have attracted significant attention due to their ability to mimic the natural skin microenvironment [38]. These three-dimensional networks consist of physically or chemically cross-linked hydrophilic polymers. They are able to bind severalfold more water than their dry weight thus maintaining significant moisture levels in the wound bed, yet they are able to retain their 3D structure and can be casted into various shapes and sizes, spray-applied to wound beds, or even solidify "in situ" [38]. One of the most promising features of hydrogels is their tailored functionality. Hydrogel properties can be modified to alter their biomechanical properties, such as stiffness or resorption rate. Furthermore, they can be modified to include cells, antibacterial agents, growth factors, nanoparticles for localized drug delivery, and even sensors for real-time feedback on healing progression [38]. Current work is being done to combine these advances with recent progress in 3D printing in order to produce site-specific, multilayered 3D-printed biological scaffolds that can be tailored to the needs of each patient [39, 40]. Together, these developments hold tremendous potential to improve patient outcomes and will likely give dermal substitutes an ever-increasing role in head and neck soft tissue reconstruction.

References

1. Debels H, Hamdi M, Abberton K, Morrison W. Dermal matrices and bioengineered skin substitutes: a critical review of current options. Plast Reconstr Surg Glob Open. 2015;3:e284. https://doi.org/10.1097/GOX.0000000000000219.
2. Griffin MF, Leung BC, Premakumar Y, Szarko M, Butler PE. Comparison of the mechanical properties of different skin sites for auricular and nasal reconstruction. J Otolaryngol Head Neck Surg. 2017;46:33. https://doi.org/10.1186/s40463-017-0210-6.
3. Duscher D, Shiffman MA. Regenerative medicine and plastic surgery elements, research concepts and emerging technologies. Cham: Springer; 2019.
4. Feinberg SE, Aghaloo TL, Cunningham LL. Role of tissue engineering in Oral and maxillofacial reconstruction: findings of the 2005 AAOMS research summit. J Oral Maxillofac Surg. 2005;63:1418–25. https://doi.org/10.1016/j.joms.2005.07.004.

5. Chua AWC, Khoo YC, Tan BK, Tan KC, Foo CL, Chong SJ. Skin tissue engineering advances in severe burns: review and therapeutic applications. Burn Trauma. 2016;4:3. https://doi.org/10.1186/s41038-016-0027-y.

6. Barillo DJ, Nangle ME, Farrell K. Preliminary experience with cultured epidermal autograft in a community hospital burn unit. J Burn Care Rehabil. 1992;13:158–65. https://doi.org/10.1097/00004630-199201000-00035.

7. Shahrokhi S, Arno A, Jeschke MG. The use of dermal substitutes in burn surgery: acute phase. Wound Repair Regen. 2014;22:14–22. https://doi.org/10.1111/wrr.12119.

8. Augustine R, Kalarikkal N, Thomas S. Advancement of wound care from grafts to bioengineered smart skin substitutes. Prog Biomater. 2014;3:103–13. https://doi.org/10.1007/s40204-014-0030-y.

9. Melville JC, Shum JW, Young S, Wong ME. Regenerative strategies for maxillary and mandibular reconstruction: a practical guide. Cham: Springer; 2019.

10. Joshi CJ, Hassan A, Carabano M, Galiano RD. Up-to-date role of the dehydrated human amnion/chorion membrane (AMNIOFIX) for wound healing. Expert Opin Biol Ther. 2020;20:1125–31. https://doi.org/10.1080/14712598.2020.1787979.

11. Davis GE, Bayless KJ, Davis MJ, Meininger GA. Regulation of tissue injury responses by the exposure of matricryptic sites within extracellular matrix molecules. Am J Pathol. 2000;156:1489–98. https://doi.org/10.1016/S0002-9440(10)65020-1.

12. Davis GE. Matricryptic sites control tissue injury responses in the cardiovascular system: relationships to pattern recognition receptor regulated events. J Mol Cell Cardiol. 2010;48:454–60. https://doi.org/10.1016/j.yjmcc.2009.09.002.

13. Ricard-Blum S, Salza R. Matricryptins and matrikines: biologically active fragments of the extracellular matrix. Exp Dermatol. 2014;23:457–63. https://doi.org/10.1111/exd.12435.

14. Halim AS, Khoo TL, Mohd. Yussof SJ. Biologic and synthetic skin substitutes: an overview. Indian J Plast Surg. 2010;43:S23–8. https://doi.org/10.4103/0970-0358.70712.

15. Girod DA, Sykes K, Jorgensen J, Tawfik O, Tsue T. Acellular dermis compared to skin grafts in oral cavity reconstruction. Laryngoscope. 2009;119:2141–9. https://doi.org/10.1002/lary.20548.

16. Alrubaiy L, Al-Rubaiy KK. Skin substitutes: a brief review of types and clinical applications. Oman Med J. 2009;24:4–6. https://doi.org/10.5001/omj.2009.2.

17. Ferreira M, Paggiaro A, Isaac C, Teixeira N, Santos G. Skin substitutes: current concepts and a new classification system. Rev Bras Cir Plást. 2011;26:696–702. https://doi.org/10.1590/S1983-51752011000400028.

18. Ehrenreich M, Ruszczak Z. Update on dermal substitutes. Acta Dermatovenerol Croat. 2006;14:172–87.

19. Fahrenbach EN, Qi C, Ibrahim O, Kim JY, Alam M. Resistance of acellular dermal matrix materials to microbial penetration. JAMA Dermatol. 2013;149:571–5. https://doi.org/10.1001/jamadermatol.2013.1741.

20. Patel S, Ziai K, Lighthall JG, Walen SG. Biologics and acellular dermal matrices in head and neck reconstruction: a comprehensive review. Am J Otolaryngol. 2022;43:103233. https://doi.org/10.1016/j.amjoto.2021.103233.

21. Motz KM, Kim YJ. Auriculotemporal syndrome (Frey syndrome). Otolaryngol Clin N Am. 2016;49:501–9. https://doi.org/10.1016/j.otc.2015.10.010.

22. Geiger SE, Deigni OA, Watson JT, Kraemer BA. Management of open distal lower extremity wounds with exposed tendons using porcine urinary bladder matrix. Wounds. 2016;28:306–16.

23. Kraemer BA, Geiger SE, Deigni OA, Watson JT. Management of open lower extremity wounds with concomitant fracture using a porcine urinary bladder matrix. Wounds. 2016;28:387–94.

24. Sebastian S. Does preoperative scalp shaving result in fewer postoperative wound infections when compared with no scalp shaving? A systematic review. J Neurosci Nurs. 2012;44:149–56. https://doi.org/10.1097/JNN.0b013e31825106d2.

25. Jeng JC, Fidler PE, Sokolich JC, Jaskille AD, Khan S, White PM, et al. Seven years' experience with Integra as a reconstructive tool. J Burn Care Res. 2007;28:120–6. https://doi.org/10.1097/BCR.0b013E31802CB83F.
26. Terino EO. Alloderm acellular dermal graft: applications in aesthetic soft-tissue augmentation. Clin Plast Surg. 2001;28:83–99. https://doi.org/10.1016/S0094-1298(20)32341-5.
27. Jansen LA, De Caigny P, Guay NA, Lineaweaver WC, Shokrollahi K. The evidence base for the acellular dermal matrix AlloDerm: a systematic review. Ann Plast Surg. 2013;70:587–94. https://doi.org/10.1097/SAP.0b013e31827a2d23.
28. Sadtler K, Sommerfeld SD, Wolf MT, Wang X, Majumdar S, Chung L, et al. Proteomic composition and immunomodulatory properties of urinary bladder matrix scaffolds in homeostasis and injury. Semin Immunol. 2017;29:14–23. https://doi.org/10.1016/j.smim.2017.05.002.
29. Paige JT, Kremer M, Landry J, Hatfield SA, Wathieu D, Brug A, et al. Modulation of inflammation in wounds of diabetic patients treated with porcine urinary bladder matrix. Regen Med. 2019;14:269–77. https://doi.org/10.2217/rme-2019-0009.
30. Zelen CM, Poka A, Andrews J. Prospective, randomized, blinded, comparative study of injectable micronized dehydrated amniotic/chorionic membrane allograft for plantar fasciitis—a feasibility study. Foot Ankle Int. 2013;34:1332–9. https://doi.org/10.1177/1071100713502179.
31. Reilly DA, Hickey S, Glat P, Lineaweaver WC, Goverman J. Clinical experience: using dehydrated human amnion/chorion membrane allografts for acute and reconstructive burn care. Ann Plast Surg. 2017;78:S19. https://doi.org/10.1097/SAP.0000000000000981.
32. Puyana S, Elkbuli A, Ruiz S, Bernal E, McKenney M, Lim R, et al. The use of dehydrated human amniotic/chorionic membrane skin substitute in the treatment of pediatric facial burn. J Craniofac Surg. 2019;30:2551. https://doi.org/10.1097/SCS.0000000000005826.
33. Lee S-H, Tseng SCG. Amniotic membrane transplantation for persistent epithelial defects with ulceration. Am J Ophthalmol. 1997;123:303–12. https://doi.org/10.1016/S0002-9394(14)70125-4.
34. Ramakrishnan KM, Jayaraman V. Management of partial-thickness burn wounds by amniotic membrane: a cost-effective treatment in developing countries. Burns. 1997;23:S33–6. https://doi.org/10.1016/S0305-4179(97)90099-1.
35. Gheorghe A, Pop M, Burcea M, Serban M. New clinical application of amniotic membrane transplant for ocular surface disease. J Med Life. 2016;9:177–9.
36. Herndon DN, Branski LK. Contemporary methods allowing for safe and convenient use of amniotic membrane as a biologic wound dressing for burns. Ann Plast Surg. 2017;78:S9. https://doi.org/10.1097/SAP.0000000000000979.
37. Kucan JO, Robson MC, Parsons RW. Amniotic membranes as dressings following facial dermabrasion. Ann Plast Surg. 1982;8:523.
38. Tavakoli S, Klar AS. Advanced hydrogels as wound dressings. Biomolecules. 2020;10:1169. https://doi.org/10.3390/biom10081169.
39. Nesic D, Durual S, Marger L, Mekki M, Sailer I, Scherrer SS. Could 3D printing be the future for oral soft tissue regeneration? Bioprinting. 2020;20:e00100. https://doi.org/10.1016/j.bprint.2020.e00100.
40. Singh D, Singh D, Han SS. 3D printing of scaffold for cells delivery: advances in skin tissue engineering. Polymers. 2016;8:19. https://doi.org/10.3390/polym8010019.

Chapter 22
The Evolution of Magnetic Resonance Neurography in Imaging of the Trigeminal Nerve

Jason Wahidi and John R. Zuniga

Historical Perspective

Injuries to peripheral nerves have been documented as early as the second century AD, with continued reports of injuries to the nerves of the jaw and face over the last three centuries. Eloquent descriptions of American Civil War injuries from SW Mitchell depict soldiers with "tingling pain" and "severe burning sensations," characteristics of nerve injuries that would go on to be verified by clinicians and neuroscientists in the coming centuries. The treatment of nerve injuries is equally storied with ablative procedures ranging from neurectomies to alcohol injections to treat trigeminal neuralgia [1]. Through a continued push toward nerve repair during the nineteenth and twentieth centuries, direct end-to-end anastomoses (neurorrhaphy) of traumatized trigeminal nerves has emerged as the most effective procedure for improving peripheral trigeminal neuropathy (PTN). Therefore, the decision of when to employ trigeminal nerve microneurosurgery necessitates timely and accurate clinical diagnosis, assessment, and surgical planning. For diagnosis, the clinical neurosensory testing (NST) algorithm was developed and first published in 1992, and its statistical power related to surgical findings was later established in 1998. It involves three levels of testing: Level A measures spatiotemporal sensory perception, Level B measures contact detection with monofilament, and Level C measures pain and threshold. The five scores of sensory impairment denote normal, mild,

J. Wahidi (✉)
Division of Oral and Maxillofacial Surgery, Department of Surgery, UT Southwestern/
Parkland Memorial Hospital, Dallas, TX, USA
e-mail: jason.wahidi@UTSouthwestern.edu

J. R. Zuniga
Division of Oral and Maxillofacial Surgery, Department of Surgery and Neurology, UT
Southwestern/Parkland Memorial Hospital, Dallas, TX, USA
e-mail: john.zuniga@UTSouthwestern.edu

J. C. Melville et al. (eds.), *Advancements and Innovations in OMFS, ENT, and Facial Plastic Surgery*, https://doi.org/10.1007/978-3-031-32099-6_22

moderate, severe, and complete loss [2]. NST testing persists today as the gold standard to confirm the diagnosis of PTN but has several shortcomings. Despite exhibiting high positive and negative predictive values for lingual nerve injuries, NST yields lower values for inferior alveolar nerve (IAN) injuries with false-positive and false-negative rates of up to 23% and 40%, respectively. In addition, the results from these tests are only accurate when delivered 1 month after the injury since they cannot distinguish levels of injury before 1 month. With higher sensory impairment scores, NST testing tends to overestimate the degree of nerve injury, and at lower sensory impairment scores, NST tends to underestimate the degree of nerve injury. The additional variability in NST scores related to age, duration of injury, and cause of injury can result in inaccuracies and delayed treatment [3]. The Medical Research Council Scale (MRCS) for sensory recovery is currently the reference standard for monitoring recovery and surgical repair outcomes. Considering that early intervention with microsurgical repair is related to better outcomes, early diagnosis of nerve injuries would be preferred. Perhaps the most significant drawback of NST testing is the inability to delineate nerve anatomy for presurgical planning. Although preoperative imaging with panoramic radiographs and computed tomography (CT) aids in identifying the expected location of the nerve based on known anatomic landmarks, these modalities again provide poor visualization of the nerve or perineural tissues. Following the first clinical uses of magnetic resonance imaging (MRI) in the 1970s, magnetic resonance neurography (MRN) was introduced in the 1980s as a noninvasive technique, without ionizing radiation, to address the shortcomings above.

Principles and Justification

MR neurography is a modification of conventional MRI techniques dedicated to imaging peripheral nerves. It can provide the surgeon with a noninvasive map of neuromuscular anatomy in multiple orthogonal planes. Like MRI, MR neurography utilizes a magnetic field and computer-generated radio waves to create detailed images of soft tissue structures. The strength of an MRI magnet is known as the "field strength" and is measured in Tesla or "T." While a conventional MRI utilizes a 1.5 T magnet, MR neurography involves "high-field-strength" imaging with a 3 T magnet. The result of using a magnet twice as strong imparts benefits such as faster scan speeds and improved image quality due to a decreased signal-to-noise (SNR) ratio. Imaging on a 3 T imaging unit is typically performed in 6–7 min. Currently, two different imaging methods are available to study peripheral nerves: anatomic MRN and diffusion-based functional MRN. Anatomic MRN can facilitate neuropathy detection by showing nerve caliber alterations, thereby providing quantitative information about nerve size. An abnormal intraneural T2 signal intensity ratio (T2SIR) can also provide qualitative nerve structure criteria. For example, a low T2SIR may indicate loss of nerve continuity, while a high T2SIR may be caused by perineural edema. Complimentary techniques such as diffusion-weighted imaging

(DWI), particularly diffusion tensor imaging (DTI), utilize the random diffusion of water within tissue to provide information about its anisotropy in different tissues. Structural components of nerve tracts, such as the high lipid content of myelin, constrain water molecules causing them to diffuse more rapidly in a direction parallel to the fiber tract rather than across it. While normal tissue typically imparts significant anisotropy of water motion, this anisotropic effect is diminished when neuronal damage is present and can be correlated with axonal degeneration and regeneration. A 2018 study by Dessouky et al. demonstrated the diagnostic accuracy of MR neurography by correlating MRN imaging with neurosensory testing and intraoperative findings. In a retrospective sample of 24 patients, 25 nerve injuries were stratified on imaging using Sunderland classification. It was shown that MRN nerve thickness measurements had a good to excellent correlation with NST and surgery classifications. As compared to NST testing and surgical findings, MRN was indeterminate in only 3/25 cases and additionally detected two nerve injuries (IAN and LN) in one case where NST recorded only one nerve injury. Though limited by a small sample size, it was concluded that MRN could provide a more accurate depiction of nerve injuries for surgical planning compared to the current standard, NST [4]. Many additional technical considerations exist when considering the imaging protocol for MRN and require close collaboration with radiologists to optimize image quality and diagnostic accuracy. The protocol utilized at the author's institution is shown in Table 22.1.

Table 22.1 MR neurography protocol on a 3-T imaging unit

Sequence	TR/TE (msec)	Section Thickness (mm)	Matrix	FOV (cm)	Comments	Acquisition time (min: sec)
Axial T2W SPAIR	2000/60	3.0	268 × 248	16	Corpus callosum to chin	5:20
Axial T1W	580/9	3.0	320 × 310	16	Corpus callosum to chin	5:10
Axial 3D balanced FFE	5.32/2.66	0.65	270 × 270	16	Corpus callosum to chin	6:00
Axial DTI	14,000/70	5.0	196 × 192	18	Skull base to chin; b values = 0 and 600 sec/mm2; 12 directions	7:00
Coronal 3D STIR	1500/78	1.5 (isotropic voxel)	–	20	Corpus callosum to chin	7:15
Coronal 3D PSIF	12/2.5	0.9 (isotropic voxel)	–	20	Corpus callosum to chin	7:30

DTI diffusion tensor imaging, *FFE* fast field echo, *FOV* field of view, *SPAIR* spectral attenuated inversion recovery, *TE* echo time, *T1W* T1-weighted, *T2W* T2-weighted, *TR* repetition time

Classification and Interpretation of Nerve Injury

Sensory innervation of the face is provided by three branches of the trigeminal nerve: the ophthalmic, maxillary, and mandibular nerves. The inferior alveolar (IAN) and lingual nerves (LN) are the most commonly injured peripheral nerves during oral and maxillofacial surgery. Among oral treatments, molar tooth extractions are very common, and up to 10 million third molars are extracted at an annual cost of over 3 billion dollars. Tooth extractions alone account for 60% of all nerve injuries in the jaw, with an incidence of permanent paresthesia and functional disability in the lip, tongue, and cheek ranging from 11,500 to 35,000 [4]. The Seddon and Sunderland grading systems have traditionally been used in classifying nerve injuries. Seddon et al. categorized nerve injuries based on severity into neurapraxia, axonotmesis, and neurotmesis. Pathologic changes in neurapraxia, the mildest type of injury, involve only the myelin sheath around the axon and are associated with an excellent prognosis. In axonotmesis, the axon suffers complete rupture resulting in Wallerian degeneration of its distal segment. However, the supporting structures, including the perineurium and epineurium, remain intact. The prognosis for recovery remains good, but time is required for axonal regeneration (approximately 1 mm per day). Neurotmesis is the most severe type of injury and refers to the complete severance of the nerve. The result is total functional loss, and unless early surgical intervention is performed, clinical recovery is not anticipated. In 1951, Sunderland further stratified the classification proposed by Seddon into the individual structures of organized nerve tissue: myelin loss, axonal loss, and endoneurial, perineurial, and epineurial injury. Despite advancements in understanding nerve injuries and microsurgical techniques and materials, the current diagnostic strategy of using NST and existing classification systems is limited. Zuniga et al. hypothesized that MR neurography could be reliably used to diagnose and classify injuries to the peripheral trigeminal nerve and performed multiple studies investigating whether MRN of peripheral trigeminal neuropathies (PTNs) could serve as a diagnostic modality by correlating NST, MRN, and surgical findings. A 2017 study by Zuniga et al. examined 60 patients with traumatic and nontraumatic peripheral trigeminal neuropathies of varying etiologies and Sunderland classifications who had undergone MRN evaluation, in addition to clinical NST and, in some cases, trigeminal nerve surgery. To test the hypothesis, two groups of patients were examined. The first were those who had a known traumatic injury of the trigeminal nerve, and the second were those without a known traumatic injury. The traumatic injuries included third molar extraction, dental implantation, mandibular surgery, and orthognathic surgery. The nontraumatic injuries included three categories of etiologies: dental injection, noninvasive endodontic treatment, and unknown sensory complaints. Patients underwent MRN imaging using 1.5 T and 3.0 T scanners, including two-dimensional and three-dimensional imaging, and two musculoskeletal radiologists read MRN findings of nerve signal and caliber alteration. A Sunderland classification was then given by the radiologists unaware of the NST grading using the

Table 22.2 Sunderland nerve classification stratified by clinical NST/MRCS grade, surgical findings, and MRN imaging

Sunderland classification	Clinical NST level and MRCS grade description	Surgical findings by direct inspection	MRN findings
1	Normal (4)/S3+ or S4 by 3 months	Intact with no internal or external fibrosis, normal mobility, and neuroarchitecture (visualized fascicles and Fanconi bands)	Anatomic: Homogenous, mild increased T2W nerve signal
2	Normal (4)/S3+ or S4 by 6 months	Intact with no internal fibrosis; external fibrosis, restricted mobility, but neuroarchitecture intact (visualized fascicles and Fanconi bands once external scar removed)	Anatomic: Homogenous increased T2W signal of nerve and mild nerve thickening or constriction; perineural fibrosis
3	Mild (3) or moderate (2)/ S2, S2+, S3 by ≥6 months	Intact with both internal and external fibrosis, restricted mobility, and disturbance of neuroarchitecture (abnormal fascicle patterns and/or Fanconi bands not visible)	Anatomic: Homogenous increased T2W signal of nerve and moderate thickening or constriction; perineural fibrosis
4	Moderate (2) or severe (1)/S1, S2, S2+ by ≥6 months	Partially transected nerve but some amount of distal nerve present with or without neuroma in continuity	Anatomic: Homogenous increased T2W signal of nerve and moderate thickening or constriction; perineural fibrosis
5	Severe (1) or complete (0)/ S0, S1 by ≥6 months	Completely transected nerve with or without amputation neuroma	Anatomic: Discontinuous nerve with end-bulb neuroma

MRCS Medical Research Council Scale, *MRN* magnetic resonance neurography, *NST* neurosensory testing, *T2W* T2-weighted
Adapted with permission from [2]

qualitative imaging criteria described in Table 22.2. Although this study had some limitations, including the lack of blinding and a control group, the utilization of descriptive statistics demonstrated that MRN has a moderate to good correlation with NST levels, MRCS grading scores, and surgical findings. Of note, in this group of patients, third molar surgery represented the most common cause of traumatic PTN [2]. Figures 22.1 and 22.2a display Sunderland Class I and II injuries, respectively, and highlight the ability of MRN to distinguish between normal and abnormal nerve morphology. Figure 22.2b displays the intraoperative, clinical correlation to a Sunderland class II injury. A Sunderland Class I injury is not an indication for surgical intervention; this important distinction may guide the surgeon in appropriate treatment planning and monitoring of nerve injuries. An additional 2018 study by Zuniga et al. aimed to evaluate the role and reliability of MRN for the diagnosis

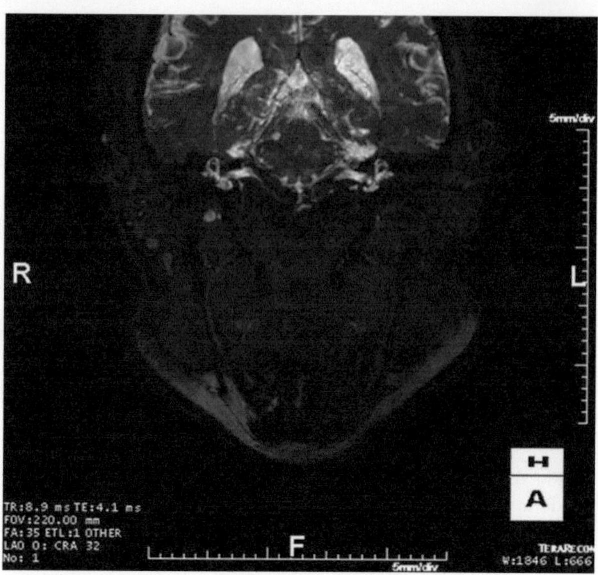

Fig. 22.1 Normal MRN: 59-year-old female with spontaneous onset of left mandibular pain (8 of 10) × 1 year with normal neurology, neurosurgery, otolaryngology, dental, and prior OMS examinations. Normal MRI brain, CT max/face, CBCT, and posterior mandible biopsy. IAN local block eliminates pain. Hemifacial numbness was reported. *NST* normal/S4 level. Findings are consistent with Class I/Normal condition. MRN findings: *Normal appearance of the maxillofacial nerves. Mild paranasal sinus mucosal disease*

of injuries to the peripheral trigeminal nerve in patients with prior molar tooth extraction to determine its accuracy with respect to the clinical and surgical staging. Twenty-four patients who exhibited NST evidence of injury of the IAN or LN were included, as well as a control group of 18 patients without symptoms of trigeminal neuralgia, recent tooth extraction, facial pain, or prior oral and maxillofacial surgery. Again, nerve measurements on MRN were read by two experienced radiologists. Patients with trigeminal neuropathy or injury showed more significant differences in nerve thickness, T2 signal intensity ratio, and contrast-to-noise ratios than control patients for the inferior alveolar nerve and lingual nerve. Figure 22.3 illustrates the correlation between MRN findings and a left IAN Sunderland Class III injury. Statistical analysis once again demonstrated that MR neurography had a moderate to good correlation with respect to clinical neurosensory testing [4]. While the studies above demonstrated that MRN has a good correlation with Sunderland classification, Zuniga et al. aimed to further correlate presurgical findings of neuroma size on MRN with the actual intraoperative neuroma or nerve gap size. It was hypothesized that presurgical MRN neuroma and abnormal nerve segment size would correlate and predict the length of the final surgical gap. Variables recorded

Fig. 22.2 (**a**) Class II Injury 49 y/o female 3 months s/p extraction teeth #19 and 20 and placement of dental implants still in pain with normal NST values with no neuropathic pain responses, consistent with Class II injury. MRN finding: *Scar entrapment of the distal left inferior alveolar nerve, immediately proximal to its ramifications into the chin and gingiva.* (**b**) Left inferior alveolar nerve exposed with high magnification showing intact fascicles

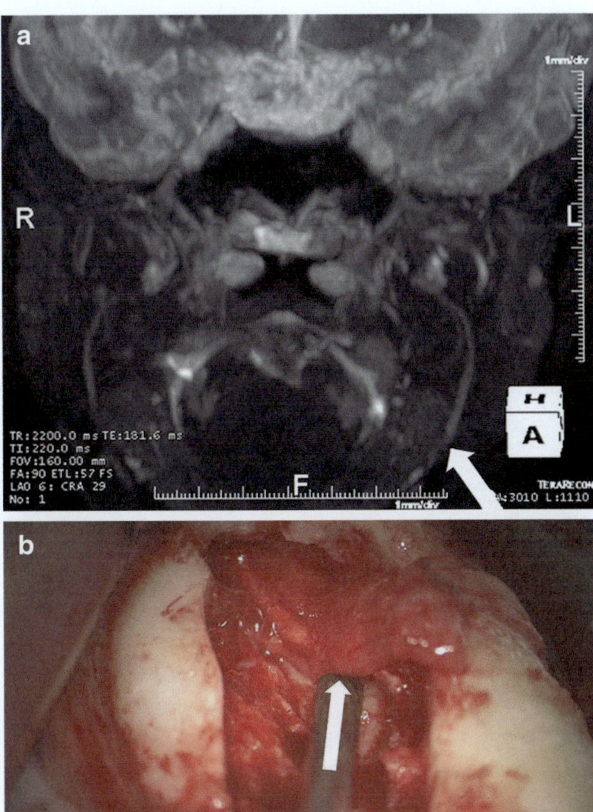

from the surgical procedures included the neuroma's length and the gap size created once normal nerve tissue was identified proximally and distally. For reference, Fig. 22.4 displays a large neuroma associated with left lingual nerve injury from a third molar extraction. The final gap size is considered the most important independent variable in microsurgical repair. If a positive correlation with presurgical MRN were to be found, the surgeon could quantitatively assess the nerve injury gap. Although limited by a small sample size, this study ultimately found no correlation between MRN neuroma length and gap size [5]. As seen in Fig. 22.5, the benefits of MRN in the early detection of nerve injury, even in the setting of negative clinical NST testing, are clear. However, while prior studies adequately demonstrated the qualitative accuracy of MRN, findings currently suggest the need for better imaging and adjunctive techniques to predict gap size for surgeons to improve presurgical planning, possibly resulting in a shorter, more predictable surgery.

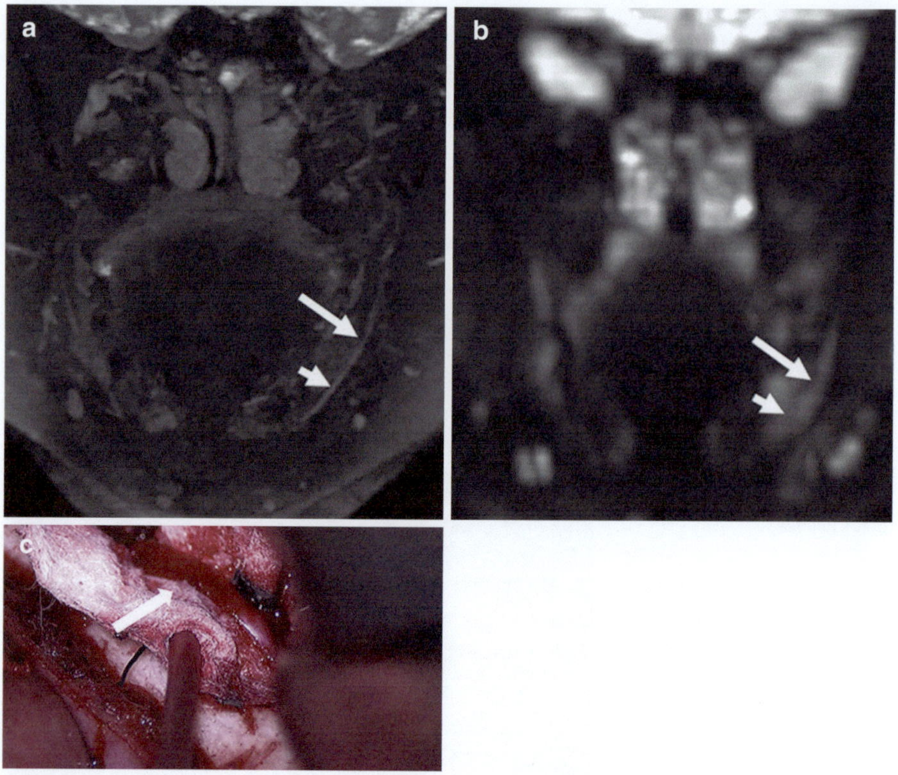

Fig. 22.3 (**a**) Class III Injury: 62-year-old female 2.5 months with painful neuropathy left IAN following dental implant #18 site with clinical NST consistent with Class III injury. MRN findings – *Left inferior alveolar neuropathy with mild scar entrapment at the prior dental extraction site.* (**b**) Diffusion tensor imaging (DTI) of the same injury showing abnormal anisotropy of the left inferior alveolar nerve. (**c**) Left inferior alveolar nerve on neuropathy showing abnormal, erythematous changes consistent with class III injury

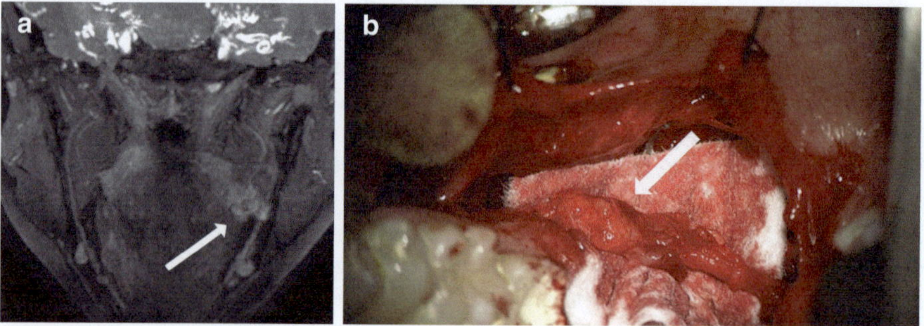

Fig. 22.4 (**a**) Class IV Injury: 45-year-old female s/p 2 months #17 extraction with severe sensory impairment, positive trigger, dystrophic ageusia, and burning, consistent with Class IV injury left lingual nerve. MRN findings: *Sunderland class IV/V injury of the left lingual nerve. Minimal hyperintensity of the left inferior alveolar nerve is probably reactive granulation tissue at the tooth extraction site.* (**b**). Left lingual nerve injury showing large neuroma with continuity consistent with a Class IV injury

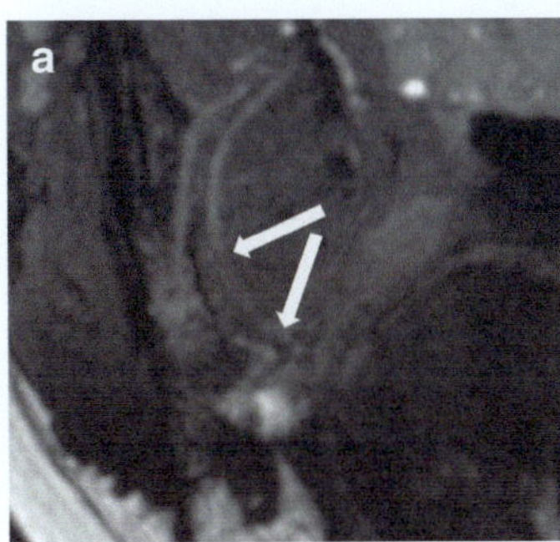
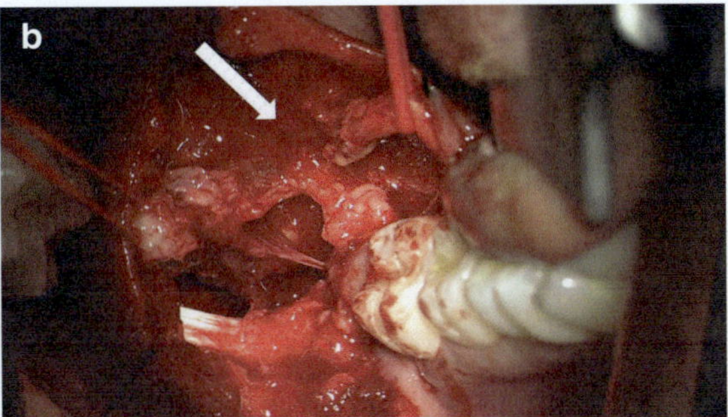

Fig. 22.5 (a) Class V Injury: 27-year-old female 1 week s/p attempted removal #32 with local, procedure aborted but complete anesthesia of right tongue reported. Unable to perform NST due to painful trismus. MRN findings: *Lingual nerve: Abnormally enlarged and hyperintense on the right without appreciable distal continuity. Sunderland class V injury of the right lingual nerve.* (b) Right lingual nerve exposure showing the proximal and distal ends separated consistent with a Class V injury

Imaging in Different Clinical Scenarios

Future Directions

As described, the application of MR neurography in oral and maxillofacial surgery can gather noninvasive, qualitative information of the IAN and LN, further augmenting the diagnostic acumen of the surgeon. It was also shown that limitations currently exist regarding the ability of MRN to provide meaningful quantitative information with nerve gap size. For surgeons to benefit from this newer imaging modality, further investigations with randomized clinical trials must be completed to solidify the relationship between MRN findings and the varying degrees of trigeminal neuropathy in the preinjury, postinjury, and post-repair state. Adjunctive MRN imaging techniques such as fractional anisotropy and diffusion coefficient alterations can aid further quantification of trigeminal neuropathy but require future study. As always, imaging findings and analysis should be an aid to surgical experience, tempered by experienced clinical judgment.

References

1. Mitchell SW, Morehouse GR, Keen WW. The classic: gunshot wounds and other injuries of nerves. Clin Orthop Relat Res. 2007;458:35–9.
2. Zuniga JR, Mistry C, Tikhonov I, Dessouky R, Chhabra A. Magnetic resonance neurography of traumatic and nontraumatic peripheral trigeminal neuropathies. J Oral Maxillofac Surg. 2018;76(4):725–36.
3. Zuniga JR, Meyer RA, Gregg JM, Miloro M, Davis LF. The accuracy of clinical neurosensory testing for nerve injury diagnosis. J Oral Maxillofac Surg. 1998;56(1):2–8.

 4. Dessouky R, Xi Y, Zuniga J, Chhabra A. Role of MR Neurography for the diagnosis of peripheral trigeminal nerve injuries in patients with prior molar tooth extraction. Am J Neuroradiol. 2017;39(1):162–9.
 5. Zuniga JR, AbdelBaky O, Alian A, Thakur U, Pezeshk P, Xi Y, Chhabra A. Does presurgical magnetic resonance neurography predict surgical gap size in trigeminal class IV and V injuries? J Oral Maxillofac Surg. 2021;79(12):2574–81.

Chapter 23
Advancements and Innovations in Office Anesthesia: Novel Drugs and Infusion Combinations for Office-Based Intravenous Sedation

Alfredo Arribas, Dominik Rudecki, Steven Hengen, and Issa Hanna

Introduction

In the field of modern dentistry and oral and maxillofacial surgery, office-based procedural sedation with modern anesthetic medications is utilized to provide patients and providers with safe and predictable outpatient anesthesia outcomes. The 2016 American Association of Oral and Maxillofacial Surgeons (AAOMS) White Paper on Office-Based Anesthesia asserts that "fearful patients, who are often in pain, are effectively, economically, and safely managed in the oral and maxillofacial surgery office with the use of deep sedation/general anesthesia that frequently incorporates agents such as propofol and/or ketamine" [1]. The AAOMS' 2017 Parameters of Care lists several goals of outpatient anesthesia including satisfactory experience for the surgeon and patient and full recovery from anesthetic effects within an appropriate time [2]. Though current day anesthetics and techniques have provided advances in successfully implementing the goals of outpatient anesthesia care, the road to present-day successes in office-based procedural sedation has been long. We owe thanks to many pioneering professionals past and present as we continually seek to improve outcomes and experiences for ourselves and our patients.

Arguably the most significant historical advancement in the management of the surgical patient has been the discovery and application of anesthesia. Boyle was first credited with the experimentation with intravenous injections in 1656 [3].

Sir Christopher Wren would later go on to write in a letter "I Have Injected Wine and Ale in a living Dog into the Mass of Blood by a Veine, in good Quantities, till I have made him extremely drunk, but soon after he Pisseth it out" [4].

A. Arribas · D. Rudecki · S. Hengen · I. Hanna (✉)
Department of Oral and Maxillofacial Surgery, UTHealth Houston, Houston, TX, USA
e-mail: alfredo.r.arribas@uth.tmc.edu; dominik.a.rudecki@uth.tmc.edu;
steven.l.hengen@uth.tmc.edu; issa.a.hanna@uth.tmc.edu

J. C. Melville et al. (eds.), *Advancements and Innovations in OMFS, ENT, and Facial Plastic Surgery*, https://doi.org/10.1007/978-3-031-32099-6_23

Two centuries later in October 1846, Boston dentist Dr. Morton was looking for alternatives to the already used nitrous oxide anesthetic. He teamed up with Massachusetts General Hospital surgeon John Collins Warren to perform the first public display of a procedure successfully completed under anesthesia. At which time history attributes Dr. Warren proclaiming "Gentlemen! this is no humbug" [5].

From the 1920s to the mid-1950s, the primary sedatives/hypnotic drugs were barbiturates [6]. Fortunately, the subsequent decades brought the anesthesia community short-acting anesthetics that included benzodiazepines like midazolam, narcotics like fentanyl, hypnotic sedatives, namely, propofol, and dissociative anesthetics, namely, ketamine. These noted agents, in some combination, have become the basis for most office-based anesthetics.

In present-day anesthesia, we now have a full array of volatile and intravenous-based anesthetics that meet specific patient needs providing therapeutic outcomes with relative safety. This chapter intends to review current anesthetic drugs, as well as anesthetic drug infusion combinations that can assist the clinician in providing safe and effective outpatient office-based anesthesia.

Remifentanil

Remifentanil is a relatively new opioid, receiving FDA approval in 1996 for applications in general anesthesia, monitored anesthesia care, and short-term postoperative analgesia in PACU. Remifentanil is a pure (mu) opioid receptor agonist, with little effect on the other opioid receptors. It is characterized by rapid onset and ultrashort, predictable duration of action. The onset of clinical effect is typically 60–90 s. The context-sensitive half-time of elimination is approximately 3 min from discontinuation, regardless of duration of infusion [7]. Remifentanil displays unique metabolism among opioids, involving rapid and uniform clearance by nonspecific blood and tissue esterases [8]. The desirable result is twofold; first, a rapid recovery, typically 5–10 min. Second, the duration of action of remifentanil does not increase with increasing duration of administration because of the lack of drug accumulation. These unique properties have made remifentanil an attractive adjunct for inpatient, outpatient, and in-office surgical procedures.

Remifentanil is packaged in 1 mg, 2 mg, and 5 mg vials which are reconstituted and diluted before administration. When used for induction of anesthesia in adult patients, remifentanil is infused at 0.5–1µg/kg/min along with a hypnotic or gas anesthetic. For maintenance of anesthesia with propofol, remifentanil is given in a continuous infusion at a rate of approximately 0.25µg/kg/min (range 0.05–2.0µg/kg/min). A 1µg/kg supplemental bolus dose can be used during episodes of intense surgical stress or in response to light anesthesia. When remifentanil is used for analgesia in the immediate postoperative period, a continuous infusion of 0.1µg/kg/min (range 0.025–0.2µg/kg/min) is appropriate [8].

While typically given in conjunction with other anesthetic agents, remifentanil's unique pharmacokinetic properties also make it an effective solo agent when given as an infusion for select conscious sedation procedures. In a study of 90 patients undergoing facial surgery, Ferraro et al. showed that remifentanil as a single agent was better tolerated, provided superior pain control, and displayed more hemodynamic stability when compared to midazolam or propofol as single agents. Their protocol included 0.08μg/kg/min of remifentanil before administration of local anesthesia and either blepharoplasty or otoplasty. Remifentanil did not cause respiratory depression in any patients, likely because this adverse effect is more likely seen with bolus administration [9].

Remifentanil's short duration of action has also made it increasingly popular for use as a single agent in emergency departments for procedures including lumbar punctures, cardioversion, orthopedic manipulation, incision and drainage, and chest tube placement [10]. Patients can rapidly undergo these procedures, recover within 10 min, and undergo a reliable neurological examination.

Adverse effects of remifentanil are similar to other opioids. Remifentanil has been shown to cause dose-dependent hypotension and bradycardia up to 2μg/kg within 3–5 min of a bolus or an infusion rate increase. When this response is clinically undesirable, it can be reversed relatively quickly by reduction of rate of infusion. Dose-dependent respiratory depression is an effect common to remifentanil and other similar opioids and is clinically relevant to the oral and maxillofacial surgeon. Recovery of respiratory drive after discontinuation of remifentanil is significantly faster than fentanyl and other opioids. After discontinuation of a 0.25μg/kg/min infusion of remifentanil, the blood level at which spontaneous respiration occurs is achieved in 2–4 min [11]. When co-administered with other anesthetic agents such as propofol, the recovery depends on the other agent. As with other opioids, chest wall rigidity is possible with the administration of remifentanil, particularly when given in boluses.

Remifentanil is an effective and efficient drug in the modern oral and maxillofacial surgeon's toolbox, most often used with other agents such as midazolam and/or propofol which will be discussed in subsequent sections.

Dexmedetomidine

Dexmedetomidine was initially approved by the Food and Drug Administration for sedation, in 1999, for use as a short-term medication (within 24 h) for analgesia and sedation in intubated and mechanically ventilated patients in an ICU setting. In 2008, the FDA approved a new indication for non-intubated patients requiring sedation before and/or during diagnostic and therapeutic procedures.

Dexmedetomidine is an intravenous α2-adrenergic receptor agonist that provides anxiolysis, sedation, and analgesia but with a decreased risk of respiratory depression [12]. The α-2 adrenergic receptor agonists were first used as nasal decongestants and soon after were used for the treatment of hypertension and withdrawal symptoms. The sedative and amnesic qualities of this drug class motivated interest in its use as an anesthetic adjuvant [12–14].

Dexmedetomidine, the pharmacologically active dextro isomer of medetomidine, has an imidazoline structure and is a potent and selective agonist of the α-2 adrenoceptor. It acts on the α-2 receptors in the locus coeruleus, in contrast to other sedatives (e.g., midazolam and propofol) which act on GABA receptors/cerebral cortex. Dexmedetomidine has a context-sensitive half-time similar to that of fentanyl, with distribution and elimination half-lives of 6 min and 2 h, respectively. It is bio-transformed in the liver and excreted primarily in urine. It shows eight times greater selectivity for α-2 than α-1 receptors and is considered a full agonist when compared to clonidine, the prototypic representative of the α-2 adrenergic receptor agonists drug class. It has demonstrated dose-dependent sympatholytic, sedative, anxiolytic, and analgesic properties in human volunteers and when administered in the perioperative period has been shown to reduce the dose requirements of other anesthetics and attenuate the sympathetic response to stressful events [15].

Its sedative actions resemble physiologic sleep and have been shown to produce sedation most similar to natural sleep. That is why stimulation facilitates awakening even during continuous administration, making dexmedetomidine a popular choice of sedative agent in the intensive care unit, allowing intubated patients to tolerate mechanical ventilation yet remain easily roused to cooperate with necessary procedures. The OMS outpatient setting involves treatment with constant stimuli making the quality of sedation with dexmedetomidine a weak point in treatment. The presence of stimuli in OMS procedures could also be the reason that intravenous sedation with dexmedetomidine alone for dental treatment may show less potent amnestic effects compared with conventional methods like benzodiazepines [16] and would explain the difficulty to evaluate sedation based on bispectral index (BIS) monitoring. Fan et al. noted that when a patient happened to doze during the loading infusion, they were often wakened by their own snoring. During the local anesthetic injections and dental extractions, however, many patients were stimulated to the point of being awake and aware, with BIS scores rapidly returning to the 90s [17].

The drug has been shown to have significant respiratory stability and preserve respiratory rate and oxygen saturation [12, 14]. Slight respiratory depression, less intense than that related to propofol, is one of its characteristics. Dexmedetomidine has proven effective in attenuating airway reflex responses and maintaining hemodynamic stability without prolonging recovery [18]. Smiley and Prior state that patients who are likely to benefit from sedation with dexmedetomidine are those who cannot tolerate respiratory depression and those who need protection from catecholamine release and the resultant tachycardia and hypertension [16].

It has been reported dexmedetomidine causes cardiovascular side effects such as hypertension and bradycardia. It induces peripheral vasoconstriction due to α-2B receptor stimulation and increases blood pressure. It has also been reported to decrease blood pressure and cause bradycardia, via inhibition of the sympathetic nervous system and activation of the parasympathetic nervous system in the presence of α-2A receptor stimulation. Increases in blood pressure can be seen on initial loading, during which the blood concentration of this agent rapidly increased. During maintenance, circulatory depression can be seen frequently. Therefore, close monitoring is needed [20].

Caution should be taken in patients with low ventricular ejection fraction ($\leq$30%) and heart block, as an episode of sinus arrest associated with dexmedetomidine use has been reported [19].

Because dexmedetomidine has no selectivity for α-2A/α-2B receptors, blood pressure changes are not constant.

The manufacturer-recommended dosage is a 1.0 µg/kg infusion over 10 min, followed by a loading dose of 0.2–0.7 µg/kg/h to maintain the required level of sedation [21]. Studies in OMS have shown multiple variations of these recommendations, where most of the studies considered the manufacturer recommended dosing, while some try higher and lower doses. Studies have used dexmedetomidine as a single agent and in combination with other sedative/analgesics [16, 20, 22, 24]. Intranasal administration is another possible and effective route that was tried in some studies but requires more research. A study comparing intranasal dexmedetomidine and midazolam used a dose of 1.5 µg/kg of dexmedetomidine with satisfactory results [24]. On sedative techniques and dosage, Smiley and Prior concluded that in the oral surgery model, in which it is impossible to shield the surgical site from the patient, the unpredictable sedative response of dexmedetomidine using fixed dosages suggests a somewhat less practical approach versus traditional sedative techniques [16].

Dexmedetomidine is difficult to evaluate by bispectral index (BIS) monitoring because during the preoperative period, patients exhibit stable sedation, but as external stimuli start, variability and overlap scores make precise measurement difficult. Due to this variability and the fact that dexmedetomidine causes decreased HR and SBP, some practitioners and studies preferred to use conventional monitoring methods to reach a more precise evaluation [25].

A systematic review by Ter Bruggen et al. showed that of the trials measuring recovery time, 5 out of 13 studies (38.5%) reported a significantly prolonged recovery time and one showed a significantly reduced recovery time with dexmedetomidine. The recovery time is reduced if the infusion is stopped at an earlier moment during the procedure. However, no differences in procedure duration were found [26].

Other experiences have shown us that the addition of midazolam to dexmedetomidine in the outpatient setting can increases the total anesthesia time and recovery time in an average of 15–20 min each [16, 22].

A systematic review by Davoudi et al. concluded that most trials in the study showed a significantly lower level of pain with dexmedetomidine and a significantly higher level of patient satisfaction with dexmedetomidine [25]. When dexmedetomidine was compared to midazolam, statistically significant amnesia and cognitive impairment were present in the midazolam group when compared to the dexmedetomidine group [23], and the patients receiving dexmedetomidine alone were more likely to report having remembered "the whole surgery" [16].

There is evidence to support dexmedetomidine as a potential sole or combination sedative agent in the OMS outpatient setting. The sedative quality of dexmedetomidine and its easy arousability makes it a popular choice for the ICU setting but might be a weakness in the OMS setting as a single agent. Patients who are likely to benefit from sedation with dexmedetomidine are those who cannot tolerate respiratory depression and those who need protection from catecholamine release and the resultant tachycardia and hypertension. For this patients, conventional monitoring is still recommended. The manufacturer recommended loading dose of 1.0 µg/kg intravenous infusion over 10 min is proven to be effective to avoid any possible side effects, like SpO2 desaturation or bradycardia [14].

Future research should examine in which procedures dexmedetomidine can be used as a sole sedative agent in preference to other sedatives [26], and in which procedures should be used as a part of a balanced sedation technique. The analgesic and amnesic features of dexmedetomidine are still in some doubt, and more studies are required to determine its effectiveness. Dexmedetomidine has remarkable sedative properties such as safety, amnesia effects, shorter recovery periods after sedation, and providing both surgeons' and patients' satisfaction [25].

Ketamine-Propofol Combination (Ketofol)

Ketamine and propofol are two sedative agents which are commonly used for procedural outpatient sedation. Both medications are routinely used either individually or with addition of other medications. More recently, ketamine and propofol admixes have been combined as "ketofol" and have been studied for their synergistic capacities and desired opposing properties.

Propofol is a sedative hypnotic agent, commonly used for induction in the operating room and as a sedative for procedural sedation or monitored anesthesia care. It has a rapid onset and short duration of action with a smooth recovery [27]. Like many general anesthetics, it acts by potentiating GABA-mediated chloride channels in the brain, increasing the inhibitory neurotransmitter effects. It can be given as a bolus or infusion or as a combination of the two. It possesses antiemetic and anxiolytic properties, which are very desirable for sedation. However, there are respiratory and hemodynamic compromises if used as a single agent. Due to a vasodilatory and cardiodepressant properties, propofol can cause hypotension and bradycardia. Also, it is associated with a dose-dependent respiratory depression, which can lead to hypoventilation and hypoxia [28].

Ketamine is a nonbarbiturate dissociative anesthetic, acting as a noncompetitive NMDA and glutamate receptor antagonist, producing profound anesthesia, amnesia, and analgesia. Ketamine is often used as a sole agent in pediatric patients for short sedation procedures. It has a short onset of action, excellent potency, and rapid recovery time. Ketamine maintains normal airway reflexes, has bronchodilatory properties, and is useful for patients with asthma or bronchospasm risk. However, its cardiostimulant properties will increase in heart rate and blood pressure [29]. Ketamine also has some additional adverse effects that are undesirable for procedural sedation. By causing hypersalivation, ketamine can put patients at greater risk of laryngospasm in an open-airway anesthesia setting. There is also an increase in emergence phenomena, especially in adults, occurring in an estimated 10–20% of sedations. Finally, there is increased incidence of nausea and vomiting with ketamine with an incidence of 5–15% in adults [30].

The mixture of propofol with ketamine has been shown to take advantage of many properties of both medications with fewer reported complications and decreased dosage requirements of each drug. Meta-analyses have shown that ketofol reduces respiratory complications, hypotension, and bradycardia [31, 32]. Ketofol has been shown to not cause an increase in nausea/vomiting or psychomimetic complications compared to propofol alone.

Although the optimal proportion of propofol with ketamine has not been determined, studies have looked at various ratios of propofol to ketamine and compared their side effects to propofol alone. A clinical trial by Cillo et al. demonstrated that a ratio of 10:1 propofol to ketamine provided the greatest benefit for continuous intravenous general anesthesia with fastest time to recovery, compared to 5:1 and 3:1 ratios [33]. Another clinical trial also demonstrated that 1:1 mixtures had the greatest number of agitation events during recovery, compared to 4:1 mixtures of propofol to ketamine [34]. These studies suggest that higher proportion of ketamine provides no advantage to the sedation and is therefore less desirable in mixture.

Thus, ketofol has shown to provide efficacious procedural sedation at lower doses of each drug. The combination of the two drugs has been shown to offset each other's undesired properties. Ketamine blunts the hemodynamic and respiratory effects of propofol, whereas propofol attenuates the nausea and sympathomimetic properties of ketamine [35].

Remifentanil-Propofol Combination (Remi-Prop)

The combination of the ultrafast-acting opioid remifentanil with the sedative-hypnotic propofol has become increasingly popular for operating room and procedural sedation applications. Remifentanil offers sedative and powerful analgesic effects with the highly desirable properties of fast onset and rapid recovery. Propofol is a versatile agent, displaying rapid onset and rapid recovery from general anesthesia in addition to its antiemetic and amnestic properties. While there are those who advocate a "propofol-only" approach to outpatient oral surgery, the most common methods involve multiple drugs. A remifentanil-propofol combination lends itself to rapid procedures common to the practice of oral and maxillofacial surgery.

Kramer et al. compared continuous infusions of propofol-remifentanil with propofol-ketamine for deep sedation of 37 patients undergoing extraction of all 4 third molars. Both groups were given 0.03 mg/kg midazolam, and the propofol-remifentanil group was given a ratio of 10 mg propofol to 5μg remifentanil per milliliter. The propofol-ketamine group was given a ratio of 10 mg propofol to 2.5 mg ketamine per milliliter. After a 500μg/kg bolus of the assigned propofol combination, both groups were infused with propofol at 100μg/kg/min. Several outcomes were measured including emergence and recovery times, hemodynamic and respiratory stability, and associated drug costs. Hemodynamic and respiratory stability was similar in the two groups, but the ketamine group had significantly longer emergence (13.6 ± 6.6 versus 7.1 ± 3.7 min) and recovery (13.6 ± 6.6 versus 7.1 ± 3.7 min) compared to the remifentanil group. The average cost of a propofol-remifentanil sedation was $4.90 more than the propofol-ketamine sedation, which could theoretically be easily offset by the difference in recovery time. In a randomized, double-blinded controlled study, Kramer et al. administered either remifentanil-propofol or ketamine-propofol to patients undergoing extraction of all third molars. Sedation parameters, hemodynamic stability, and respiratory stability were similar. The ketamine-propofol group required nearly twice as long for both emergence and recovery [36].

Remifentanil-propofol also has applications in pediatric deep sedation. In a randomized clinical trial, Seol et al. sedated 1–3-year-olds undergoing burn dressing changes with propofol (2 mg/kg) and either ketamine (1 mg/kg) or remifentanil (0.1µg/kg + 0.5µg/kg/min infusion). The primary outcome was recovery time, as defined by achieving a Steward Recovery Score of 6. They found that remifentanil-propofol resulted in a significantly shorter recovery time (10.3 min versus 22.5 min). There were no events of significant hypotension or bradycardia during the procedures [27].

Remifentanil complements propofol with its strong analgesic effects. Haytural et al. compared the effects of propofol alone versus propofol in combination with either remifentanil or fentanyl for patients undergoing endoscopic retrograde cholangiopancreatography. Ninety patients were divided into three groups. The first group was given propofol (1.5 mg/kg) loading dose followed by a 1 mg/kg/h. infusion. The second group was loaded with remifentanil (0.05µg/kg) and propofol (1.5 mg/kg) and given the same 1 mg/kg/hr. infusion of propofol thereafter. The third group was loaded with fentanyl (1µg/kg) and propofol (1.5 mg/kg) and given the same infusion of propofol as the other groups. In order to maintain sedation at between 3 and 4 on the Ramsey Sedation Scale, members of each group were given 0.5 mg/kg boluses of propofol. The propofol-fentanyl group was also given 0.01 mg/kg boluses of fentanyl concomitantly. The study measured the amount of propofol needed to maintain an appropriate level of sedation as well as the patient's pain levels. There was no difference in procedure time. The propofol-only group as a whole required a total of 375 mg of propofol. The propofol-remifentanil group required 150 mg, while the propofol-fentanyl group required 245 mg of propofol. The pain levels of the propofol-remifentanil group were significantly lower than each of the other two groups while requiring less propofol and no significant difference in hemodynamic stability or respiratory drive.

While fast and effective, the major downside of a remifentanil-propofol anesthetic technique is respiratory depression and potential desaturation. This is not uncommon for oral surgery procedures as a whole and can be attenuated by lowering infusion rates or administering smaller boluses [37]. These changes often take a minute or less to take effect. In a prospective study implementing a propofol-remifentanil target-controlled infusion (TCI) sedation technique for patients undergoing dental extractions, Nagels et al. showed the number of oxygen-desaturation events (ODE) to be associated with BMI and male sex. At a fixed BMI, the odds of at least one ODE were 2.6 greater for males than females [38].

Remimazolam

Benzodiazepines, specifically midazolam, are one of the most commonly used medications for outpatient anesthesia [39]. Favorable properties of midazolam include anxiolytic and amnestic properties while providing a relatively short half-life and minimal respiratory depression [40]. Compared to other anesthetics, midazolam has a relatively favorable onset of action of 3–5 min and a relatively short elimination half-life of 1.5–2.5 h [47]. Though optimal drug pharmacokinetics for outpatient sedations would include the absence of an active metabolite, midazolam only elicits 10% of the drug activity from the active metabolite alpha-1 hydroxymidazolam [42]. It is also important to note that metabolism of midazolam is dependent on liver function as it is primarily hepatically metabolized, via CYP450, to hydroxylated metabolites that are conjugated and renally excreted [41, 42]. Though this may not be a significant issue in most healthy individuals, it does play a role in the variability of the pharmacokinetics and clinical outcomes of this drug. In the application of outpatient anesthesia, an optimal drug profile might include nonorgan-dependent metabolism, fast onset with quick recovery, and a good safety profile. Remimazolam, FDA approved for us in the USA in 2020, seems to fit these optimal profiles.

Remimazolam was developed to take advantage of esterase pharmacology that has been successfully used in the opioid remifentanil [39]. Remimazolam's esterase pharmacology allows for more precise control of infusion and bolus titration while providing rapid recovery after termination of drug administration [40]. When compared to midazolam, which is dependent CYP450 metabolism in the liver, the ester moiety of remimazolam is a substrate for nonspecific tissue esterase enzymes and is not dependent on specific organ metabolism [39]. Morimoto reported that remimazolam has an onset of sedation within 60 s of administration [43].

Doi et al. in multicenter, single-blind, randomized trial looked at the efficacy and safety of remimazolam vs. propofol as an induction agent and as a continued infusion for anesthesia maintenance. The trial randomized 375 patients to either the remimazolam group or propofol group. They measured primary endpoints of efficacy which included BIS score for depth of sedation, need for rescue sedative medication, and body movement. Remimazolam and propofol treatment groups were noted to have a 100% efficacy. The number of adverse events including hypotensive events and pain at injection site was statistically greater in the propofol group when compared to the remimazolam cohorts. The propofol group experienced 61.3% adverse drug reaction (ADR) versus 41.0% for the remimazolam patients. The most frequent ADR was decreased blood pressure and pain at injections site, with propofol patients experiencing these events 49.3% and 18.7%, respectively, and the remimazolam patients 22% and 0%, respectively.

Morimoto in his paper looked at remimazolam efficacy and safety for short procedural sedation. He reviewed three clinical trials and specifically noted that at the time of publication there were no clinical studies that evaluated remimazolam and short procedural sedations. In the first trial reviewed, a phase Ib study [44], participants undergoing a colonoscopy procedure were cohorted to remimazolam 0.04 mg/kg, 0.075 mg/kg, or 0.1 mg/kg bolus with each group receiving a standard 50 µg of fentanyl. In all cohorts, >70% of the patients were well sedated and awake within 10 min after administration. Additionally, there were no reports of adverse events. Morimoto looked at phase IIa study of patients undergoing upper endoscopy, comparing remimazolam at three bolus doses of 0.1 mg/kg, 0.15 mg/kg, and 0.2 mg/kg with a fourth arm of midazolam 0.075 mg/kg. Each arm had 825 participants. The remimazolam groups had a shorter onset to sedation of 1.5–2.5 min when compared to 5 min for the midazolam group. Yet procedural success rates were only 32%, 56%, and 64%, respectively, for the remimazolam groups and 44% for the midazolam group. A third, phase III study evaluated patients undergoing a colonoscopy. The study enrolled 461 patients and had 3 arms: 5 mg dose of remimazolam followed by an additional 2.5 mg dose of remimazolam, placebo, and a single midazolam dose of 1.75 mg. Successful endoscopy was performed in 91.3%, 1.7%, and 25.2% of the patients, respectively [45]. The incidence of hypoxia was low, 1%, for either remimazolam or midazolam patients. Remimazolam patients did have a quicker recovery of neuropsychiatric function and discharge criteria earlier.

The clinical trials show that remimazolam is more useful for short procedural sedation cases such as colonoscopy [43, 45, 46]. Morimoto in his personal experience utilizing remimazolam in his anesthesia practice over a 1-year period noted its effect varied between patients. He also noted that elderly patients were more sensitive to its effects and that remimazolam should be used with caution in this patient population.

Remimazolam is a novel short-acting, esterase-metabolized benzodiazepine that can be in used in place of the more commonly used midazolam or at times in place of propofol in anesthetic cases. Though both clinical retrospective and prospective data are very limited at this time, current data available does show that it may have future usefulness.

Conclusion

We owe gratitude to those in the past who pioneered the discovery of anesthetic medications and their application. Their discoveries have provided us a foundation for the discovery of new anesthetic medications and the understanding how we can implement these medications into providing safe outpatient anesthesia.

In the field of modern dentistry and oral and maxillofacial surgery, office-based procedural sedation with modern anesthetic medications is utilized to provide patients and providers with safe and predictable outpatient anesthesia outcomes.

Newer anesthesia medications which provide innovative mechanisms of metabolism (remimazolam and remifentanil) and medications that function by targeting historically nontargeted receptors (Dexmedetomidine) have proven effective in providing safe outpatient anesthesia. Esterase-metabolized anesthesia medications, specifically remimazolam and remifentanil, provide a "fast on-fast off" anesthetic that allows for effective titration of medication and a shortened recovery time. Both are amicable attributes for outpatient sedation anesthesia.

Additionally, infusion anesthesia medication combinations, combining medications with varied targeted mechanisms (remifentanil-propofol, ketamine-propofol, midazolam-remifentanil), have also proven an effective model in providing safe outpatient anesthesia. Such drug combinations help limit the need for larger doses of single mechanism anesthetics and help achieve an anesthesia goal by reducing the amount of a single therapeutic target.

When determining what drugs to choose, or what combination to utilize, it is always important to remember that patients can have varied responses to medications, and individual assessment of the patient and medical history is needed to help tailor the anesthetic approach.

Independent of your anesthetic drug model, it is always the anesthesiologist or anesthetist's responsibility to choose the anesthetic drugs, drug combinations, and drug doses that are effective and safe for an individual patient, including accounting for the type of procedure and procedure duration.

It is the responsibility of the practitioner to understand, in depth and detail, the anesthesia drugs and drug combinations that they chose when implementing safe and effective outpatient anesthesia. Utilizing evidence-based data, in combination with clinical experience, the provider should develop the skill set and comfort in providing effective and safe outpatient sedation to their patient population.

References

1. Office based anesthesia provided by the oral and maxillofacial surgeon. White Paper. American Association of Oral and Maxillofacial Surgeons (AAOMS); 2016.
2. Anon. Parameters of care for oral and maxillofacial surgery. A guide for practice, monitoring and evaluation. American Association of Oral and Maxillofacial Surgeons. J Oral Maxillofac Surg. 1992;50(7 Suppl 2):i–xvi, 1–174.
3. Bause GS. Boyle, a most skeptical chemist. Anesthesiology. 2009;110:610.
4. Bennet JA. A Study of Parentalia, with two unpublished letters of Sir Christopher Wren. Ann Sci. 1973;30:129–47. Bergman NA: Early intravenous anesthesia: An eyewitness account. Anesthesiology 1990; 72:185–6. (Anesthesiology October 2009, Vol. 111, 923–924.)
5. Haridas RP. "Gentlemen! This is no humbug": did John Collins Warren, M.D., proclaim these words on October 16, 1846, at Massachusetts General Hospital, Boston? Anesthesiology. 2016;124(3):553–60.
6. Lehmann HE, Ban TA. Pharmacotherapy of tension and anxiety. Springfield: Charles C Thomas; 1970.
7. Egan TD, Lemmens HJ, Fiset P, et al. The pharmacokinetics of the new short-acting opioid remifentanil (GI87084B) in healthy adult male volunteers. Anesthesiology. 1993;79:881–92.

8. Ultiva label. https://www.accessdata.fda.gov/drugsatfda_docs/label/2016/020630s016lbl.pdf.
9. Ferraro GA, Corcione A, Nicoletti G, et al. Blepharoplasty and otoplasty: comparative sedation with remifentanil, propofol, and midazolam. Aesthet Plast Surg. 2005;29(3):181–3.
10. Kisilewicz M, Rosenberg H, Vaillancourt C. Remifentanil for procedural sedation: a systematic review of the literature. Emerg Med J. 2017;34(5):294–301.
11. Cohen J, Royston D. Remifentanil. Curr Opin Crit Care. 2001;7(4):227–31.
12. Hall JE, Uhrich TD, Barney JA, et al. Sedative, amnestic, and analgesic properties of small-dose dexmedetomidine infusions. Anesth Analg. 2000;90:699.
13. Ebert TJ, Hall JE, Barney JA, et al. The effects of increasing plasma concentrations of dexmedetomidine in humans. Anesthesiology. 2000;93(2):382–94.
14. Belleville JP, Ward DS, Bloor BC, et al. Effects of intravenous dexmedetomidine in humans. I: sedation, ventilation, and metabolic rate. Anesthesiology. 1992;77:1125–33.
15. Nelson LE, Lu J, Guo T, et al. The alpha2-adrenoceptor agonist dexmedetomidine converges on an endogenous sleep promoting pathway to exert its sedative effects. Anesthesiology. 2003;98:428.
16. Smiley MK, Prior SR. Dexmedetomidine sedation with and without midazolam for third molar surgery. Anesth Prog. 2014;61:3–10.
17. Fan TW, Ti LK, Islam I. Comparison of dexmedetomidine and midazolam for conscious sedation in dental surgery monitored by bispectral index. Br J Oral Maxillofac Surg. 2013;51:428.
18. Yacout AG, Osman HA, Abdel-Daem MH, et al. Effect of intravenous dexmedetomidine infusion on some proinflammatory cytokines, stress hormones and recovery profile in major abdominal surgery. Alexandria J Med. 2012;48:3–8.
19. Aksu R, Akin A, Biçer C, et al. Comparison of the effects of dexmedetomidine versus fentanyl on airway reflexes and hemodynamic responses to tracheal extubation during rhinoplasty: a double-blind, randomized, controlled study. Curr Ther Res Clin Exp. 2009;70:209–20.
20. Taniyama K, Oda H, Okawa K, et al. Psychosedation with dexmedetomidine hydrochloride during minor Oral surgery. Anesth Prog. 2009;56:75–80.
21. Hospira Inc. Precedex. (dexmedetomidine hydrochloride) Injection: prescribing information. http://www.accessdata.fda.gov/drugsatfda_docs/label/2010/021038s017lbl.pdf.
22. Taylor DC, Ferguson HW, Stevens M, et al. Does including dexmedetomidine improve outcomes after intravenous sedation for outpatient dentoalveolar surgery? J Oral Maxillofac Surg. 2020;78:203–13.
23. Sivasubramani S, Pandyan DA, Ravindran C. Comparison of vital surgical parameters, after Administration of Midazolam and Dexmedetomidine for conscious sedation in minor oral surgery. Ann Maxillofac Surg. 2019;9:283–8.
24. Hiwarkar S, Kshirsagar R, Singh V, et al. Comparative evaluation of the intranasal spray formulation of midazolam and dexmedetomidine in patients undergoing surgical removal of impacted mandibular third molars: a split mouth prospective study. J Maxillofac Oral Surg. 2018;17(1):44–51.
25. Davoudi A, Attar BM, Shadmehr E. Risks and benefits of pre-operative dexmedetomidine in oral and maxillofacial surgeries: a systematic review. Expert Opin Drug Saf. 2017;16(6):711–20.
26. Ter Bruggen FJ, Eralp I, Jansen CK, et al. Efficacy of Dexmedetomidine as a sole sedative agent in small diagnostic and therapeutic procedures: a systematic review. Pain Pract. 2017;17(6):829–84.
27. Seol T-K, Lim J-K, Yoo E-K, Min S-W, Kim C-S, Hwang J-Y. Propofol-ketamine or propofol-remifentanil for deep sedation and analgesia in pediatric patients undergoing burn dressing changes: a randomized clinical trial. Paediatr Anaesth. 2015;25(6):560–6.
28. Folino TB, Muco E, Safadi AO, et al. Propofol. [Updated 2021 Jul 31]. In: StatPearls [Internet]. Treasure Island, FL: StatPearls Publishing; 2022. https://www.ncbi.nlm.nih.gov/books/NBK430884/.

29. Rosenbaum SB, Gupta V, Palacios JL. Ketamine. [Updated 2021 Nov 20]. In: StatPearls [Internet]. Treasure Island, FL: StatPearls Publishing; 2022. https://www.ncbi.nlm.nih.gov/books/NBK470357/.
30. Abu-Laban RB, Zed PJ, et al. Ketamine-propofol combination (Ketofol) versus propofol alone for emergency department procedural sedation and analgesia: a randomized double-blind trial. Ann Emerg Med. 2012;59(6):504–512.e2.
31. Jalili M, Bahreini M, Doosti-Irani A, et al. Ketamine-propofol combination (ketofol) vs propofol for procedural sedation and analgesia: systematic review and meta-analysis. Am J Emerg Med. 2016;34(3):558–69.
32. Ferguson I, Bell A, Treston G, et al. Propofol or ketofol for procedural sedation and analgesia in emergency medicine—the POKER study: a randomized double-blind clinical trial. Ann Emerg Med. 2016;68(5):574–582.e1.
33. Cillo JE. Analysis of propofol and low-dose ketamine admixtures for adult outpatient dentoalveolar surgery: a prospective, randomized, positive-controlled clinical trial. J Oral Maxillofac Surg. 2012;70(3):537–46.
34. Miner JR, Moore JC, Austad EJ, et al. Randomized, double-blinded, clinical trial of propofol, 1:1 propofol/ketamine, and 4:1 propofol/ketamine for deep procedural sedation in the emergency department. Ann Emerg Med. 2014;65(5):479–88.
35. Yan JW, McLeod SL, Iansavitchene A, et al. Ketamine-propofol versus propofol alone for procedural sedation in the emergency department: a systematic review and meta-analysis. Acad Emerg Med. 2015;22(9):1003–13.
36. Kramer KJ, Ganzberg S, Prior S, et al. Comparison of propofol-remifentanil versus propofol-ketamine deep sedation for third molar surgery. Anesth Prog. 2012;59(3):107–17.
37. Park S, Choi SL, Nahm FS, et al. Dexmedetomidine-remifentanil vs propofol-remifentanil for monitored anesthesia care during hysteroscopy. Medicine. 2020;99(43):e22712.
38. Nagels AJ, Bridgman JB, Bell SE, et al. Propofol-remifentanil TCI sedation for oral surgery. N Z Dent J. 2014;110(3):85–9.
39. Noor N, Legendre R, Cloutet A, et al. A comprehensive review of remimazolam for sedation. Health Psychol Res. 2021;9(1):24514.
40. Sneyd JR, Rigby-Jones AE. Remimazolam for anaesthesia or sedation. Curr Opin Anaesthesiol. 2020;33(4):506–11.
41. Midazolam product insert—Fresnius Kabi. www.fresenius-kabi.us. Accessed Mar 2017.
42. Lingamchetty TN, Hosseini SA, Saadabadi A. Midazolam [Updated 2021 Aug 6]. In: StatPearls [Internet]. Treasure Island, FL: StatPearls Publishing; 2022. https://www.ncbi.nlm.nih.gov/books/NBK537321/.
43. Morimoto Y. Efficacy and safety profile of remimazolam for sedation in adults undergoing short surgical procedures. Ther Clin Risk Manag. 2022;18:95–100.
44. Worthington MT, Antonik LJ, Goldwater DR, et al. A phase Ib. dose-finding study of multiple doses of remimazolam (CNS 7056) in volunteers undergoing colonoscopy. Anesth Analg. 2013;117:1093–100.
45. Rex DK, Bhandari R, Desta T, et al. A phase III study evaluating the efficacy and safety of remimazolam (CNS 7056) compared with placebo and midazolam in patients undergoing colonoscopy. Gastrointest Endosc. 2018;88:427–37.
46. Doi M, Morita K, Takeda J, et al. Efficacy and safety of remimazolam versus propofol for general anesthesia: a multicenter, single-blind, randomized, parallel-group, phase IIb/III trial. J Anesth. 2020;34:545–53.
47. Borkett KM, Riff DS, Schwartz HI, et al. A phase IIa, randomized, double-blind study of remimazolam (CNS 7056) versus midazolam for sedation in upper gastrointestinal endoscopy. Anesth Analg. 2015;120:771–80.

Chapter 24
Advancements in Transoral Robotic Surgery and the Treatment of Oropharyngeal Cancer

Garren Michael Iida Low and Jo-Lawrence Martinez Bigcas

Introduction

Traditionally, the approach to tumors of the oropharynx was dichotomous depending on location and size of primary tumor. For easily accessible, small T-stage tumors, many were amenable to removal with a headlight under direct line of sight. Approach to the base of tongue and to larger T-stage tumors was performed transcervical, often including lip-split mandibulotomy with releasing incisions along the floor of mouth musculature. This provides excellent access to the structures of the oropharynx at the risk of significant surgical morbidity. In addition to soft tissue derangement, the facial nerve would be placed at risk laterally, and the bone of the mandible was prone to infection given the need for hardware repair in a field soon to be radiated. The application of the surgical robot for use in the head and neck provided an alternate access strategy to the pharynx. Several robotics systems have been used in the United States, but the current leader in market share, and only Federal Drug Administration-approved system for transoral robotic surgery (TORS), is the da Vinci Surgical System (Intuitive Surgical, Sunnyvale, CA). In addition to the robotic unit itself, multiple oral retractors have been created to allow

G. M. I. Low
Department of Otolaryngology Head and Neck Surgery, Drexel University College of
Medicine, Pittsburgh, PA, USA

Department of Otolaryngology Head and Neck Surgery, Allegheny Health Network,
Pittsburgh, PA, USA
e-mail: Garren.Low@ahn.org

J.-L. M. Bigcas (✉)
Department of Otolaryngology Head and Neck Surgery, Kirk Kerkorian School of Medicine
at the University of Nevada Las Vegas, Las Vegas, NV, USA
e-mail: Jo-Lawrence.Bigcas@unlv.edu

© The Author(s), under exclusive license to Springer Nature
Switzerland AG 2023
J. C. Melville et al. (eds.), *Advancements and Innovations in OMFS, ENT, and
Facial Plastic Surgery*, https://doi.org/10.1007/978-3-031-32099-6_24

line-of-sight access to the pharynx. The robot has been adapted to many other uses in head and neck surgery, such as robotic thyroidectomy and laryngectomy. However, none of these approaches have found as wide of an audience as surgery of the oropharynx. TORS has reintroduced surgery as a viable and valuable primary modality for treating tumors of the oropharynx, especially in the era of HPV-related disease. Since both surgery and concurrent chemotherapy and radiation provide a high rate of cure in this disease, TORS plays a central role in the many de-escalation trials focused on reducing the side effects of cancer treatment.

Robotic Surgery of the Oropharynx Using da Vinci Surgical Systems

Robotic surgical systems are designed to be physician extenders. The tools are adaptations of older technologies with the goal of flattening the learning curve for the surgeon. An endoscopic camera is utilized in each system, analogous to a Hopkins rod telescope. The view and surgical anatomy are not significantly different from previously utilized surgical approaches. The angled camera allows better visualization around corners in the oropharynx and posterior oral cavity than transoral direct visualization. The magnification and quality of this camera are powerful enough that the National Comprehensive Cancer Network (NCCN) guidelines for workup of an unknown primary cancer believed to be in the oropharynx include an option to use TORS simply for visualization and biopsy [1].

The surgical arms of the robot were created such that motion rotates around an "elbow" and a "wrist." The arms were designed to mimic natural movements of the human hand and arm. The movements of the robotic instruments then mimic the mechanics of the surgeon hand controls in the operating console.

Da Vinci Si

The first iteration of the da Vinci Surgical System used widely in the head and neck was the Si. This system is built with a high-resolution, 3D camera which provides a magnified view of the field and three arms which can accommodate multiple devices. During use in the head and neck, the Si system is used with only two arms. The third arm would usually be left unused with no instrument engaged due to lack of space in the oral cavity. The arms are frequently outfitted with a spatula tip monopolar Bovie electrocautery and a fenestrated grasper or Maryland dissector with integrated bipolar cautery. After insertion of the mouth gag and placing the patient in suspension, the camera and both arms are docked individually in the oropharynx, and the surgeon then moves to the console to begin the operation. There, the surgeon would use the hand controls to operate the arms and move the camera of the robot.

The Si, which has now been sunsetted, had several advantages when operating in the oropharynx. The shaft of the EndoWrist instruments was only 5 mm in diameter, allowing for good use of the space in the oropharynx. The instruments, a grasper and spatula tip Bovie, were familiar to the open head and neck surgeon, and thus the learning curve proved to be more approachable [2].

There were several parts of the Si system that were felt to be awkward or otherwise areas for improvement. The system was equipped with three arms, which were all used in abdominal surgery. However, in the oropharynx, there was insufficient space to use a third arm. The wrists and elbows were also relatively proximal on the shaft. These distances were more appropriate for abdominal surgery, and movement at the elbow could be awkward in the oropharynx. Despite these criticisms, the Si system was used successfully for many years as the only TORS system in the oropharynx.

Da Vinci Xi

The Xi system is the next iteration in the da Vinci lineup of machines. The endoscope is smaller, 8 mm as opposed to 12 mm in the Si system, which increased operating space in the oropharynx and reduced the number of collisions with the camera. The camera itself also underwent an upgrade with higher definition picture. The robotic arms, external to the patient, are longer and thinner than on the Si, reducing the frequency of collisions of the arms themselves. Despite these advances, the Xi system, as of this writing, is not FDA-approved for surgery in the oropharynx, and thus data is limited on its use. Additionally, the EndoWrist instruments are only provided with 8 mm shafts in the Xi system. The 5 mm shafts used in the Si system had comparatively improved mobility in the oral cavity and oropharynx. There are reports of the larger Xi EndoWrist instruments causing more issues with maneuvering and collisions between instruments [3].

Despite slow uptake of TORS using the Xi in the United States, there have been several recent manuscripts detailing its successful use. As the system remains non-FDA approved, much of this data comes from the international TORS community. A Korean group has published a cadaveric proof-of-concept study that showed the Xi system could be used successfully in the oropharynx, supraglottis, and hypopharynx [3]. In Belgium, a series of 59 patients was reported on with good outcomes. The majority of the patients in this series had oropharynx primaries; however, seven patients had laryngeal cancers, and four had hypopharynx cancers [4].

A recent systematic review and meta-analysis looked at the Xi system as utilized in TORS and compared to the previous Si model. They found a total of 74 patients with a 1.35% rate (1 patient) of positive margins and 2 additional patients with "uncertain" margins. They compared this group of patients as operated on by the Xi system with 128 patients operated on by the older Si robot. The Si group had zero cases with positive margins and three patients (2.34%) with uncertain margins. They noted the same structural concerns with the da Vinci Xi, such as the 8 mm EndoWrist instruments. Regardless, the Xi system will likely never be widely used for TORS without FDA approval and industry backing in creating smaller EndoWrist instruments [5].

Da Vinci SP

The single-port (SP) system is the newest in the line of da Vinci robotic surgical systems. It provides several mechanical improvements that are advantageous to the transoral robotic surgeon. Like the two systems that preceded it, the SP has a high-definition camera and three wristed instrument arms with interchangeable tips. The camera and all three instruments are delivered through a single 25 mm cannula, creating a drastic change in deployment. This cannula was designed to be placed through a single trocar or maneuvered to deliver the instruments transorally. Because of the tighter delivery mechanism, this allows simultaneous use of the third arm for the first time in TORS. The deployment of the instruments directly into the oral cavity also allows for placement of the wrist and elbow of the instrument deeper in the oropharynx. This allows the surgeon greater mobility when operating on deeper structures such as the hypopharynx and larynx. Early data has shown similar rates of complications and margin status as compared to the Si system [6, 7] (Fig. 24.1).

Fig. 24.1 EndoWrist instruments extending from trocar in da Vinci SP Surgical System (figure reproduced from the Intuitive Da Vinci SP product website (https://www.intuitive.com/en-us/products-and-services/da-vinci/systems/sp))

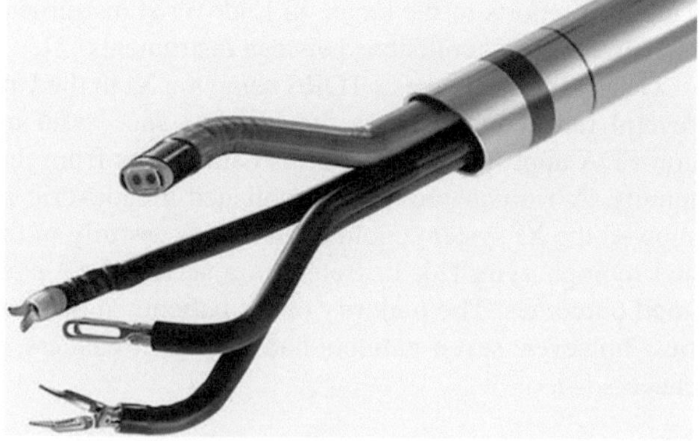

Retractor Systems

While robotic technology addresses limitations of minimally invasive non-robotic surgery, such as field of view and optimizing the use of limited surgical space, the feasibility of transoral robotic surgery is often restricted by impediments to surgical site exposure. TORS technology requires the development of innovative retractor systems to improve the interface between the robot and the surgical site.

Tonsillectomy is the most common ablative oropharyngeal surgery performed. Mouth gags commonly used in oropharyngeal surgery—the McIvor, Crowe-Davis, and Dingman retractors—have been adapted for use in robotic surgery. Most widely used retractor systems resemble the Dingman retractor, which was developed at the University of Michigan in the 1960s. Like the McIvor and Crowe-Davis retractors, it has a tongue blade to displace the oral tongue inferiorly. Its extended closed frame includes buccal retractors that improve the field of view and allow more light into the operative field (Fig. 24.2).

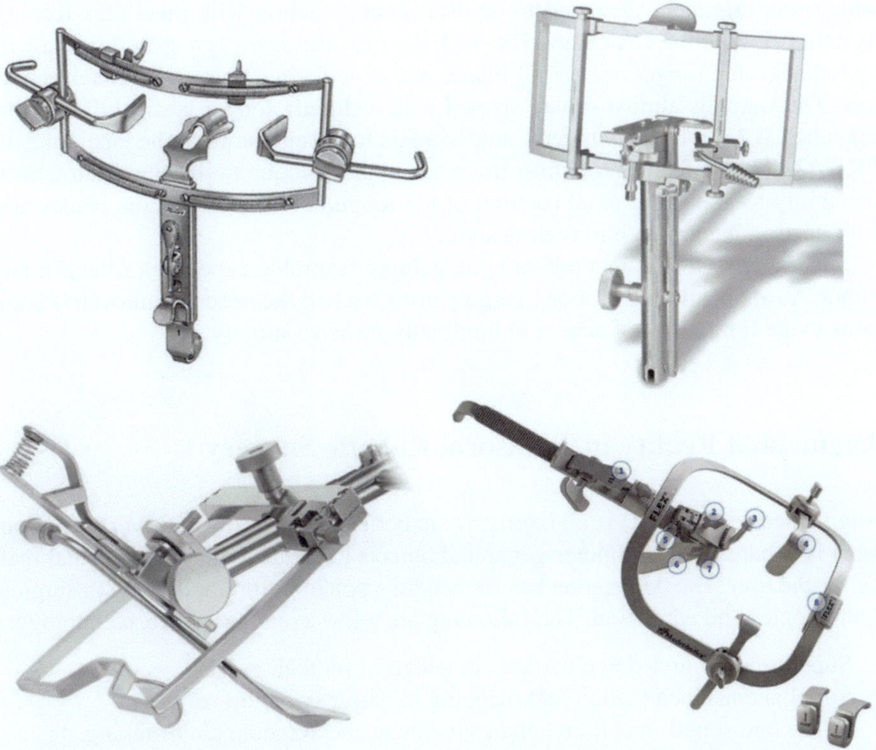

Fig. 24.2 Retractor systems commonly used in oropharyngeal robotic surgery. (Top left) Dingman retractor. (Top right) Laryngeal Advanced Retractor System (LARS). (Bottom left) FK-WO retractor system. (Bottom right) Flex retractor system (figure adapted from catalog photos from vendors of each retractor)

The first retractor system adapted for use in TORS is the Feyh-Kastenbauer (FK) (Gyrus Medical Inc., Tuttlingen, Germany). It is a closed-frame, rectangular-shaped retractor with a wide variety of tongue blades. Its unique tongue-retracting blades are designed to improve distal access to the tongue base and beyond. It also offers optional use of articulating cheek retractors that can be fixed to the frame. The original FK retractor was further modified by Weinstein and O'Malley. It may also be referred to as the FK-WO retractor system. The modifications of the FK-WO system optimize the interface with the da Vinci robot, and the system also includes a variety of tongue blades to extend use to the larynx and hypopharynx.

The Laryngeal Advanced Retractor System (LARS) (Fentex, Tuttlingen, Germany) was introduced by Remacle et al. in 2011 [8]. This closed-frame, rectangular-shaped retractor has a wider horizontal dimension than the FK-WO system, which is more vertically oriented. The LARS framework also has bended curves that can aid in preventing contact with the robotic arms. It also comes with a variety of blades which make this retractor system amenable to surgery in the oral cavity, oropharynx, larynx, hypopharynx, and cervical esophagus.

Medrobotics Corporation (Raynham, MA, USA) designed the Flex Retractor, which was originally designed to be used in conjunction with their Flex Robotic System [9]. Like the LARS and FK-WO, the Flex Retractor is a closed frame with interchangeable tongue-retracting blades and articulating clamps for cheek retractors. The frame is almost square shaped with a slightly longer vertical dimension. Like the LARS, it has a rounded frame to adapt to the curvature of the face. Like the FK-WO, it has a feature to adjust the blade angle. Unique to the Flex Retractor is the ability to adjust the axial rotation of the tongue blade. The tongue blades also have suction integrated into their design.

Success in TORS is incumbent upon gaining favorable exposure of the primary tumor. As applications of robotic surgery grow, so will the need for innovative solutions to the limitations of access in minimally invasive surgery.

Augmented Reality in Transoral Robotic Surgery

Augmented reality (AR) is an interactive experience where the real-world environment is enhanced by computer-generated objects to create a mixed perceptual reality for the user. The AR market has tremendous potential for application in surgical technologies and education. The following are a few examples of AR technology:

- Superimposed first-down markers in televised football games.
- Simultaneous localization and mapping in map/navigation software.
- Filters and superimposition enhancements in social media photo-taking.
- Online furniture stores using cell phone cameras to show potential customers how a particular piece would fit and look in their home or office before purchasing.
- Online clothing stores using camera technology to show how their product would look on potential customers.

There are different types of augmented reality. The types of AR that have applications in robotic surgery include location-based AR, projection-based AR, and superimposition/overlay AR. Location-based AR interweaves virtual 3D objects in physical space. In this type of augmented reality, virtual objects are tied to real-world physical locations. When the camera points at that location, the virtual object is projected on the camera. This is different from projection-based augmented reality. Projection-based AR uses machine vision technology, which may combine visible light cameras with 3D-sensing systems to project images onto actual physical objects. The projections are visible to all the people in that physical space. In overlay AR, the physical object is seen by the user as replaced by a virtual object.

With the surgical robotic system as the interface between the surgeon and the surgical site, augmented reality (AR) technologies can provide additional information, cues, and alarms to improve surgeon performance. Forte and Kuckenbecker classified five tool categories for AR in robotic surgery [10].

- Virtual markers.
- Computational tools.
- Rehearsal of procedure.
- Visual alarms.
- Viewing patient data.

Within otolaryngology, augmented reality technologies seem to be gaining popularity as power users find more applications. Wong et al. found that publications outlining AR technologies in otolaryngology have increased between 1997 and 2018 [11]. In their study, they found 23 articles representing 18 AR platforms. Most were in the rhinology subspecialty (52%), followed by head and neck (30%) and otology (26%). The most common use was intraoperative guidance (55%), followed by surgical planning (24%) and procedural simulation (9%). Visual input was mostly from endoscopes (50%), eyewear (22%), and microscopes (4%). Endoscopic sinus surgery lends itself well to augmented reality use cases because of its foundation in endoscopes and the prolific use of intraoperative navigation. Robotic head and neck surgery has similar application potential, yet research and applications are still nascent.

In traditional open head and neck surgery, surgeons rely on experience, vision, and tactility. The robot, however, creates an altered depth of field, and the visual input interfaces with the surgeon's eyes through the endoscope. The robot also does not provide the surgeon with tactile information or haptic feedback. Robotic surgeons learn to overcome the sensory deficits inherent to robotic surgery and rely more heavily on high-definition 3D vision. These are opportunities to implement AR tools that can augment robotic surgery, which in turn create a safer operating environment for the surgeon and the patient. One such example is intraoperative navigation. In sinus surgery, intraoperative navigation is a widely used technology. It not only facilitates the procedure but also helps identify structures to avoid, such as the skull base and the orbit. It also is a powerful intraoperative educational tool for trainees and educators. Integration of image overlay to augment robotic surgery has been described. Tsang et al. performed a cadaveric study to demonstrate the potential for intraoperative navigation during robotic nasopharyngectomy [12]. The technology is still in its infancy and application, and use cases are likely to expand.

For trainees, surgical simulation can provide additional repetitions of transoral robotic surgery. Preoperatively, there are opportunities for rehearsing procedures and using imaging that can be integrated for intraoperative navigation to avoid structures like the carotid arteries. Intraoperative information about the patient, such as their imaging, can be available on-screen and integrated into the visual experience of the surgeon. Tools to measure depth or distance can have potential application in AR-assisted robotic surgery. Catastrophic bleeding is the most feared complication in transoral robotic surgery. It is a common practice to ligate branches of the external carotid artery and/or the external carotid artery itself to avoid such a bleed [13]. Visual markers, alarms, and superimposition AR can potentially herald avoidable structures relative to your specimen and current location in the operative field. Liu et al. described various applications of augmented reality for in vivo tumor resection [14]. Chan et al. described a cadaver experiment where they were able to perform image-guided robotic surgery in soft tissue [15]. A major issue in intraoperative navigation for neck surgery is the lack of constant landmarks and deformable nature of soft tissue. They were able to register a 3D virtual model of the cadaver to maxillary dentition, which allowed them to overlay the course of the internal carotid artery (Fig. 24.3).

Augmented reality is an early technology with numerous applications. With the robotic technology at the interface between the surgeon and the surgical site, surgeons can continue to develop tools to augment the surgical experience.

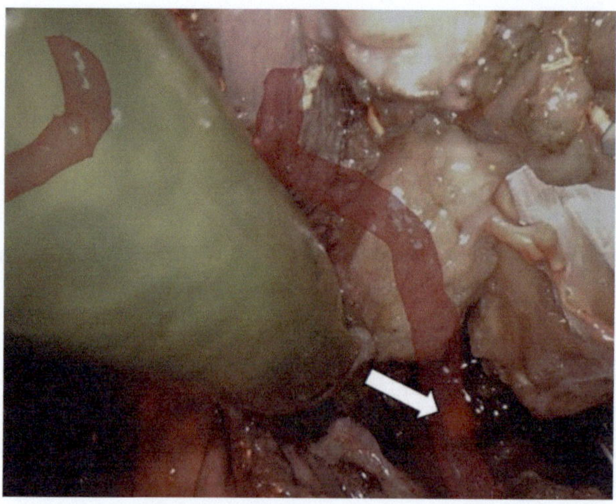

Fig. 24.3 Figure adapted from Chan et al. demonstrating superimposition augmented reality of the location of the internal carotid artery (white arrow) within soft tissue [15]

Extended Applications of Robotic-Assisted Surgery in the Head and Neck

Hypophyarynx

Cancer of the hypopharynx has a particularly poor prognosis within head and neck cancer, and surgery in this area has largely been the realm of open surgery due to the difficulty of access through the natural orifice pathway. A recent systematic review looked at TORS approaches to the hypopharynx and found that robotic surgery was used successfully for tumor extirpation in this site; however, the robot was utilized primarily for lower T-stage disease. Cumulative survival was found to be 85.5% (95% CI 55.8%–96.5%). The single-port robot has been utilized more extensively for hypopharynx tumors due to greater mobility of the wristed instruments [16].

Larynx

From the beginnings of robotic-assisted surgery, head and neck surgeons have used the robot to access tumors of the larynx, utilizing the superior optics to help visualize tumors both supraglottic and endolaryngeal. TORS approaches have been used in endoscopic partial laryngectomy with good results. However, even with the smaller instruments of the single-port model, the robot has increased bulk compared to transoral laser microsurgery (TLM) approaches, and proponents of TLM will be quick to point out the technique's greater versatility and long track record of use in the supraglottis and glottis. Despite this, the utility of the robot for this area continues to grow as techniques improve and adapt to use in the larynx. For example, the use of a wide, flat tongue retractor in the FK-WO retractor system can be used to move a significant amount of tongue out of the way and improves access of the instruments to the larynx [17] (Fig. 24.4).

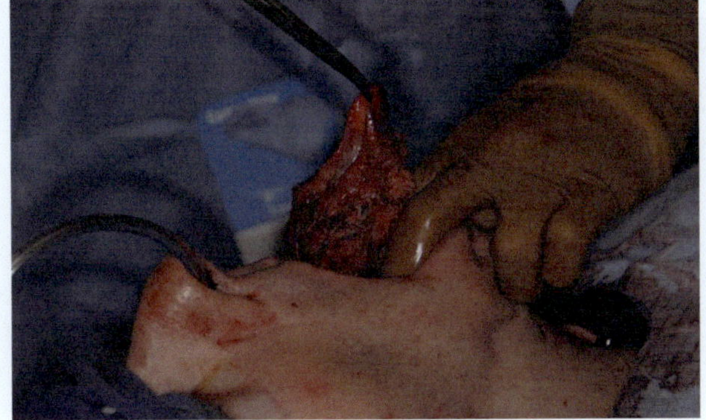

Fig. 24.4 Larynx specimen being removed from oral cavity during robot-assisted transoral total laryngectomy (figure reproduced from Smith et al. [18])

Robotic total laryngectomy has been performed and published in several small case series. The surgery adds significant operative time and still requires a small external incision for formation of the tracheostoma. The surgery itself builds from the techniques of endoscopic partial laryngectomy and is an interesting technical application of the da Vinci robot. Patient selection, as is the case for all TORS patients, is key, and at this time, only salvage laryngectomy patients not requiring neck dissection have undergone robotic total laryngectomy in the literature [18].

Thyroid

Remote access thyroidectomies have been performed as early as the late 1990s. However, the use of the robot to assist in visualization was first adopted in 2005. At that time, access was through the axilla, using the Si iteration of the da Vinci robot. Other techniques described include a retro-auricular approach and, most recently, a transoral approach. Intraoperative nerve monitoring is recommended for each of these approaches.

The American Thyroid Association notes that remote access thyroid surgery should only be performed in extremely high-volume remote access thyroidectomy centers, and they have published very strict guidelines for patient selection. Importantly, surgery should only be performed on the least complicated subjects, avoiding large nodules, abnormal anatomy, prior thyroiditis, or prior surgery. Even in optimal cases, each approach carries additional risks that are not present with traditional open thyroidectomy. Transaxillary approaches have resulted in brachial plexus injuries. Temporary injury to the greater auricular and marginal mandibular nerves has been reported with the retroauricular approach. Injuries to the mental nerves have been reported in the transoral approach. Routine postoperative antibiotics are recommended after the transoral approach, as compared to no antibiotics being recommended with open thyroidectomy. All remote access thyroidectomy techniques have an increased operative time and increased cost. However, for the patient who is interested in scarless or remote scarring after thyroidectomy, these costs may be worth it as assessed on a case-by-case basis [19].

Parotid

The use of the robot has also been explored for a reduction in postoperative skin scar appearance after parotidectomy. A series of 40 superficial parotidectomies were performed by a group from Seoul. Thirty-two of these tumors were benign, and 8 were malignant. Some of these procedures were accompanied by robotic neck dissection. Mean operative time for these surgeries was 226 min for parotidectomy and 375 min for parotidectomy with neck dissection. There were three patients with a transient (<1 month) facial weakness in their series but no cosmetic deficits at 6 months. As with other robotic-assisted surgeries utilized for cosmesis, robotic parotidectomy with or without neck dissection provides a smaller skin incision in exchange for a significantly longer operative time. Like robotic thyroidectomy approaches, concerns remain regarding learning curve and iatrogenic morbidity during the learning period [20].

Nasopharynx

Just as the robot allows for surgery "around the corner" into the hypopharynx, studies have shown proof of concept for use in the nasopharynx. Using a transoral approach, preclinical studies have shown the ability for the robot to be used in extirpation of nasopharynx tumors with or without division of the soft palate. Tumors of the nasopharynx traditionally respond well to radiotherapy, and thus surgery is usually utilized in the setting of recurrent or persistent disease. The limitations previously discussed (cost, operative time, size mismatch of instruments to operating space) all also apply to robotic surgery of the nasopharynx [21].

Robotic-Assisted Reconstructive Surgery

One of the downsides of robotic oropharyngectomy over a large open procedure is the increased difficulty in reconstructing a large defect. Smaller defects can be left to heal by secondary intention, and patients tolerate this moderately with minimal scar formation albeit with significant postoperative pain. Traditionally, a large open ablation of the oropharynx would be closed with a free flap reconstruction. Inset into this area has been performed with the assistance of the robot with good success. This does increase surgical time significantly, but with good patient selection, there is a significant reduction in morbidity [22]. A group in Taiwan has also successfully performed robotic-assisted microvascular anastomoses for their free flap reconstructions with good success [23].

Robotic Surgery in De-escalation Therapy for Oropharyngeal Cancer

Traditional open approaches to the oropharynx are complicated and carry major comorbid risk. These approaches include lip-split mandibulotomy and pharyngotomy. A study by Parsons et al. [24] compiled data from 51 studies from 1970 to

2000, looking at outcomes of over 6400 oropharyngeal cancer cases, comparing surgery +/− adjuvant radiotherapy to definitive radiotherapy +/− posttreatment neck dissection and found that the overall survival between the two groups was the same, but severe and fatal complications were significantly higher in the surgery group. Naturally, practitioners during that period shifted to paradigms favoring radiation over surgery. From 1985 to 2000, primary chemoradiation doubled in the United States, while surgery and primary radiation declined. Primary chemoradiation became the gold standard for treating oropharyngeal cancer.

Advancements in the understanding of human papillomavirus (HPV)-driven oropharyngeal cancer led to further considerations for de-escalation therapies. Compared to HPV-negative disease, HPV-positive squamous cell carcinoma was found to have a much better prognosis. In a multi-institutional study by Ang et al., they examined the outcomes of radiotherapy on a 323-patient cohort of advanced oropharyngeal squamous cell carcinoma—206 with HPV-positive disease [25]. Three-year survival was 82% in the HPV-positive group versus 57% for the HPV-negative group. There was a 58% reduction in risk of death for HPV-positive disease. As more patients survive the epidemic of p16+ oropharyngeal cancer, they also must live with the complications of radiation therapy, including lymphedema, radiation scarring, trismus, xerostomia, and dysphagia. As our understanding of oropharyngeal cancer and its treatment continues to evolve, what is the appropriate amount of treatment? Can we optimize survival and decrease morbidity?

Robotic surgery has become a centerpiece in the era of new de-escalation paradigms for oropharyngeal cancer. There are four basic categories of treatment de-escalation:

- Reduction in radiation doses and volume.
- Alterations in chemotherapy dose and frequency.
- Chemoradiation-combined de-escalation.
- Upfront surgery +/− adjuvant radiation.

Particularly for early stage (low T, low N) oropharyngeal cancers, TORS has become a widely accepted alternative to radiation. Studies have shown similar survival outcomes comparing radiation to TORS for HPV-positive disease. Not surprisingly, there is evidence to suggest that TORS for HPV-negative disease has superior outcomes [26] to radiation. In the appropriately selected patient, TORS is a minimally invasive technology that can achieve similar results to open approaches to the oropharynx with less morbidity and operating room time. Avoiding a mandibulotomy or pharyngotomy—procedures rife with potential for immediate and long-term complications—is, in some ways, a form of surgical de-escalation. Since the first descriptions of TORS by O'Malley and Weinstein in 2005, its adoption has increased, while a concomitant decrease in primary radiation therapy has been observed in early stage T1/T2 oropharyngeal cancers [27] (Fig. 24.5).

In the ideal TORS patient, a cure is possible with surgery alone and no need for adjuvant radiation or chemotherapy. Surgery consists of resection of the primary tumor with the indicated neck dissection. Histopathologic analysis of the tumor and neck dissection specimens identifies adverse features where adjuvant therapy may

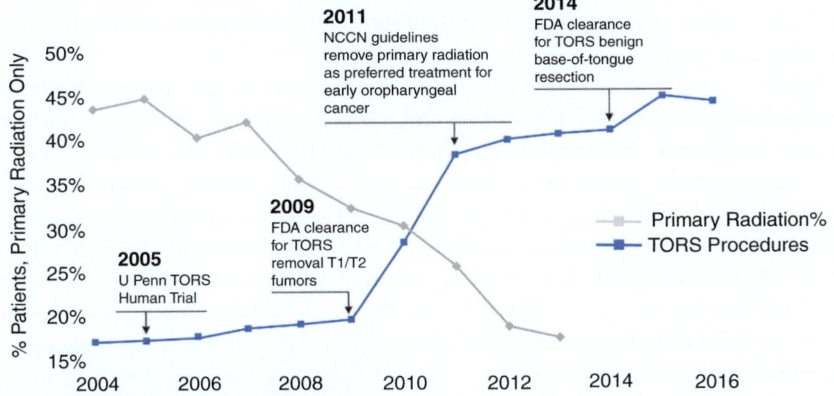

Note: TORS procedure frends come from Infuitive Surgical internalsales data
Primary radiation data is limited to the timeframe between 2004 and 2013.
[1]Cracchiolo, J., Baxi, S., Morris, L., Ganly, I., Patel, S., Cohen, Roman, B. (2016). Increase in primary surgical freatment of T1 and T2 oropharyngeal squamous cell carcinoma and rates of adverse pathologic features: features: National Cancer Data Base, 122(10): 1523-1532

Fig. 24.5 This figure from Cracchiolo et al. demonstrates the shift paradigm of TORS adoption for early-stage oropharyngeal cancer [27]

provide some survival advantage. These features include close or positive margins, perineural invasion, lymphovascular invasion, extranodal extension, large positive lymph node(s), multiple positive nodes, and atypical metastatic pattern. The indications for adjuvant chemotherapy or radiotherapy may vary among practitioners. Though the intent may be to achieve single modality surgical cure, there is always the possibility for strongly recommended adjuvant therapy in the form of radiation or chemoradiation. There is a growing body of literature demonstrating that upfront surgery can achieve comparable results with lower-dose, de-escalated adjuvant radiation compared to full-dose adjuvant radiation.

Randomized trials comparing TORS to radiation and their respective functional outcomes and survivals are sparse. The ORATOR study, published in 2019, is one such study [28]. Sixty-eight patients with T1–T2 N0–2 were randomized to either TORS with neck dissection (with or without adjuvant chemoradiation based on histopathologic features) or radiation therapy (70 Gy, with chemotherapy if N1–2). While there were expected higher rates of neutropenia, hearing loss, and tinnitus in the radiation group, the surgical group had higher rates of trismus. Interestingly, MD Anderson Dysphagia Index (MDADI) scores were higher in the radiation group (86.9 with SD 11.4) than the surgery group (80.1 with SD 13.0). Clinically meaningful change in MDADI score is detected when a 10-point difference occurs between groups. Thus, the difference between groups does not qualify as meaningful clinical change in quality of life 1-year posttreatment. The study's 3-year follow-up update again demonstrates improved dysphagia in the RT arm over surgery. However, the differences in MDADI scores between groups are of a smaller magnitude than at the 1-year posttreatment time point. The researchers also strongly recommended tracheostomy to every TORS patient following a postoperative death due to oropharyngeal bleeding. The presumed high prevalence of tracheostomies in the TORS group is an additional confounder for mild dysphagia in the immediate postoperative period.

National Comprehensive Cancer Network guidelines outline paradigms for radiation dosing; however, local radiation and medical oncology paradigms vary from practice to practice. Pertinent to TORS, postoperative radiation therapy or concurrent chemoradiation is recommended within 6 weeks of surgery, and the indications are based on histopathology. For high-risk cancers with adverse features, the recommended dose of adjuvant radiation is 60–66 Gy (2.0 Gy per fraction for 6–6.5 weeks). For low or intermediate risk, the dosing recommendation can vary from 44 to 50 Gy in 3D-CRT to 54–63 Gy for IMRT. While the ideal TORS patient is still a clinical T1 or small-T2 primary tumor with single nodal disease with no radiologic or clinical evidence of extracapsular spread, it seems that there has been a shift away from primary radiation and toward more surgery. Surgery provides invaluable staging and histopathologic information that can spare or decrease the need for high-dose radiation or chemoradiation. In an early study of TORS-inspired de-escalation, Weinstein, Quon et al. applied postoperative radiation at 54 Gy in 24 patients (12 with radiation alone and 12 indicated for chemoradiation) [29]. They had one recurrence in an unoperated contralateral neck. As we learn more about behaviors of oropharyngeal cancers, we can investigate to pursue lower doses of adjuvant radiation. Three large, randomized trials are currently deployed looking at postoperative de-escalation paradigms—ECOG 3311, ADEPT, and PATHOS.

ECOG 3311 is a study currently in follow-up that examines de-escalated adjuvant treatment in patients receiving TORS. The study design includes 511 patients with AJCC seventh edition stage III-IV HPV-positive oropharyngeal cancer who underwent TORS and stratified them based on risk. There is a low-risk arm, which included pT1–T2 N0–1 with >3 mm margins, and they receive no adjuvant therapy. Intermediate risk patients (close margin, < 1 mm ENE, 2–4 metastatic nodes, perineural or lymphovascular invasion) were randomized into two groups—one receiving 50 Gy and the other receiving 60 Gy. The high-risk group (positive margins, > 1 mm ENE, > 4 positive nodes) underwent chemoradiation with radiation dosed to 66 Gy. Three-year survival update was given at ASCO in 2021 [30]. All four arms of the study had greater than 90% progression-free survival (PFS). The low-risk group had similar survivals to both randomized intermediate-risk groups. Within the randomized intermediate-risk groups, functional outcomes were better in the lower dose treatment arm. Patients who received radiation alone had better swallowing outcomes compared to the triple-modality treatment received by the high-risk group. Though the data of this phase 2 study should be interpreted with caution, it heralds a victory for de-escalation.

The ADEPT trial (NCT01687413) is a phase III trial out of Washington University School of Medicine. This study examines adjuvant therapy in p16-positive oropharyngeal cancer ($n = 496$) where TORS achieved negative margins and the neck dissection demonstrates extracapsular extension. The adjuvant arms include chemoradiation (60 Gy + weekly cisplatin 40 mg/m^2) versus radiation alone (60 Gy), looking at PFS and disease-free survival (DFS). The results of this trial are not yet available.

The PATHOS trial looks at T1-T3, N0-N2b tumors treated by TORS with neck dissection and stratifies them based on histopathologic features [31]. The low-risk arm is observed without any adjuvant therapy. The high-risk group (positive margins and/or extracapsular spread) is randomized to either radiation (60 Gy) alone or chemoradiation (60 Gy + cisplatin). The intermediate group (PNI, LVI, close margins) is randomized among two radiation-only dosing paradigms of 50 Gy versus 60 Gy. The question being asked in the PATHOS trial is whether long-term dysphagia (measured by the MDADI) can be reduced through less intense adjuvant radiation treatment without an adverse clinical outcome. The results of this trial are not yet available.

A clinical trial known as DART-HPV or MC-1675 (NCT02908477) looks at a significantly de-escalated adjuvant radiation therapy (DART) protocol of hyperfractionated 30–36 Gy [32]. The significant decrease in radiotherapy dose compared to other trials draws from successful treatment of HPV-related anorectal cancers with a similar dosing regimen. Inclusion criteria for the trial include having undergone TORS and having one of the following risk factors indicating adjuvant treatment: lymph node >3 cm, two or more positive lymph nodes, perineural invasion, lymphovascular invasion, T3 or T4 primary disease (with gross total resection within two attempts), or extranodal extension (ENE). 194 patients were recruited into the study. Intermediate-risk patients were randomized 2:1 to DART (30 Gy/1.5 Gy BID + docetaxel 15 mg/m^2 on day 1 and 8) or standard of care (60 Gy +/− weekly cisplatin 40 mg/m^2). Risk stratification was based on the presence of extranodal extension and smoking history. The high-risk group received 36 Gy/1.8 Gy BID or standard of care. The endpoints of the trial are treatment toxicity, overall survival, and quality of life. The study is still ongoing, currently with a median follow-up of just over 2 years as of July 2021. Compared to the standard-of-care arm, the DART arm has demonstrated less toxicity, less need for feeding tubes, improved swallowing function, and better quality-of-life indices. Regarding survival, 2-year follow-up statistics show similar PFS in DART versus standard of care, except in the subset of the high-risk ENE+ DART group where their N-stage was pN2. Otherwise, DART compared to standard-of-care adjuvant chemoradiation, the data is promising for de-escalation.

Conclusion

Progress in the treatment of oropharyngeal cancer continues to improve as we refine our understanding of the disease, introduce new technologies, and rigorously question the dogma that drives our practices. As oncologists, we are tasked to find the best treatment plan for our patients—one that maximizes survival and minimizes long-term undesired secondary effects. In the epidemic of HPV-related oropharyngeal cancer, transoral robotic surgery has undoubtedly become a powerful weapon. As a technology, it has opened opportunities to advance its own agenda. From the first iterations of the da Vinci Si, the need for more access, applications, and safety has not only driven its own evolution, but it has also created industries to support it. This is seen in innovations in retractor systems, endoscopes, camera technologies, and the development of augmented reality tools. As the indications for robotic head and neck surgery continue to expand so will the need for more solutions.

Robotic surgery has given head and neck surgeons a powerful weapon that not only de-escalates traditional approaches to the oropharynx but may also empower radiation oncologists and medical oncologists to de-escalate their therapies. In some patients, TORS provides a minimally invasive means for achieving the same end results as primary radiation, with less radiation-driven toxicity. This is not to say that surgery is without risk; it certainly carries its own set of risks, complications, and morbidity. Surgery does, however, provide invaluable histopathologic information, which may indicate the need for postoperative chemoradiation. As we continue to investigate what is the appropriate amount of treatment, TORS has made it possible to pursue multimodal paradigms of de-escalation.

References

1. Patel SA, Magnuson JS, Holsinger FC, Karni RJ, Richmon JD, Gross ND, et al. Robotic surgery for primary head and neck squamous cell carcinoma of unknown site. JAMA Otolaryngol Head Neck Surg. 2013;139(11):1203–11.
2. Hans S, Delas B, Gorphe P, Menard M, Brasnu D. Transoral robotic surgery in head and neck cancer. Eur Ann Otorhinolaryngol Head Neck Dis. 2012;129(1):32–7.
3. Kim DH, Kim H, Kwak S, Baek K, Na G, Kim JH, et al. The settings, pros and cons of the new surgical robot da Vinci xi system for transoral robotic surgery (TORS): a comparison with the popular da Vinci si system. Surg Laparosc Endosc Percutan Tech. 2016;26(5):391–6.
4. Meulemans J, Vanermen M, Goeleven A, Clement P, Nuyts S, Laenen A, et al. Transoral robotic surgery (TORS) using the da Vinci xi: prospective analysis of feasibility, safety, and outcomes. Head Neck. 2022;44(1):143–57.
5. Fiacchini G, Vianini M, Dallan I, Bruschini L. Is the da Vinci xi system a real improvement for oncologic transoral robotic surgery? A systematic review of the literature. J Robot Surg. 2021;15(1):1–12.
6. Orosco RK, Arora A, Jeannon JP, Holsinger FC. Next-generation robotic head and neck surgery. ORL J Otorhinolaryngol Relat Spec. 2018;80(3–4):213–9.
7. Van Abel KM, Yin LX, Price DL, Janus JR, Kasperbauer JL, Moore EJ. One-year outcomes for da Vinci single port robot for transoral robotic surgery. Head Neck. 2020;42(8):2077–87.
8. Remacle M, Matar N, Lawson G, Bachy V. Laryngeal advanced retractor system: a new retractor for transoral robotic surgery. Otolaryngol Head Neck Surg. 2011;145(4):694–6.
9. Hasskamp P, Lang S, Holtmann L, Stuck BA, Mattheis S. First use of a new retractor in transoral robotic surgery (TORS). Eur Arch Otorhinolaryngol. 2016;273(7):1913–7.
10. Forte M, Kuchenbeker K. Interactive augmented reality for robot-assisted surgery. Montréal, QC: SAGES 2017 Annual Meeting; 2017.
11. Wong K, Yee HM, Xavier BA, Grillone GA. Applications of augmented reality in otolaryngology: a systematic review. Otolaryngol Head Neck Surg. 2018;159(6):956–67.
12. Tsang RK, Sorger JM, Azizian M, Holsinger CF. Real-time navigation in transoral robotic nasopharyngectomy utilizing on table fluoroscopy and image overlay software: a cadaveric feasibility study. J Robot Surg. 2015;9(4):311–4.
13. Gleysteen J, Troob S, Light T, Brickman D, Clayburgh D, Andersen P, et al. The impact of prophylactic external carotid artery ligation on postoperative bleeding after transoral robotic surgery (TORS) for oropharyngeal squamous cell carcinoma. Oral Oncol. 2017;70:1–6.

14. Liu WP, Richmon JD, Sorger JM, Azizian M, Taylor RH. Augmented reality and cone beam CT guidance for transoral robotic surgery. J Robot Surg. 2015;9(3):223–33.
15. Chan JYK, Holsinger FC, Liu S, Sorger JM, Azizian M, Tsang RKY. Augmented reality for image guidance in transoral robotic surgery. J Robot Surg. 2020;14(4):579–83.
16. De Virgilio A, Iocca O, Malvezzi L, Di Maio P, Pellini R, Ferreli F, et al. The emerging role of robotic surgery among minimally invasive surgical approaches in the treatment of Hypopharyngeal carcinoma: systematic review and meta-analysis. J Clin Med. 2019;8(2):256.
17. Smith RV. Transoral robotic surgery for larynx cancer. Otolaryngol Clin North Am. 2014;47(3):379–95.
18. Smith RV. Transoral robotic total laryngectomy. Oper Tech Otolaryngol Head Neck Surg. 2013;24(2):92–8.
19. Kandil E, Attia AS, Hadedeya D, Shihabi A, Elnahla A. Robotic thyroidectomy: past, future, and current perspectives. Otolaryngol Clin North Am. 2020;53(6):1031–9.
20. Park YM, Kim DH, Kang MS, Lim JY, Kim SH, Choi EC, et al. Real impact of surgical robotic system for precision surgery of parotidectomy: retroauricular parotidectomy using da Vinci surgical system. Gland Surg. 2020;9(2):183–91.
21. Tsang RK, Holsinger FC. Transoral endoscopic nasopharyngectomy with a flexible next-generation robotic surgical system. Laryngoscope. 2016;126(10):2257–62.
22. Tsai YC, Liu SA, Lai CS, Chen YW, Lu CT, Yen JH, et al. Functional outcomes and complications of robot-assisted free flap oropharyngeal reconstruction. Ann Plast Surg. 2017;78(3 Suppl 2):S76–82.
23. Lai CS, Lu CT, Liu SA, Tsai YC, Chen YW, Chen IC. Robot-assisted microvascular anastomosis in head and neck free flap reconstruction: preliminary experiences and results. Microsurgery. 2019;39(8):715–20.
24. Parsons JT, Mendenhall WM, Stringer SP, Amdur RJ, Hinerman RW, Villaret DB, et al. Squamous cell carcinoma of the oropharynx: surgery, radiation therapy, or both. Cancer. 2002;94(11):2967–80.
25. Ang KK, Harris J, Wheeler R, Weber R, Rosenthal DI, Nguyen-Tan PF, et al. Human papillomavirus and survival of patients with oropharyngeal cancer. N Engl J Med. 2010;363(1):24–35.
26. Mahmoud O, Sung K, Civantos FJ, Thomas GR, Samuels MA. Transoral robotic surgery for oropharyngeal squamous cell carcinoma in the era of human papillomavirus. Head Neck. 2018;40(4):710–21.
27. Cracchiolo JR, Baxi SS, Morris LG, Ganly I, Patel SG, Cohen MA, et al. Increase in primary surgical treatment of T1 and T2 oropharyngeal squamous cell carcinoma and rates of adverse pathologic features: national cancer data base. Cancer. 2016;122(10):1523–32.
28. Nichols AC, Theurer J, Prisman E, Read N, Berthelet E, Tran E, et al. Radiotherapy versus transoral robotic surgery and neck dissection for oropharyngeal squamous cell carcinoma (ORATOR): an open-label, phase 2, randomised trial. Lancet Oncol. 2019;20(10):1349–59.
29. Weinstein GS, Quon H, O'Malley BW Jr, Kim GG, Cohen MA. Selective neck dissection and deintensified postoperative radiation and chemotherapy for oropharyngeal cancer: a subset analysis of the University of Pennsylvania transoral robotic surgery trial. Laryngoscope. 2010;120(9):1749–55.
30. Ferris RL, Flamand Y, Weinstein GS, Li S, Quon H, Mehra R, et al. Phase II randomized trial of transoral surgery and low-dose intensity modulated radiation therapy in resectable p16+ locally advanced oropharynx cancer: an ECOG-ACRIN cancer research group trial (E3311). J Clin Oncol. 2022;40(2):138–49.
31. Owadally W, Hurt C, Timmins H, Parsons E, Townsend S, Patterson J, et al. PATHOS: a phase II/III trial of risk-stratified, reduced intensity adjuvant treatment in patients undergoing transoral surgery for human papillomavirus (HPV) positive oropharyngeal cancer. BMC Cancer. 2015;15:602.
32. Ma DM, Price K, Moore EJ, Patel SH, Hinni ML, Fruth B, et al. MC1675, a phase III evaluation of De-escalated adjuvant radiation therapy (DART) vs. standard adjuvant treatment for human papillomavirus associated oropharyngeal squamous cell carcinoma. Int J Radiat Oncol Biol Phys. 2021;111(5):1324.

Chapter 25
Cold Ablation Robot-Guided Laser Osteotome (CARLO®): Technology and Clinical Application in Maxillofacial Surgery and Reconstruction

Tobias Ettl, Marta Morawska, and Philipp Jürgens

Introduction

Bone osteotomy is a major component of many cranio- and maxillofacial (CMF) interventions for corrective or reconstructive intent.

For decades, osteotomies were performed by mechanical instruments as saws and drills with well-known collateral effects. The vibrations and heat generated by those mechanical tools provoke damage of soft tissue and delayed healing process for the cut area. During the last two decades, the piezoelectric surgery has gained great popularity for its ability to precisely cut bone structures without causing injuries to soft tissue and providing accelerated bone healing [1, 2].

Laser radiation can be used to cut, shape, treat, and remove soft tissues. A variety of laser wavelengths have been analyzed and suggested for cutting cortical bone [3]. This thermal mechanism of bone ablation results in coagulation, carbonization, and vaporization of living tissues. Laser osteotomy offers the potential advantage of high precision and reduced collateral damage to surrounding tissues. Other advantages include high productivity, narrow kerf (kerf is the gap between the cut

T. Ettl (✉)
Department of Oral and Maxillofacial Surgery, University Medical Centre Regensburg, Regensburg, Germany
e-mail: tobias.ettl@ukr.de

M. Morawska
Department of Cranio-Maxillofacial Surgery, Advanced Osteotomy Tools (AOT) AG, Basel, Switzerland
e-mail: marta.morawska@aot.swiss

P. Jürgens
Department of Cranio-Maxillofacial Surgery, Leading Medical Center (LMC) Munich, Munich, Germany
e-mail: pj@mkg-arabellapark.de

J. C. Melville et al. (eds.), *Advancements and Innovations in OMFS, ENT, and Facial Plastic Surgery*, https://doi.org/10.1007/978-3-031-32099-6_25

surfaces) width, low roughness of cut surfaces, and minimum distortion. The two main obstacles faced with laser osteotomy are thermal damage and residual char formation of adjacent tissues and its potential impact on healing [4, 5]. Thermal damage greatly depends on the laser settings, such as wavelength, power, and pulse duration [4, 6, 7]. The selection of appropriate settings has proven to lead to clean, non-carbonized cuts with similar bone-healing profiles compared to ones obtained using piezoelectric device [8]. However, despite the promising outcomes of studies, the majority of research in laser surgery relies on handheld lasers, which outcomes depend on the manual skills of the surgeon and cannot fully utilize digitalized workflows for preoperative planning.

Cold Ablation Robot-Guided Laser Osteotomy

CARLO® (Cold Ablation Robot-guided Laser Osteotome) (Fig. 25.1a, b) represents a surgical robotic platform, which uses cold laser ablation for bone cutting. An erbium-doped yttrium aluminum garnet (Er:YAG) laser emits radiation at 2.94 µm, and so it can be used for thermal bone ablation due to water exhibiting a strong absorption coefficient at this wavelength. The water molecules selectively absorb the energy, thereby increasing the internal pressure in the form of steam, which causes the explosive destruction of inorganic substances [7]. Potential thermal damage to the surrounding tissues is eliminated by spraying water into the surgical field [3]. In contrast to conventional rotating instruments and piezoelectric surgery, laser-induced thermal bone ablation does not create a smear layer on the osteotomy edges. This results in a channeled scaffold that preserves the trabecular ridges, which allows the passage of cells to the site of injury, therefore potentially benefiting bone healing [8] (Fig. 25.1c, d).

Several preclinical and clinical studies have shown that the healing outcome when using an Er:YAG laser with water cooling is comparable to that of conventional mechanical osteotomy and piezoelectric surgery [8–10]. The described technique is currently available by the start-up company Advanced Osteotomy Tools (AOT AG, Basel, Switzerland) as miniaturized ablation laser with an optical system in a compact casing and mounted on a tactile surgical robot (KUKA Light Weight medical grade Robot, Augsburg, Germany), which is controlled by a navigation system.

The laser head of the system hosts the ablation laser and, additionally, a visualization laser for enhanced safety, which is coaxially bundled. The low-power continuous-wave Class I green visualization laser indicates the osteotomy path at all times. The so-called CARLO® enables exact contact- and debris-free osteotomies according to a preoperative virtual planning without the need for cutting guides and independent of surgeon's individual maneuvers. This device offers the possibility of a total digital workflow that allows the direct transfer of the virtual planning into the operating room. The potential of the CARLO® device has been confirmed

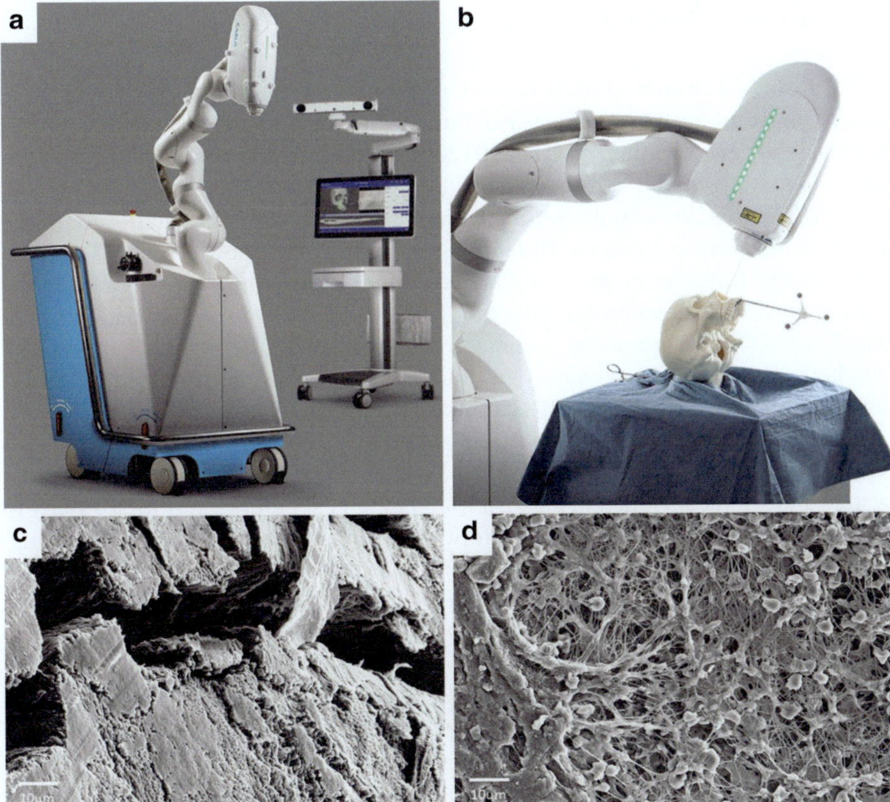

Fig. 25.1 The Cold Ablation Robot-guided Laser Osteotome (CARLO primo). (**a, b**) CARLO® trolley with navigation camera. (**c**) Bone surface cut with piezoelectric device. (**d**) Bone surface cut with CARLO primo at x1000 magnification. Note the preserved bone structure after CARLO cut resembling natural bone ((**c–d**) *adapted from Baek* et al., *2015*) [9]

previously in in vivo animal studies that compared piezoelectric surgery and the CARLO® device in minipig mandibles and sheep skulls. The results showed that the osteotomies had similar durations but higher accuracies and a tendency of faster bone healing when the CARLO® device was employed [8–10].

Applications in Craniomaxillofacial Surgery

The feasibility of the CARLO® device for craniomaxillofacial interventions has been demonstrated in a first-in-man (FiM) study [9, 10], in daily clinical use for midface osteotomies and on human cadavers by successfully performing mandible split osteotomies and fibula osteotomies with various designs [10].

Orthognathic Surgery

In 2019 the first-in-man clinical multicenter study to evaluate the safety and accuracy of linear midface osteotomies performed with the CARLO® device was started (ClinialTrials.gov Identifier: NCT03901209). 28 patients were enrolled across multiple sites (Allgemeines Krankenhaus der Stadt Wien (AKH Wien), Austria; Universitätsklinikum Hamburg-Eppendorf, Germany; Kantonsspital Aarau AG, Switzerland; Universitätsspital Basel, Switzerland). It was shown that cold ablation robot-guided laser osteotomy could successfully be performed with no intraoperative complications or technical failure [11, 12]. In addition, these publications mention CARLO® as a promising technical innovation with the potential to set new standards for accuracy and safety in craniomaxillofacial interventions. CARLO® device was granted CE-1250 certification for midface osteotomies in January 2021.

Since the certification, the CARLO® system is routinely used in Paracelsus-Klinik in Munich, Germany (Fig. 25.2). First 50 patients were operated using the system and will be included in the Post Market Clinical Follow-up (PMCF) study to confirm that CARLO® can be used safely and efficiently in routine clinical setting. The study so far revealed no safety issues or side effects associated with the use of CARLO®, confirming the findings from FiM study.

Although the current CE certification includes only upper jaw, recent studies aim at extending the indication to full orthognathic surgery. In 2021, a study using human cadavers aimed at assessing safety and efficacy of CARLO® for performing Bilateral Sagittal Split Osteotomy (BSSO) [13]. The study utilized the possibility of

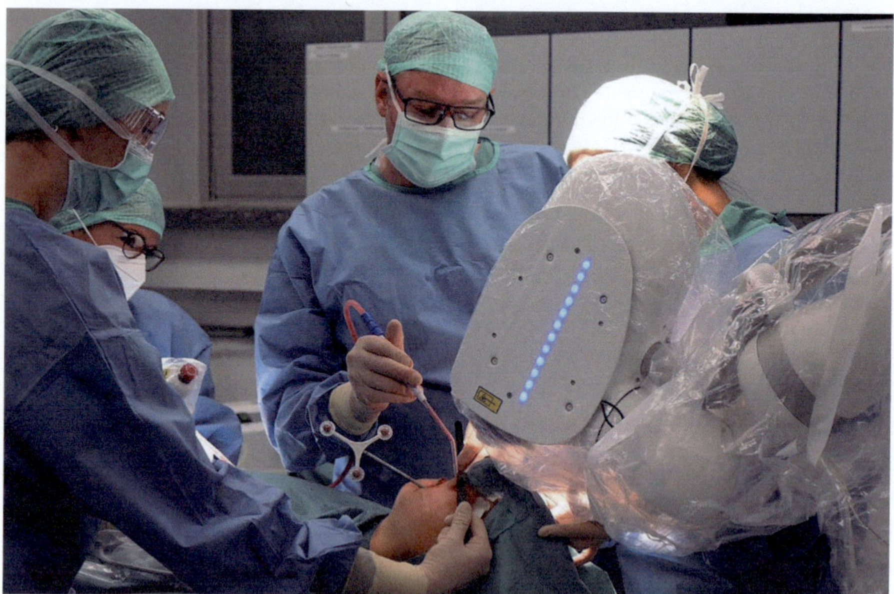

Fig. 25.2 CARLO being used in daily clinical practice in Paracelsus-Klinik in Munich, Germany

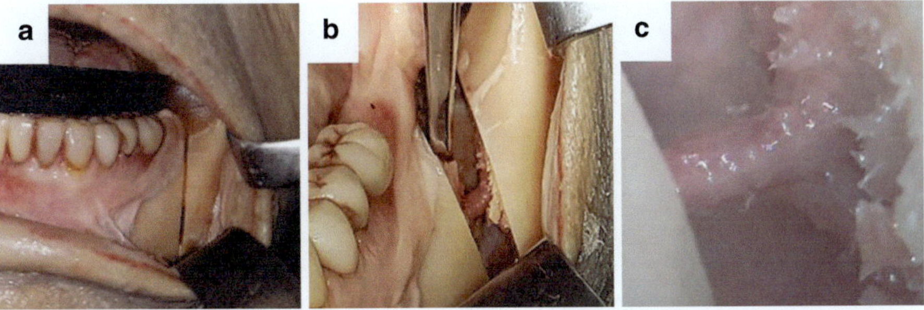

Fig. 25.3 Cadaver study bilateral sagittal split osteotomy (BSSO). (**a**) Initial cut with CARLO® prior to fracturing. Note the cortex is still intact after application of five pulses. (**b**) Osteotomy site after successful fracturing with intact nerve. (**c**) 20x magnification of the intact nerve following the fracturing

protecting vulnerable structures, such as nerves, by creating "risk zones" over the inferior alveolar nerve (IAN). During CARLO® surgery, these risk zones translate into risk segments, where a limited number of laser pulses is used, to cut through the cortex without compromising the IAN canal walls. During the study, 30 osteotomies were performed with 100% success rate for primary end point (no damage to IAN), verifying the safety of the device (Fig. 25.3). The secondary end point (no malfracture) was achieved with 97% success rate, which is consistent with the rate reported in clinical practice [14]. What is more, CARLO® cut was associated with high accuracy (defined as max. 2 mm discrepancy between planned and executed cut) and no observed carbonization. However, the duration of surgery was slightly longer then when using piezoelectric tool, but comparable to standard techniques [15].

In addition to BSSO, a pilot study with three cadavers was conducted to assess CARLO® use for surgically assisted rapid palatal expansion (SARPE). Following the use of CARLO, there was no visible damage of the soft tissue on the hard palate in any of the studied cephali. In addition, no damage was observed to teeth roots and upper alveolar ridge. The average accuracy was kept within the required 2 mm from the planned cut. Overall, the studies showed that CARLO® is ready to perform the full workflow of orthognathic surgery safely and efficiently, possibly offering a safer and more precise alternative to standard surgical techniques.

Mandibular Reconstruction

The initial feasibility of free fibula flap reconstruction of the mandible using CARLO was successfully proven in a pilot study using human cadaver (Fig. 25.4a–d).

There are several clinical patient benefits in using CARLO® for mandibular reconstruction with free fibula graft, such as high accuracy of the osteotomies and hence, high fitting of the graft, and higher primary stability than conventional tools would allow. When functional geometries are performed with CARLO®, the contact

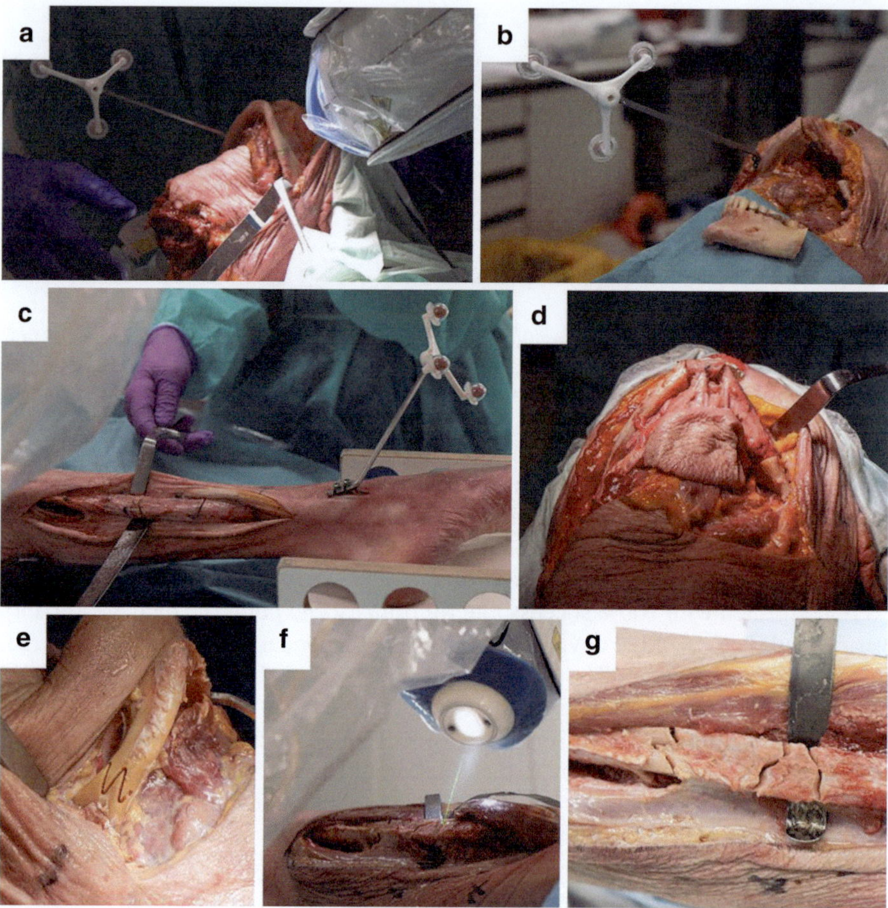

Fig. 25.4 Pilot cadaver study. Mandible reconstruction with free fibula graft using CARLO®. (**a**) CARLO® performing mandibular defect. The marker is fixed to the mandible for permanent registration. (**b**) Clean straight cut of the mandible using CARLO®. (**c**) Clean straight cut in the fibula using CARLO®. (**d**) Reconstructed mandible with skin paddle. (**e**) Functional mandible defect with sinusoidal geometry. (**f**) CARLO® laser osteotome performing functional cut in a cadaver fibula. (**g**) Functional cut in the fibula with sinusoidal geometry

area between bone segments is increased which will imply accelerated bony ossification and a reduction of load-bearing osteosynthesis material (Fig. 25.4e–g).

Another big advantage would be the omission of cutting guides, resulting in time-saving, cost-saving, and removing of fabrication errors and mispositioning of the template during the surgery. The time needed for performing full surgical workflow for CARLO® device, including planning and execution, would be substantially less than in computer-assisted template-guided reconstruction, allowing fast treatment, which would be especially beneficial for cancer patients. At best, adaption of osteotomy planning and CARLO® execution according to the extent of cancer resection will be possible within surgery. Overall, the combination of high precision, advantages of functional cuts, and time-saving in comparison to conventional state-of-the-art techniques could prove highly beneficial to patients.

Further CMF Indications

Several other promising CMF indications for CARLO® use are currently under investigation. Of course, orthognathic CARLO® surgery could be extended to Le Fort II and III osteotomies in patients with midfacial hypoplasia, and also fronto-orbital advancements in craniosynostosis seem to be a good indication for safe CARLO® performance. Besides, osteonecrosis of the jaw is a fairly common problem among oncology patient population, being as high as 18.6% [16]. A number of studies explored the use of laser surgery in the treatment of osteonecrosis of the jaw, with a great success [17]. CARLO® could offer advancements in the treatment of osteonecrosis not only for a precise resection of the lesion, based on presurgical planning, but also for ad hoc surface ablation, which is currently performed with a bur [18]. It is conceivable that resulting preservation of the cancellous bone structure with CARLO® ablation, in contrast to more closed structure when using mechanical instruments, could result in better healing outcomes in the treatment of osteonecrosis.

On the other hand, the possibility of resecting free-form shapes could be a promising approach in resection of craniofacial tumors and deformities, particularly bone tumors. The tumor shape can be segmented and mapped preoperatively, resulting in a very precise resection. Additionally, the use of CARLO® allows for very precise reconstruction of missing bone fragments using autograft approaches, such as calvarial or iliac crest bone [19]. This may be interesting for preimplant augmentation using autogeneous bone in contrast to the increasing use of freeze-dried bone allografts. In a pilot study, the zygomatic bone was traced in a virtual model, and its shape was precisely resected from the cranium. This free-shape approach could be used not only for a precise fit of the graft to the resection site but possibly also for increased stability of the construct and lower use of osteosynthesis material, when specific cutting geometries are used. The custom cut could be particularly useful for stock temporomandibular joint (TMJ) prosthesis preparation to adapt cranial fossa and the ramus for better fit and load-bearing.

Overall, clinical practice and recent studies highlight the promising features of CARLO® system, including preservation of natural bone surface while cutting, precision independent from individual surgeon's skill, the possibility of geometric cuts, and the potential to utilize digital presurgical planning strategies, which could revolutionize the future of CMF surgery.

Outlook

Technology Development

Of course, there are some major challenges for the future. Currently, there is no CE-certified presurgical planning software that is compatible with CARLO® device. The surgeries can be planned in commercial software, such as Mimics® (Materialize, Belgium) or IPS CaseDesigner (KLS Martin, Germany) and exported as Standard Tessellation Language (.stl) files, where CARLO® planning can be superimposed on the preplanned surfaces (Fig. 25.5).

In future, dedicated software for planning orthognathic surgeries, tumor resections and reconstruction, and other indications will be developed to fully digitalize CARLO® workflow and save time between the planning and surgery. With intra-surgical 3D scans and navigation, ad hoc planning and execution seems possible in the near future.

Another limitation is high data volumes generated by the CARLO® device. CARLO® uses the optical coherence tomography (OCT) system to control cutting depth for prevention of injury of surrounding tissues. This real-time monitoring generates gigabytes of data within seconds. Thus, processing of these high data rates is an enormous challenge. However, the OCT system can have other uses than just measurement of cutting depth. Besides cutting, light also offers diagnostic possibilities. As it has no mass, it can be coupled into the same optical path as the cutting laser giving unparalleled live information about the surgery and the tissue being cut. OCT is one of the techniques that may be integrated into CARLO for real-time

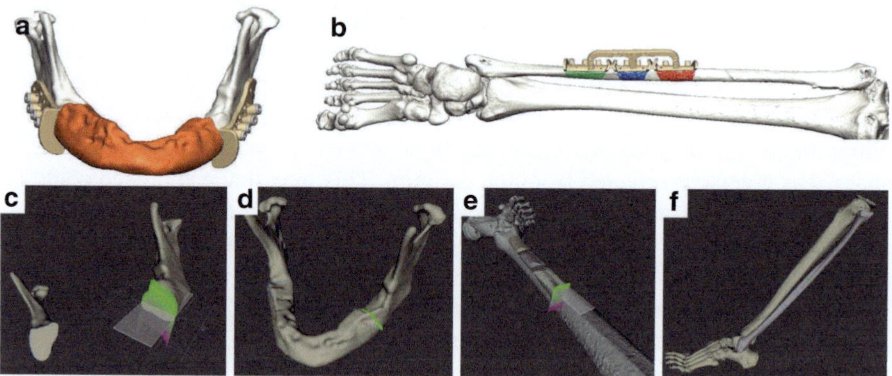

Fig. 25.5 Virtual planning executed with commercial planning platform transferred to CARLO®. (**a**) Mandibular resection determined by cutting guides. (**b**) Fibular resection determined by cutting guides. (**c**) Resected mandible is exported as .stl files and loaded to CARLO® planning software. The start and end point of the cut as well as support point defining the plane are placed. The cutting path can be adjusted so that it fits perfectly on the surface of the fragment. (**d**) Next, resected mandible is replaced with the whole mandible. (**e**) Resected fibula fragments together with tibia for orientation are exported as .stl files and loaded to CARLO® planning software. The start and end point of the cut as well as support point defining the plane are placed. (**f**) Resected fibula is replaced with the whole fibula

diagnostics during surgery. One of the most promising techniques in intra-surgical cancer diagnostics is laser-induced plasma spectroscopy (LIBS), where short laser pulses (<10 ns) applied to the tissue of interest vaporize a very small volume of the tissue, generating a hot plasma cloud, in which basic elements can be analyzed [20]. It has already been shown that LIBS can be used to distinguish different tissue types [21]. Furthermore, other studies show that the LIBS method can distinguish between benign and malignant cells [22]. While the idea of using LIBS for cancer is known for a long time, major progress for tissue differentiation has happened mainly during the last years. This work takes major advantage of the high robustness against environmental influences. Its advantages in combination with an Er:YAG laser were also proven, making this diagnostic technique a promising candidate for integration into CARLO® device, a step toward autonomous diagnostic-surgical complex.

Future Indications

The ongoing technological will allow future expansion of indications beyond CMF. Improved depth control with more efficient processing of OCT data combined with geometrical cuts already available in CARLO® will allow precise adjustment of bone length and corrections of malunions in extremities without the use of patient-specific cutting guides.

The technology can also be used in neurosurgical indications. Currently, trials are underway to test the use of CARLO® for stereoelectroencephalography (sEEG) [23]. The use of CARLO® would allow a precise placement of electrode channels based on imaging data, allowing omission of the stereotactic frame during surgery. The same techniques could be used for a less invasive and more precise brain biopsies [24]. With development of faster laser, additional neurosurgical indications that require longer cutting path and higher cutting depth, e.g., craniotomies, will be possible.

Overall, the ongoing technological advancements and research into additional indications could allow CARLO® to be used not only to cut virtually any bone in the body but also differentiate between tissues, diagnose potential tumors, and map their margins. The potential of replacing multiple software and devices with CARLO® could eventually prove to be cost-effective and time-saving, placing CARLO® as an important element of the OR of the future.

References

1. Kirpalani T, Dym H. Role of piezo surgery and lasers in the oral surgery office. Dent Clin N Am. 2020;64(2):351–63.
2. Costa DL, Thomé de Azevedo E, Przysiezny PE, Kluppel LE. Use of lasers and piezoelectric in intraoral surgery. Oral Maxillofac Surg Clin North Am. 2021;33(2):275–85.
3. Rajitha Gunaratne GD, Khan R, Fick D, Robertson B, Dahotre N, Ironside C. A review of the physiological and histological effects of laser osteotomy. J Med Eng Technol. 2017;41(1):1–12.

4. Stübinger S, Nuss K, Pongratz M, Price J, Sader R, Zeilhofer HF, et al. Comparison of Er:YAG laser and piezoelectric osteotomy: an animal study in sheep. Lasers Surg Med. 2010;42(8):743–51.

5. Nelson JS, Orenstein A, Liaw LH, Berns MW. Mid-infrared erbium:YAG laser ablation of bone: the effect of laser osteotomy on bone healing. Lasers Surg Med. 1989;9(4):362–74.

6. Walsh JT Jr, Flotte TJ, Deutsch TF. Er:YAG laser ablation of tissue: effect of pulse duration and tissue type on thermal damage. Lasers Surg Med. 1989;9(4):314–26.

7. Hibst R. Mechanical effects of erbium:YAG laser bone ablation. Lasers Surg Med. 1992;12(2):125–30.

8. Baek KW, Dard M, Zeilhofer HF, Cattin PC, Juergens P. Comparing the bone healing after cold ablation robot-guided Er:YAG laser osteotomy and piezoelectric osteotomy-a pilot study in a minipig mandible. Lasers Surg Med. 2021;53(3):291–9.

9. Baek KW, Deibel W, Marinov D, Griessen M, Dard M, Bruno A, et al. A comparative investigation of bone surface after cutting with mechanical tools and Er:YAG laser. Lasers Surg Med. 2015;47(5):426–32.

10. Augello M, Baetscher C, Segesser M, Zeilhofer HF, Cattin P, Juergens P. Performing partial mandibular resection, fibula free flap reconstruction and midfacial osteotomies with a cold ablation and robot-guided Er:YAG laser osteotome (CARLO(®))—a study on applicability and effectiveness in human cadavers. J Craniomaxillofac Surg. 2018;46(10):1850–5.

11. Holzinger D, Ureel M, Wilken T, Müller AA, Schicho K, Millesi G, et al. First-in-man application of a cold ablation robot guided laser osteotome in midface osteotomies. J Craniomaxillofac Surg. 2021;49(7):531–7.

12. Ureel M, Augello M, Holzinger D, Wilken T, Berg BI, Zeilhofer HF, et al. Cold ablation robot-guided laser osteotome (CARLO(®)): from bench to bedside. J Clin Med. 2021;10(3):450.

13. Koehnke R, Assaf AT, Helmbold K. Cold Ablation Robot-guided Laser Oateotome on simulated bilateral sagittal split osteotomy in a cadaveric model. Submitted to Int J Oral Maxillofac Surg 2023.

14. Posnick JC, Choi E, Liu S. Occurrence of a 'bad' split and success of initial mandibular healing: a review of 524 sagittal ramus osteotomies in 262 patients. Int J Oral Maxillofac Surg. 2016;45(10):1187–94.

15. Köhnke R, Kolk A, Kluwe L, Ploder O. Piezosurgery for sagittal Split osteotomy: procedure duration and postoperative sensory perturbation. J Oral Maxillofac Surg. 2017;75(9):1941–7.

16. Khan A, Morrison A, Cheung A, Hashem W, Compston J. Osteonecrosis of the jaw (ONJ): diagnosis and management in 2015. Osteoporos Int. 2016;27(3):853–9.

17. Rupel K, Ottaviani G, Gobbo M, Contardo L, Tirelli G, Vescovi P, et al. A systematic review of therapeutical approaches in bisphosphonates-related osteonecrosis of the jaw (BRONJ). Oral Oncol. 2014;50(11):1049–57.

18. Ristow O, Otto S, Troeltzsch M, Hohlweg-Majert B, Pautke C. Treatment perspectives for medication-related osteonecrosis of the jaw (MRONJ). J Craniomaxillofac Surg. 2015;43(2):290–3.

19. Elsalanty ME, Genecov DG. Bone grafts in craniofacial surgery. Craniomaxillofac Trauma Reconstr. 2009;2(3):125–34.

20. Fortes FJ, Moros J, Lucena P, Cabalín LM, Laserna JJ. Laser-induced breakdown spectroscopy. Anal Chem. 2013;85(2):640–69.

21. Rohde M, Mehari F, Klämpfl F, Adler W, Neukam FW, Schmidt M, et al. The differentiation of oral soft- and hard tissues using laser induced breakdown spectroscopy—a prospect for tissue specific laser surgery. J Biophotonics. 2017;10(10):1250–61.

22. Moon Y, Han JH, Choi JH, Shin S, Kim YC, Jeong S. Mapping of cutaneous melanoma by femtosecond laser-induced breakdown spectroscopy. J Biomed Opt. 2018;24(3):1–6.

23. Winter F, Winter T, Bammerlin M, Shawarba J, Dorfer C, Roessler K. Navigated, robot-driven laser craniotomy for SEEG application using optical coherence tomography in an animal model. Front Robot AI. 2021;8:695363.

24. Ha TT, Thieringer FM, Bammerlin M, Cordier D. High precision bone cutting by Er:YAG lasers might minimize the invasiveness of navigated brain biopsies. Front Oncol. 2022;11(5456):690374.

Chapter 26
Motor Nerve Reconstruction of the Facial Nerve

Jeffrey T. Gu, Natalie A. Krane, Myriam Loyo, Allison Slijepcevic, and Mark K. Wax

Introduction

Facial palsy (FP), a disorder in which movement of the muscles innervated by the facial nerve are negatively impacted, is a devastating condition with functional and aesthetic consequences and is often associated with depression, social isolation, and poor quality of life (QOL) [1, 2, 3]. Facial asymmetry from facial palsy may lead to displays of incongruent emotional expression, which may be misinterpreted and make social interaction more challenging. Facial expression plays an essential role in human communication by allowing us to convey emotions and provide nonverbal cues. Functionally, facial paralysis may significantly impair eyelid closure secondary to paralytic lagophthalmos, result in collapse of the external nasal valve causing nasal obstruction, and impair oral competence and speech. Facial paralysis can result from central or peripheral etiologies depending upon where the injury has occurred along the facial motor pathway. Etiologies are myriad and include idiopathic (i.e., Bell's palsy), stroke, congenital abnormalities, infectious, autoimmune, traumatic, iatrogenic, and neoplastic causes.

J. T. Gu · M. Loyo · M. K. Wax (✉)
Department of Otolaryngology-Head and Neck Surgery, Oregon Health and Science University, Portland, OR, USA
e-mail: guj@ohsu.edu; loyo@ohsu.edu; waxm@ohsu.edu

N. A. Krane
Division Facial Plastic and Reconstructive Surgery, Department of Otolaryngology-Head and Neck Surgery, Oregon Health and Science University, Portland, OR, USA
e-mail: krane@ohsu.edu

A. Slijepcevic
Department of Otolaryngology-Head and Neck Surgery, Atrium Wake Forest Baptist, Wake Forest, NC, USA
e-mail: aslijepc@wakehealth.edu

J. C. Melville et al. (eds.), *Advancements and Innovations in OMFS, ENT, and Facial Plastic Surgery*, https://doi.org/10.1007/978-3-031-32099-6_26

Reanimation of facial expression is equally as diverse and may be achieved by restoring continuity of the nerve-muscle network using techniques for nerve repair or substitution to facilitate neurotization of the distal facial nerve, or with techniques to substitute muscle function through muscle transfer. In this chapter, we provide a framework of options for motor nerve reconstruction of the facial nerve. Discussion of repair options is organized by size and extent of the defect and varies from primary repair of the transected nerve to cable graft repair of the resected nerve, as well as different nerve transfer procedures, cross-facial nerve grafts, and free gracilis muscle transfer for reanimation of the paralyzed face.

Timing of Repair and Outcomes

Duration of denervation and status of the facial musculature are among the most important factors when determining the potential for treating facial paralysis. Reversibly paralyzed facial muscles with potential for spontaneous recovery have physiologically viable fibers with intact motor units that will respond to ingrowing axons. Flaccid facial paralysis with atrophic or fibrotic facial muscles are irreversibly paralyzed and will not respond to reinnervation due to mechanical and physiologic barriers to incoming axons and therefore require functional muscle to replace the denervated facial muscles. Facial muscles completely denervated for less than 1 year have been shown to respond to nerve transfer [1]. Evidence from case series suggest that patients who undergo nerve repair within 1 year after onset of FP were more likely to achieve a House-Brackmann (HB) grade of three or better compared to patients who underwent neurorrhaphy longer than 1 year from onset [4]. Although optimal timing for nerve transfer remains a topic in need of further study, repairs performed beyond 12 months from injury are less likely to succeed than procedures performed earlier than 12 months. However, facial musculature may remain receptive to reinnervation for periods up to 24 months following denervation in adults [5, 6].

Jowett et al. proposed a classification system to categorize FP into five management domains based on timing of presentation and status of the facial nerve and facial musculature: (1) acute flaccid FP, (2) flaccid FP with potential for spontaneous recovery, (3) flaccid FP with viable facial musculature and low potential for spontaneous recovery, (4) flaccid FP without viable facial musculature, and (5) post-paralytic FP [7].

When considering timing and options for repair, using the aforementioned classification system may help guide treatment considerations. When the facial nerve has incurred transection, prompt tension-free repair at the time of injury is the best treatment option to prevent flaccid FP. In cases of complete facial paralysis with an anatomically intact facial nerve, the timing of repair is less clear given potential for spontaneous recovery. Previously for patients who developed acute flaccid FP following cerebellopontine angle (CPA) resections with an intact nerve, it was common practice to observe for spontaneous recovery for a period of 1 year prior to any intervention. However, this approach results in delay of intervention in the subset of patients who do not recover spontaneously. Recovery patterns of FP following resection of CPA masses suggest that satisfactory recovery of facial functional is unlikely to occur when there is no clinical evidence of facial movement within the first 6 months [8]. Thus, recovery at 6 months following CPA resection can be used to reliably predict outcomes after 1 year. In patients with an anatomically intact facial nerve and HB grade V or worse who do not show improvement of at least one HB grade after 6 months of observation, the probability of ultimate recovery of meaningful expression is less than 10% [9]. Therefore, the risk of facial nerve exploration is minimal, and nerve transfer to one midfacial branch can be safely pursued prior to 1 year following nerve injury.

In cases where the facial nerve has been transected and minimal improvement in facial function is seen 6–12 months after onset, there is a low potential for spontaneous recovery of facial motion, but viable facial musculature remains. Since facial musculature may remain receptive to reinnervation procedures up to 12 months after denervation, nerve repair and transfers are indicated within this timeframe. Interposition graft repair may be indicated to restore neural continuity at the time of injury when a tension-free repair is not possible. In cases where interposition graft repair is not feasible, or when no recovery is noted within the first 12 months, a nerve transfer procedure to the main trunk of the facial nerve can be considered. Volitional expressions may be restored through targeted nerve transfers in this timeframe, such as masseter or hypoglossal nerve transfer to lower branches of the facial nerve for smile reanimation, or cross facial nerve grafting to upper branches for blink restoration.

In situations of flaccid FP without viable native musculature, such as following resection or congenital absence, or unlikely to be receptive to reinnervation (e.g., denervation period exceeding 24 months), nerve repair or transfers are no longer indicated. In such cases, surgical interventions including static facial suspensions and free muscle transfers should be considered. Dynamic smile reanimation may be achieved through temporalis muscle transfer (e.g., lengthening temporalis myoplasty or minimally invasive coronoid transposition) or neurotized free muscle transfer.

Factors Affecting Reconstruction

In addition to timing considerations regarding duration of denervation and status of the facial musculature, it is important to also consider patient factors, including age and history of prior radiation. Historically, elderly patients in their seventh and eighth decades of life were often excluded from the option of dynamic facial reanimation [10]. Prior reports examining rodent and human models of axonal load suggested axonal regeneration and total axon counts in peripheral and central nerves can decrease with age, which were thought to contribute to worse outcomes of cross-facial grafting in the aging population [11]. Improved outcomes in general have been found to be associated with increased axonal load and specifically with the presence of greater than 900 axons in the donor nerve when a cross-facial nerve graft is used [12]. More recently, findings from human cadaveric studies suggest there is a high likelihood that a zygomatic branch of the nerve would have over 900 axons at its last intra-parotid point and that age may not always correlate with axonal counts [13]. Furthermore, several clinical series examining outcomes of facial reanimation in patients 60 years of age or older have shown good outcomes without significant differences in morbidity from dynamic facial reanimation using nerve transfers or free functional gracilis flaps [10, 14, 15]. Therefore, age alone should not preclude the consideration of dynamic facial reanimation in elderly patients.

At the younger end of the spectrum, etiologies of pediatric facial palsy are equally varied and can be generalized into congenital and acquired causes. Congenital causes of pediatric facial palsy include birth trauma, Moebius syndrome, congenital unilateral lower lip paralysis, hemifacial macrosomia, CHARGE, and other syndromes. Most cases of acquired pediatric facial palsy arise from infectious etiologies but can also be due to intracranial masses, iatrogenic injury, or trauma. The most common cause of pediatric facial palsy is Bell's palsy, which accounts for 40–50% of all pediatric cases and usually presents unilaterally. Most cases of Bell's palsy recover full facial function and do not require surgical intervention. In cases that do require surgical intervention, free muscle transfer with cross facial nerve grafting allows for functional reanimation. Children are more capable of cerebral plasticity, and, therefore, a robust and sustainable dynamic reconstruction should be the goal whenever possible to optimize facial movement and psychosocial interactions in children. Excellent long-term functional outcomes with improvement in smile, facial asymmetry, and QOL have been reported in children following free gracilis muscle transfer (FGMT) [16, 17].

The effect of high-dose radiation therapy on facial nerve grafts was previously thought to be detrimental, which led many surgeons to prefer static or dynamic slings over facial nerve grafts in patients undergoing postoperative radiation therapy. However, outcomes from dynamic or static slings are commonly inferior to that after facial nerve grafting or free muscle transfer. Results from animal models comparing facial nerve cable autografts with and without prior radiation treatment have not demonstrated any significant differences in clinical appearance or axon counts [18, 19]. In human cohort studies, radiotherapy with mean doses of 6000 cGy has not been found to be a significant negative prognostic factor in best facial nerve function achieved, especially when normal or near-normal function is present preoperatively [20, 21]. In a retrospective case study of 55 patients, long-term outcomes in patients observed over a 10-year period after facial nerve grafting have demonstrated successful reinnervation in the group receiving postoperative radiation, with no significant differences in success rates when compared to nonirradiated patients [22]. Altogether, these results suggest that patients requiring radiation therapy should not be precluded from dynamic reanimation procedures with facial nerve grafting. Perioperative consideration and optimization of comorbidities that affect wound healing and microvasculature, including nutritional status, tobacco use, and other modifiable factors, should be addressed, although these factors and their impact on outcomes in facial reanimation procedures have not specifically been studied.

Primary Repair and Outcomes

In the case of the transected nerve, such as from iatrogenic nerve sectioning, nerve resection during tumor resection, or penetrating trauma, primary repair of the nerve allows for the best chance for return of nerve function. Primary repair offers a single neurorrhaphy, as opposed to multiple sites of neurorrhaphy with cable grafting repair. Evidence from histologic studies has demonstrated decreasing number of viable axons at each neurorrhaphy. Electrophysiologic studies have also shown better outcomes from axonal regeneration with end-to-end suture repair [23]. Two conditions must be met for primary neurorrhaphy to result in successful outcomes: both proximal and distal nerve ends must exist, and direct nerve coaptation must be performed in the absence of tension. Tension leads to diminished perfusion and neural regeneration [24]. A defect of up to 18 mm of missing nerve can be repaired primarily, although this may necessitate mastoidectomy and rerouting of the nerve to achieve a tension-free repair. If the repair is under tension, it is likely to be unsuccessful, and nerve grafting would be a better option to consider [5, 23, 25]. Timing of repair in traumatic nerve transections is critical and should be performed as early as possible. Wallerian degeneration begins within 24 h and is complete at 72 h. During the first 72 h after injury, the nerve segments can be stimulated intraoperatively, and identification of branches is easier in the unscarred environment. The axons regenerate at a rate of about 1 mm per day allowing for axonal growth to eventually reach the neuromuscular junction.

For primary repair of the transected nerve, the severed nerve ends are first fully mobilized to allow for tension-free neurorrhaphy and then debrided under microscopic magnification to remove devitalized tissue. A contrasted background may be helpful for improving visualization, and 8–0 or 9–0 polypropylene suture is used for the anastomosis to bring together the epineurium. Placement of fascicular or perineural sutures is challenging to perform and may place the nerve substance at greater risk. Two or three well-placed sutures should be sufficient to reapproximate the segments [23]. Measurements of objective facial functioning have been reported in the literature using the Sunnybrook facial grading system (SFGS), which consists of three parts evaluating resting symmetry, symmetry of voluntary movement, and synkinesis. Subjective facial functioning and patient satisfaction have been reported using the facial disability index, which is a brief self-reported questionnaire of physical disability and psychosocial factors related to facial neuromuscular function with physical function and social/well-being function subscales. Long-term follow-up of primary repair after traumatic facial nerve injuries has shown adequate objective facial functioning as measured by the SFGS (mean score 74/100, range 40–96), and good subjective functional and emotional outcomes as measured by the mean facial disability index (FDI) physical and social scores (mean FDI physical function score 86, range 50–100; mean FID social/well-being function score 81, range 40–100) [25].

Cable Repair and Outcomes

When tension-free neurorrhaphy cannot be achieved despite mobilization of the facial nerve, an interposition or cable graft is the best option for repair. The options for nerve grafting are numerous. Careful consideration of the accessibility of the nerve, donor site morbidity, and surgeon experience should guide decision-making to determine the optimal donor nerve. When only a single nerve branch needs repair, the great auricular nerve (GAN) may be used as it is usually within the same operative field (Fig. 26.1a, b). When multiple branches need repair, a longer nerve such as the sural nerve may be considered as it would provide additional graft material. Grafts are directed preferentially toward the midfacial branches to restore smile. Other commonly used sensory nerves harvested for facial nerve grafting include the medial or lateral antebrachial cutaneous nerves, which may be considered if reconstruction with a radial forearm free tissue transfer is planned [23]. Currently, there is no consensus on whether sensory or motor nerve grafts provide the best outcomes for patients requiring cable grafting, and overall there does not appear to be any significant differences noted within the literature regarding polarity of the graft [23, 26]. Patients with cancer and perineural spread at the margin of resection have been shown to have successful reinnervations with immediate facial nerve grafting [27]. Return of facial function should be expected no sooner than 6 months after nerve repair or grafting and can commonly take between 12 and 18 months for maximal recovery. Patients who undergo surgery can expect a HB grade III as the best possible outcome [28]. Compared to primary nerve repair, cable grafting has a slower return of nerve function and an increased rate of synkinesis [29].

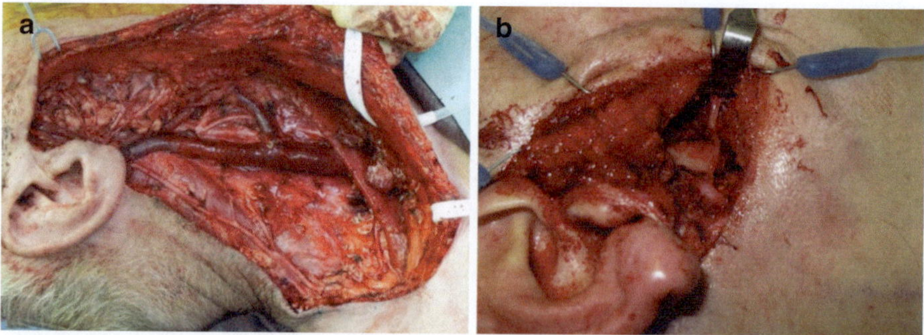

Fig. 26.1 Cable graft repair using the greater auricular nerve (GAN) within the same operative field. (**a**) Dissection of the GAN is visualized at the posterior aspect of the surgical field. (**b**) Cable graft using GAN to buccal branch (images courtesy of Mark K. Wax, MD)

Sural Nerve

The sural nerve is a useful cable graft in situations requiring longer lengths of graft material, or if several branches require repair. Grafts of up to 40 cm can be obtained, which can then be divided into several longitudinal nerve segments. If a size mismatch exists, the sural nerve can usually be safely neurolyzed along its fascicles for relatively long distances to provide several fascicles of decreased diameter for better size match. The sural nerve branches off the tibial nerve in the popliteal fossa and passes along two heads of the gastrocnemius muscle and courses posterior to the lateral malleolus next to the lesser saphenous vein. Although morbidity from harvesting the sural nerve is quite low, patients should be counseled preoperatively regarding the resulting numbness to the lower lateral leg and lateral aspect of the dorsum of the foot (Fig. 26.2a). Early techniques involved a lengthy continuous lower-leg incision extending from just posterior to the lateral malleolus to the midcalf region (Fig. 26.2b). Newer techniques have evolved utilizing a series of stair-step incisions, as well as endoscopic approaches and single incision techniques [30]. Care should be taken to place the incision for the donor site away from areas of contact with footwear to avoid irritation of the scar. The sural nerve graft is then sutured in an end-to-end fashion to allow for tension-free neurorrhaphy (Fig. 26.2c). In a case series reviewing patients with sural nerve graft over a 10-year period, more than half of patients had a HB grade III or IV [22].

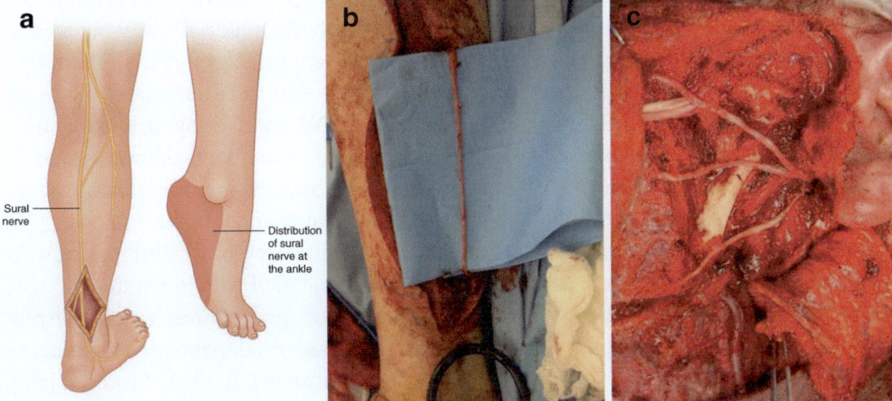

Fig. 26.2 Sural nerve graft. (**a**) The sural nerve can be found using surface landmarks. It is found posterior to the lateral malleolus. Patients should be counseled regarding numbness to the lateral aspect of the dorsum of the foot. (**b**) Dissection of the sural nerve via a continuous lower-leg incision. (**c**) Sural nerve cable graft repair of the upper division branches (illustrations courtesy of Natalie A. Krane, MD; Images courtesy of Mark K. Wax, MD)

Great Auricular Nerve (GAN)

Conley first described the concept of cable grafting in 1955, using the GAN as the donor nerve [31]. The GAN has the advantage less morbidity, as it does not typically require an additional donor site. The GAN is also of a similar caliber to the facial nerve and provides an excellent size match, and up to 10 cm of length may be harvested (Fig. 26.1a). The GAN can be located by drawing a line from the angle of the jaw to the mastoid tip. The nerve will bisect this line as it passes parallel and posterior to the external jugular vein and over the sternocleidomastoid muscle (SCM). The nerve should be dissected free and can be followed proximally around the SCM to obtain extra length. The spinal accessory nerve is close by when performing proximal dissection near Erb's point and should be preserved. Patients should be counseled to expect numbness of the ear lobe and postauricular skin if the GAN is harvested [23].

Acellular Nerve Allografts

Acellular nerve allografts such as the Avance nerve graft by AxoGen, Inc. (Alachua, FL) can be used in place of a nerve autograft to minimize donor site morbidity, or in cases where donor nerve options are limited, although autografts remain the gold standard. AxoGen nerve grafts are made from cadaveric human tissue that has been decellularized in order to render it nonimmunogenic. It is available in various diameters and lengths and provides an infrastructure to support nerve regeneration and allow for tension-free repair [32, 33]. Additional synthetic materials may be used as artificial conduits for interposition grafting, such as caprolactone (Polyganics BC, Groningen, Netherlands), polyglycolic acid (Synovis Micro Companies), and collagen type 1 (Integra LifeSciences Co., Plainsboro, NJ and Collagen Matrix, Inc., Franklin, TN) [34]. Outcomes of acellular allografts have been demonstrated in peripheral nerve repair and have been shown to be successful in restoring nerve function; however, there are little data regarding outcomes in facial nerve repair [35, 36]. There have been no human trials evaluating the efficacy of acellular allografts in facial nerve reanimation. Further investigation is needed to understand the role these materials may play in facial nerve reinnervation procedures, as the current data on peripheral nerve repair propose potential limitations dependent on the nerve grafted and when acellular nerve grafts longer than 15 mm in length are required [37].

Nerve Transfer

When the proximal end of the facial nerve is not available for reanastomosis, but distal nerve branches and facial muscles are viable, nerve transfer is indicated. Many donor sources have been described, including spinal accessory nerve, phrenic nerve, contralateral facial nerve, hypoglossal nerve, and the masseteric motor branch of the trigeminal nerve [38]. The most commonly used nerve substitutions for treatment of facial paralysis include the masseteric and hypoglossal nerves. Ideally, nerve transfer should be performed within 1 year of facial nerve injury, as this has been shown to have the most predictable results [39]. If the facial nerve is known to be transected or resected, then nerve transfer should be considered as soon as possible. Patients who are 6–18 months out from onset of facial paralysis without electrical evidence of nerve recovery may also be considered. Successful reinnervation in patients over 24 months out from initial injury is rare [40].

Masseteric Nerve Transfer

Masseteric nerve transfer for facial reanimation was first described by Spira in 1978 in order to address lower facial paralysis [41]. The masseteric nerve has many advantages including its close proximity to recipient facial nerve branches, low morbidity to chewing function, large number of motor axons, and rapid reinnervation times [42]. Limitations of masseteric nerve transfer include lack of satisfactory facial resting tone, and inability to produce a spontaneous emotive smile, although more recent literature have shown that a spontaneous smile may be present in 23% of patients [43].

The masseteric nerve is a motor branch of the anterior division of the trigeminal nerve. It exits from the cranial cavity through the foramen ovale and passes over the lateral pterygoid muscle and through the sigmoid notch to enter the posterior surface of the masseter muscle near its origin. It can be reliably exposed by dissecting the area between the inferior border of the zygomatic arch and the mandibular arch. This area has been described as the "subzygomatic triangle," which is bounded by the inferior border of the zygomatic arch superiorly, the vertical border of the temporomandibular joint posteriorly, and the frontal branch of the facial nerve inferiorly and anteriorly. The masseteric nerve can be found within the subzygomatic triangle by following a line bisecting the angle formed by the temporomandibular joint and the zygomatic arch as it crosses the midpoint of the triangle base formed by the frontal branch of the facial nerve. The location of the masseteric nerve has also been described as 3 cm anterior to the tragus and 1 cm inferior to the zygomatic arch [40, 44]. A nerve stimulator can be used to confirm the identity of the masseteric nerve by visualizing contraction throughout the entire masseter muscle. The nerve is then traced out distally until there is enough length to perform a tension-free anastomosis to the buccal branch of the facial nerve. The masseteric nerve is then transected distally and neurorrhaphy to the cut end of the facial nerve is performed with two to three stitches through the epineurium (Fig. 26.3a).

Outcomes for masseteric nerve transfer for facial reanimation have traditionally been reported in terms of the HB grading scale. However, since the masseteric nerve transfer technique is only intended to improve specific areas of facial dysfunction, and the HB lacks specificity and reliability, newer outcome measures such as the

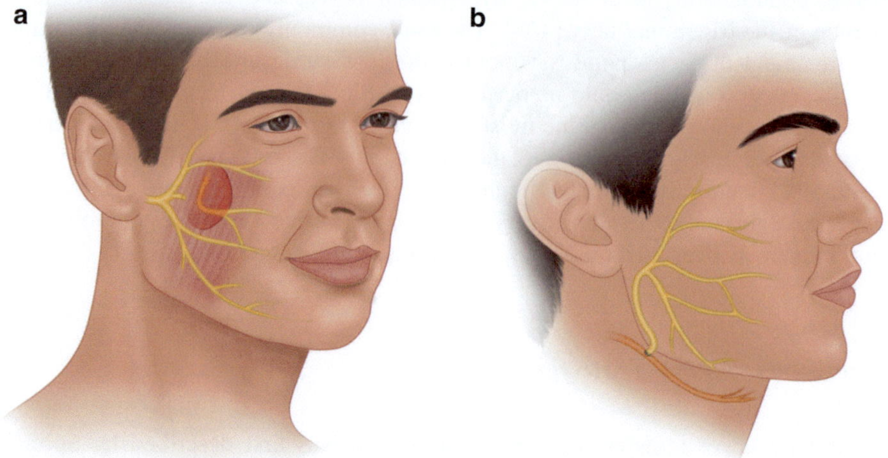

Fig. 26.3 Nerve transfer procedures. (**a**) Masseteric nerve transfer. Blue arrow depicts neuror-rhaphy between masseteric nerve and facial nerve. (**b**) Hypoglossal nerve transfer. Purple segment depicts cable graft connecting main trunk of facial nerve to hypoglossal nerve (illustrations courtesy of Natalie A. Krane, MD)

facial asymmetry index (FAI) and Sunnybrook facial nerve grading scale (SFGS) have become more widely adopted. Several studies in the literature have sought to report more specific outcomes examining improvement in oral commissure symmetry and length of time from reanimation to facial movement [40, 45]. A recent meta-analysis of 71 studies reported improvement in oral commissure symmetry by 3.62 ± 2.7 mm, with time to first movement of 4.6 ± 2.6 months. Patients undergoing direct masseteric nerve transfer had earlier time to first movement than patients with an interposition graft (3.9 ± 2.6 months vs. 6.6 ± 3.9 months) [38]. A recent study examined using FAI to measure the difference in distance between the medial canthus and oral commissure in healthy and paralyzed sides of the face and found that preoperative FAI was a significant predictive factor of improvement in commissure symmetry at rest. For each 1.0 mm of worse preoperative oral commissure asymmetry, the resulting postoperative improvement was 0.6 mm; therefore, masseteric to facial nerve transfer may yield a 60% correction in oral commissure asymmetry [46]. Complications from masseteric nerve transfer are typically rare but most commonly include masseter atrophy (1.9%) and sialocele (0.5%) [38, 46].

Hypoglossal Nerve Transfer

Hypoglossal nerve transfer was first performed in 1904 by Korte and later was popularized by Conley and Baker. The hypoglossal nerve provides motor innervation to all extrinsic and intrinsic muscles of the tongue, excluding the palatoglossus. It emerges beneath the posterior belly of the digastric muscle and, at the level of the digastric muscle tendon, turns anteriorly toward the tongue. Hypoglossal nerve transfer can restore resting tone; however, the appearance of the smile may not be as natural as is seen with masseteric nerve transfer or cross-facial nerve grafting, as the patient must subtly move the tongue to contract the zygomaticus major muscle [47].

The location of the hypoglossal nerve prevents direct coaptation to the facial nerve without a cable graft or splitting and transposing the hypoglossal nerve (Fig. 26.3b). Early techniques for hypoglossal nerve transfer proposed complete sectioning of the nerve with subsequent anastomosis to the main trunk of the facial nerve, which resulted in recovery of facial tone and some recovery of volitional movement [48]. However, complete sectioning of the nerve lead to significant morbidity to speech and swallowing due to hemiatrophy and dysfunction of the tongue. Partial neurotomy techniques of the hypoglossal nerve became popularized in an effort to minimize donor site morbidity. Techniques to split the hypoglossal nerve along its length and transposing a split segment for end-to-end coaptation to the facial nerve, or use of an end-to-side interpositional graft between a partially sectioned hypoglossal nerve and the main facial nerve trunk, have been shown to be successful with reduced rates of hemiglossal atrophy [49]. Additional techniques have proposed mobilization of the intratemporal segment of the facial nerve to provide additional length for direct end-to-end coaptation of the hypoglossal to the facial nerve [48].

Similar to outcomes reporting for masseteric nerve transfer, specific measures such as oral commissure excursion, oral commissure symmetry at maximum smile and at rest, and the Sunnybrook Facial Nerve Grading Scale (SFGS) have been used, in addition to the HB grading scale. In a recent meta-analysis of 71 studies, oral commissure symmetry at maximum smile and at rest after hypoglossal nerve transfer was noted to be 3.09 ± 3.2 mm and 2.22 ± 1.6 mm, respectively. Time to first movement with hypoglossal nerve transfer was 6.3 ± 1.3 months, with the subset who received an interposition graft taking longer to achieve movement at 6.9 ± 3.2 months [38]. A retrospective cohort study examining face-specific QOL outcomes noted improved postoperative Facial Clinimetric Evaluation (FaCE) and Facial Disability Index scores following hypoglossal nerve transfer [50]. Another retrospective cohort study examined objective outcomes using FACE-gram and Emotrics software to measure oral commissure excursion, symmetry of excursion and angle, with notable postoperative improvements after nerve transfer procedures [51]. The most common complication reported is dysphagia/dysarthria (4.1%), followed by tongue numbness, hypogeusia, infection, and graft separation (less than 0.5%) [38].

Cross-Facial Nerve Graft (CFNG)

The cross-facial nerve graft (CFNG) was first introduced by Scaramella [52] and involves the use of the main peripheral branches of the contralateral functioning facial nerve to innervate corresponding branches and muscle groups on the paralyzed side of the face, thereby allowing for the potential of a spontaneous smile. An interposition nerve graft, most commonly the sural nerve given its length, is tunneled across the face. A buccal branch of the contralateral facial nerve is used as the donor nerve because of the redundant innervation to this area of the face, thereby reducing the risk of facial weakness on the donor side of the face. Multiple segmental branches can be used to power several distal paralyzed branches [53]. The CFNG can be used in patients within 2 years of facial nerve injury, prior to muscle atrophy and fibrosis of the motor end plates [54].

CFNG can be performed as either a single-stage or a two-stage procedure. The single-stage operation coapts the donor facial nerve branch to the paralyzed side at the same operation through the CFNG. Advantages of the single-stage procedure are primarily that it avoids a second procedure. In the two-stage procedure, the nerve graft is sutured to the contralateral facial nerve, tunneled to the paralyzed side, and left there until the graft shows evidence of nerve regeneration. Tinel's sign, which can be elicited as a tingling sensation by percussing along the path of the CFNG, can be used to follow axonal ingrowth, which occurs at a rate of about 1 mm per day. The second stage is usually performed 6–12 months later, and the CFNG is sutured to the distal branches of the facial nerve on the paralyzed side. The two-stage approach allows for the surgeon to ensure that axonal load grows exclusively from the healthy side to the affected side and may have the advantage of a more predictable result [55]. When considering repair after 6 months from initial facial nerve injury, a "babysitter" procedure with a partial hypoglossal to facial nerve transfer, along with a CFNG, can be considered. The babysitter procedure is typically performed as a two-stage procedure, wherein a hypoglossal to facial nerve transfer is first performed to prevent muscle atrophy and loss of motor end plates while allowing axonal growth through the CFNG. Six months later, the CFNG is then connected to distal facial nerve branches on the paralyzed side [54].

The main disadvantages of the CFNG include an additional site of morbidity from sural nerve harvest, and potential for suboptimal reinnervation. In either the single- or two-stage approach, there is potential for atrophy and fibrosis of the denervated recipient muscles prior to reinnervation through the CFNG. As the axons grow through the CFNG, they must pass through two sites of coaptation, and growth through the CFNG may be slow and unpredictable. The two-stage approach has the disadvantage of requiring an additional procedure [43, 56].

Outcomes of the CFNG have been promising in terms or producing a spontaneous emotive smile; however, results may take up to 9 months for axons to cross the long interposition graft, and up to only half of the axons may ultimately reach the distal nerve branches [57]. A study comparing CFNG with masseteric nerve transfer found that facial motor recovery was less symmetric, commissural displacement and contraction velocity were lower, and spontaneity was higher in CFNG compared to masseteric nerve transfer [43]. Complications from CFNG include facial weakness on the donor side, nerve graft harvest donor site morbidity, and graft separation [53, 58].

Free Gracilis Muscle Transfer (FGMT)

The free gracilis muscle transfer (FGMT) was introduced in 1976 by Harii [59] and has become the gold standard for dynamic facial reanimation in cases of prolonged FP (Fig. 26.4a). Regional muscle transpositions (e.g., digastric, masseter, or temporalis) often do not provide sufficient oral commissure excursion and may result in an unnatural smile vector [54, 60]. The nerve transfers discussed earlier in this chapter may provide excellent results, however, depend on the presence of viable mimetic muscles and motor end plates, and, therefore, are no longer suitable options after 2 years of facial paralysis.

The gracilis muscle is one of the most superficially located thigh adductors (Fig. 26.4b, c). It arises from the medial margin of the lower half of the body of the pubic symphysis and from the upper half of the pubic arch. It runs vertically

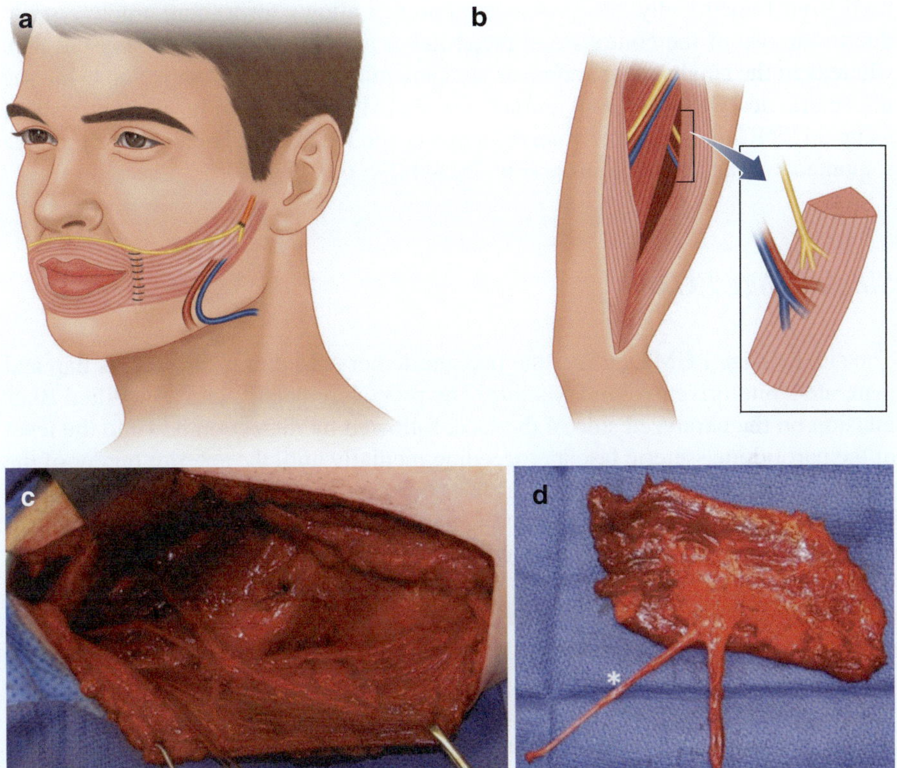

Fig. 26.4 Free gracilis muscle transfer. (**a**) Graphical depiction of FGMT with dual innervation from a CFNG and masseteric nerve transfer. (**b**) Graphical depiction of the gracilis muscle donor site. (**c**) Intraoperative gracilis muscle harvest and dissection of pedicle. (**d**) The gracilis muscle is narrowed and thinned until its weight is between 15 and 25 g prior to inset. * *Obturator nerve* (illustrations courtesy of Natalie A. Krane, MD; Images courtesy of Mark K. Wax, MD)

downward and forms a round tendon, which passes beneath the tendon of the sartorius to insert into the medial surface of the upper end of the tibia. The main vascular supply and venous outflow from the gracilis muscle emerge directly from the profunda femoris vessels and then pass between the adductor longus and adductor brevis muscles to enter the gracilis from the lateral side. The main motor innervation of the gracilis is from the obturator nerve, which emerges from the obturator foramen and divides into anterior and posterior branches under the pectineus muscle. The anterior branch descends between the adductor brevis and adductor longus muscles, providing motor branches to these muscles prior to entering the lower part of the upper third of the gracilis.

FGMT may be performed in one or two stages. The single-stage procedure involves utilizing the masseteric nerve to innervate the free muscle flap. The two-stage approach utilizes a CFNG, which is performed 6–12 months prior to free muscle transfer. The likelihood of obtaining a nearly normal spontaneous smile approaches 85% if the patient is <50 years of age and a cross-facial nerve graft is used [61]. Functionally, the two-stage approach allows for a more emotive smile due to the use of the contralateral facial nerve to control the gracilis muscle flap, whereas in the single-stage approach, the patient controls the gracilis flap using the masseteric nerve to voluntarily initiate a smile [61]. More recently, dual innervation using a CFNG and masseteric nerve to power the FGMT has been used to produce a spontaneous and reliable smile (Fig. 26.4a) [62, 63].

Single-Stage FGMT

The single-stage FGMT utilizes the masseteric nerve to power the gracilis flap and generate a bite-driven voluntary smile. The procedure begins with a modified Blair incision on the paralyzed side of the face, followed by dissection down to the level of the parotidomasseteric fascia proceeding medially until the anterior border of the parotid is exposed. The FGMT may be neurotized with the masseteric nerve or through a CFNG. If using the masseteric nerve, the masseteric nerve is identified on the deep surface of the masseter muscle (as previously discussed), and, once isolated, transection of the masseteric nerve is performed as distally as possible for eventual coaptation with the obturator nerve. Alternatively, a single-stage CFNG can be performed to coapt the donor facial nerve branch to the obturator nerve at the same operation through the CFNG [62].

The gracilis donor site landmarks are the medial condyle of the tibia inferiorly and the insertion of the adductor tendons onto the superior pubic ramus and symphysis superiorly. A line is drawn between these points, and an incision is made parallel to it about 1–2 cm medially. Dissection proceeds through subcutaneous fat toward the muscle belly, taking care to avoid the great saphenous vein. The best way to identify the gracilis muscle is to identify the vascular pedicle. The gracilis branch of the adductor artery travels between the adductor longus anteriorly and adductor magnus posteriorly before entering the gracilis at a right angle. The gracilis artery is accompanied by two venae comitantes and the pedicle enters the anterior aspect of the deep surface of the gracilis, roughly 8 cm below the pubic tubercle. The anterior branch of the obturator nerve supplies the gracilis and enters it 1–2 cm superior to the point where the vascular pedicle enters. Dissection of the gracilis itself begins inferior to the pedicle, followed by developing a plane between the adductor magnus and longus muscles. The total length of harvested gracilis should exceed the distance between the tragus and the corner of the mouth by 2 cm. About 40–50% of the anteroposterior width of the muscle is divided. To provide the longest possible neural pedicle, the obturator nerve is dissected proximally until other branches are encountered, after which it is divided. The pedicle is then dissected and methodically ligated. Before the gracilis flap is inset, it must be narrowed and thinned until its weight is between 15 and 25 g, commensurate with the body habitus of the patient (Fig. 26.4d). The muscle is oriented with the neurovascular pedicle emerging on the inferior edge, and its cut edges are sutured to the orbicularis oris inferiorly. The vessels are then anastomosed under the operating microscope. The lateral inset of the muscle is performed by suspending the muscle to the temporalis fascia, taking care to lateralize the oral commissure by approximately 50% of the anticipated smile excursion [61].

Single-stage FGMT powered by the masseteric nerve has been shown to have excellent reliability with up to 95% of patients producing a smile after surgery. However, although these patients have a voluntary smile, there is a relatively lower success rate at producing a spontaneous smile [64]. In a retrospective cohort study comparing single- and two-stage FGMT, patients who underwent single-stage FGMT powered by the masseteric nerve had a greater smile excursion than in two-stage FGMT powered by a cross-face nerve graft [65]. The most common complications of FGMT are hematoma, infection, vascular compromise, lateralization of the nasolabial fold, and excessive bulk of the gracilis flap. Hematomas should be treated aggressively to prevent accumulation of blood and subsequent pressure and inflammation, leading to possible flap compromise. Wound infections are uncommon, especially with perioperative antibiotic prophylaxis [61]. Vascular compromise is most commonly due to venous obstruction and can be detected when severe induration develops in the muscle over a short period of time [61].

Two-Stage FGMT

O'Brien expanded upon the initial technique proposed by Harii to include a CFNG to power the FGMT. In the first stage, a sural nerve is harvested to be used as a CFNG and then coapted to the distal buccal branches of the unaffected facial nerve. After 6–9 months of axonal regrowth, the second stage is performed to harvest and inset the FGMT and perform a neurorrhaphy between the CFNG to the obturator nerve of the FGMT. Compared with other donor sources, the CFNG in combination with a FGMT provides the greatest degree of spontaneity in facial expression [66].

Outcomes from two-stage FGMT have been successful in restoring spontaneous mimetic smile. Bhama and colleagues examined a cohort of 154 FGMT over 10 years, noting smile length symmetry, as well as spontaneity, to be greater in patients who received a two-stage FGMT with CFNG. Onset of movement was noted to occur within 6–9 months, with smile outcomes optimized with facial nerve physical therapy [67]. QOL following FGMT was also noted to be significantly improved [65, 68]. However, a more recent meta-analysis of FGMT powered by CFNG compared to masseteric nerve demonstrated improved oral commissure excursion in FGMT powered by the masseteric nerve [69]. The most common complications after two-stage FGMT are similar to those of single-stage FGMT and include hematoma, vascular compromise, infection, lateralization of the nasolabial fold, and excessive bulk of the gracilis flap.

Facial Nerve Rehabilitation

Although significant advances in surgical technique to restore facial animation have been made, optimal outcomes still depend on diligent facial rehabilitation postoperatively. Physical therapy exercises, such as active assistive movement exercises, may help strengthen facial muscles. Patients with the ability to initiate slight movement may benefit from soft tissue mobilization with massage and neuromuscular retraining by performing slow, controlled graded facial expressions with visual feedback in front of a mirror [70]. The facial grading scale (FGS) has been used to quantify facial function after facial nerve injury and has been shown to improve significantly after treatment with facial rehabilitation exercises. In a study of 76 patients with chronic facial paralysis (>12 months from onset) of varying etiologies, all patients had improvement in FGS scores with facial rehabilitation. Significant improvement in FGS was associated with number of therapy sessions and lower starting FGS score [71]. Significant improvements have been shown with postoperative rehabilitation to promote motor relearning of facial expression after hypoglossal to facial nerve transfer [72].

Conclusion

Surgical techniques and management of facial palsy have come a long way in advancing and improving outcomes in facial reanimation. Motor nerve reconstruction of the facial nerve may be achieved through primary repair of the transected nerve, cable graft repair of the resected nerve, as well as nerve transfer, cross-facial nerve grafts, and free gracilis muscle transfer. Surgeons and patients should consider and balance expected outcomes with functional donor site morbidity when deciding on the reconstructive approach. Additionally, postoperative facial rehabilitation is an essential aspect of recovery to achieve optimal outcomes.

References

1. Boahene K. Reanimating the paralyzed face. F1000Prime Rep. 2013;5:1–10.
2. Occhiogrosso J, Derakhshan A, Hadlock TA, Shanley KM, Lee LN. Dermal filler treatment improves psychosocial well-being in facial paralysis patients. Facial Plast Surg Aesthet Med. 2020;22:370–7.
3. Dusseldorp JR, van Veen MM, Mohan S, Hadlock TA. Outcome tracking in facial palsy. Otolaryngol Clin North Am. 2018;51:1033–50.
4. Gao Z, et al. Neurorrhaphy for facial reanimation with interpositional graft: outcome in 23 patients and the impact of timing on the outcome. World Neurosurg. 2019;126:e688–93.
5. Wu P, et al. Key changes in denervated muscles and their impact on regeneration and reinnervation. Neural Regen Res. 2014;9:1796–809.
6. Zhang S, Hembd A, Ching CW, Tolley P, Rozen SM. Early masseter to facial nerve transfer may improve smile excursion in facial paralysis. Plast Reconstr Surg Glob Open. 2018;6:1–9.
7. Jowett N. A general approach to facial palsy. Otolaryngol Clin North Am. 2018;51:1019–31.
8. Albathi M, et al. Early nerve grafting for facial paralysis after cerebellopontine angle tumor resection with preserved facial nerve continuity. JAMA Facial Plast Surg. 2016;18:54–60.
9. Rivas A, et al. A model for early prediction of facial nerve recovery after vestibular schwannoma surgery. Otol Neurotol. 2011;32:826–33.
10. Hembd A, et al. Facial reanimation in the seventh and eighth decades of life. Plast Reconstr Surg. 2018;141:1239–51.
11. Hembd A, et al. Correlation between facial nerve axonal load and age and its relevance to facial reanimation. Plast Reconstr Surg. 2017;139:1459–64.
12. Terzis JK, Wang W, Zhao Y. Effect of axonal load on the functional and aesthetic outcomes of the cross-facial nerve graft procedure for facial reanimation. Plast Reconstr Surg. 2009;124:1499–512.
13. Hembd A, et al. Facial nerve axonal analysis and anatomical localization in donor nerve: optimizing axonal load for cross-facial nerve grafting in facial reanimation. Plast Reconstr Surg. 2017;139:177–83.
14. Lee AH, et al. Free functional Gracilis flaps for facial reanimation in elderly patients. Facial Plast Surg Aesthet Med. 2021;23:180–6.
15. Banks CA, Jowett N, Iacolucci C, Heiser A, Hadlock TA. Five-year experience with fifth-to-seventh nerve transfer for smile. Plast Reconstr Surg. 2019;143:1060e–71e.
16. Deramo PJ, Greives MR, Nguyen PD. Pediatric facial reanimation: an algorithmic approach and systematic review. Arch Plast Surg. 2020;47:382–91.
17. Greene JJ, Tavares J, Mohan S, Jowett N, Hadlock T. Long-term outcomes of free gracilis muscle transfer for smile reanimation in children. J Pediatr. 2018;202:279–284.e2.
18. McGuirt WF. Effect of radiation therapy on facial nerve cable autografts. Trans Sect Otolaryngol Am Acad Ophthalmol Otolaryngol. 1976;82:ORL 486.
19. Zhu Y, et al. Effects of postoperative radiotherapy on vascularized nerve graft for facial nerve repair in a rabbit model. J Oral Maxillofac Surg. 2019;77:2339–46.
20. Brown PD, Eshleman JS, Foote RL, Strome SE. An analysis of facial nerve function in irradiated and unirradiated facial nerve grafts. Int J Radiat Oncol Biol Phys. 2000;48:737–43.
21. Gidley PW, et al. The impact of radiotherapy on facial nerve repair. Laryngoscope. 2010;120:1985–9.
22. Leong SC, Lesser TH. Long-term outcomes of facial nerve function in irradiated and nonirradiated nerve grafts. Ann Otol Rhinol Laryngol. 2013;122:695–700.
23. Humphrey CD, Kriet JD. Nerve repair and cable grafting for facial paralysis. Facial Plast Surg. 2008;24:170–6.
24. Terzis J, Faibisoff B, Williams B. The nerve gap: suture under tension vs. graft. Methods Mol Biol. 1975;56:166–70.
25. Frijters E, Hofer SOP, Mureau MAM. Long-term subjective and objective outcome after primary repair of traumatic facial nerve injuries. Ann Plast Surg. 2008;61:181–7.

26. Hoshal SG, Solis RN, Bewley AF. Nerve grafts in head and neck reconstruction. Curr Opin Otolaryngol Head Neck Surg. 2020;28:346–51.
27. Wax MK, Kaylie DM. Does a positive neural margin affect outcome in facial nerve grafting? Head Neck. 2007;29:546–9.
28. Darrouzet V, et al. Management of facial paralysis resulting from temporal bone fractures: our experience in 115 cases. Otolaryngol Head Neck Surg. 2001;125:77–84.
29. Owusu JA, Truong L, Kim JC. Facial nerve reconstruction with concurrent masseteric nerve transfer and cable grafting. JAMA Facial Plast Surg. 2016;18:335–9.
30. Azizzadeh B, et al. Single-incision sural nerve harvest: technical considerations for cross-facial nerve grafting. Laryngoscope. 2019;129:2464–6.
31. Conley JJ. Facial nerve grafting in treatment of parotid gland tumors: new technique. AMA Arch Surg. 1955;70:359–66.
32. Robinson J, Fisher D. Facial nerve reconstruction using acellular nerve allograft. J Craniofac Surg. 2021;33:1–2.
33. Hu M, Xiao H, Niu Y, Liu H, Zhang L. Long-term follow-up of the repair of the multiple-branch facial nerve defect using acellular nerve allograft. J Oral Maxillofac Surg. 2016;74(218):e1–218.e11.
34. Safa B, Buncke GA, Substitutes. Conduits and processed nerve allografts. Hand Clin. 2016;32:127–40.
35. Brooks DN, et al. Processed nerve allografts for peripheral nerve reconstruction: a multi-center study of utilization and outcomes in sensory, mixed, and motor nerve reconstructions. Microsurgery. 2011;32:1–14.
36. Moore AM, et al. Acellular nerve allografts in peripheral nerve regeneration: a comparative study. Muscle Nerve. 2011;44:221–34.
37. Gaudin R, et al. Approaches to peripheral nerve repair: generations of biomaterial conduits yielding to replacing autologous nerve grafts in craniomaxillofacial surgery. Biomed Res Int. 2016;2016:1.
38. Urban MJ, et al. Hypoglossal and masseteric nerve transfer for facial reanimation: a systematic review and meta-analysis. Facial Plast Surg Aesthet Med. 2021;24:1–8.
39. Yang SF, Kim JC. Reinnervation with selective nerve grafting from multiple donor nerves. Facial Plast Surg Clin North Am. 2021;29:389–96.
40. Bayrak SB, Kriet JD, Humphrey CD. Masseteric to buccal branch nerve transfer. Curr Opin Otolaryngol Head Neck Surg. 2017;25:280–5.
41. Spira M. Anastomosis of masseteric nerve to lower division of facial nerve for correction of lower facial paralysis: preliminary report. Plast Reconstr Surg. 1978;61:330–4.
42. Cassoni A, et al. Masseter-facial neurorrhaphy for facial palsy reanimation: what happens after masseter denervation? Histomorphometric and stomatognathic functional analysis. J Craniomaxillofac Surg. 2020;48:680–4.
43. Hontanilla B, Olivas J, Cabello Á, Marré D. Cross-face nerve grafting versus masseteric-to-facial nerve transposition for reanimation of incomplete facial paralysis: a comparative study using the FACIAL CLIMA evaluating system. Plast Reconstr Surg. 2018;142:179E–91E.
44. Collar RM, Byrne PJ, Boahene KDO. The subzygomatic triangle: rapid, minimally invasive identification of the masseteric nerve for facial reanimation. Plast Reconstr Surg. 2013;132:183–8.
45. Murphey AW, Clinkscales WB, Oyer SL. Masseteric nerve transfer for facial nerve paralysis a systematic review and meta-analysis. JAMA Facial Plast Surg. 2018;20:104–10.
46. Nina Lu G, Han R, Lee E, Byrne P, Boahene K. Predicting resting oral commissure tone outcomes following masseter nerve transfer in facial reanimation. Facial Plast Surg Aesthet Med. 2021;23:249–54.
47. Joseph AW, Kim JC. Management of flaccid facial paralysis of less than two years' duration. Otolaryngol Clin North Am. 2018;51:1093–105.
48. Kochhar A, et al. Transposition of the intratemporal facial to hypoglossal nerve for reanimation of the paralyzed face: the VII to XII transposition technique. JAMA Facial Plast Surg. 2016;18:370–8.

49. Campero A, Socolovsky M. Facial reanimation by means of the hypoglossal nerve: anatomic comparison of different techniques. Neurosurgery. 2007;61:41–50.
50. Volk GF, et al. Functional outcome and quality of life after hypoglossal-facial jump nerve suture. Front Surg. 2020;7:1–9.
51. Krane NA, et al. Early outcomes in an emerging facial nerve center: the Oregon Health and Science University (OHSU) experience. Ann Otol Rhinol Laryngol. 2021;130:459–66.
52. Scaramella LF. Anastomosis between the two facial nerves. Laryngoscope. 1975;85:1359–66.
53. Jandali D, Revenaugh PC. Facial reanimation: an update on nerve transfers in facial paralysis. Curr Opin Otolaryngol Head Neck Surg. 2019;27:231–6.
54. Chan JYK, Byrne PJ. Management of facial paralysis in the 21st century. Facial Plast Surg. 2011;27:346–57.
55. Lee EI, Hurvitz KA, Evans GRD, Wirth GA. Cross-facial nerve graft: past and present. J Plast Reconstr Aesthet Surg. 2008;61:250–6.
56. Faris C, Lindsay R. Current thoughts and developments in facial nerve reanimation. Curr Opin Otolaryngol Head Neck Surg. 2013;21:346–52.
57. Kim L, Byrne PJ. Controversies in contemporary facial reanimation. Facial Plast Surg Clin North Am. 2016;24:275–97.
58. Daeschler SC, Zuker R, Borschel GH. Strategies to improve cross-face nerve grafting in facial paralysis. Facial Plast Surg Clin North Am. 2021;29:423–30.
59. Harii K, Ohmori K, Torii S. Free gracilis muscle transplantation, with microneurovascular anastomoses for the treatment of facial paralysis: a preliminary report. Plast Reconstr Surg. 1976;57:133–43.
60. Militsakh ON, Sanderson JA, Lin D, Wax MK. Rehabilitation of a parotidectomy patient-a systematic approach. Head Neck. 2013;35:1349–61.
61. Hohman MH, Hadlock TA. Microneurovascular free gracilis transfer for smile reanimation. Oper Tech Otolaryngol Head Neck Surg. 2012;23:262–7.
62. Boonipat T, et al. Dual innervation of free gracilis muscle for facial reanimation: what we know so far. J Plast Reconstr Aesthet Surg. 2020;73:2196–209.
63. Klebuc MJ, Xue AS, Doval AF. Dual innervation of free functional muscle flaps in facial paralysis. Facial Plast Surg Clin North Am. 2021;29:431–8.
64. Miller MQ, Hadlock TA. Lessons from gracilis free tissue transfer for facial paralysis: now versus 10 years ago. Facial Plast Surg Clin North Am. 2021;29:415–22.
65. Bhama PK, et al. Objective outcomes analysis following microvascular gracilis transfer for facial reanimation: a review of 10 years' experience. JAMA Facial Plast Surg. 2014;16:85–92.
66. Azizzadeh B, Pettijohn KJ. The gracilis free flap. Facial Plast Surg Clin North Am. 2016;24:47–60.
67. Jowett N, Hadlock TA. Free gracilis transfer and static facial suspension for midfacial reanimation in long-standing flaccid facial palsy. Otolaryngol Clin North Am. 2018;51:1129–39.
68. Lindsay RW, Bhama P, Weinberg J, Hadlock TA. The success of free gracilis muscle transfer to restore smile in patients with nonflaccid facial paralysis. Ann Plast Surg. 2014;73:177–82.
69. Vila PM, Kallogjeri D, Yaeger LH, Chi JJ. Powering the gracilis for facial reanimation: a systematic review and meta-analysis of outcomes based on donor nerve. JAMA Otolaryngol Head Neck Surg. 2020;146:429–36.
70. Lindsay RW, Robinson M, Hadlock TA. Comprehensive facial rehabilitation improves function in people with facial paralysis: a 5-year experience at the Massachusetts eye and ear infirmary. Phys Ther. 2010;90:391–7.
71. Karp E, et al. Facial rehabilitation as noninvasive treatment for chronic facial nerve paralysis. Otol Neurotol. 2019;40:241–5.
72. Negley KJ, Rasool A, Byrne PJ. Motor relearning after hypoglossal-facial nerve anastomosis. Am J Phys Med Rehabil. 2021;100:E85–8.

Chapter 27
Pearls and Pitfalls in Microvascular Reconstructive Fellowships

Mark K. Wax, Arshad Kaleem, Daniel Petrisor, and Steve Cannady

American Board of Facial Plastic Reconstructive Surgery Certification

The Department of Otolaryngology Head Neck Surgery at OHSU began its foray into microvascular reconstruction in the late 1990s. At that time, the department utilized the services of the plastic surgery department to facilitate integration of free tissue transfer into the reconstructive paradigm. It soon became apparent that timing, coordination, and an understanding of the particular reconstructive needs for the head and neck patient required a more integrated service line. Thus, a dedicated head and neck microvascular reconstructive surgeon was added to the oncologic program. It was clear from the start that a high-volume microvascular reconstructive service could expand the frontiers not just of the otolaryngologists but also other various subspecialties whose needs required a dedicated service. Once the service

M. K. Wax (✉)
Department of Otolaryngology-Head and Neck Surgery, Oregon Health and Science University, Portland, OR, USA
e-mail: waxm@ohsu.edu

A. Kaleem
Head and Neck Oncology/Microvascular Reconstructive Surgery, High Desert Oral and Facial Surgery, El Paso, TX, USA

D. Petrisor
Head and Neck Oncologic and Microvascular Reconstructive Surgery, Department of Oral and Maxillofacial Surgery, Oregon Health and Science University, Portland, OR, USA
e-mail: petrisor@ohsu.edu

S. Cannady
Division Chief for Head and Neck Surgery, Department of Otorhinolaryngology, University of Pennsylvania, Philadelphia, PA, USA
e-mail: steven.cannady@pennmedicine.upenn.edu

J. C. Melville et al. (eds.), *Advancements and Innovations in OMFS, ENT, and Facial Plastic Surgery*, https://doi.org/10.1007/978-3-031-32099-6_27

was established, it became evident that the microvascular program could provide adjunct subspecialty training in the field of otolaryngology. The volume and multidisciplinary nature of the program was felt capable of providing the expertise for advanced training. Simultaneously, the need for dedicated microvascular reconstructive surgeons across the nation was increasing.

A fellowship was established through the American Academy of Facial Plastic Reconstructive Surgery (AAFPRS), which in turn enabled subspecialty certification by the American Board of Facial Plastic Reconstructive Surgery (ABFPRS). At the time the fellowship was established, there were two methods of providing reconstructive services to the otolaryngology patient. This was either by the head and neck ablative team or by a dedicated reconstructive individual from the facial plastic team. Our department was a recognized leader in the country for facial plastic and reconstructive services. Thus, expansion into the microvascular field was felt to be best performed by affiliation with the AAFPRS. This would lead to board specialty certification by the ABFPRS.

The introduction of a fellow brings a tremendous amount of angst to any training program. There is grave concern on behalf of the residents that cases will be "stolen" and/or the surgical and educational experience will be diluted. There is also concern on behalf of other faculty that the fellow will not have the same technical or academic skill set of other attendings. All of these issues need to be addressed in a proactive fashion prior to bringing on the fellow. We accomplish this through multiple meetings with the residents and the faculty. We had buy-in from all parties concerned.

Perhaps most important was the continued attention paid to the interaction between the fellow and the resident service. It is very easy to drift from a congenial cooperative relationship to hidden anxiety, uncomfortableness, and resentment. Fortunately, as program director, I was able to meet with the residents on a quarterly basis and ascertain where the relationship with the fellow was sitting. Over the years, the issue has become more not that the fellow infringes on their training but more that occasionally we will take on a fellow whose technical and academic skill set is not equivalent to the graduates of our program and that their contribution to the residency education is not as great as what others have been in the past. A constant finger on the pulse allows one to navigate this.

As with most microvascular services, there is a perception that takes backs, failures, and complications come in batches. You can have a long period where everything is smooth and then a month where everything goes south. During one of these episodes, I must've been grumbling about fellows when my fellow informed me that "you should've known if you took a fellow that you would have more complications and more issues"; this in fact has not proven to be true. We have recently undertaken a multi-institutional review of programs that have fellows, and the "July affect" does not exist. Morbidity and complications are spread evenly through the year. They do not change on a year-to-year basis.

Taking on a fellow has had many upsides. Our institution has been able to attract fellows of a diverse nature. They have lent an extra facet and perspective to the residency program. Their integration into the teaching environment has been a definite plus to all concerned. Perhaps most stimulating has been the ability to interact with someone who is totally interested in what goes on in the field. The constant stimulation and conversation that happens during the case keeps everyone on their toes. An additional benefit is that the fellows allow "one point" of contact with multiple other services such as neurosurgery, oculoplastic, orthopedics, and OMFS. It allows for better integration into a seamless care paradigm.

The most stressful issue for the program director arises during the selection process for the next year. The facial plastics and reconstructive matching program is predominantly geared for reconstructive and cosmetic surgery, not so much for microvascular reconstruction. Being able to parse out the individuals whose true interest lies in microvascular reconstructive surgery as a major component of the fellowship can be the hardest part. Many applicants are attracted by the facial plastics experience. It does dramatically decrease the number of candidates in the pool. But once you have parsed out of those individuals, the interest level is immensely high. The ability to allow the fellow to seek expertise and knowledge in other areas that interest them has been a very satisfying experience.

Overall, the addition of a fellowship program run through the facial plastic and reconstructive program required a fair amount of work upfront to ensure integration into the academic milieu of a residency program. The added benefits are immense.

Microvascular Training: The Oral Maxillofacial Experience

Free tissue transfer utilizing microvascular anastomosis started in the early to mid-70s and has evolved into a very reliable and dependable method of reconstruction, with the development of centers for training across different specialties. In the United States, most of these centers of advanced training in microvascular reconstruction have been limited to otolaryngology-head and neck surgery and plastic surgery. In the United Kingdom and most European Oral Maxillofacial Surgery (OMFS) programs, microvascular reconstruction has been an integral component of OMFS training for a long time. In the United States, it was not until the 1990s that there was a dedicated push to integrate microvascular reconstruction fellowships into OMFS.

The impetus for free tissue transfer and primary reconstruction of major maxillofacial defects arose from expanded scope OMFS practitioners who subspecialized head and neck oncology. By 1990, a renaissance of interest in oral/head and neck oncologic surgery in OMFS was underway at several sites within the US Dr. Robert Ord, who was trained in the United Kingdom, joined the OMFS faculty of the University of Maryland in 1989 and began treating oral cancer patients along with his OMFS residents. At about the same time, Bryce Potter and Eric Dierks jointly formed Head and Neck Surgical Associates and began an active head and neck cancer service at Emanuel and Providence Hospitals in Portland, Oregon, that more extensively involved the OHSU OMFS residents. Joseph Helman joined the faculty at the University of Michigan in 1994 and began an oral cancer service. In Miami,

Robert Marx was well along in his evolution to integrate oral/head and neck cancer in his program.

Major primary reconstruction of the head and neck requiring free tissue transfer was done in collaboration with plastics and ENT services. In OMFS, the first two-surgeon team in which one of the surgeons was also a microvascular reconstructive surgeon was developed at the University of Maryland in 1998 when Remy Blanchaert returned to Baltimore from his microvascular training in Portland and Seattle to join his mentor, Robert Ord. This created the model for many to follow. There are approximately 12 fellowship programs that provide oral/head and neck oncologic and microvascular training. Most of the (OMFS) fellowships are a 2-year program with first year of fellowship dedicated to ablative surgery and the second year of the fellowship to microvascular reconstructive surgery. Fellows are selected through a match process conducted by the American Academy of Craniomaxillofacial Surgery (AACMFS).

At the University of Miami, Robert Marx DDS established a very vigorous fellowship training in ablative maxillofacial surgery but then expanded the program as he felt the need for a dedicated OMFS microvascular surgeon. As a result, he hired one of his fellows, Ramzey Tursun DDS, who did his microvascular fellowship training under a plastic surgeon, Jaime Flores MD. In 2013, microvascular training became part of the 2-year fellowship at the University of Miami. Maxillofacial reconstruction became a major part of the fellowship, and over 4 years, another microvascular surgeon was added to the faculty.

The fellowship program at the University of Miami has certainly helped the residency program as it is considered a training program with the broadest scope in the country. This attracts candidates from a variety of backgrounds and interests and in particular those residents who are interested in advanced training in microvascular surgery. The fellows bring their own experiences with them that is an added advantage for the fellowship program. The key for a successful fellowship year is finding fellows who want to learn and then inspire others and teach others. Our most successful graduates have gone on to join academic programs where they are involved in active practice of microvascular reconstruction and teaching residents and fellows.

Bringing a new fellow each year with a different training background can be a challenge to integrate in the program. This becomes an issue when training someone who has never been under the microscope or has never done a major head and neck reconstructive surgery as part of their residency training. However, most of the fellows who match into the fellowship quickly learn the skills needed for microvascular surgery. OMFS trained fellows do well in head and neck reconstruction because of their knowledge of head and neck anatomy and relationship of the jaws and occlusion. I believe that most OMFS programs should hire fellowship trained microvascular faculty to ensure that all residents have exposure to microvascular techniques and major maxillofacial reconstruction. Furthermore, I have found that high-volume free flap programs benefit from having two microvascular trained surgeons on staff. This supports faculty in better handling the stress of a heavy fellowship training, and the fellows benefit by learning from two different mentors.

One of the challenges of having a fellowship program in a residency is that it could be seen as a "very busy" program by applicants who are not interested in major head and neck oncologic and reconstructive surgery. Having a fellowship program can also be seen as a "diluting" factor in residency training as it takes away the operating opportunities from the residents. This is a delicate matter for every fellowship director to manage. At our program, we address this by setting up clear expectations and responsibilities. We make sure that the fellow is seen as a senior partner by the residents whose primary focus is to learn microvascular surgery. The residents help in flap checks, but the fellows are ultimately responsible for the care of free flap patients.

Having strong relationships with other services is beneficial for the training of fellows and residents. At the University of Miami, plastic surgery residents rotate through our service to get exposure to head and neck reconstruction. In addition, we have a collaborative relationship with the head and neck service and are working to further strengthen this collaboration by doing two team surgeries with them. I believe there should be opportunities for the fellows for cross specialty training among OMFS and ENT. There are areas that ENT can provide experience from their training, and similarly we can provide training and services that are not common to head neck service such as jaw in day or any reconstruction involving major dental rehabilitation. Such cross-specialty training will diversify the training of the fellows of both specialties. This collaboration can be beneficial not just in training the fellows but also in providing multidisciplinary care.

Overall, having a microvascular fellowship has a positive impact on the residency training, and OMFS-based microvascular fellowships provide a pathway for OMFS residents to pursue microvascular training that builds on their expertise and training especially as it relates to the maxillofacial region.

American Head and Neck Surgery Fellowship Experience

Over the past 15–20 years, the number of otolaryngology fellowship programs in microvascular surgery has expanded from less than 10 to well over 50. There have been multiple routes taken to establishing a strong training experience for fellows, while some programs expanding their head and neck programs have started fellowship programs de novo, and others have wrestled with how to incorporate this aspect of training into an existing fellowship program. The expansion of training programs has ultimately led to many options for trainees wishing to acquire this training and, therefore, practice.

Over this same time period, otolaryngology has increasingly taken over more of the reconstructive aspects of head and neck cases volume as opposed to other service lines (i.e., plastic surgery) performing this portion. In a recent study, single institution, plastics fellowship program surveys, and national quality improvement project (NSQIP) data all showed increases of otolaryngology head and neck surgery (OHNS) case share, while increasing numbers of microvascular cases were observed. The single institution was in fact our institution and observed the period of time after microvascular surgeon number in OHNS increased from one to five surgeons; this led to increasing case numbers from 59 to 227, while increasing case share from 81.4 to 94% (effectively increasing OHNS performed micro cases from 48 to 213). Over the same study period (2011–2016), survey data indicated that OHNS programs performing over 100 microvascular surgeries increased from 40 to 73%. Lastly, NSQIP data over the same period indicate a 134% increase in OHNS performed head and neck microvascular cases [1]. Currently, our colleagues in oral maxillofacial surgery (OMFS) are increasingly entering into the oral oncology field and similarly performing reconstructions. In our current field, we are now seeing growth in a multidisciplinary head and neck reconstructionist paradigm. I will describe below our experience as we grew our team, brought our fellows an expanded microvascular experience, and welcomed our OMFS team as major contributor to head and neck surgery and education in microvascular head and neck surgery.

Expanding the Microvascular Team

Prior to 2013, our institution had a large plastic surgery (PS) microvascular team of which several performed *some* head and neck reconstruction. We also had an established AHNS surgeon that performed microvascular surgery. Given the direction of national trends, the decision was made to expand microvascular surgery capacity within our department, ultimately going from one to five micro trained surgeons. This had the impact of expanding our overall microsurgery numbers from 19 to 240 cases. This demonstrates that expanding a team can lead to overall growth and that no surgeon's volume decreased over this time. On average, even the busiest reconstruction surgeons stayed busy or increased volume.

The growth of our team had a direct impact on microvascular training at our institution. Prior to 2013, our fellowship was attracting candidates primarily interested in ablative surgery. In addition, the PS fellowship attracted surgeons interested in head and neck microvascular experiences. After the expansion of OHNS offered microvascular experience, we began to attract microvascular candidates. Admittedly, this trend may not all be attributable to our capacity and volume change, as general interest in becoming a microvascular surgeon has risen among OHNS as well as has general head and neck cancer surgery interest. However, at least in part, I would suggest that busier programs do attract interest of candidates.

OMFS Collaborative Expansion

Given the interest, expertise, and talents of OMFS trained colleagues, it is not surprising that fellowship training programs in head and neck surgery (HNS) have also expanded for this specialty. Traditionally, our specialties have overlapped on benign and malignant disease treatment in the head and neck. Thus, our approach was collaborative from the onset of the shared space and disease line that is head and neck cancer. We brought a fellowship trained OMFS microvascular surgeon onto our disease service line several years ago. He is involved in resident and fellow training for both OMFS and OHNS and clinically operates within our head and neck disease team. As more training programs for OMFS emerge, more collaboration between our specialties are eminent. We have seen the skills sets of both services compliment each other and enhance the care of head and neck cancer. Furthermore, the differences in training lead to shared teaching benefits for fellows trained by programs that integrate OMFS and OHNS expertise. In essence, the more we have grown our team and welcomed capable interested individuals into the clinical program and training program, the busier and more successful our team has become. I often discuss with fellows that "good is good," and we want good and interested talent on our teams. So it matters less the training discipline or background than it does the skills of the individuals. The transition from PS to OHNS- or OMFS-based reconstruction likely represented a surge in interest from our fields rather than a change needed based on skill. And, I believe that as we move toward a shared future, I would expect both OHNS and OMFS to thrive together to continue to improve the quality and capacity of head and neck reconstruction.

References

1. Kozak GM, Katzel EB, Rose JF, Nathan SL, Wu LC. An analysis of specialty-specific microsurgical head and neck reconstruction: a look at a single institution and national trends over a decade. Ann Plast Surg. 2020;84(4):413–7. https://doi.org/10.1097/SAP.0000000000002082.

Chapter 28
Advancements in Plastic Surgery: Face Transplant

Ricardo Rodriguez Colon, Daniel Boczar, Hilliard T. Brydges, and Eduardo D. Rodriguez

Facial transplantation (FT), first performed in 2005, is indicated in patients living with functional and aesthetic deficits unamenable to conventional reconstructive techniques. Mechanisms of injury for the 48 FTs performed to date have included burns, and ballistic injury, among others [1]. The extent of tissue transplanted varies and can include full or partial facial soft tissue, along with varying portions of the craniofacial skeleton. Currently, no widely accepted criteria exist, with recipient selection being largely patient and transplant team specific. Our FT patient cohort outcomes are displayed in Fig. 28.1.

R. R. Colon · D. Boczar · H. T. Brydges · E. D. Rodriguez (✉)
Hansjörg Wyss Department of Plastic Surgery, New York University Langone Health, New York, NY, USA
e-mail: Ricardo.Rodriguezcolon@nyulangone.org; Daniel.Boczar@nyulangone.org; Hilliard.Brydges@nyulangone.org; Eduardo.Rodriguez@nyulangone.org

J. C. Melville et al. (eds.), *Advancements and Innovations in OMFS, ENT, and Facial Plastic Surgery*, https://doi.org/10.1007/978-3-031-32099-6_28

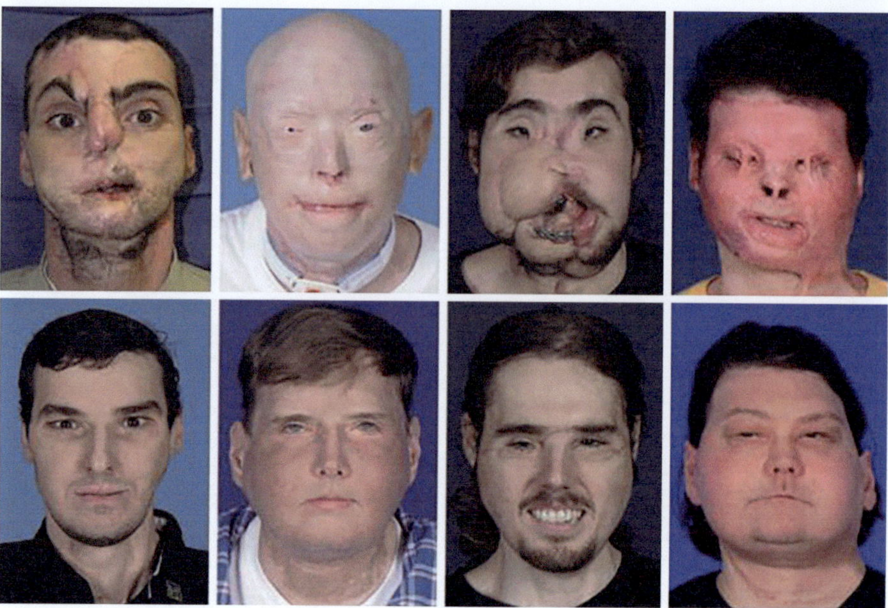

Fig. 28.1 Pre- and postoperative pictures of patients who received facial transplantation by Dr. Eduardo D. Rodriguez and his team (printed with permission and copyrights retained by Eduardo D. Rodriguez, M.D., D.D.S)

Preoperative Considerations

Patient Evaluation and Selection

Patient selection is paramount to success, as the immediate posttransplant rehabilitation and lifelong maintenance require significant commitment by recipients and their families. A multidisciplinary team evaluation is performed to evaluate medical, psychosocial, and functional considerations. Important considerations to elucidate are patients' functional status, associated injuries/deficits, medical history—including chronic conditions and history of malignancy—social support, and psychiatric conditions.

Initial evaluation includes determining if the patient's deficits could be sufficiently addressed with conventional autologous reconstructive methods. If so, these should be employed and have demonstrated favorable cosmetic and functional outcomes. Those considered suitable candidates should receive vascular imaging and detailed immunologic evaluation before FT. Lastly, salvage reconstructive options should be available if the transplant procedure fails or if the allograft necessitates removal.

Indications and Contraindications

Although no consensus inclusion or exclusion criteria exist, there are some generally aggreged upon indications, and relative contraindications, all of which remain transplant center specific. FT is typically indicated in patients with functional and aesthetic deficits unamenable to conventional reconstructive techniques. These include extensive facial soft tissue injury with or without damage to the underlying craniofacial skeleton.

Relative contraindications focus on medical, psychosocial, and psychiatric considerations. Medically, patients should be screened for infectious diseases—particularly human immunodeficiency virus (HIV)—hepatitis, active or prior malignancy, and immunologic or hematologic derangements. Given the lifelong immunosuppression and medical care required following FT and the assistance needed in the early postoperative periods, medical noncompliance and lack of appropriate social support are often considered exclusion criteria for FT. At our institution, caregiver support is required for FT candidacy. FT should be avoided in those with active psychiatric disorders, namely, depression and substance use disorder.

One controversial consideration in FT candidacy is that of blindness. Opponents of FT in blind patients cite the inability to self-visualize the allograft, thereby prohibiting the identification of signs of potential transplant rejection, including edema and erythema, and the inability for blind patients to fully comprehend appreciate the aesthetic outcomes and consequently achieve the psychosocial benefit. However, two transplants have been performed on blind patients, with proponents citing ethical concerns in excluding blind patients from FT. Early psychosocial and transplant outcomes in these patients appear promising [2–4].

Patient-Specific Planning

The 48 FTs reported in the literature have varied in the extent of tissue transplanted with varying amounts of soft tissue and bone included, along with specialized structures, such as the tongue. Patient injuries and missing facial structures guide tissue inclusion. For example, a patient with an intact upper facial third would receive an allograft limited to the middle and lower facial thirds. Important soft tissue structures that can be included to varying degrees include the nose, ears, eyelids, and oral mucosa. Bony structures can be included in the allograft to address severely damaged or missing segments of the craniofacial skeleton. Restoration of the craniofacial structure, namely, the vertical and horizontal buttresses, is vital to functional and aesthetic recovery. Prior FTs have included zygomatic arches, maxillae, mandible, nasal bones, and orbital floors [1, 5]. Of note, a classification system on the soft tissue and bony defects for FT has been described (Fig. 28.2).

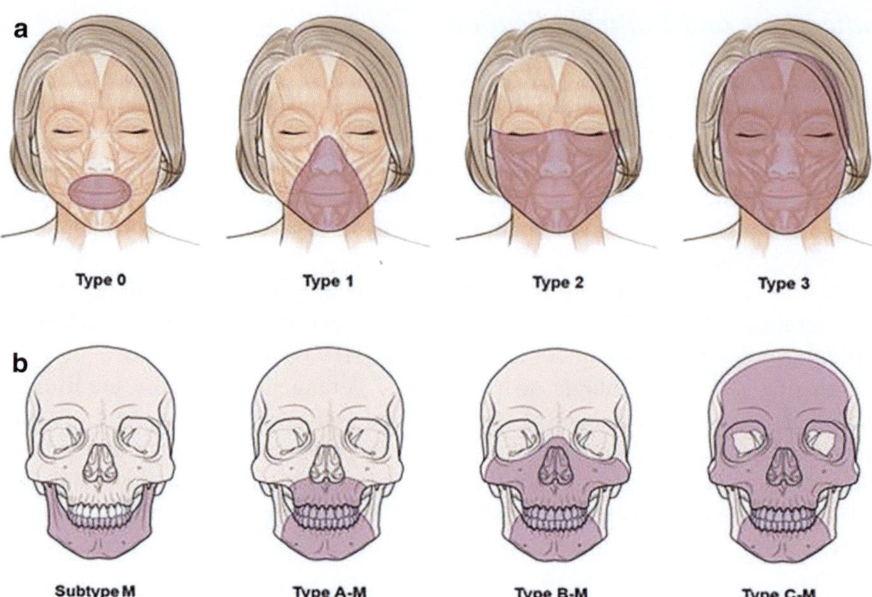

Fig. 28.2 (**a**) Soft-tissue defect classification system for facial transplantation. Type 0, oral, includes upper lip, lower lip, and oral commissures; Type 1, oral-nasal includes nasal soft-tissue structures with or without type 0; Type 2, oral-nasal-orbital includes infraorbital and malar regions with or without Type 1; Type 3, full facial includes forehead, supraorbital, and preauricular and may include all facial soft tissues; (**b**) skeletal tissue defect classification for facial transplantation. Type A, Le Fort I-type, includes partial or complete maxilla; Type B, Le Fort III-type, includes maxilla, inferomedial orbital, and zygomatic bones with or without nasal, vomer, and ethmoid bones; Type C, monobloc type, includes frontal and supraorbital bones with or without facial bones in the other types of defects; Subtype M includes partial or complete mandible (printed with permission and copyrights retained by Eduardo D. Rodriguez, M.D., D.D.S)

Donor Selection

Donor selection contributes significantly to aesthetic, functional, and immuno-logic outcomes. FT donors require additional screening compared to solid organ donors, beyond immunologic and serologic matching, which includes skin tone, hair color, and facial structure. The transplant team dictates the extent of immu-nologic and serologic matching needed, with some centers accepting more mis-match than others. Viral serology matching should also be carefully considered, as an FT recipient transplanted with Epstein-Barr virus mismatch developed mono-clonal B-cell lymphoma [6].

Immunosuppression Therapy

FT recipients require lifelong immunosuppression, and centers vary in their induction and maintenance therapy approach. Although induction regimens vary, they often consist of antithymocyte globulin (ATG) or anti-IL-2 receptor antibody, along with a combination of tacrolimus, mycophenolate mofetil (MMF), and steroids [7, 8]. Maintenance immunosuppression regimens are less variable, generally consisting of triple therapy with tacrolimus, mycophenolate mofetil, and a steroid taper [9]. Our current immunosuppressive regimen includes steroids, ATG, anti-CD20 for induction immunosuppression, and steroids, tacrolimus, and MMF for maintenance therapy.

The need to prevent rejection must be balanced with the potential complications of long-term immunosuppression, including kidney damage, metabolic derangements, malignancy, and opportunistic infections [5, 9]. However, this is a delicate and challenging balance, and much research focuses on safer immunosuppressive therapies and inducing donor-specific tolerance.

Preparation and Planning

Facial Transplantation Team

Due to its novelty, FT requires an interdisciplinary group of highly skilled experts. From preoperative evaluation to long-term follow-up, care of FT patients necessitates physical and occupational therapists, psychiatrists or psychologists, radiologists, nurses, transplant surgeons, and reconstructive surgeons, among others. Additional groups that facilitate FT success include but are not limited to organ procurement organizations, local legislative bodies, medical center administration, and support staff. The collaborative effort between these stakeholders has led to the development of algorithms for transferring donors to recipient institutions and facilitated simultaneous procurement of solid organs.

Cadaveric Rehearsals

Given the complexities and coordination required for successful FT, cadaveric rehearsals should be performed, and if possible, with the entire surgical team together. These rehearsals allow the team to plan for patient-specific operative considerations that would have been identified during recipient evaluation. Additionally, algorithms and perioperative checklists should be developed to ensure uniformity and reduce error through this process.

Imaging

Preoperative imaging of the recipient and donor should be performed through CT angiography and formal angiography. The benefits are twofold: ensuring vessel patency and identifying anatomic variants that could have potentially catastrophic outcomes. Ophthalmic artery variants have been described, where the ophthalmic branches of the external carotid.

Additional Preparation

Importantly, to respect the donor and their families, the donor's facial integrity should be restored. This can be achieved through either a 3-D printed or a plaster mask and allows for any desired end-of-life rituals to be performed.

Surgical Considerations

FT is a challenging procedure because of the unique nature of each patient's defect and technical details of the operation. Facial procurement and recipient procedures are performed simultaneously, and several surgical approaches have been described in the past 16 years. Prior to transplantation, the donor and recipient should both receive a tracheostomy.

The procedure starts with careful neck dissection elevating a subplatysmal flap, followed by circumferential exposure of the key anatomical structures such as the veins (internal jugular and facial veins), arteries (common carotid artery, external and internal carotid arteries, facial artery, occipital artery, and lingual artery), and the nerves (facial nerves and hypoglossal nerves). Next, periorbital structures are dissected carefully to avoid ocular complications such as ectropion, lid retraction, and loss of blink reflex. Finally, excision of the parotid and submandibular glands is performed to prevent sialoceles.

Osteotomies on both donor and recipient are guided by CAD/CAM cutting guides to maximize cephalometric and occlusal relationships between the recipient and donor skeletons [10]. Two patients of our FT cohort received tooth-bearing maxillomandibular transplants to address ballistic composite midface injuries [10]. Both cases included bilateral mandibular sagittal split osteotomies and Le Fort III osteotomies to incorporate the mandibular and maxillary teeth while reestablishing facial structure and projection. Skeletal inset and fixation were executed before the vascular anastomoses to prevent kinking of the vascular pedicles. Computer-aided intraoperative surgical navigation was employed to project a virtual surgical plan on the recipient's skeletal defect, increasing the accuracy of allograft inset [10] (Figs. 28.3 and 28.4). Bony alignment and appropriate skeletal fixation are confirmed using intraoperative CT.

Adequate vascular perfusion is vital for successful transplantation, so we advocate for a bilateral arterial supply using the external carotid arteries and corresponding veins. Vascular anastomoses are executed using an operating microscope to increase precision. Indocyanine green fluorescence angiography is used to confirm allograft perfusion prior to disconnecting the allograft from the donor's major vessels and following vascular anastomoses in the recipient [11] (Fig. 28.5). To prevent synkinesis, the allograft facial nerve branches are anastomosed distally, in proximity to the target muscles. Sensory nerve coaptation is executed when possible.

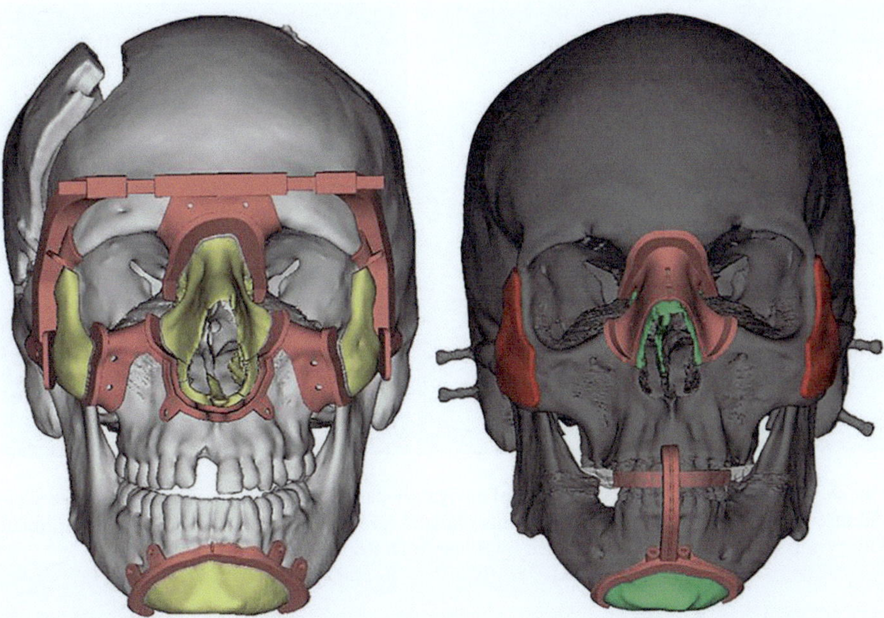

Fig. 28.3 Computer-aided design and manufacturing of patient-specific skeletal cutting guides. The allograft included skeletal subunits to augment facial projection while preserving retaining ligaments and muscular insertion sites. Donor (left) and recipient (right) planned osteotomies and custom cutting guides (printed with permission and copyrights retained by Eduardo D. Rodriguez, M.D., D.D.S)

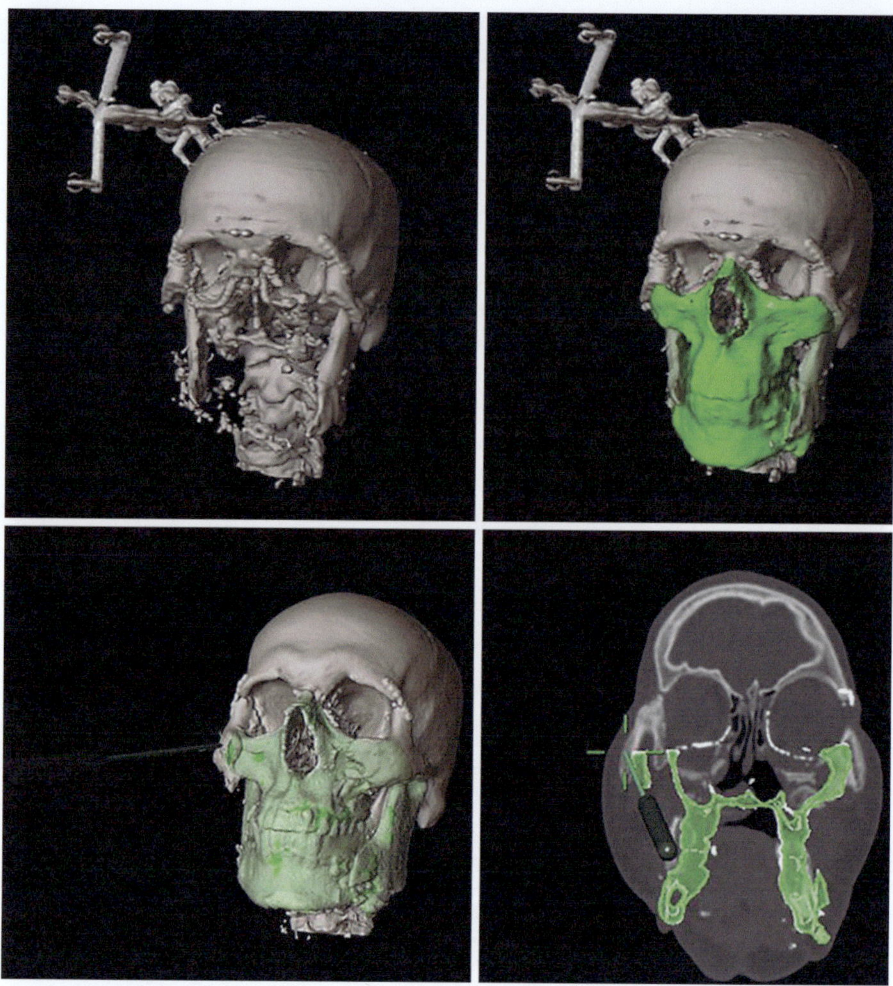

Fig. 28.4 Real-time intraoperative surgical navigation can be leveraged to confirm accurate skeletal inset and compare the skeletal segments planned (green) with actual (gray) position (printed with permission and copyrights retained by Eduardo D. Rodriguez, M.D., D.D.S)

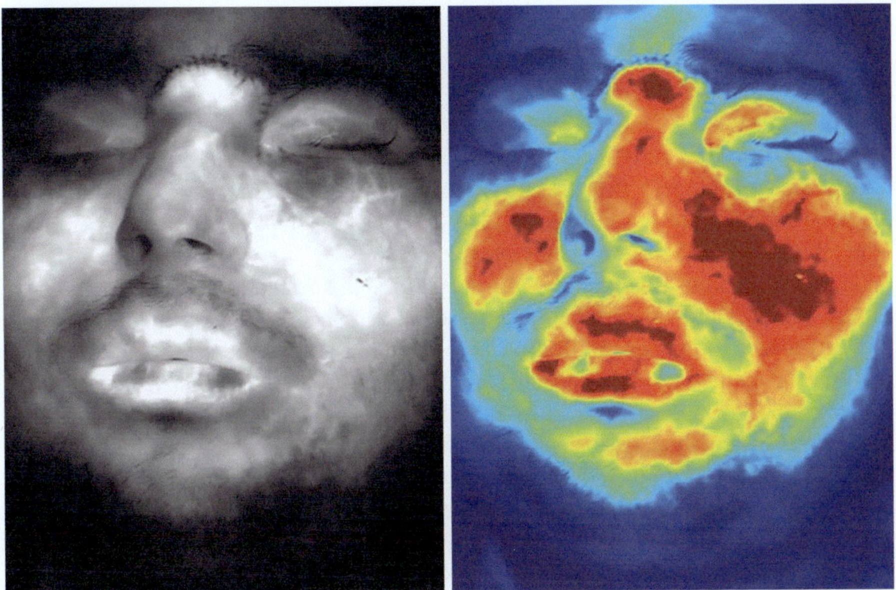

Fig. 28.5 Indocyanine green fluorescence angiography to verify appropriate allotransplant arterial perfusion and venous outflow (printed with permission and copyrights retained by Eduardo D. Rodriguez, M.D., D.D.S)

Postoperative Considerations

Outcomes

48 FT have been performed to date. Few reports on long-term outcomes are available, but the available data demonstrates the procedure's favorable functional, aesthetic, and psychosocial outcomes. Motor and sensory recovery occurs primarily in the first year post-surgery [12]. Motor function is generally apparent around postoperative month (POM) 6 to 8 but may be present earlier [13]. Patients report satisfactory recovery of speech, lip competence, facial expression, and swallowing. Sensory recovery generally begins around POM 3, even in patients where sensory nerve coaptation was not conducted. At POM 8, patients report two-point discrimination and recovery of light touch, pain, and thermal sensation [13].

Rejection

Allograft acute and chronic immunologic rejection is an expected complication following FT. Most patients have experienced at least one acute rejection episode, which presents clinically as erythema and swelling of the facial allograft. On the other hand, chronic rejection presents as premature aging, leukoderma, and mucosal dryness secondary to tissue fibrosis [14]. To date, no FT patients have experienced hyperacute rejection or graft-versus-host disease.

Routine skin biopsies are the current gold standard for rejection surveillance. Tissue samples are histologically assessed using the Banff classification, which grades inflammatory cell infiltration and epithelial involvement [15]. Noninvasive monitoring methods and blood biomarkers have attracted interest from the VCA centers; however, their use remains experimental [1]. Once a diagnosis of allograft rejection is established, treatment should be initiated as soon as possible. Treatment usually consists of IV pulse dose corticosteroids, adjustment of maintenance immunosuppressants, and plasmapheresis if needed [13].

Other Complications

Close postoperative follow-up is crucial to detect immunologic and operative complications. Postoperative CT and angiography are performed early in the postoperative course to evaluate the technical success and detect complications.

Palatal and floor of the mouth wound dehiscence, necrosis, and fistula formation have been documented in approximately half of the FT patients to date [10]. They generally manifest at the recipient–donor suture lines and could happen even in the presence of an adequate palatal blood supply. Sialocele is another common complication, which may occur even if major salivary glands are excluded from the allograft and can be treated with drainage and botulinum toxin injections [10, 16]. Regular assessment of dental and periodontal health is crucial to avoid dental caries, tooth loss, periodontal disease, and infections.

Skeletal stability is affected by the dynamic forces on the bone-to-bone interface during functional recovery. One of our patients presented with mandibular nonunion on postoperative day (POD) 108, possibly due to a fibrous contracture at the proximal mandibular segment. This complication was managed with open reduction and internal fixation with a titanium plate [10]. Postoperative malocclusion is a frequent complication among maxillomandibular containing FTs, even in patients who presented a Class I occlusion immediately after surgery [10]. The absence of motor tone and proprioceptive feedback during recovery of speech and mastication in the first 6 to 9 months posttransplantation is likely associated with progressive development of malocclusion [17]. Close patient follow-up is crucial to avoid and manage postoperative malocclusion. A revisional Le Fort advancement can also be employed. However, we advocate for a preemptive application of orthodontic elastics immediately following transplantation to avoid the need for malocclusion revision surgery.

Revision Surgeries

Revision surgery plays an important role in the management of FT patients. Most FT recipients undergo follow-up procedures, which can be aimed at addressing facial soft tissue, craniofacial skeleton, dentition, oronasal cavity, salivary glands, and periorbital tissue [18]. The average time to first revision surgery is 149 ± 179 days, and patients receive on average 4.8 revision procedures. The combined experience of VCA centers has demonstrated the safety of revision surgeries performed at diverse time points. Our center's experience demonstrates that revision surgery to address malocclusion and loss of the donor-recipient intraoral interface integrity can be performed without compromising the allograft [18]. A facial re-transplantation was recently performed in a patient to address chronic allograft rejection, demonstrating the feasibility of this approach as a salvage option [19].

Future Directions

Since the first successful transplant in 2005, significant advances have been made in the field, allowing for the first successful combined VCA transplantation. A combined face and bilateral hand transplantation was performed on a severe burn victim by our institution in 2020. As of the time of publication, the patient is progressing well clinically and psychosocially.

The FT donor pool is an important limitation to the procedure. Current legislation for VCA donation requires additional consent beyond solid organ donation protocols. Efforts should be made to amend the policy to include VCA. The expansion of online resources regarding the procedure is crucial to increase public awareness and approval. It is our hope that policy changes and increasing awareness will lead to increased donor supply, thereby increasing the opportunity for those in need. Further, a larger donor pool will improve immune matching, leading to better overall outcomes. Cross-sex donation is a potential avenue for increasing the available donor pool.

As lifelong immunosuppression to avoid rejection is associated with significant complications, VCA centers continue to explore multiple venues for donor-specific tolerance induction [20, 21]. Lastly, topical/local immunosuppression and stem cell therapies have shown promise in preclinical studies and can potentially contribute to safer immunosuppressive regimens [22].

Acknowledgments The authors would like to acknowledge the donor patients and families for selflessly donating the gift of life and the recipient patients and families.

References

1. Diep GK, Berman ZP, Alfonso AR, Ramly EP, Boczar D, Trilles J, et al. The 2020 facial transplantation update: a 15-year compendium. Plast Reconstr Surg Glob Open. 2021;9(5):e3586.
2. Carty MJ, Bueno EM, Lehmann LS, Pomahac B. A position paper in support of face transplantation in the blind. Plast Reconstr Surg. 2012;130(2):319–24.
3. Hendrickx H, Blondeel PN, Van Parys H, Roche NA, Peeters PC, Vermeersch HF, et al. Facing a new face: an interpretative phenomenological analysis of the experiences of a blind face transplant patient and his partner. J Craniofac Surg. 2018;29(4):826–31.
4. Lemmens GM, Poppe C, Hendrickx H, Roche NA, Peeters PC, Vermeersch HF, et al. Facial transplantation in a blind patient: psychologic, marital, and family outcomes at 15 months follow-up. Psychosomatics. 2015;56(4):362–70.
5. Kantar RS, Alfonso AR, Diep GK, Berman ZP, Rifkin WJ, Diaz-Siso JR, et al. Facial transplantation: principles and evolving concepts. Plast Reconstr Surg. 2021;147(6):1022e–38e.
6. Petruzzo P, Kanitakis J, Testelin S, Pialat JB, Buron F, Badet L, et al. Clinicopathological findings of chronic rejection in a face grafted patient. Transplantation. 2015;99(12):2644–50.
7. Rifkin WJ, David JA, Plana NM, Kantar RS, Diaz-Siso JR, Gelb BE, et al. Achievements and challenges in facial transplantation. Ann Surg. 2018;268(2):260–70.
8. Kollar B, Pomahac B, Riella LV. Novel immunological and clinical insights in vascularized composite allotransplantation. Curr Opin Organ Transplant. 2019;24(1):42–8.
9. Rifkin WJ, Manjunath AK, Kantar RS, Jacoby A, Kimberly LL, Gelb BE, et al. A comparison of immunosuppression regimens in hand, face, and kidney transplantation. J Surg Res. 2021;258:17–22.
10. Ramly EP, Kantar RS, Diaz-Siso JR, Alfonso AR, Shetye PR, Rodriguez ED. Outcomes after tooth-bearing Maxillomandibular facial transplantation: insights and lessons learned. J Oral Maxillofac Surg. 2019;77(10):2085–103.
11. Sosin M, Ceradini DJ, Levine JP, Hazen A, Staffenberg DA, Saadeh PB, et al. Total face, eyelids, ears, scalp, and skeletal subunit transplant: a reconstructive solution for the full face and total scalp burn. Plast Reconstr Surg. 2016;138(1):205–19.
12. Tasigiorgos S, Kollar B, Turk M, Perry B, Alhefzi M, Kiwanuka H, et al. Five-year follow-up after face transplantation. N Engl J Med. 2019;380(26):2579–81.
13. Khalifian S, Brazio PS, Mohan R, Shaffer C, Brandacher G, Barth RN, et al. Facial transplantation: the first 9 years. Lancet. 2014;384(9960):2153–63.
14. Krezdorn N, Lian CG, Wells M, Wo L, Tasigiorgos S, Xu S, et al. Chronic rejection of human face allografts. Am J Transplant. 2019;19(4):1168–77.
15. Cendales LC, Kanitakis J, Schneeberger S, Burns C, Ruiz P, Landin L, et al. The Banff 2007 working classification of skin-containing composite tissue allograft pathology. Am J Transplant. 2008;8(7):1396–400.
16. Frautschi R, Rampazzo A, Bernard S, Djohan R, Papay F, Gharb BB. Management of the salivary glands and facial nerve in face transplantation. Plast Reconstr Surg. 2016;137(6):1887–97.
17. Krezdorn N, Alhefzi M, Perry B, Aycart MA, Tasigiorgos S, Bueno EM, et al. Trismus in face transplantation following ballistic trauma. J Craniofac Surg. 2018;29(4):843–7.
18. Diep GK, Ramly EP, Alfonso AR, Berman ZP, Rodriguez ED. Enhancing face transplant outcomes: fundamental principles of facial allograft revision. Plast Reconstr Surg Glob Open. 2020;8(8):e2949.
19. Diaz-Siso JR, Borab ZM, Plana NM, Parent B, Stranix JT, Rodriguez ED. Vascularized composite Allotransplantation: alternatives and catch-22s. Plast Reconstr Surg. 2018;142(5):1320–6.
20. Lellouch AG, Ng ZY, Rosales IA, Schol IM, Leonard DA, Gama AR, et al. Toward development of the delayed tolerance induction protocol for vascularized composite allografts in nonhuman primates. Plast Reconstr Surg. 2020;145(4):757e–68e.
21. Leonard DA, Kurtz JM, Cetrulo CL Jr. Achieving immune tolerance in hand and face transplantation: a realistic prospect? Immunotherapy. 2014;6(5):499–502.
22. Safi AF, Kauke M, Nelms L, Palmer WJ, Tchiloemba B, Kollar B, et al. Local immunosuppression in vascularized composite allotransplantation (VCA): a systematic review. J Plast Reconstr Aesthet Surg. 2021;74(2):327–35.

Index